Stroke: An Issue of Neurology Clinics

Stroke: An Issue of Neurology Clinics

Edited by Edie Lane

AMERICAN
MEDICAL PUBLISHERS
www.americanmedicalpublishers.com

American Medical Publishers,
41 Flatbush Avenue,
1st Floor, New York,
NY 11217, USA

Visit us on the World Wide Web at:
www.americanmedicalpublishers.com

ISBN: 978-1-63927-329-4

Cataloging-in-Publication Data

Stroke : an issue of neurology clinics / edited by Edie Lane.
p. cm.
Includes bibliographical references and index.
ISBN 978-1-63927-329-4
1. Cerebrovascular disease. 2. Cerebrovascular disease--Diagnosis. 3. Cerebrovascular disease--Patients. 4. Neglect (Neurology). 5. Brain--Diseases. 6. Neurological emergencies. 7. Neurologists. I. Lane, Edie.
RC388.5 .S77 2022
616.81--dc23

Table of Contents

Preface

A medical condition in which the poor blood flow towards the brain causes cell death is known as a stroke. The two main types of stroke include ischemic and hemorrhagic. Ischemic stroke occurs due to insufficient blood flow to the brain to meet metabolic demands that lead to cerebral hypoxia and causes the death of the brain tissues. Hemorrhagic stroke is a condition where bleeding occurs within the skull. A stroke could occur due to different reasons such as a blood clot around atherosclerotic plaques, arterial embolism, reduction of blood flow due to heart failure and hypertension. The most common signs and symptoms of a stroke include an inability to move or feel on one side of the body, problems in understanding or speaking, loss of vision to one side and dizziness. This book presents researches and studies performed by experts across the globe. Coherent flow of topics, student-friendly language and extensive use of examples make this book an invaluable source of knowledge. This book will also provide interesting topics for research which interested readers can take up.

This book has been the outcome of endless efforts put in by authors and researchers on various issues and topics within the field. The book is a comprehensive collection of significant researches that are addressed in a variety of chapters. It will surely enhance the knowledge of the field among readers across the globe.

It gives us an immense pleasure to thank our researchers and authors for their efforts to submit their piece of writing before the deadlines. Finally in the end, I would like to thank my family and colleagues who have been a great source of inspiration and support.

Editor

1

In vivo TSPO and cannabinoid receptor type 2 availability early in post-stroke neuroinflammation in rats

Teruyo Hosoya[1], Dai Fukumoto[2], Takeharu Kakiuchi[2], Shingo Nishiyama[2], Shigeyuki Yamamoto[2], Hiroyuki Ohba[2], Hideo Tsukada[2], Takatoshi Ueki[1], Kohji Sato[1] and Yasuomi Ouchi[3*]

Abstract

Background: Upregulated levels of 18-kDa translocator proteins (TSPO) and type 2 endocannabinoid receptors (CB2) are considered to reflect different aspects of microglia-related neuroinflammatory responses in the brain. Relative to the increase in the TSPO expression that occurs slightly later during neuroinflammation in a proinflammatory fashion, CB2 activation is considered to relate to the neuroprotective responses that occurs predominantly at an early stage of brain disorders. These findings, however, were deduced from studies with different animal samples under different experimental settings. Here, we aimed to examined the differences in TSPO binding and CB2 availability at an early stage of stroke in the same animal using positron emission tomography (PET).

Methods: We used a total of eight Sprague-Dawley rats that underwent photothrombotic stroke surgery. The binding levels of a TSPO tracer [^{11}C](*R*)PK11195 and a CB2 tracer [^{11}C]NE40 were measured at 24 h after the surgery in the same animal using PET in combination with immunohistochemistry for CB2 and several other markers. A morphological inspection was also performed with X-ray computed tomography for small animals.

Results: The levels of [^{11}C]NE40 binding potential (BP_{ND}) were significantly higher in the cerebral cortical region on the lesion side than those on the non-lesion side, whereas no difference was found in the levels of [^{11}C](*R*)PK11195 BP_{ND} between hemispheres. The tracer influx index (R1) data were all reduced on the lesion side irrespective of tracers. This increase in [^{11}C]NE40 BP_{ND} was concomitant with an elevation in CB2 expression mainly within the microglia in the peri-infarct area, as shown by immunohistochemical examinations with Iba-1, CD11b/c+, and NG2+ staining.

Conclusions: The present results provide in vivo evidence of different responses of microglia occurring in the acute state of stroke. The use of the CB2 tracer [^{11}C]NE40 allows us to evaluate the roles played by the neuroprotective aspect of microglia in acute neuroinflammatory processes.

Keywords: Microglia, Cannabinoid receptor type 2, Translocater protein, Neuroinflammation, Positron emission tomography, Immunostaining, Early stroke

* Correspondence: ouchi@hama-med.ac.jp
[3]Department of Biofunctional Imaging, Preeminent Medical Photonics Education & Research Center, Hamamatsu University School of Medicine, 1-20-1 Handayama, Higashi-ku, Hamamatsu 431-3192, Japan
Full list of author information is available at the end of the article

Background

Microglia change morphologically and functionally from their resting state to their activated state in response to several neuroinflammatory and neurodegenerative diseases. In other words, microglial activation accompanies any damage to the brain environment. This is one reason why activated microglia represent an important marker of neuroinflammation [1]. Specifically, noninvasive imaging of activated microglia is a useful tool to detect in vivo neuroinflammatory disease. To date, the first-generation translocator protein 18 kDa (TSPO) marker [^{11}C](*R*)PK11195 has been widely used as a PET radioligand for that purpose. PET studies using [^{11}C](*R*)PK11195 have been carried out on patients with several neuroinflammatory diseases such as Alzheimer's disease (AD) [2], Parkinson's disease (PD) [3], and Huntington's disease [4]. In addition, ischemic stroke causes direct insults to brain tissue and the immediate activation of microglia, which can also be visualized on PET with [^{11}C](*R*)PK11195 [5]. This is an experimental advantage in studies on time course changes in microglial activation, unlike animal models for chronically developed neurodegenerative brain disorders. Specifically, since stroke is a sudden onset disease, an early depiction of the extent at which the brain is compromised is important for treatment to delay the disease progression. In this context, TSPO imaging may be preferable. To date, it is well documented that the accumulation of [^{11}C](*R*)PK11195 or the second-generation tracer [^{18}F]DPA714 is reported to occur relatively later after brain injury resulting from toxin injection [6] or traumatic insults [7, 8].

The imaging of endocannabinoid receptor type 2 (CB2) has recently been considered to be an alternative method for targeting activated microglia using PET imaging. The endocannabinoid system in the central nervous system has been identified to provide neuroprotective effects following brain injury. In particular, CB2 is upregulated in microglia during neurodegenerative and neuroinflammatory diseases such as AD [9–11], multiple sclerosis [12], PD [13] and ischemia [14–17], and is associated with microglial activity [18]. Moreover, the administration of a selective CB2 agonist reduced infarct volume and improved motor function scores [16]. Recently, a PET tracer that binds specifically to CB2 was developed to illustrate CB2 availability in vivo [19]. Although it was reported that the binding of [^{11}C]NE40 24 h after ischemic injury using a photochemically induced thrombosis (PIT) technique failed to increase [20], six out of nine PET data were not corrected for the attenuation of radioactivity, and the correction is critical for the quantification of PET data. Considering the early-developed neuroprotective role of microglia, a failure to detect the elevation of [^{11}C]NE40 uptake in AD patients [21] is understandable because the activated microglia during the chronic state of neurodegeneration are considered to be acting as proinflammatory agents [22]. Therefore, the stroke model might be suitable for evaluating the early response of microglia because the insult can be controlled purposefully.

In neuroinflammation, microglia are considered to play a dual role in their function. Classically activated M1 phenotype microglia release proinflammatory mediators, whereas alternatively activated M2 phenotype microglia enhance phagocytic activity and reduce the production of inflammatory mediators [23, 24]. In our previous study, we demonstrated that neuronal damage occurred on days 1, 3, 7, and 14 after PIT using [^{11}C](*R*)PK11195 [25]. The uptake peak of [^{11}C](*R*)PK11195 was found on day 7 after PIT treatment and overlapped with the high immunoreactivity area of microglial marker Ibal, suggesting that the uptake of [^{11}C](*R*)PK11195 reflects microglial activity. However, it is difficult to distinguish between neurotoxic M1 and neuroprotective M2 microglia phenotypes on PET imaging with [^{11}C](*R*)PK11195. Then, we focused on [^{11}C]NE40, which targets CB2, with the goal of observing neuroprotective microglia at an acute stage of brain injury.

Therefore, the purpose of the present study was to focus on the early phase of stroke and to elucidate the different binding patterns of CB2 and TSPO tracers in a very acute stage of brain insult, such as stroke, by comparing the levels of [^{11}C]NE40 binding with those of [^{11}C](*R*)PK11195 binding in rats after PIT surgery. These in vivo data were evaluated with immunohistochemistry for CB2, TSPO, and several cell type-specific markers after completion of the PET measurements, resulting in cessation of the in vivo study with the same animals.

Methods

Animals

Eight 8-week-old male Sprague-Dawley rats (250–300 g) purchased from the SLC Company (Hamamatsu, Japan) were used in this study. They were housed in cages with free access to food and water. All animal protocols and the following experiments were approved by the Ethics Committees of the Central Research Laboratory at Hamamatsu Photonics and Hamamatsu University School of Medicine. In addition, all applicable institutional and/or national guidelines for the care and use of animals were followed.

The PIT procedure was performed as reported previously [26]. Briefly, the rats were anesthetized and maintained with 2% halothane in a mixture of 70% room air and 30% O_2 throughout the following procedure. After the insertion of an infusion line into the tail vein, the scalp and temporal muscle were flipped, and then a subtemporal craniotomy was performed. The main trunk of the left middle cerebral artery (MCA) was observed through the dura mater under an operating microscope through a window that was anterior to the foramen of the mandibular nerve. After the intravenous infusion of 20 mg/kg of rose bengal (Wako Pure Chemical Industry, Osaka, Japan), photoillumination was performed utilizing a green light at 540 nm (model L4887, Hamamatsu Photonics, Hamamatsu, Japan), which was delivered to the MCA through the dura mater for 10 min using a 3-mm optic fiber placed onto the window within the skull base. After confirming thrombotic occlusion of the MCA, the incision was closed. The animals were then allowed to awake from anesthesia and were returned to their cages.

PET measurements

We utilized a high-resolution animal PET scanner (SHR-38000, Hamamatsu Photonics, Japan) under an axial field of view (FOV) of 330 mm, a transaxial FOV of 108 mm, and a transaxial spatial resolution of 2.3 mm in the center. Eight animals were scanned twice a day using PET with $[^{11}C](R)$PK11195 and $[^{11}C]$NE40 beginning 24 h after PIT. The interval between the two scans was set to 2 h, and the order of the scans was counterbalanced. The animals were anesthetized using an initial dose of chloral hydrate (400 mg/kg, i.p.) followed by a continuous infusion of chloral hydrate (100 mg/kg/h, i.v.) during the entire imaging experiment. They were placed in the prone position on a fixation plate and then set within the gantry hole of the PET scanner. After a 15-min transmission scan utilizing an external $^{68}Ge/^{68}Ga$ rod source (67 MBq) for attenuation correction, a serial emission scan that lasted for 60 min was performed immediately following each tracer injection of $[^{11}C](R)$PK11195 or $[^{11}C]$NE40 at a dose of 48 MBq/kg; tracers were injected intravenously through the cannula that was inserted into the tail vein. The specific activity of each tracer used was above 50 GBq/μmol. No arterial sampling was conducted. The PET data were reconstructed using 3D DRAMA (iteration 2, gamma 0.1) with a Gauss filter of 1.0 mm in full width at half maximum (FWHM), yielding a voxel size of 0.65 × 0.65 × 1.0167 mm for the reconstructed image. To obtain the anatomical information, X-CT scans were performed immediately following PET measurement using a ClairvivoCT (Shimadzu Corporation, Kyoto, Japan).

Data analysis and statistics

Using an image analysis software (PMOD, version 3.1; PMOD Technologies Ltd, Zurich, Switzerland), we estimated the levels of BP_{ND} (an availability of TSPO and CB2) and R1 (a tracer influx index according to blood flow: a ratio of K1/K′1, or an influx in target of interest/an influx in reference of interest) for $[^{11}C](R)$PK11195 and $[^{11}C]$NE40 based on a simplified reference tissue model [27, 28] and then created the parametric brain images of BP_{ND} and R1 (a tracer uptake index). During this process, the time-activity curve from the bilateral cerebellar cortex was used as a reference input function because the infratentorial brain region might be less affected by the MCA occlusion event; however, functional connection emerging as diaschisis could be a possibility of the confounding factor. The selection of the intact contralateral cortical region as a reference region as conducted elsewhere [20] seems inadequate because the numbers of the CD11b+/CD3+ cells (for microglia) were comparable in ischemia-affected and non-affected hemispheres 24 h after stroke [29].

As described elsewhere [30, 31], the elliptical regions of interest (ROIs), ranging from 12 to 24 mm^2 wide, were symmetrically placed in the bilateral brain regions covering the peri-infarct area mainly in the frontal and parietal cortices by referring to the X-CT images, on which the coronal slices of the frontal and parietal cortices were determined according to the Paxinos rat brain stereotactic atlas [32] (see Additional file 1: Figure S1).

Student's t test statistics were used to compare the conditions and the significance level was set at $p < 0.05$ with a correction for multiple comparisons because multiple loci were chosen.

Immunohistochemistry

The rats were anesthetized with chloral hydrate (400 mg/kg) and then transcardially perfused with saline followed by 4% paraformaldehyde (PFA) (pH 7.4). The brains were removed, post-fixed in 4% PFA, and immersed in cryoprotectant solution (30% sucrose in 0.1 M phosphate buffer) until the tissue sank. Tissues were frozen in dry ice and stored at −80 °C until they were used. Twenty-micrometer frozen coronal sections were cut using a cryostat. The slides were blocked with 5% goat serum in PBS containing 0.1% Triton X-100 for 1 h at room temperature (RT) and then incubated with primary antibodies for 2 h at RT. After being washed, the slides were then incubated for 2 h at RT with secondary antibodies. The following primary antibodies were used in this study: mouse anti-GFAP (1:500, Millipore), rabbit anti-Iba1 (1:1000, Wako), mouse anti-CD11b/c (1:500, DB Pharmingen), mouse anti-NG2 (1:200, Millipore), rabbit anti-cannabinoid receptor 2 (1:100, Abcam), and rabbit anti-rat TSPO (1:200, Biobyt). The following secondary antibodies were used in this study: Alexa Fluor 488 anti-rabbit-IgG and Alexa Fluor 594 anti-mouse-IgG (1:500, Invitrogen).

Results

PET findings

The Student's t test showed a significantly higher level of $[^{11}C]$NE40 BP_{ND} in the affected regions of the frontal cortex ($t = 3.54$, $p < 0.05$ corrected for multiple comparisons) and parietal cortex on the lesion side ($t = 3.21$, $p < 0.05$ corrected) than $[^{11}C](R)$PK11195 BP_{ND} (Table 1, Fig. 1a, b). In

Table 1 Differences in the levels of BP_{ND} and RI values

	Region	[11C]NE40		[11C](*R*)PK11195	
		Lesion	Contralateral	Lesion	Contralateral
BP_{ND}	Frontal	1.79 ± 0.99*	0.51 ± 0.48	1.07 ± 1.20	1.47 ± 0.90
	Parietal	1.27 ± 0.77*	0.63 ± 0.51	0.60 ± 0.56	0.73 ± 0.58
R1	Frontal	0.73 ± 0.74	0.87 ± 0.31	0.68 ± 0.80	0.80 ± 0.34
	Parietal	0.68 ± 0.27	1.02 ± 0.30	0.47 ± 0.31	0.73 ± 0.27

*$p < 0.05$ vs contralateral (non-lesion) side

contrast, the R1 value that reflects the degree of tracer influx depending on regional blood flow was frequently observed to be low in the MCA territory, regardless of the tracer used (Fig. 1c, d), suggesting that the influxes of these two different tracers might be equally damaged in this experimental setting. An additional examination using tracer-summation PET images (standardized uptake value, SUV) failed to show this significance although the similar trend was found (Additional file 2: Figure S2).

As shown in Fig. 2, higher uptake of [11C]NE40 was observed in the peri-infarct region (penumbra, arrow) than the [11C](*R*)PK11195. Although the difference in time course of the tracer uptake (the tissue time-activity curve, TAC) was small between [11C]NE40 and [11C](*R*)PK11195, there was a gradual increase in [11C]NE40 TAC on the ipsilateral (infarct) side later during the scan, while no difference was observed in [11C](*R*)PK11195 TACs on either side.

Immunohistochemical findings

The brain section images revealed that large ischemic lesions occurred from the striatum to the cortical region in our experimental model. Within the infarct core, only cell debris was observed (Additional file 3: Figure S3). As shown in Additional file 3: Figure S3 and Fig. 3, Iba-1-positive cell and CD11b/c+ cell regions were predominantly found within the peri-infarct region, while GFAP-positive astrocytes were found to be scattered throughout the brain.

Co-staining for CB2 and the microglial marker CD11b/c showed that CD11b/c+ microglia in the contralateral (non-lesion) area were in their resting state with ramified processes, while they were negative for CB2 on day 1 after PIT treatment (Fig. 3). It appeared that microglial processes surrounded the CB2+ cells. In the peri-infarct area, some CD11b/c+ cells were co-labeled with CB2; their form exhibited a round shape (Fig. 3, arrowhead). Co-staining for TSPO and CD11b/c shows that microglia did not express TSPO (Fig. 3).

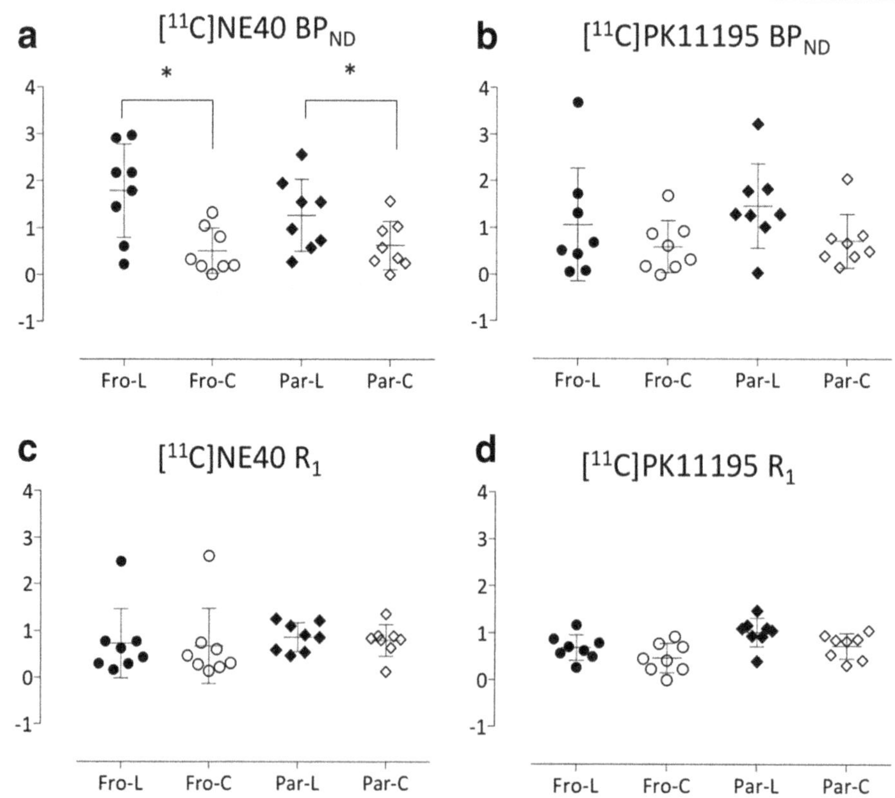

Fig. 1 The levels of BP_{ND} (**a**, **b**) and R1 (**c**, **d**) in each brain region in [11C]NE40 and [11C](R)PK11195 studies, respectively. Only BP_{ND} of [11C]NE40 was significantly higher in the affected cortical regions compared to the intact regions (*$p < 0.05$)

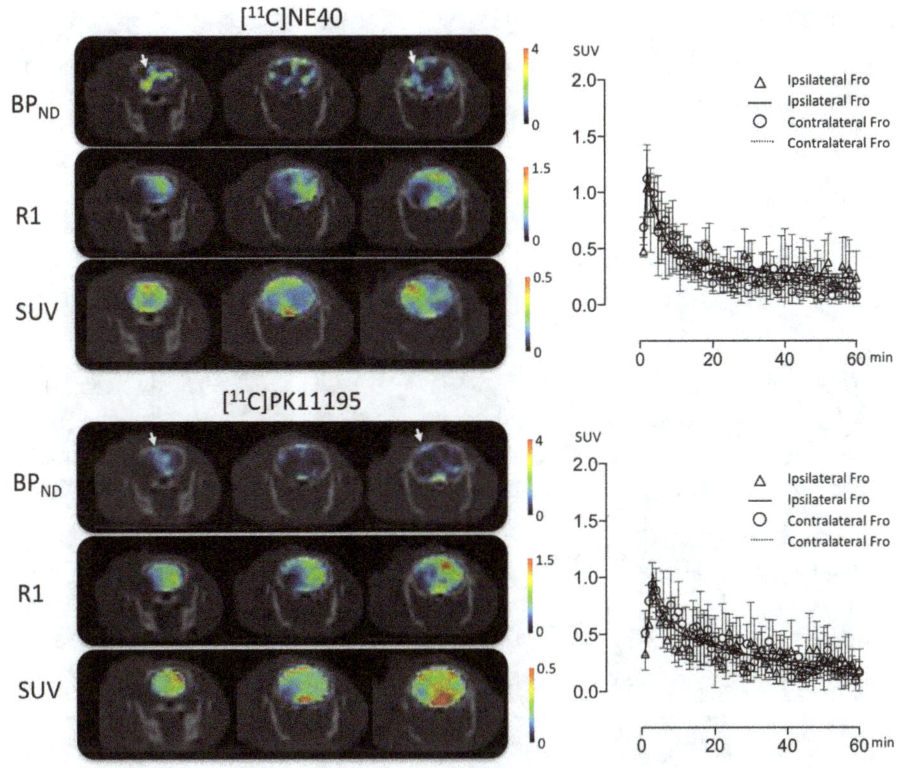

Fig. 2 Coronal parametric images of BP_{ND}, R1, and SUV (standardized uptake value) superimposed on X-CT images in [^{11}C]NE40 and [^{11}C](R)PK11195 studies. A SUV image was generated as a summation of tracer uptake during 40–60 min post-injection. The *arrows* indicate the peri-infarct region (penumbra). Mean tissue time-activity curves with standard deviations of each tracer on both frontal cortices are shown in different panels. Ipsilateral, lesion side; contralateral, non-lesion side

TSPO was negative in all areas. Because no GFAP-positive astrocytes were co-labeled with CB2, GFAP+ cells were unlikely to be associated with CB2+ cells (Fig. 4).

Because NG2 (neural/glial antigen 2) was reported to be highly expressed at an early state after brain injury [33] and in the activated microglia and infiltrated macrophages in brain insults [34–37], we also performed co-staining for CB2 and NG2 to determine whether CB2 in the peri-infarct area was expressed by activated NG2+ cells. The NG2 signal was very strong in regions adjacent to the infarct area and some NG2-positive cells were co-labeled with CB2 (Fig. 4). Notably, CB2+/NG2+ cells were round in shape (Fig. 4, arrow head) and CB2−/NG2+ cells exhibited a ramified form with thin processes (Fig. 4, arrow).

Co-staining with CB2 and the neural marker NeuN showed that some NeuN+ cells in the contra- and ipsilateral cortices were weakly co-labeled with CB2 (Fig. 5). However, in the peri-infarct area, no NeuN+ cells were co-labeled with CB2. Therefore, the uptake of [^{11}C]NE40 in the contralateral cortex might reflect some degree of its binding to CB2 on neurons.

Discussion

Microglial activation detection using the CB2 tracer

We found an increase in [^{11}C]NE40 binding and elevated CB2 availability specifically in the peri-infarct area at an early stage after ischemic injury induced by the PIT method. This finding was consistent with our immunohistochemical results that showed co-localization of CD11b/c+ and CB2-positive cells exhibiting microglia with a round shape, suggesting that some CD11b/c+ cells expressed CB2 in regions adjacent to the infarct area. This immunohistochemical finding is also in line with the previous observation that a number of CD11b+/CD3+ cells (for microglia) were found in ischemia-affected areas 24 h after stroke [29]. A previous report suggested that CB2 can be detected in the "responsive" and "primed" states but not in the "resting" state of microglia in vitro [38]. Thus, microglia on day 1 after PIT treatment might be at an early stage in the inflammatory process, being in either the "responsive" or "primed" state in vivo. In contrast, the binding of [^{11}C](*R*)PK11195 was not co-localized in areas with high [^{11}C]NE40 binding. Because TSPO tracers such as [^{11}C](*R*)PK11195 are considered to be PET probes of delayed microglial activation as shown in literature [22],

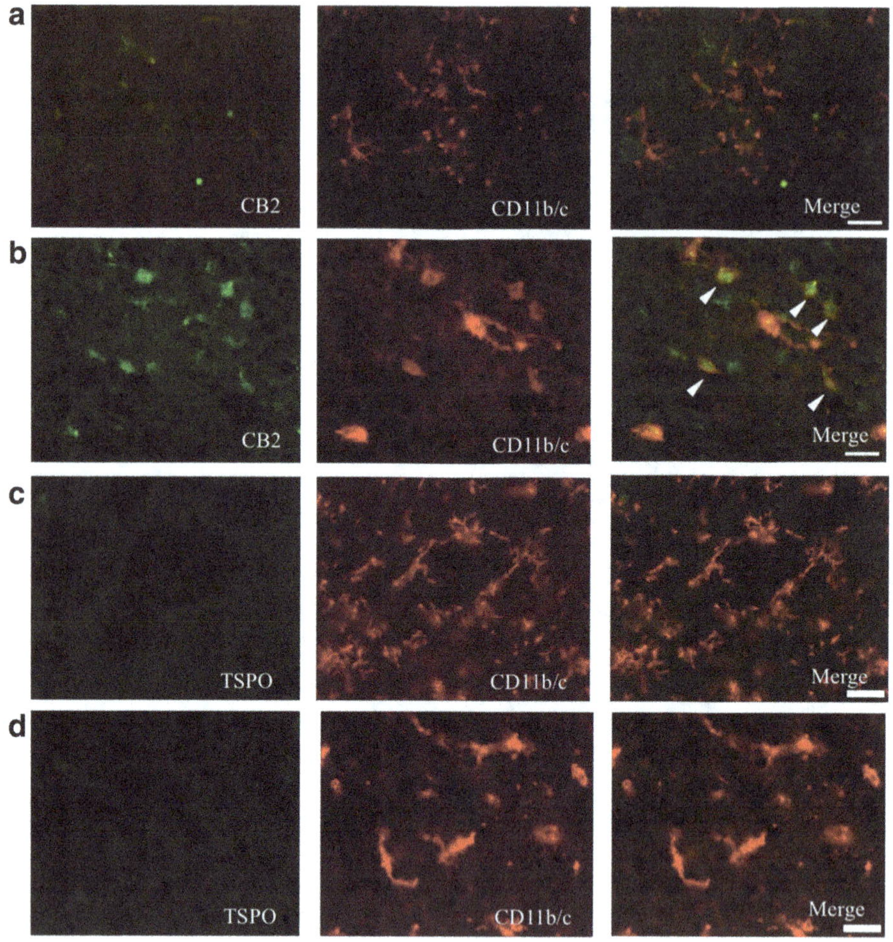

Fig. 3 Double-immunostaining for CB2 and CD11b/c in the contralateral (non-lesion) (**a**) and the peri-infarct (**b**) areas and for TSPO in the contralateral (**c**) and peri-infarct (**d**) areas on day 1 after PIT treatment. Several microglia were co-stained for CB2 and CB11b/c (*arrowhead*). *Scale bar*, 25 μm

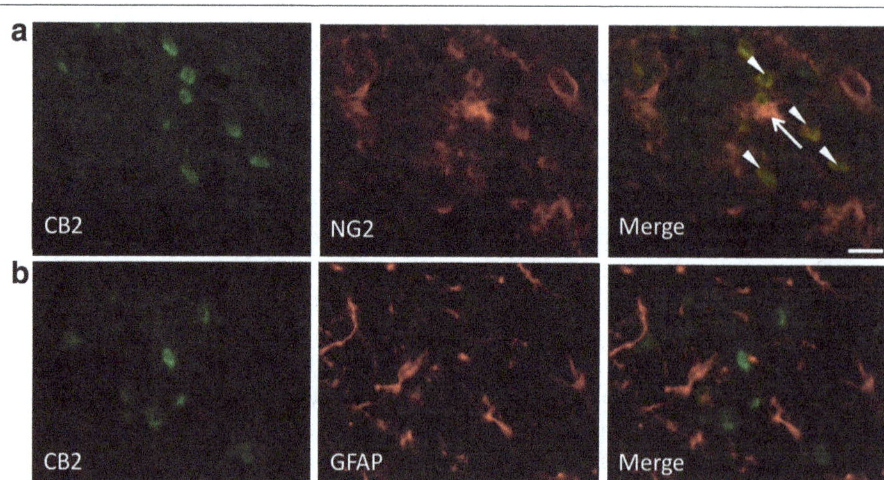

Fig. 4 Double-immunostaining for CB2 (*green*) and GFAP (*red*) in the peri-infarct area (**a**). NG2+/CB2+ cells were round (*arrowhead*) and NG2 +/CB2− cells were in a ramified form (*arrow*). **b** Double-immunostaining for CB2 (*green*) and NG2 (*red*) in the peri-infarct area on day 1 post PIT treatment. *Scale bar*, 25 μm

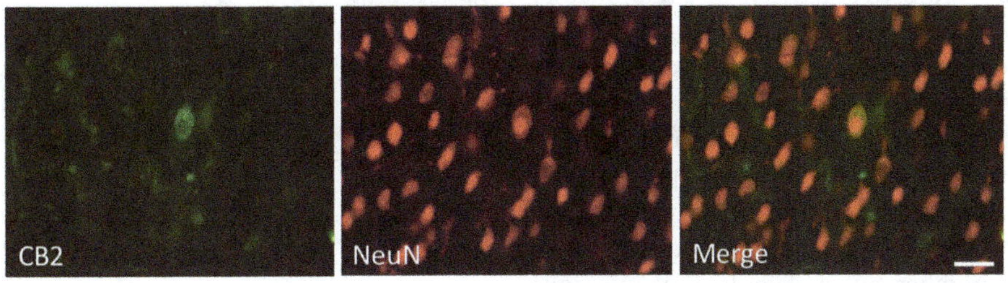

Fig. 5 Double-immunostaining for CB2 and NeuN in the contralateral cortex. Some NeuN+ cells were weakly co-labeled with CB2. *Scale bar*, 25 μm

the presence of [^{11}C]NE40 uptake along with a lack of [^{11}C](*R*)PK11195 uptake suggests that CB2 may be more implicated than TSPO during the early-phase activation of microglia in the post-stroke brain region.

Differences in binding of TSPO and CB2 tracers

In our previous study, we utilized [^{11}C](*R*)PK11195 and studied its uptake at several time points in the PIT model; furthermore, by utilizing immunostaining for Iba1, high [^{11}C](*R*)PK11195-uptake areas appeared to correspond to high microglial activity areas on day 7 after PIT treatment [25]. In this study, we demonstrated that [^{11}C]NE40 is a suitable target for a PET tracer detecting neuroinflammation developed soon after brain ischemic insult because the uptake of [^{11}C]NE40 is higher than that of [^{11}C](*R*)PK11195 1 day after PIT treatment. To date, [^{11}C](*R*)PK11195 has primarily been used for the imaging of inflammatory conditions such as neurodegenerative diseases. In the chronic stage of inflammation [6], neurotoxic M1 phenotype microglia are dominant and the TSPO tracer [^{11}C](*R*)PK11195 reflects inflammatory rather than anti-inflammatory microglial activity [22]. To support this contention, we recently showed an elevation in the second-generation TSPO tracer [^{11}C]DPA713 for illustrating chronically activated microglia under inflammatory circumstances [39].

Role of microglia in activation

Some studies have indicated that microglial CB2 is neuroprotective both in vivo and in vitro. The administration of the CB2 agonist JWH-133 in an ischemic rat brain model reduced ischemic volume, promoted the production of anti-inflammatory mediators, and suppressed the release of inflammatory mediators and Iba1 expression in microglia [15]. In an in vitro experiment, the administration of anandamide (a kind of endocannabinoids) to lipopolysaccharide-treated microglia reduced the activation of M1 phenotype microglia and elevated anti-inflammatory factors [40]. Overexpression of CB2 causes mice to have resistance to depression after stress [41] and intraperitoneal administration of a CB2 agonist can ameliorate anxiolytic effects [42]. Thus, the present PET data that show a higher accumulation of [^{11}C]NE40 and lower binding of [^{11}C](*R*)PK11195 at an early stage after PIT-induced stroke indicate possibly different roles of microglia in terms of neuroprotective or neuroinflammatory content during early brain injury.

Immunostaining and PET findings

The current immunohistological study showed that the CB2+ cells were surrounded by microglial processes and some CD11b/c+ cells with a round morphology were co-labeled with CB2 in the peri-infarct area. In addition, CB2-positive cells were weakly co-labeled with NeuN in the contralateral cortex and CB2+/NeuN+ neurons were surrounded by CB2+ cell processes. The latter finding might induce a slight upregulation of [^{11}C]NE40 on the contralateral side, which might explain why no GFAP+ cells were co-labeled with CB2. The immunostaining finding that CB2-colabelled NG2+ cells were found to be round in shape suggested that they were monocytes and played a protective role [43]. In contrast, NG2+ cells without co-labeling with CB2 were thought to be oligodendrocyte precursor cells insensitive to CB2. It appears that astrocytes are not associated with CB2 1 day after PIT treatment, even though GFAP+ cells were co-labeled with CB2 on day 3 after ischemic injury [44]. Day 1 after injury may be too early for astrocytes to respond because the activation of astrocytes is considered to occur at a late stage of the inflammatory process. Although the TSPO tracer [^{11}C](*R*)-PK11195 is believed to bind not only to activated microglia but also to activated astrocytes, either [^{11}C]NE40 or [^{11}C](*R*)PK11195 may not have captured astrocyte activation during the early stages of injury in the current experiment. Incompatible with the low level of [^{11}C](*R*)-PK11195 binding, the TSPO immunohistochemical staining exhibited a negligible level of TSPO expression in microglia in the ipsilateral lesion area.

Limitations

First, we measured changes in the uptake of both [^{11}C]NE40 and [^{11}C](*R*)PK11195 24 h after surgery. These data cannot elucidate the timing of the state switch, dominancy, protective activity, or inflammatory processes of microglia. Different methods for acute stroke (transient or permanent ischemia) would generate different outcomes in the ischemic region with regard to inflammatory substances and cells as shown previously [29, 44]. According to these reports, the present PIT technique, one of the permanent stroke models, would yield less damage than transient, reperfusion model. As for microglia, not number but morphology of microglia was reportedly changed 1 day after permanent stroke [44]. Despite these findings, further study is needed to address changes in time course of inflammatory events after stroke. Second, because the cerebellum was chosen as the reference region to calculate BP_{ND} in this study, vascular injury may affect each region of the brain on the theory of diaschisis. However, the cerebellar PET counts were averaged between both sides in this study to minimize these possible diaschisis effects. Therefore, the estimated BP_{ND} values could reflect tissue tracer binding at target regions. Third, because the spatial resolution of the PET scanner used was relatively large (2.3 mm), there might be an effect of partial volume on the results. To reduce this effect, we tried to set ROIs that measured areas twice as large as the FWHM of the scanner, or we may choose autoradiography instead of PET although the parameters changing in the same animal cannot be obtained in autoradiography.

Conclusions

The present increase in [^{11}C]NE40 binding, but not [^{11}C](*R*)PK11195 binding concomitant with a higher CB2 immunochemical expression within the microglia over the peri-infarct region early after PIT injury, indicates that acutely activated microglia in early-stage ischemic stroke might be involved in the neuroprotective process of neuroinflammation. While a recent new CB2 tracer [^{11}C]A836339 has been reported to exceed the sensitivity of [^{11}C]NE40 to bind to CB2 under the chronic state of neurodegeneration in vivo [9], the present result suggests that [^{11}C]NE40 might be adequate for depicting activated microglia at a very early stage of brain disorders.

Additional files

Additional file 1: Figure S1. CT images and regions of interest. Frontal, −2 mm from the olfactory-frontal cortex junction (nearly 3 mm from the bregma). Parietal, −6 mm from the junction (nearly −1 mm from the bregma). Blue, lesion side; light blue, contralateral (non-lesion) side.

Additional file 2: Figure S2. The levels of SUV in each brain region. No significant difference was found in either [^{11}C]NE40 or [^{11}C](R)PK11195 SUV levels.

Additional file 3: Figure S3. Immunohistochemical results one day after photochemically induced thrombosis (PIT). Iba-1- and GFAP-positive regions are scattered around the infarct core.

Abbreviations

^{11}C-(*R*)PK11195: (*R*)-*N*-(11)C-Methyl-*N*-(1-methylpropyl)-1(2-chlorophenyl)isoquinoline -3-carboxamide; ^{11}C-DPA713: *N*,*N*-Diethyl-2-[2-(4-methoxyphenyl)-5,7-dimethylpyrazolo[1,5-a]pyrimidin-3-yl]acetamide; ^{11}C-NE40: 2-Oxo-7-[11C]methoxy-8butyloxy-1,2-dihydroquinoline-3-carboxylic acid cyclohexylamide; AD: Alzheimer's disease; BPND: Binding potential non-displaceable; CB2: Type 2 endocannabinoid receptor; CD11b: An integrin family member; GFAP: Glial fibrillary acidic protein; MCA: Middle cerebral artery; NeuN: Neuronal nuclei; NG2: Neural/glial antigen 2; PD: Parkinson's disease; PET: Positron emission tomography; PFA: Paraformaldehyde; PIT: Photochemically induced thrombosis; R1: Tracer influx index; RT: Room temperature; TAC: Time-activity curve; TSPO: Translocator protein

Acknowledgements

The authors would like to thank Dr. Norihiro Harada (Hamamatsu Photonics KK) and Drs. Sumiko Mikawa and Hiromu Furukawa (Department of Neuroanatomy and Neuroscience, Hamamatsu University School of Medicine) for their excellent support.

Funding

This work was supported by grants from the Japanese Ministry of Education, Culture, Sports, Science and Technology, from the JSPS KAKENHI with Grant Numbers 26293263 and 26670538, and from the Takeda Science Foundation.

Authors' contributions

TH and YO designed, analyzed, and wrote the paper. TH, DF, TK, SY, and HO performed the research. SN and HT synthesized the tracers. TU and KS evaluated and advised the design. All authors have seen and agreed with the content of the manuscript.

Competing interests

We declare that this work is free from any limitation by financial or any other relationship that might lead to a conflict of interest. The authors declare that they have no competing interests.

Consent for publication

Not applicable. The study involves no human materials.

Author details

[1]Department of Neuroanatomy and Neuroscience, Hamamatsu University School of Medicine, 1-20-1 Handayama, Higashi-ku, Hamamatsu 431-3192, Japan. [2]Central Research Laboratory, Hamamatsu Photonics KK, 5000 Hirakuchi, Hamakita-ku, Hamamatsu 434-8601, Japan. [3]Department of Biofunctional Imaging, Preeminent Medical Photonics Education & Research Center, Hamamatsu University School of Medicine, 1-20-1 Handayama, Higashi-ku, Hamamatsu 431-3192, Japan.

References

1. Venneti S, Wiley CA, Kofler J. Imaging microglial activation during neuroinflammation and Alzheimer's disease. J Neuroimmune Pharmacol. 2009;4:227–43.
2. Yokokura M, Mori N, Yagi S, et al. In vivo changes in microglial activation and amyloid deposits in brain regions with hypometabolism in Alzheimer's disease. Eur J Nucl Med Mol Imaging. 2011;38:343–51.

3. Ouchi Y, Yoshikawa E, Sekine Y, et al. Microglial activation and dopamine terminal loss in early Parkinson's disease. Ann Neurol. 2005;57:168–75.
4. Venneti S, Lopresti BJ, Wiley CA. The peripheral benzodiazepine receptor (translocator protein 18 kDa) in microglia: from pathology to imaging. Prog Neurobiol. 2006;80:308–22.
5. Pappata S, Levasseur M, Gunn RN, et al. Thalamic microglial activation in ischemic stroke detected in vivo by PET and [11C]PK1195. Neurology. 2000; 55:1052–4.
6. Shukuri M, Takashima-Hirano M, Tokuda K, et al. In vivo expression of cyclooxygenase-1 in activated microglia and macrophages during neuroinflammation visualized by PET with 11C-ketoprofen methyl ester. J Nucl Med. 2011;52:1094–101.
7. Wang Y, Yue X, Kiesewetter DO, Niu G, Teng G, Chen X. PET imaging of neuroinflammation in a rat traumatic brain injury model with radiolabeled TSPO ligand DPA-714. Eur J Nucl Med Mol Imaging. 2014; 41:1440–9.
8. Israel I, Ohsiek A, Al-Momani E, Albert-Weissenberger C, Stetter C, Mencl S, Buck AK, Kleinschnitz C, Samnick S, Siren AL. Combined [(18)F]DPA-714 micro-positron emission tomography and autoradiography imaging of microglia activation after closed head injury in mice. J Neuroinflammation. 2016;13:140.
9. Wu J, Bie B, Yang H, et al. Activation of the CB2 receptor system reverses amyloid-induced memory deficiency. Neurobiol Aging. 2013;34:791–804.
10. Martín-Moreno AM, Reigada D, Ramírez BG, et al. Cannabidiol and other cannabinoids reduce microglial activation in vitro and in vivo: relevance to Alzheimer's disease. Mol Pharmacol. 2011;79:964–73.
11. Savonenko AV, Melnikova T, Wang Y, et al. Cannabinoid CB2 receptors in a mouse model of Aβ amyloidosis: immunohistochemical analysis and suitability as a PET biomarker of neuroinflammation. PLoS One. 2015;10:e0129618.
12. Palazuelos J, Davoust N, Julien B, et al. The CB(2) cannabinoid receptor controls myeloid progenitor trafficking: involvement in the pathogenesis of an animal model of multiple sclerosis. J Biol Chem. 2008;283:13320–9.
13. Concannon RM, Okine BN, Finn DP, Dowd E. Differential upregulation of the cannabinoid CB_2 receptor in neurotoxic and inflammation-driven rat models of Parkinson's disease. Exp Neurol. 2015;269:133–41.
14. Ashton JC, Rahman RMA, Nair SM, et al. Cerebral hypoxia-ischemia and middle cerebral artery occlusion induce expression of the cannabinoid CB2 receptor in the brain. Neurosci Lett. 2007;412:114–7.
15. Zarruk JG, Fernández-López D, García-Yébenes I, et al. Cannabinoid type 2 receptor activation downregulates stroke-induced classic and alternative brain macrophage/microglial activation concomitant to neuroprotection. Stroke. 2012;43:211–9.
16. Zhang M, Martin BR, Adler MW, et al. Cannabinoid CB2 receptor activation decreases cerebral infarction in a mouse focal ischemia/reperfusion model. J Cereb Blood Flow Metab. 2007;27:1387–96.
17. Fernández-López D, Faustino J, Derugin N, et al. Reduced infarct size and accumulation of microglia in rats treated with WIN 55,212-2 after neonatal stroke. Neurosci. 2012;207:307–15.
18. Benito C, Tolón RM, Pazos MR, et al. Cannabinoid CB2 receptors in human brain inflammation. Br J Pharmacol. 2008;153:277–85.
19. Evens N, Vandeputte C, Coolen C, et al. Preclinical evaluation of [11C]NE40, a type 2 cannabinoid receptor PET tracer. Nucl Med Biol. 2012;39:389–99.
20. Vandeputte C, Casteels C, Struys T, et al. Small-animal PET imaging of the type 1 and type 2 cannabinoid receptors in a photothrombotic stroke model. Eur J Nucl Med Mol Imaging. 2012;39:1796–806.
21. Postnov A, Ahmad R, Evens N, et al. Quantification of 11C-NE40, a novel PET radioligand for CB2 receptor imaging. J Nucl Med. 2013;54:188. abstract.
22. Banati RB, Newcombe J, Gunn RN, et al. The peripheral benzodiazepine binding site in the brain in multiple sclerosis: quantitative in vivo imaging of microglia as a measure of disease activity. Brain. 2000;123:2321–37.
23. Hu X, Li P, Guo Y, et al. Microglia/macrophage polarization dynamics reveal novel mechanism of injury expansion after focal cerebral ischemia. Stroke. 2012;43:3063–70.
24. Wang G, Zhang J, Hu X, et al. Microglia/macrophage polarization dynamics in white matter after traumatic brain injury. J Cereb Blood Flow Metab. 2013;33:1864–74.
25. Fukumoto D, Hosoya T, Nishiyama S, et al. Multiparametric assessment of acute and subacute ischemic neuronal damage: a small animal positron emission tomography study with rat photochemically induced thrombosis model. Synapse. 2011;65:207–14.
26. Umemura K, Nakashima M. A new model of middle cerebral artery thrombosis in rats. Japanese J Psychopharmacol. 1993;13:9–17.
27. Lammertsma AA, Hume SP. Simplified reference tissue model for PET receptor studies. NeuroImage. 1996;4:153–8.
28. Gunn RN, Lammertsma AA, Hume SP, Cunningham VJ. Parametric imaging of ligand-receptor binding in PET using a simplified reference region model. NeuroImage. 1997;6:279–87.
29. Lehmann J, Härtig W, Seidel A, et al. Inflammatory cell recruitment after experimental thromboembolic stroke in rats. Neurosci. 2014;279:139–54.
30. Ouchi Y, Tsukada H, Kakiuchi T, et al. Changes in cerebral blood flow and postsynaptic muscarinic cholinergic activity in rats with bilateral carotid artery ligation. J Nucl Med. 1998;39:198–202.
31. Shimizu Y, Yamamoto S, Fukumoto D, et al. Loud noise exposure during activity and neurogenesis in the living rat brain: preliminary study. J Neurol Neurophysiol. 2014;5:6.
32. Levine JM. Increased expression of the NG2 chondroitin-sulfate proteoglycan after brain injury. J Neurosci. 1994;14:4716–30.
33. Matsumoto H, Kumon Y, Watanabe H, et al. Accumulation of macrophage-like cells expressing NG2 proteoglycan and Iba1 in ischemic core of rat brain after transient middle cerebral artery occlusion. J Cereb Blood Flow Metab. 2008;28:149–63.
34. Bu J, Akhtar N, Nishiyama A. Transient expression of the NG2 proteoglycan by a subpopulation of activated macrophages in an excitotoxic hippocampal lesion. Glia. 2001;34:296–310.
35. Jones LL, Yamaguchi Y, Stallcup WB, Tuszynski MH. NG2 is a major chondroitin sulfate proteoglycan produced after spinal cord injury and is expressed by macrophages and oligodendrocyte progenitors. J Neurosci. 2002;22:2792–803.
36. Smirkin A, Matsumoto H, Takahashi H, et al. Iba1(+)/NG2(+) macrophage-like cells expressing a variety of neuroprotective factors ameliorate ischemic damage of the brain. J Cereb Blood Flow Metab. 2010;30:603–15.
37. Paxinos G, Watson C. The rat brain in stereotaxic coordinates/George Paxinos, Charles Watson, 2nd edn. Academic Press; 1986.
38. Cabral GA, Raborn ES, Griffin L, et al. CB2 receptors in the brain: role in central immune function. Br J Pharmacol. 2008;153:240–51.
39. Yokokura M, Terada T, Bunai T, et al. Depiction of microglial activation in aging and dementia: positron emission tomography with [11C]DPA713 versus [11C](R)PK11195. J Cereb Blood Flow Metab. 2017;37:877–89.
40. Malek N, Popiolek-Barczyk K, Mika J, et al. Anandamide, acting via CB2 receptors, alleviates LPS-induced neuroinflammation in rat primary microglial cultures. Neural Plast. 2015;2015:130639.
41. Garcia-Gutierrez MS, Perez-Ortiz JM, Gutierrez-Adan A, Manzanares J. Depression-resistant endophenotype in mice overexpressing cannabinoid CB(2) receptors. Br J Pharmacol. 2010;160(7):1773–84.
42. Bahi A, Al Mansouri S, Al Memari E, Al Ameri M, Nurulain SM, Ojha S. beta-Caryophyllene, a CB2 receptor agonist produces multiple behavioral changes relevant to anxiety and depression in mice. Physiol Behav. 2014; 135:119–24.
43. Moransard M, Dann A, Staszewski O, et al. NG2 expressed by macrophages and oligodendrocyte precursor cells is dispensable in experimental autoimmune encephalomyelitis. Brain. 2011;134:1315–30.
44. Schmidt W, Schäfer F, Striggow V, et al. Cannabinoid receptor subtypes 1 and 2 mediate long-lasting neuroprotection and improve motor behavior deficits after transient focal cerebral ischemia. Neurosci. 2012;227:313–26.

2

The splenic response to stroke: from rodents to stroke subjects

Hilary A. Seifert[1,2] and Halina Offner[1,2,3*]

Abstract

Background: Stroke is the fifth leading cause of death and the leading cause of long-term disability in the USA, costing $40.2 billion in direct and indirect costs. Globally, stroke is the second leading cause of death and has a higher prevalence in lower- and middle-income countries compared to high-income countries.
The role of the spleen in stroke has been studied in rodent models of stroke and is seen as a major contributor to increased secondary neural injury after stroke. Splenectomy 2 weeks prior to ischemic and hemorrhagic stroke in mice and rats shows decreased infarct volumes. Additionally, the spleen decreases in size following stroke in rodents. Pro-inflammatory mediators are also increased in the spleen and subsequently the brain after stroke. These data in preclinical models of stroke have led stroke neurologists to look at the splenic response in stroke subjects. The outcomes of these studies suggest the spleen is responding in a similar manner in stroke subjects as it is in animal models of stroke.

Conclusion: Animal models demonstrating the detrimental role of the spleen in stroke are providing strong evidence of how the spleen is responding during stroke in human subjects. This indicates treatments targeting the splenic immune response in animals could provide useful targets and treatments for stroke subjects.

Keywords: Stroke, Splenectomy, Immune response, Clinical studies, Animal models

Background

Stroke is the leading cause of disability and the fifth leading cause of death in the USA. Each year, 42.4 million strokes occur globally. The most common type is ischemic stroke resulting from a clot occluding a cerebral vessel [1]. While advancements have been made in treating the clot and restoring blood flow to the brain, there are still many factors that influence infarct size and the resulting disability. The immune system has been shown to play a detrimental role after stroke [2–4]. The spleen is a storage site for immune cells [5] and has been shown in animal models to play a role in increasing neural injury after experimental stroke [6–10]. This review will examine the spleen's role in animal models of stroke and how these studies have translated into examining the spleens in stroke subjects.

* Correspondence: offnerva@ohsu.edu
[1]Neuroimmunology Research R&D-31 Veterans Affairs Portland Health Care System, 3710 SW US Veterans Hospital Rd, Portland, OR 97239, USA
[2]Department of Neurology, Oregon Health and Science University, Portland, OR, USA
Full list of author information is available at the end of the article

Stroke statistics

Stroke is the fifth leading cause of death in the USA and second leading cause of death around the world. In the USA, 795,000 strokes occur annually resulting in the largest cause of long-term disability and costing $40.1 billion in direct and indirect costs. Globally 42.4 million strokes occur each year, with high-income countries seeing a decrease in the incidence of ischemic and hemorrhagic stroke compared to low and middle income countries. Of the two main stroke subtypes, ischemic and hemorrhagic, ischemic strokes account for 87% of strokes while hemorrhagic strokes make up 13%. There are racial differences in stroke risks and outcomes. American Indian/Alaska Natives and non-Hispanic blacks have higher stroke prevalence compared to non-Hispanic whites, Hispanics, and Asians/Pacific Islanders (~ 4.5 vs. ~ 2%, respectively). Additionally there are differences between men and women with regards to stroke risk, incidence, and outcomes. Overall women have a higher lifetime risk of stroke than men, and 55,000 more women than men experience a stroke each year. Men are at a slightly higher risk for stroke in younger and middle-aged groups but women have a much greater risk for stroke later in life and are more likely to die from a stroke. Women accounted for 58% of stroke deaths in the USA in 2015 [1].

The spleen

The spleen is a secondary immune organ that is part of the immune system. The spleen acts as a filter for the blood to remove any dying red blood cells, antibody coated cells, and bacterial pathogens. Additionally, the spleen serves as a communication hub for various immune cells to interact with each other, including T cells, B cells, macrophages/monocytes, and dendritic cells to initiate adaptive immune responses. The spleen is divided between the red and white pulp. The red pulp contains macrophages that filter the blood as it passes through the spleen and antibody producing B cells that allow for rapid delivery of antibodies into circulation. The white pulp has concentrated areas of lymphocytes. The close proximity of these cells allows for easy interaction of T cells and B cells to mount adaptive responses and allows macrophages and dendritic cells easy access to lymphocytes. T cells are concentrated around arterioles and make up periarteriolar lymphoid sheaths. This allows T cells to be in close proximity to the blood supply that allows dendritic cells easy access to naïve T cells, which once activated leave the spleen. B cells are organized to form B cell follicles. B cell follicles are where B cell responses are honed with isotype switching and increasing antigen specificity. These processes require T cells. The highly specific structure of the spleen allows for all these cells to be in close proximity to each other [5].

Peripheral immune response to stroke

Numerous studies have demonstrated the role the immune system plays in increasing neural injury follow stroke. Mice lacking lymphocytes, both $Rag^{-/-}$ [2] and SCID mice [3], have decreased infract volumes compared to wild type mice following middle cerebral artery occlusion (MCAO). An additional study showed peripheral immune cells in the stroked brain hours to days after the initial insult [4]. The spleen, which is a reservoir of immune cells, is of interest in secondary neural injury following stroke. Splenocytes have been found in the brain in only the injured hemisphere at 48 and 96 h following MCAO [11], a rodent model of stroke.

Splenic response to ischemia/reperfusion injuries

The spleen's involvement is well documented to enhance inflammation in ischemia/reperfusion (IR) injuries to various organs. The liver was the first organ where splenectomy was shown to decrease injury from the IR and blunt the inflammatory response triggered by IR [12]. Splenectomy also protected the intestines [13] and the kidneys [14] from IR injury. The injury in all three organs is believed to be mediated by monocytes in the spleen that activate Kupffer cells in the liver. Removing the spleen and splenic monocytes prevents activation of Kupffer cells, resulting in less inflammation and a reduction in tissue damage, as does blocking Kupffer cell activation with gadolinium chloride. Splenic monocytes were also found to play a detrimental role following IR injury to the heart, since splenectomy was protective against IR injury in that organ [15].

Splenic response to stroke in rodents

Rodent spleens show a decrease in size after MCAO that appears to be catecholamine (CA)-mediated, but the reason for the change in spleen size after stroke varies between rats and mice. The splenic capsule of rat spleens expresses α_1 adrenergic receptors that cause splenic contraction when activated [16]. Following permanent MCAO (pMCAO) in rats, circulating CAs cause a transient decrease in spleen size. While the spleen is highly innervated by sympathetic neural networks [17], denervation of the spleen prior to pMCAO did not prevent the spleen from contracting. However, blocking the α_1 receptors with prazosin or carvedilol did block splenic contraction, whereas propranolol did not block contraction. Carvedilol also decreased infarct size [18]. Additionally, rat spleens demonstrated a transient decrease in size with the smallest size detected 48 h after pMCAO but a return to pre-stroke size by 72 h. During splenic contraction, splenocytes were released into the systemic circulation and traveled to the injured hemisphere of the brain. Innate splenocytes were found in the brain as early as 48 h, whereas adaptive splenocytes appeared at 96 h following pMCAO [11]. Generally, there was a negative correlation between spleen size and infarct volume [19]. Mice also exhibit a significant loss of cells and decreased spleen size following transient MCAO (tMCAO) that persists over time. This loss of splenocytes appears to be due to apoptosis of the splenocytes and loss of splenic structures, including B cell follicles. At 96 h after tMCAO, mice show a 90% reduction in splenocyte numbers compared to sham-operated mice. The greatest effect is on B cells, while T cell numbers appear to increase, specifically regulatory T cells [20]. An additional study showed that mouse spleens continued to decrease in size through day 7 post-tMCAO [21]. Mouse spleens are extensively innervated like rat spleens and also appear to highly express α_1-adenergic receptors on the splenic capsule [22]. Unlike rats, mouse spleens do not contract, but the catecholaminergic innervation of immune cells appears to negatively impact some of these cells resulting in cell death.

In addition to the cellular responses in the spleen to stroke, there are also changes in cytokine and chemokine responses. In mouse spleens, there is an increase by 22 h after tMCAO in TNFα, interferon gamma (IFNγ), IL-6,

MCP-1, and IL-2, all of which are pro-inflammatory mediators [23]. One pro-inflammatory cytokine of interest is IFNγ, since IFN$\gamma^{-/-}$ mice have smaller infarcts than wild-type mice [2]. In rats, splenic increases in IFNγ production as early as 24 h after pMCAO results in a delayed increase in IFNγ in the injured brain at 72 h. This early transient increase in IFNγ in the spleen is likely connected to the later increase in IFNγ in the brain, since splenectomy decreases the IFNγ expression in the brain [7]. Similar results were found in mice after tMCAO such that IFNγ was increased at 72 h in the brain and splenectomy significantly decreased IFNγ levels within the brain [8]. IFNγ also initiated the expression of the pro-inflammatory chemokine interferon inducible protein 10 (IP-10) in both the spleen and the brain after pMCAO. Splenectomy prior to pMCAO or treatment with an IFNγ neutralizing antibody after pMCAO reduced IP-10 levels in the brain and subsequent T cell recruitment to the brain [24].

Splenectomy in rodent models of stroke

Splenectomy carried out 2 weeks prior to initiating MCAO in mice or intracerebral hemorrhage (ICH) in rats afforded protection in the brain. Initial studies found that splenectomy 2 weeks prior to pMCAO in rats decreased infarct volume by 80% and reduced immune cell infiltration into the brain [6]. Subsequently, a study found that splenectomy significantly decreased edema and water content in a rat model of ICH [10]. In mice, splenectomy prior to tMCAO was first carried out only in males and showed a significant reduction in infarct volume [8]. Additional studies in mice again showed that male mice were protected from stroke after splenectomy but that the protective effect was lost in female mice [9]. It was found that female mice had more regulatory lymphocytes in their spleens than male mice and the loss of these regulatory cells in female mice resulted in the loss of protection from stroke [9, 25]. Additionally, male mice had more activated T cells in their spleens after tMCAO compared to female mice [26]. A study in older mice demonstrated that splenectomy decreased infarct volume in older male mice, improved behavioral outcomes, and decreased immune cell infiltration into the brain [27]. A more recent study in rats showed splenectomy immediately following tMCAO significantly decreased infarct volume and improved behavioral deficits [28]. Other studies have concluded that splenectomy does not protect mice or rats from tMCAO although it was noted that the MCAO surgery was performed immediately after the splenectomy surgery [29, 30]. Splenectomy is a major surgery, and the body compensates for the loss of the spleen by transiently increasing circulating immune cells over the course of a week (data not published). Additionally, the body is also responding to the surgical insult of removing the spleen. Therefore, splenectomy should be performed 2 weeks prior to the MCAO surgery to allow the animal's body to recovery from the splenectomy surgery. Another study investigating the role the spleen plays in enhancing neural injury used splenic irradiation in place of splenectomy as a noninvasive way to blunt the splenic responses. Rats received targeted splenic irradiation 3 or 4 h after tMCAO, and this significantly decreased infarct size but did not damage the spleen or surrounding organs or lead to immune suppression or increased infections [31].

Neuroprotective therapies also involve the spleen

Various therapies that protect the brain after stroke interact with the spleen. Some therapies interact with splenocytes or travel to the spleen. Others prevent the decrease in spleen size seen after tMCAO. Stem cells from various sources protect the brain after stroke and also travel to the spleen. Human umbilical cord blood (HUCB) cells reduce infarct after pMCAO in rats and restore spleen size at 48 h post-pMCAO [19, 32]. HUCB cells protected gray and white matter [33] in rats when administered 24 h after MCAO and reduced behavioral deficits. Additionally, HUCB cells saved the spleen weight [19], were found in the injured brain and the spleen [34], and allowed splenocytes to respond normally when stimulated with concanavalin A when the cells were administered intravenously [19]. Studies with human bone marrow stem cells (hBMSC) found these cells decreased infarct volume in rats and migrated to the spleen when administered intravenously [35]. The previous two examples were immune cell derived stem cells that migrated to the spleen after stroke to help reduce the infarct. A study in a model of ICH used neural stem cells and found these cells were more effective at reducing edema and brain water content after ICH when injected intravenously compared to direct injection into the brain. In addition, it was reported that neural stem cells in the spleen were in direct contact with the splenic monocytes. The spleen was also found to be necessary for neural stem cells to provide protection since protection was lost when the rats underwent splenectomy 2 weeks prior to ICH and neural stem cell administration [10].

Other therapies save spleen size and reduce infarct. One such therapy is treatment with recombinant T cell receptor ligands (RTL), which are partial major histocompatibility complex II molecules covalently bound to myelin peptides. After tMCAO in mice, RTL administration reduced infarct size by 50%, reduced the recruitment of immune cells to the brain, and prevented the reduction in spleen size seen in mice. This effect was only seen in mice given the RTL with a myelin peptide [36–38]. Another therapy, carvedilol—a pan adrenergic blocker, also reduced infarct size in rats with pMCAO and prevented splenic contraction [18].

The splenic response in stroke subjects

The initial pilot study in stroke subjects used ultrasound to evaluate at the spleen size in 30 stroke subjects with ischemic stroke that were at the hospital within 6 h after onset of symptoms. This study found that the spleen size of subjects initially decreased and if the subject continued to decline on the NIH Stroke Severity (NIHSS) score then their spleens continued to decrease in size. However, in some subjects, the NIHSS score decreased as the spleen size began to increase until it surpassed the initial ultrasound reading [39]. Another study used a retrospective approach looking at CT scans of 82 stroke subject spleens. This study included both ischemic and hemorrhagic stroke subjects. The study concluded that the spleen undergoes a biphasic response to stroke characterized by a transient decrease in spleen size reaching its smallest size at 48 h post stroke. There were gender differences in spleen size after stroke, but no difference between stroke subtypes [40]. A larger study derived from the initial pilot study was expanded to include both ischemic and hemorrhagic stroke subjects and a cohort of healthy control subjects to establish a baseline spleen size. The 158 healthy controls underwent an ultrasound of their spleen for 5 consecutive days. Based on these data, significant differences were found between gender, height, weight, and body surface area (BSA). To evaluate if there was any splenic contraction in stroke subjects, their spleen volumes were compared to healthy controls based on gender and BSA. A spleen was considered to be contracted if it was 20 cm^3 smaller than their gender and BSA matched healthy controls. This study found that 40.5% of stroke subjects had a contracted spleen. Individuals were at a significantly higher risk for splenic contraction if they were African American, over the age of 75, had a more severe stroke, or had a history of stroke. There were no differences between genders, types of stroke, or admission NIHSS score. Plasma cytokines were also analyzed in a subset of subjects and individuals with splenic contraction had significantly elevated levels of IFNγ, IL-6, IL-12, and IL-10 [41]. In an expansion of the previous study, a retrospective looked at only ischemic stroke subjects to determine if there was an association between splenic contraction and systemic inflammatory response syndrome (SIRS). SIRS is an inflammatory process that is detrimental to stroke recovery and independent of an infection. SIRS was considered present if two of the following were present: elevated heart rate, changes in body temperature, elevated respiratory rate, or changes in white blood cell counts. Non-infectious SIRS is associated with longer hospital stays and poorer functional outcomes. Splenic contraction was not associated with the development of early SIRS. African Americans and individuals aged over 75 were at a significantly higher risk of splenic contraction following a stroke. African Americans had a 92.3% chance of developing SIRS within the first 48 h of stroke if they had splenic contraction compared to a 62.5% chance of developing SIRS with splenic contraction in other races. In individuals over the age of 75, there was a negative correlation with splenic contraction and the

Table 1 Studies looking at the splenic response to stroke

		Species	Type	Duration	Citation
Observations	Splenocyte apoptosis	Mus	tMCAO	96 h	[20]
	Increased IFNg levels	Mus	tMCAO	96 h	[8]
		Rat	pMCAO	96 h	[7, 24]
	Splenic contraction	Rat	pMCAO	96 h	[7]
	Change in spleen size	Hu	Ischemic	Variable	[39]
		Hu	Ischemic hemorrhagic	Variable	[40]
	Splenic contraction (some subjects)	Hu	Ischemic hemorrhagic	Variable	[41]
	SIRS with splenic contraction (some subjects)	Hu	Ischemic	Variable	[42]
Pre-treatment	Splenectomy protection (males only)	Mus	tMCAO	96 h	[9]
	Splenectomy protection	Mus	tMCAO	96 h	[8]
		Rat	pMCAO	96 h	[6]
		Rat	ICH	72 h	[10]
	Carvedilol	Rat	pMCAO	48 h	[18]
Post-treatment	RTL	Mus	tMCAO	96 h	[36–38]
	Splenic irradiation	Rat	tMCAO	48 h, 7 days	[31]
	HUCBC's	Rat	pMCAO	48 h, 96 h	[19, 32–34]
	NSC	Rat	ICH	72 h	[10]

This table summarizes experiments that involve the splenic response in stroke. Some observational studies, some pre-treatment studies, some post-treatment studies. Studies with mice, rats, and human stroke subjects are included

development of SIRS at 72 h post stroke, while there was no significant connection between splenic contraction and SIRS in the younger age groups. In stroke subjects over the age of 75, the development of SIRS was higher in individuals without splenic contraction compared to those subjects with splenic contraction (71.4 vs. 46.1, respectively) [42].

Conclusion

The importance of the spleen in contributing to increased neural damage following a stroke is becoming increasing evident in stroke subjects. Changes that were seen in preclinical models of stroke in rodents are similar to the data being collected in stroke subjects. While there are limitations to all animal models of human diseases, the role of the spleen in stroke from preclinical models so far has provided some insight into the disease process of human stroke. Not only has the spleen been shown to decrease in size following stroke there is also an increase in IFNγ in subjects with splenic contraction (Table 1). This could lead to biomarkers for stroke outcomes or targets to treat stroke in certain subsets of subjects (Fig. 1).

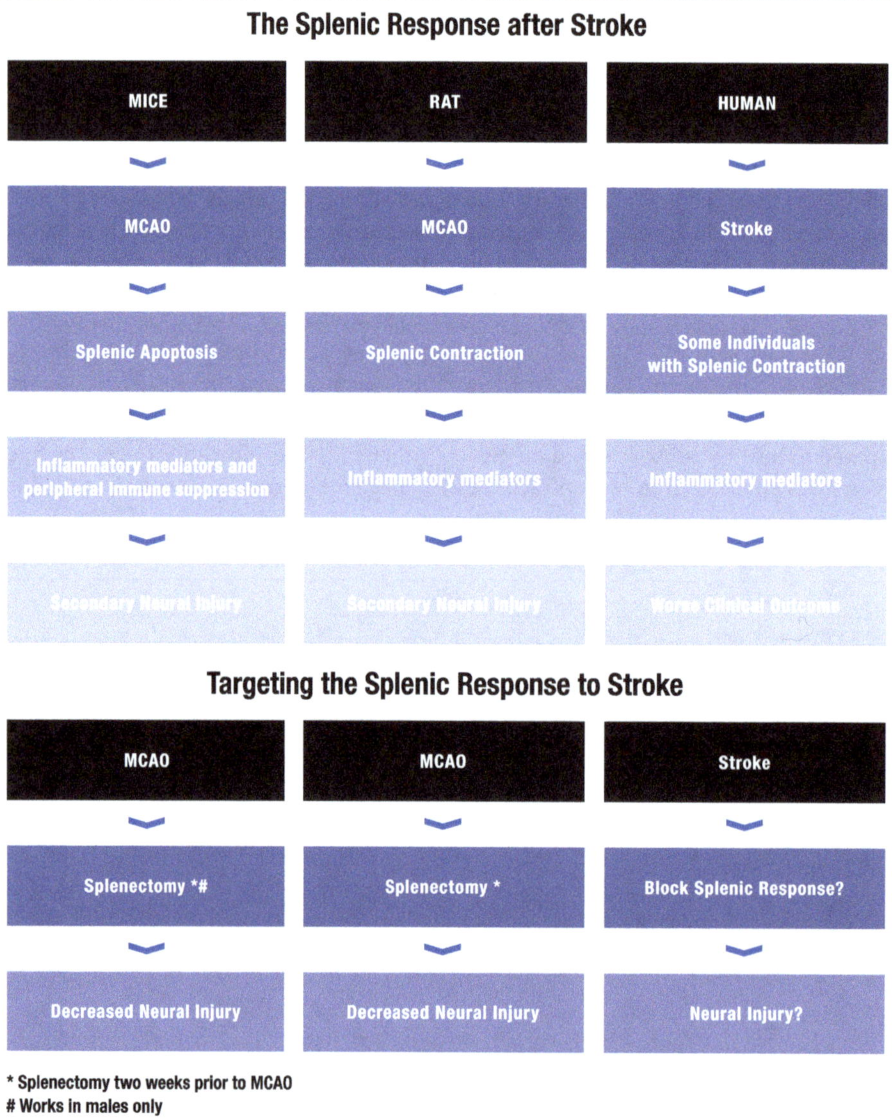

Fig. 1 The splenic immune response to stroke. The spleen responds to stroke in mice, rats, and humans after cerebral ischemia. In experimental models with mice and rats using MCAO as a model for ischemic stroke, the spleen decreases in size. In mice, this is due to splenic apoptosis and loss of cells. In rats, the spleen contracts and releases immune cells into circulation. In stroke subjects, the spleen contracts in some individuals. The spleen's involvement in post-stroke events contributes to secondary neural injury and worse outcomes. When the spleen is targeted in animal models of stroke, using splenectomy, this decreases neural injury in mice and rats. Can targeting the spleen in humans improve clinical outcomes by decreasing neural injury? * indicates splenectomy 2 weeks prior to MCAO. # splenectomy only works in male mice

Abbreviations

BSA: Body surface area; CA: Catecholamine; hBMSC: Human bone marrow stem cells; HUCB: Human umbilical cord blood; ICH: Intracerebral hemorrhage; IFNγ: Interferon gamma; IP-10: Interferon inducible protein 10; IR: Ischemia/reperfusion; MCAO: Middle cerebral artery occlusion; NIHSS: NIH stroke severity; NSC: Neural stem cells; pMCAO: Permanent MCAO; RTL: Recombinant T cell receptor ligands; SIRS: Systemic inflammatory response syndrome; tMCAO: Transient MCAO

Acknowledgements

The authors thank Gail Kent for assistance with manuscript preparation and submission.

Funding

This work was supported by American Heart Association grants 17GRNT33220001 and NIH/NINDS R01NS076013, and R01NS080890 (Halina Offner). This material is the result of work supported with resources and the use of facilities at the VA Portland Health Care Center in Portland, OR. The contents do not represent the views of the US Department of Veterans Affairs or the United States Government.

Authors' contributions

HS and HO wrote and edited the review. Both authors read and approved the final manuscript.

Consent for publication

Not applicable.

Competing interests

HO and OHSU have a significant financial interest in Artielle ImmunoTherapeutics, Inc., a company that may have a commercial interest in the results of the research and technology involving RTL. This potential conflict of interest has been reviewed and managed by the OHSU and VA Portland Health Care System Conflict of Interest in Research Committees. HS declares no conflicts of interest.

Author details

[1]Neuroimmunology Research R&D-31 Veterans Affairs Portland Health Care System, 3710 SW US Veterans Hospital Rd, Portland, OR 97239, USA. [2]Department of Neurology, Oregon Health and Science University, Portland, OR, USA. [3]Department of Anesthesiology and Perioperative Medicine, Oregon Health and Science University, Portland, OR, USA.

References

1. Benjamin EJ, et al. Heart disease and stroke statistics-2018 update: a report from the American Heart Association. Circulation. 2018;137(12):e67–e492.
2. Yilmaz G, et al. Role of T lymphocytes and interferon-gamma in ischemic stroke. Circulation. 2006;113(17):2105–12.
3. Hurn PD, et al. T- and B-cell-deficient mice with experimental stroke have reduced lesion size and inflammation. J Cereb Blood Flow Metab. 2007; 27(11):1798–805.
4. Stevens SL, et al. The use of flow cytometry to evaluate temporal changes in inflammatory cells following focal cerebral ischemia in mice. Brain Res. 2002;932(1–2):110–9.
5. Mebius RE, Kraal G. Structure and function of the spleen. Nat Rev Immunol. 2005;5(8):606–16.
6. Ajmo CT Jr, et al. The spleen contributes to stroke-induced neurodegeneration. J Neurosci Res. 2008;86:2227–34.
7. Seifert HA, et al. The spleen contributes to stroke induced neurodegeneration through interferon gamma signaling. Metab Brain Dis. 2012;27(2):131–41.
8. Jin R, et al. Simvastatin attenuates stroke-induced splenic atrophy and lung susceptibility to spontaneous bacterial infection in mice. Stroke. 2013;44(4): 1135–43.
9. Dotson AL, et al. Splenectomy reduces infarct volume and neuroinflammation in male but not female mice in experimental stroke. J Neuroimmunol. 2015;278:289–98.
10. Lee ST, et al. Anti-inflammatory mechanism of intravascular neural stem cell transplantation in haemorrhagic stroke. Brain. 2008;131(Pt 3):616–29.
11. Seifert HA, et al. A transient decrease in spleen size following stroke corresponds to splenocyte release into systemic circulation. J Neuroimmune Pharmacology. 2012;7(4):1017–24.
12. Okuaki Y, et al. Splenectomy-reduced hepatic injury induced by ischemia/ reperfusion in the rat. Liver. 1996;16(3):188–94.
13. Savas MC, et al. Splenectomy attenuates intestinal ischemia-reperfusion-induced acute lung injury. J Pediatr Surg. 2003;38(10):1465–70.
14. Jiang H, et al. Splenectomy ameliorates acute multiple organ damage induced by liver warm ischemia reperfusion in rats. Surgery. 2007;141(1):32–40.
15. Leuschner F, et al. Angiotensin-converting enzyme inhibition prevents the release of monocytes from their splenic reservoir in mice with myocardial infarction. Circ Res. 2010;107(11):1364–73.
16. Aboud R, Shafii M, Docherty JR. Investigation of the subtypes of alpha 1-adrenoceptor mediating contractions of rat aorta, vas deferens and spleen. Br J Pharmacol. 1993;109(1):80–7.
17. Felten DL, et al. Noradrenergic and peptidergic innervation of lymphoid tissue. J Immunol. 1985;135(2 Suppl):755s–65s.
18. Ajmo CT Jr, et al. Blockade of adrenoreceptors inhibits the splenic response to stroke. Exp Neurol. 2009;218(1):47–55.
19. Vendrame M, et al. Infusion of human umbilical cord blood cells in a rat model of stroke dose-dependently rescues behavioral deficits and reduces infarct volume. Stroke. 2004;35(10):2390–5.
20. Offner H, et al. Splenic atrophy in experimental stroke is accompanied by increased regulatory T cells and circulating macrophages. J Immunol. 2006; 176(11):6523–31.
21. Bao Y, et al. A role for spleen monocytes in post-ischemic brain inflammation and injury. J Neuroinflammation. 2010;7:92.
22. Grisanti LA, Perez DM, Porter JE. Modulation of immune cell function by alpha(1)-adrenergic receptor activation. Curr Top Membr. 2011;67:113–38.
23. Offner H, et al. Experimental stroke induces massive, rapid activation of the peripheral immune system. J Cereb Blood Flow Metab. 2006;26(5):654–65.
24. Seifert HA, et al. Pro-inflammatory interferon gamma signaling is directly associated with stroke induced neurodegeneration. J NeuroImmune Pharmacol. 2014;9(5):679–89.
25. Seifert HA, et al. Sex differences in regulatory cells in experimental stroke. Cell Immunol. 2017;318:49–54.
26. Banerjee A, et al. Phenotypic changes in immune cell subsets reflect increased infarct volume in male vs. female mice. Transl Stroke Res. 2013;4(5):554–63.
27. Chauhan A, et al. Splenectomy protects aged mice from injury after experimental stroke. Neurobiol Aging. 2018;61:102–11.
28. Belinga VF, et al. Splenectomy following MCAO inhibits the TLR4-NF-kappaB signaling pathway and protects the brain from neurodegeneration in rats. J Neuroimmunol. 2016;293:105–13.
29. Kim E, et al. Role of spleen-derived monocytes/macrophages in acute ischemic brain injury. J Cereb Blood Flow Metab. 2014;34(8):1411–9.
30. Zierath D, et al. Splenectomy does not improve long-term outcome after stroke. Stroke. 2017;48(2):497–500.
31. Ostrowski R, et al. Acute splenic irradiation reduces brain injury in the rat focal ischemic stroke model. Transl Stroke Res. 2012;3:473–81.
32. Vendrame M, et al. Anti-inflammatory effects of human cord blood cells in a rat model of stroke. Stem Cells Dev. 2005;14:595–604.
33. Rowe DD, et al. Cord blood administration induces oligodendrocyte survival through alterations in gene expression. Brain Res. 2010;1366:172–88.
34. Vendrame M, et al. Cord blood rescues stroke-induced changes in splenocyte phenotype and function. Exp Neurol. 2006;199(1):191–200.
35. Acosta SA, et al. Intravenous bone marrow stem cell grafts preferentially migrate to spleen and abrogate chronic inflammation in stroke. Stroke. 2015;46(9):2616–27.
36. Subramanian S, et al. Recombinant T cell receptor ligand treats experimental stroke. Stroke. 2009;40(7):2539–45.
37. Dziennis S, et al. Therapy with recombinant T-cell receptor ligand reduces infarct size and infiltrating inflammatory cells in brain after middle cerebral artery occlusion in mice. Metab Brain Dis. 2011;26(2):123–33.

38. Akiyoshi K, et al. Recombinant T cell receptor ligands improve outcome after experimental cerebral ischemia. Transl Stroke Res. 2011;2(3):404–10.
39. Sahota P, et al. Changes in spleen size in patients with acute ischemic stroke: a pilot observational study. Int J Stroke. 2013;8(2):60–7.
40. Chiu NL, et al. The volume of the spleen and its correlates after acute stroke. J Stroke Cerebrovasc Dis. 2016;25(12):2958–61.
41. Vahidy FS, et al. Acute splenic responses in patients with ischemic stroke and intracerebral hemorrhage. J Cereb Blood Flow Metab. 2016;36(6):1012–21.
42. Zha A, et al. Association between splenic contraction and the systemic inflammatory response after acute ischemic stroke varies with age and race. Transl Stroke Res. 2017;27:1–9.

3

Homocysteine exaggerates microglia activation and neuroinflammation through microglia localized STAT3 overactivation following ischemic stroke

Shuang Chen, Zhiping Dong, Man Cheng, Yaqian Zhao, Mengying Wang, Na Sai, Xuan Wang, Huan Liu, Guowei Huang and Xumei Zhang*

Abstract

Background: Elevated plasma homocysteine (Hcy) levels have been indicated as a strong and modifiable risk factor of ischemic stroke; the previous studies have shown that exposure to Hcy activates cultured microglia. However, whether neurotoxicity of Hcy involves microglia activation following brain ischemia and the underlying mechanisms remains incompletely understood.

Methods: The cerebral damage was evaluated by staining with 2,3,5-triphenyltetrazolium chloride, hematoxylin-eosin, and Fluoro Jade B. The activation state of microglia was assessed via immunoreaction using the microglial markers Iba1 and OX-42. Then, the inflammatory factors such as tumor necrosis factor α (TNF-α), interleukin 6 (IL-6), and phosphorylated signal transducer and activator of transcription 3 (pSTAT3) were examined by Western blot analysis and fluorescence immunohistochemistry.

Results: Elevated Hcy level augmented brain damage and neural cell toxicity in the brain cortex and the dentate gyrus region of the hippocampus after cerebral ischemia/reperfusion. Meanwhile, Hcy activated microglia and induced the expression of the inflammatory factors such as TNF-α and IL-6. Moreover, Hcy caused an increase in pSTAT3 expression which occurs in microglial cells. AG490, a JAK2-STAT3 inhibitor, effectively inhibited the phosphorylation of STAT3, microglial cell activation and the secretion of IL-6, TNF-*α* raised by Hcy treatment.

Conclusions: STAT3 signaling pathway located in microglia plays a critical role in mediating Hcy-induced activation of microglia and neuroinflammation in rat MCAO model. This suggests the feasibility of targeting the JAK2/STAT3 pathway as an effective therapeutic strategy to alleviate the progression of Hcy-associated ischemia stroke.

Keywords: Homocysteine, Microglial cell, Inflammation, Ischemic brain, Signal transducers and activators of transcription 3

Background

Ischemic stroke is one of the most frequent causes of injury to the central nervous system (CNS). Complex pathological mechanisms are involved in brain injury after cerebral ischemia. Inflammatory processes have a fundamental role in the pathophysiology of ischemic injury stroke. Microglial cells, which are rapidly and time-dependently activated after ischemia, are considered as the major cellular contributors to post-injury inflammation [1, 2]. Stroke-induced microglial activation causes release of a variety of inflammatory mediators many of which are cytotoxic and/or cytoprotective. Emerging evidence demonstrates that alternatively activated microglia promotes tissue repair by secreting anti-inflammatory mediators and growth factors [3, 4]. In contrast, overactivated microglia following ischemia stroke can secrete a wide range of inflammatory factors and neurotoxic compounds, including nitric oxide, tumor necrosis factor (TNF)-α, interleukin (IL)-6, and reactive oxygen species (ROS), which are deleterious to bystander neurons and impact their processes [5]. As a result of

* Correspondence: zhangxumei@tmu.edu.cn
Department of Nutrition and Food Science, School of Public Health, Tianjin Medical University, Tianjin 300070, China

findings such as these, it is increasingly well-accepted that microglia activation has been known to exert dual effects on ischemic injury. An improved understanding of the mechanisms underlying microglial activation and their functional modulation by the local microenvironment is likely to advance our knowledge of many CNS pathological states.

Homocysteine (Hcy) is an intermediate sulfhydryl-containing amino acid derived from methionine. It has been proved that patients suffering with severe hyperhomocysteinemia manifest typical clinical cardiovascular symptoms as well as neurological disorders, such as cerebral atrophy, dementia, and seizures [6]. The mechanism underlying Hcy mediated-pathogenesis of nervous system disorders is not yet fully understood. The toxicity of Hcy to CNS neurons is widely recognized affecting both the neuronal survival rate and the ability of neurons to transmit signal and thus to form functional neural networks [7]. Moreover, Hcy is deemed to affect microglia proliferation in vitro [8]. However, whether microglia activation and microglia-mediated inflammatory responses involve neurotoxicity of Hcy remains largely unknown.

The signal transducer and activator of transcription 3 (STAT3), a member of the STAT protein family of transcription factors, has been extensively described as a central signaling molecule that controls cellular adaption in response to environmental stimuli or stress. Several groups have shown that the STAT3 is activated in vitro and in vivo experimental models of stroke and subsequently activated STAT3 promotes numerous genes responsible for many cellular functions that may play a critical role in both neural injury and repair [9, 10]. There are conflicting data whether this pathway activation leads to improved neurological recovery. Some findings suggest that treatments that activate the STAT3 signaling after experimental stroke may lead to improved functional performance and/or decreased cell death [11]. On the contrary, accumulating evidence suggests that activation of STAT3 leads to decreased cerebral recovery and that blocking this pathway leads to better neurological outcomes [12]. Thus, the precise contribution of STAT3 activation after stroke remains incompletely understood. On the other hand, STAT3, an important regulator of inflammatory gene expression, has been shown to play an important regulatory role in microglial reactivity to various stimuli and mediate pro-inflammatory responses in microglia in response to various CNS insults. Activated STAT3 can promote the transcription and expression of many genes that encode proinflammatory mediators, including cytokines, chemokines, adhesion molecules, and inflammatory enzymes [2]. In addition, it has been demonstrated that neuroinflammatory processes after cerebral ischemia involve aberrantly activated STAT3. The strong induction of pSTAT3 is predominantly localized in the macrophages/microglia in the post-ischemic brain [12]. Given the importance of STAT3 in activating microglia and inducing cytokine/chemokine expression, we investigated whether Hcy activates STAT3 in microgla and whether STAT3 is involved in the Hcy-induced inflammatory responses.

Accordingly, the present study was designed to elucidate the molecular mechanism of neurotoxicity by Hcy in relation to microglial-mediated neuroinflammation and microglial STAT3 overactivation using a rat model of transient focal cerebral ischemia. This study demonstrates for the first time that STAT3 overactivation located in microglia cells plays an important role in Hcy-induced microglia activation and the inflammatory responses both in the brain cortex and the dentate gyrus (DG) region of the hippocampus following ischemic injury.

Methods

Experimental animals and administration

One hundred adult male Sprague-Dawley rats (180–220 g) (Grade SPF, Certificate Number SCXK (jing) 2012–0001) were purchased from Vital River Laboratory Co. Ltd. (Beijing, China). The experimental protocols were approved by the Tianjin Medical University Animal Ethics Committee and performed in compliance with institutional guidelines under approved protocols. The rats were randomly allocated into six groups: SHAM operation control group (SHAM), middle cerebral artery occlusion reperfusion group (MCAO), Hcy-treated SHAM group (SHAM + Hcy), Hcy-treated MCAO group (MCAO + Hcy), Hcy combined with AG490(α-cyano-(3,4-dihydroxy)-N-benzyl-cin-namide)-treated SHAM group (SHAM+ Hcy + AG490), and Hcy combined with AG490-treated MCAO group (MCAO + Hcy + AG490). Hcy (1.6 mg/kg/day, Sigma-Aldrich, St. Lous, Mo, USA) was administered by tail vein injection (Additional file 1: Video S1) for 21 days prior to SHAM or MCAO operation. The AG490 (3 mg/kg, Abcam, Cambridge, MA, USA) was administered by intraperitoneal injection before 1 h of SHAM or MCAO operation.

Induction of focal cerebral ischemia-reperfusion

The MCAO rats were induced by using the intraluminal filament technique as we described previously [13]. A nylon thread was advanced by the left common carotid artery, through the left internal carotid artery and into the origin of the middle cerebral artery. Two hours after cerebral ischemia, the thread was carefully withdrawn to establish reperfusion. Animals assigned to SHAM operation were treated similarly, except that the thread was not advanced to the origin of the middle cerebral artery.

Measurement of infarct volume

At 24 h after reperfusion, three rats in each group were euthanized and the brains were rapidly removed and frozen at −20 °C for 15 min. Serial coronal brain slices with a 2 mm thickness each were stained with 2% 2,3,5-triphenyltetrazolium chloride (TTC) at 37 °C for 15 min followed by fixation with 4% paraformaldehyde for 24 h. Infarct volume measurements were carried out by an investigator blinded to the treatment groups as previously described [14].

Hematoxylin and eosin (HE) staining

Rats were euthanized at 72 h after the MCAO operation for HE staining. Left brains were quickly removed and further fixed using 4% paraformaldehyde overnight. Then brain tissues were equilibrated in a phosphate-buffered 30% sucrose solution, embedded in paraffin, and cut into 6-μm coronal sections.

Three rats of each group were assigned to HE staining. Sections of brain tissues embedded in paraffin were stained with HE for routine histological examinations and the morphological changes were observed under a light microscope (IX81; Olympus, Tokyo, Japan).

Fluoro-jade B staining

Fluoro-Jade B is a high affinity fluorescent marker for the localization of neuronal degeneration. Fluoro-Jade B staining was performed using a modification of a previously published procedure [15]. Briefly, the sections were immersed in a solution containing 1% sodium hydroxide in 80% alcohol for 5 min, followed by 2 min in 70% alcohol and 2 min in distilled water. The slides were then transferred to a solution containing 0.06% potassium permanganate for 10 min, then incubated in the staining solution of Fluoro-Jade B (Millipore, Chemicon, USA) for 20 min. After washing 3 times in distilled water, the sections were allowed to dry, immersed in xylene, coverslipped, and examined using a fluorescence microscope with 450–490 nm excitation light.

Immunofluorescence analysis

Immunofluorescence analysis of the paraffin embedded tissues was performed using standard protocols provided by the antibody manufacturers. Briefly, sections were fixed in 4% paraformaldehyde, blocked with 10% normal goat serum, and then incubated overnight at 4 °C with the primary antibodies: rabbit anti-TNF-α (Abcam, Cambridge, MA; 1:200), mouse anti-Iba1 (Abcam; 1:100), mouse anti-IL-6 (Abcam; 1:200,), mouse anti-OX-42 (Abcam; 1:100), rabbit anti-pSTAT3 (Cell Signaling Technology, Danvers, MA, USA; 1:100). Thereafter, sections were briefly washed with PBS and incubated for 1 h at room temperature with appropriate secondary antibodies (tetramethylrhodamine -conjugated anti-mouse IgG; fluorescein isothiocyanate -labeled anti-rabbit IgG; Abcam; 1:100). 4′, 6-diamidino-2- phenylinedole (DAPI; Solarbio, Beijing, China; 1 μg/ml) was used to dye the nuclei before 10 min of mounting. The sections were then analyzed with an Olympus IX81 microscope (Olympus, Tokyo, Japan) and Image-Pro Plus 6.0 software.

Western Blot assay

The protein levels of pSTAT3, two microglia markers Iba1and OX-42, and proinflammatory cytokines TNF-α and IL-6 in the ipsilateral ischemic hemisphere (including brain cortex and hippocampus) were measured by Western blot. The protein concentration in the supernatant was measured with the bicinchoninic acid (BCA) protein assay Kit (Pierce, Rockford, IL, USA). Equivalent amounts of protein were separated on 10% sodium dodecyl sulfate-polyacrylamide gel electrophoresis. The electrophoretic transfer of proteins from polyacrylamide gels to nitrocellulose blotting membranes (Millipore, Bedford, MA, USA) was performed according to the wet electrical transfer method. The membranes were blocked with 5% non- fat dry milk in tris-buffered saline and tween 20 (TBST) and subsequently incubated with mouse anti-STAT3 antibody (Cell Signaling Technology; 1:1000), rabbit anti-phosphorylated STAT3 at Tyr705 (1:1000, Cell Signaling Technology), Mouse anti- Iba-1 (Abcam; 1:1000), mouse anti- OX-42 (Abcam; 1:1000), and mouse anti-β-actin (Cell Signaling Technology; 1:2000). After washing in TBST, immunoblots were incubated with horseradish peroxidase-conjugated secondary antibodies (HRP-linked anti-rabbit IgG; HRP-linked anti-mouse IgG; Cell Signaling Technology; 1:2000) for 1 h at room temperature. The immunoblots were developed with chemiluminescence reagents (Millipore, Bedford, MA), and then observed using the ChemiDoc™ XRS+ Imaging System (Bio-Rad, Hercules, California, USA). The densities of the immunobands were quantitated by Image J 1.4.3.67.

Statistical analysis

Data were expressed as mean ± S.D. Variance was analyzed by a one-way ANOVA followed by Student-Newman-Keuls test. Statistical analysis was performed with SPSS v.16.0. Values of $p < 0.05$ were considered statistically significant.

Results

Effects of Hcy on brain infarction and neural cell injury

First, we explored the possible neurotoxic effects of Hcy in the MCAO rat model. TTC-stained brain sections were evaluated 24 h after MCAO and reperfusion. As shown in Fig. 1, no infarct area was found in the sham-operated group, because the rats in this group

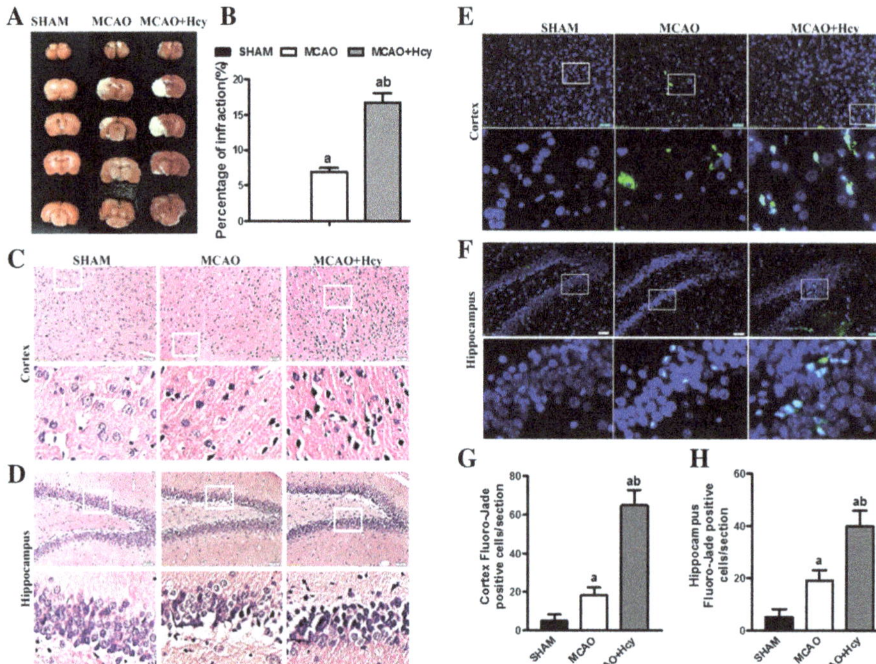

Fig. 1 Effect of homocysteine on cerebral infarct volume and neural cell morphological structure in the rats at 72 h post-MCAO. **a** Representative photographs of TTC-stained brain coronal sections showing the increase in infarct (white) by Hcy treatment. **b** Bar graph showing the infarct volume expressed as the percentage of the whole brain volume. Treatment with Hcy greatly increased the infarct volume compared with the MCAO group. The data are expressed as the means ± SD (n = 3 each group). $^{a}p < 0.05$ vs. the SHAM group, $^{b}p < 0.05$ vs. the MCAO group. **c**, **d** Cell histopathological changes in the cerebral cortical and DG region of the hippocampus by HE staining. Bar = 50 μm. **e**, **f** Representative microphotographs by fluorescent microscopy show Fluoro Jade B+ (green)-labeled neurodegeneration in the brain cortex and hippocampus. Quantitative analysis of Fluoro-Jade B+ positive cells in the brain cortex (**g**) and hippocampus (**h**) was shown. Data are presented as the mean ± SD for 6 animals in each group (8–10 histological sections per brain). Bar = 50 μm. DAPI (blue) a nuclear marker

underwent a similar surgical procedure but were not subjected to MCAO. In the MCAO rats; however, the unstained white infarct zone was visible in the ipsilateral ischemic hemisphere, with an infarct volume of 6.9 ± 0.5% of the entire brain volume. Hcy treatment markedly enlarged the infarct volume to 16.8 ± 1.3%, compared with the MCAO group ($p < 0.05$; Fig. 1a, b).

Neuronal morphology of the brain cortex and the DG region of the hippocampus after cerebral ischemia/reperfusion was observed by HE staining72 h after reperfusion. In the SHAM group, most neurons were arranged in a regular pattern and contained the large and round nuclei. In the MCAO group, neurons were disarranged, many nuclei have become pyknotic (shrunken and dark), and they were surrounded by swollen cellular processes in the brain cortex and the DG region of the hippocampus after cerebral ischemia/reperfusion. Compared with the MCAO group, the pathological changes of the MCAO + Hcy group were magnified (Fig. 1 c, d).

Next, we tested neuronal degeneration by the Fluoro-Jade B assay 24 h post-ischemia. Few Fluoro-Jade B-labeled cells were detected in ipsilateral SHAM-controlled animals. However, in MCAO group, the number of the positive cells was significantly increased, compared to SHAM group. Furthermore, the fluorescence intensity of Fluoro-Jade B staining was notably higher in cerebral cortex and hippocampus in MCAO + Hcy group compared to the MCAO group ($p < 0.05$; Fig. 1 e–h).

In addition, Fluoro-Jade B staining was also used to detect whether Hcy or AG490 themselves caused cell injury in control animals. The results showed that few and sparse positive cells could be found in cerebral cortex and hippocampus in SHAM, SHAM + Hcy and SHAM + Hcy + AG490 groups. No differences were observed among the three experimental groups (data not shown). Thus, it is evident that Hcy or AG490 themselves did not significantly affect the uninjured brains. This suggested that Hcy may enhance the vulnerability of neuronal cells to the ischemic injury.

Hcy raised MCAO-induced microglial activation

To determine whether cortical and hippocampal microglia are capable of responding to Hcy, immunostaining for Iba1 and OX-42, two microglia specific markers, was performed to assess the pathological changes of microglia in the ipsilateral hemisphere. Figure 2 shows that

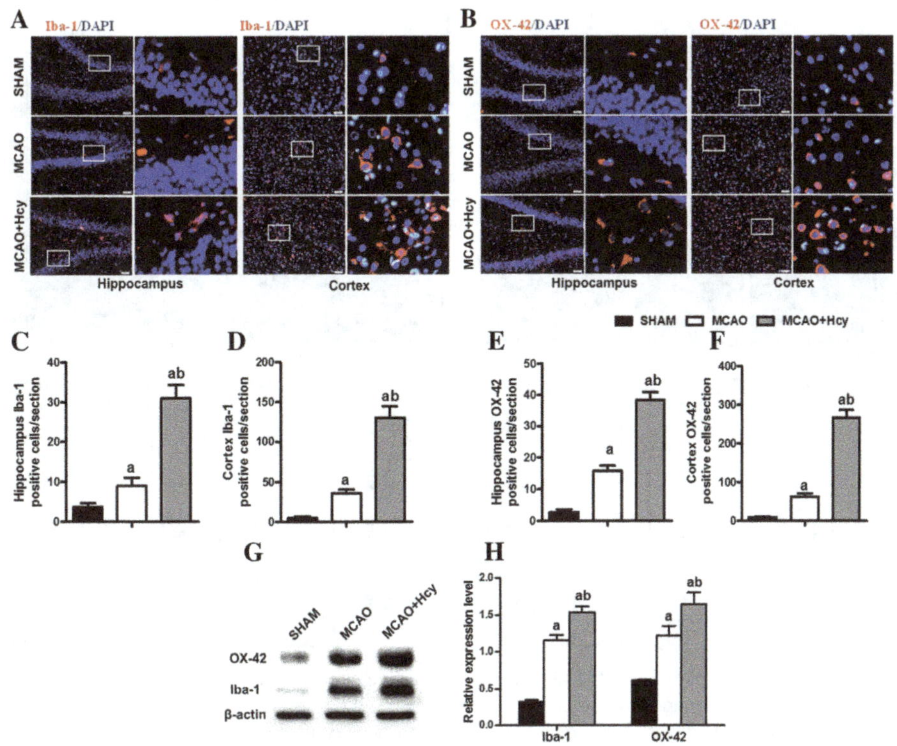

Fig. 2 Hcy raised the MCAO-induced expression of Iba1 and OX-42 in the ipsilateral ischemic hemisphere. **a, b** Immunofluorescence analysis of Iba1 and OX-42 (two microglia markers) 24 h following MCAO injury. Representative images of Iba1 (red) and OX-42 (red) staining in DG area of the hippocampus and the cerebral ischemic cortex. Nuclei are stained with 4, 6-diaminido-2-phenylindole (DAPI, blue). Overlays demonstrate the colocalization of Iba1 (or OX-42) and DAPI. Each right-hand column depicts a magnified image of the rectangular region of the corresponding image in the left column. Bar = 50 μm. **c, d** Quantification of Iba1-positive cells in the post-ischemic hippocampus and cerebral cortex. **e, f** Quantification of OX-42-positive cells in the post-ischemic hippocampus and cerebral cortex. The data are presented as the mean ± SD. Six rats in each group and 10 fields for each rat were examined. **g** The expression of Iba1or OX-42 was detected by Western blot. Representative Western blot showing the activation of microglia in the ipsilateral ischemic hemisphere extracts using an Iba-1(or OX-42) antibody. **h** The levels of Iba1 and OX-42 proteins were quantified and normalized to ß-actin levels. The data are presented as the mean ± SD (n = 5 each group). $^{a}p < 0.05$ vs. the SHAM group, $^{b}p < 0.05$ vs. the MCAO group

there were only a few Ibal (OX-42)-immunoreactive cells in the cerebral cortex and hippocampus in the sham-operated group. The strikingly increased number of Ibal (OX-42)-positive cells was observed in the cortical ischemic penumbra and hippocampus, which were further raised by Hcy treatment compared with the MCAO group ($p < 0.05$; Fig. 2a–f).

These results were also confirmed by western blot analysis. We assessed Ibal (OX-42) protein expression of the ipsilateral ischemic hemisphere extracts by Western Blot. The results showed that Ibal (OX-42) protein expression increased after Hcy treatment for 24 h, compared with MCAO group ($p < 0.05$; Fig. 2g, h).

Next, we examine the effect of Hcy on the microglial changes in the contralateral non-ischemic side. As shown in Fig. 3, a statistically significant increase in the number of Ibal or OX-42 positive cells was detected in the contralateral hippocampus and cortical region in MCAO group, compared to SHAM group ($p < 0.05$). In MCAO + Hcy group, a slight increase, but not significant, in the number of positive cells was visible within the contralateral hippocampus ($p > 0.05$). In contrast, the number of Ibal or OX-42 positive cells in the contralateral brain cortex was more significantly increased in Hcy-treated group ($p < 0.05$), compared to MCAO group, although this increase was not significant in the hippocampus.

Hcy exposure induced IL-6 and TNF-α cytokine secretion in ischemic brains

Proinflammatory mediators (such as IL-6 family of cytokines and TNF-α) have been implicated in a variety of neurotoxic conditions, often in association with the activation of microglia [16–18]. To assess the effect of Hcy on the neuroinflammatory response induced by MCAO, immunostaining was used to detect the levels of TNF-α and IL-6 production in DG area of the hippocampus and the cerebral ischemic cortex. As shown in Fig. 4a–f, the proinflammatory cytokines TNF-α and IL-6 was not significantly detected in the sham-operated group, whereas

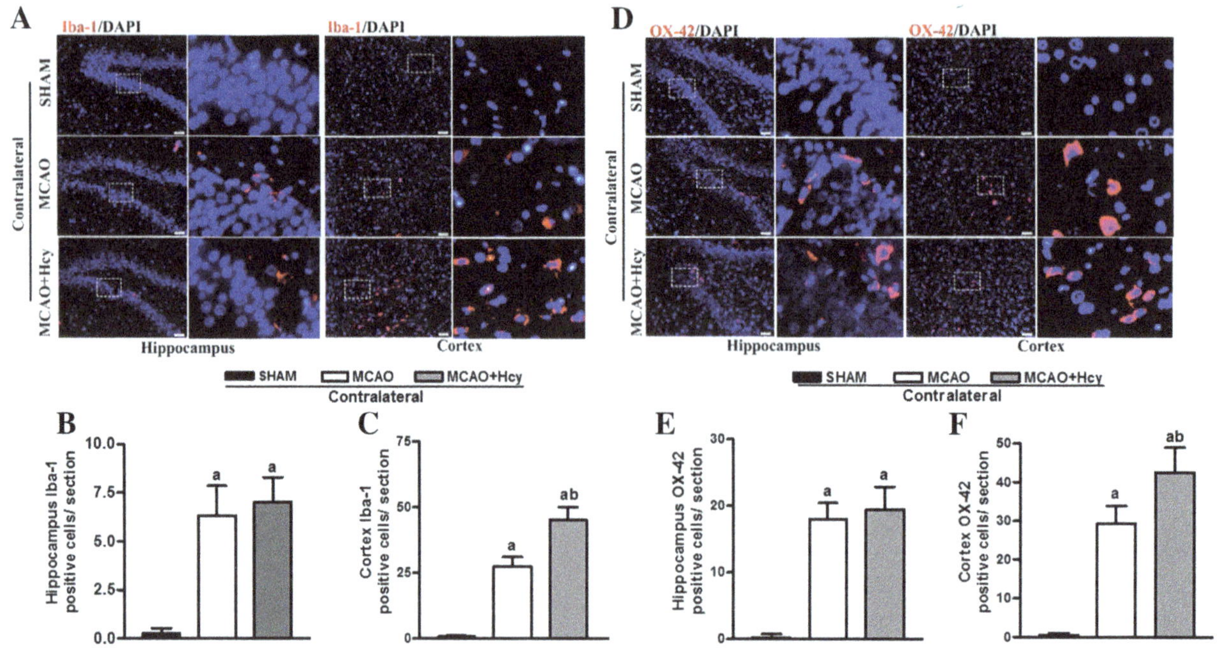

Fig. 3 The effect of Hcy on the expression of Iba1 and OX-42 in the contralateral nonischemic side. **a**, **d** Representative images of Iba1 (red) and OX-42 (red) staining in DG area of the hippocampus and the cerebral ischemic cortex. The blue staining represents DAPI. Overlays demonstrate the colocalization of Iba1 (or OX-42) and DAPI. Each right-hand column depicts a magnified image of the rectangular region of the corresponding image in the left column. Bar = 50 μm. **b**, **c** Quantification of Iba1-positive cells in the post-ischemic hippocampus and cerebral cortex. **e**, **f** Quantification of OX-42-positive cells in the post-ischemic hippocampus and cerebral cortex.The data are presented as the mean ± SD. Five rats in each group and 10 fields for each rat were examined. $^{a}p < 0.05$ vs. the SHAM group, $^{b}p < 0.05$ vs. the MCAO group

their immunoreactivities strongly increased in the cerebral ischemic cortex and hippocampus compared with the sham-operated group ($p < 0.05$). After treatment with Hcy, TNF-α and IL-6 secretion was further elevated, compared with the MCAO group ($p < 0.05$).

Coincident with the change in Iba1-positive (or OX-42) cells in the cerebral ischemic cortex and the hippocampus, Western Blot analysis also showed that the protein expressions of TNF-α and IL-6 were significantly augmented in the ipsilateral ischemic hemisphere extracts after Hcy treatment ($p < 0.05$, Fig. 4g, h). These results suggest that Hcy can upregulate MCAO-induced neuroinflammation.

Phosphorylation of STAT3 in microglia was upregulated by Hcy exposure

The STAT3 signaling pathway has been suggested to play a critical role in neuroinflammation and the activation of microglia following neurotoxic insults and stroke. To investigate whether the STAT3 signal is involved in Hcy-induced the activation of microglia, we co-stained for pSTAT3 and for two microglia markers: Iba1 and OX-42. Double immunofluorescence demonstrates that pSTAT3-labeled cells were colocalized with Iba-1 or OX-42 antigen. The immunoreactivity of pSTAT3 in microglia was not significantly detected in the sham-operated group, which was strongly increased both in the brain cortex and the DG region of the hippocampus in MCAO group (Fig. 5a, b). Injections of Hcy further significantly increased the number of pSTAT3 and Iba1 (OX-42) double positive cells in the hippocampus (Fig. 5 c, e, $p < 0.05$) and the cerebral ischemic cortex (Fig. 5d, f, $p < 0.05$). Furthermore, the Western Blot results revealed the increased level of pSTAT3 in brain tissue extracts in MCAO group compared with the sham-operated group. Hcy treatment further increased the phosphorylation of STAT3 compared with the MCAO group ($p < 0.05$), despite the fact that the total levels of STAT3 were not altered in microglia (Fig. 5l, n).

The Janus family of tyrosine kinase 2 (JAK2), an upstream kinase, mediates STAT3 phosphorylation at Tyr-705 site. Numerous studies have shown that specific inhibition of STAT3 activation by JAK2-specific inhibitor AG490 blocked STAT3 phosphorylation [19, 20]. Both Western Blot and immunofluorescence analysis revealed that AG490 treatment abolished the increase in Hcy-induced phosphorylation of STAT3 (Fig. 5).

JAK2 inhibitor, AG490, partially attenuated microglia activation induced by Hcy treatment

To further assess the potential role of the STAT3 pathway in Hcy-induced activation of microglia, we next examined whether a specific JAK2 inhibitor AG490 could

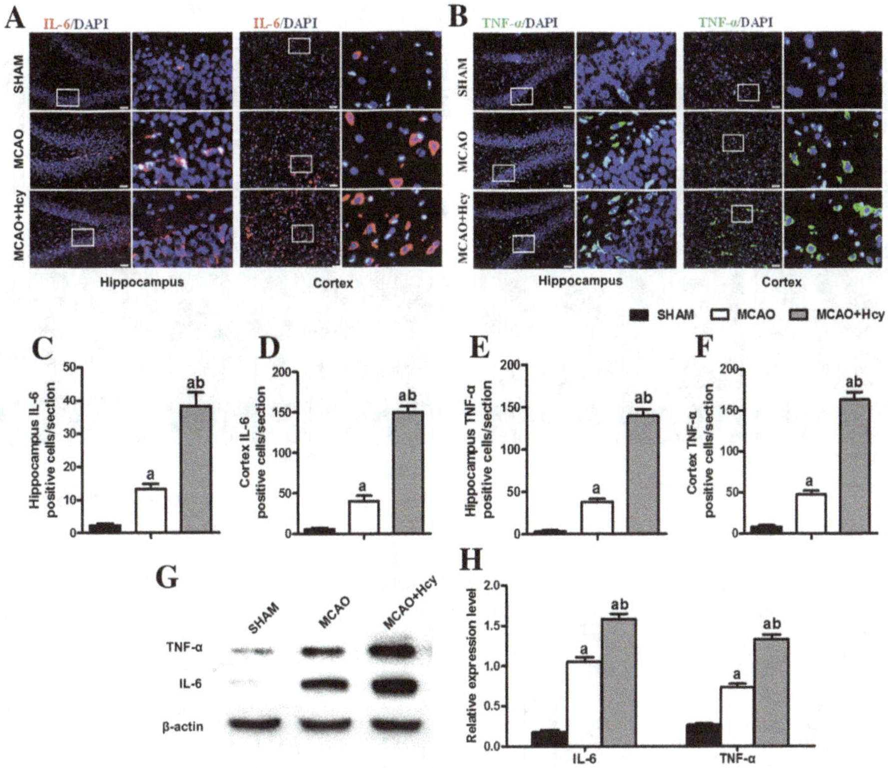

Fig. 4 Hcy induced the secretion of proinflammatory cytokines TNF-α and IL-6 in ischemic brain injury. **a, b** Representative photomicrographs of the immunofluorescence staining of IL-6 (red) and TNF-α (green) in DG area of the hippocampus and the cerebral ischemic cortex. Nuclei are stained blue with DAPI. Each right-hand column depicts a magnified image of the rectangular region of the corresponding image in the left column. **c-f** Bar graphs show semi-quantification of fluorescence intensity for TNF-α and IL-6. Values are mean ± SD. Six rats in each group and 10 fields for each rat were examined. Bar = 50 μ m. **g, h** Western Blot analysis of TNF-α and IL-6. β-actin protein was used here as an internal control. The data are presented as the mean ± SD for five independent experiments. $^{a}p < 0.05$ vs. the SHAM group, $^{b}p < 0.05$ vs. the MCAO group

affect Hcy-induced increase of Iba1 and OX-42 protein expression in the cerebral cortex and the hippocampus. The immunofluorescence analysis showed that the number of Iba1 (OX-42)-positive cells raised by Hcy was significantly decreased by AG490 administration compared with the MCAO group ($p < 0.05$, Fig. 5h–k). Similarly, Western Blot showed that AG490 partially blocked the expression of Iba1 (OX-42) in brain tissue extracts after Hcy treatment, compared with the MCAO group ($p < 0.05$, Fig. 5m, o). It suggested that Hcy-induced microglial activation may be mediated, at least in part, by JAK2-STAT3 signaling pathway.

AG490 partially attenuated Hcy-induced TNF-α and IL-6 production

The functional association between cytokine signaling and JAK-STAT signaling prompted us to examine the involvement of STAT3 in Hcy-induced inflammatory responses. We explored the effects of AG490 on Hcy-induced release of cytokines TNF-α and IL-6 by immunofluorescence staining and Western Blot analysis. Immunohistochemical analysis revealed that the decrease in the number of TNF-α-positive and IL-6-positive cells was observed in the hippocampus DG region and the cerebral ischemic cortex of the rats receiving AG490 and Hcy combined treatment compared with those of MCAO rats treated with Hcy alone (Fig. 6a–f).

Consistent with immunofluorescence staining results, Western Blot analysis showed that the expression of TNF-α and IL-6 in Hcy-injected rats was significantly higher than the expression in the ischemic brains but these elevations were remarkably inhibited by the AG490 treatment (Fig. 6g, h). Thus, the above results demonstrated that AG490 partially abolished the increase in Hcy-induced TNF-α and IL-6 production.

Discussion

The ischemic stroke is one of the common causes of morbidity and mortality worldwide. There are many causes of ischemic stroke, and hyperhomocysteinemia is one of the documented causes. Hyperhomocysteinemia originates from a deviation in the methionine-homocysteine metabolism including disturbances of enzymes, vitamin deficiencies, and different other factors [21, 22]. Although it has been shown that Hcy has a neurotoxic effect on ischemic brains, its roles in modulating

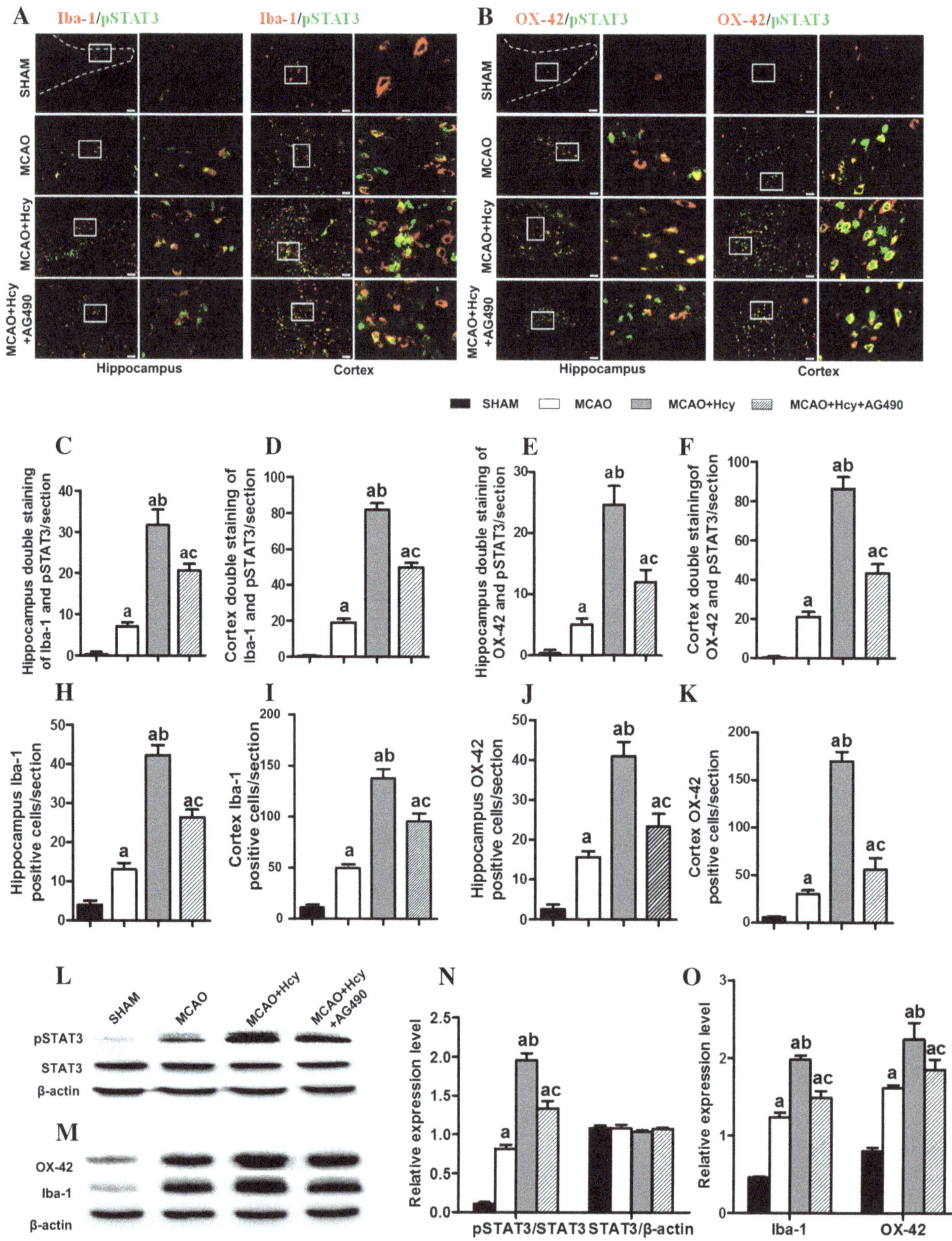

Fig. 5 (See legend on next page.)

(See figure on previous page.)
Fig. 5 Hcy activates microglia by regulating STAT3 signaling pathway which occurs in microglia following stroke. **a, b** Representative photomicrographs of double immunofluorescence staining of pSTAT3 (green) with Iba-1 (red) or OX-42 (red), the markers of activated microglia, in the DG region of the rat hippocampus and the cerebral ischemic cortex. Overlays demonstrate the colocalization of pSTAT3 and Iba-1 (or OX-42). Each right-hand column depicts a magnified image of the rectangular region of the corresponding image in the left column. Scale bars =50 μm. **c-f** Quantitative assessment of pSTAT3/Iba-1 (or OX-42) double positive cells in the rat brain hippocampus and the cortex (n = 6, 10 fields/brain). **h-k** Quantitative assessment of Iba-1 (or OX-42) positive cells in the rat bran hippocampus and cortex (n=6, 10 fields/brain). **l** The phosphorylated and total protein expression of STAT3 was detected by Western Blot assay. **m** Representative western blot for Iba-1 (or OX-42). **n** Bar graphs show semiquantitative levels of pSTAT3/STAT3 and STAT3/ß-action as determined by band density analysis. **o** Semiquantitative analysis of Iba-1/ß-action and OX-42/ß-action, respectively. The data are presented as means ± SD from three independent experiments. $^{a}p < 0.05$ vs. the SHAM group, $^{b}p < 0.05$ vs. the MCAO group, $^{c}p < 0.05$ vs. the MCAO + HCY group

microglial activation and inducing inflammation have not been documented. The present study reveals that Hcy treatment enhanced brain injury, induced activation of microglia, and triggered the expression of pro-inflammatory cytokines in the brain cortex and the DG region of the hippocampus using a rat MCAO model. Moreover, to our best knowledge, this is the first study to provide evidence that changes of STAT3 activities located in microglia involve Hcy-induced microglia activation and inflammation responses following stroke.

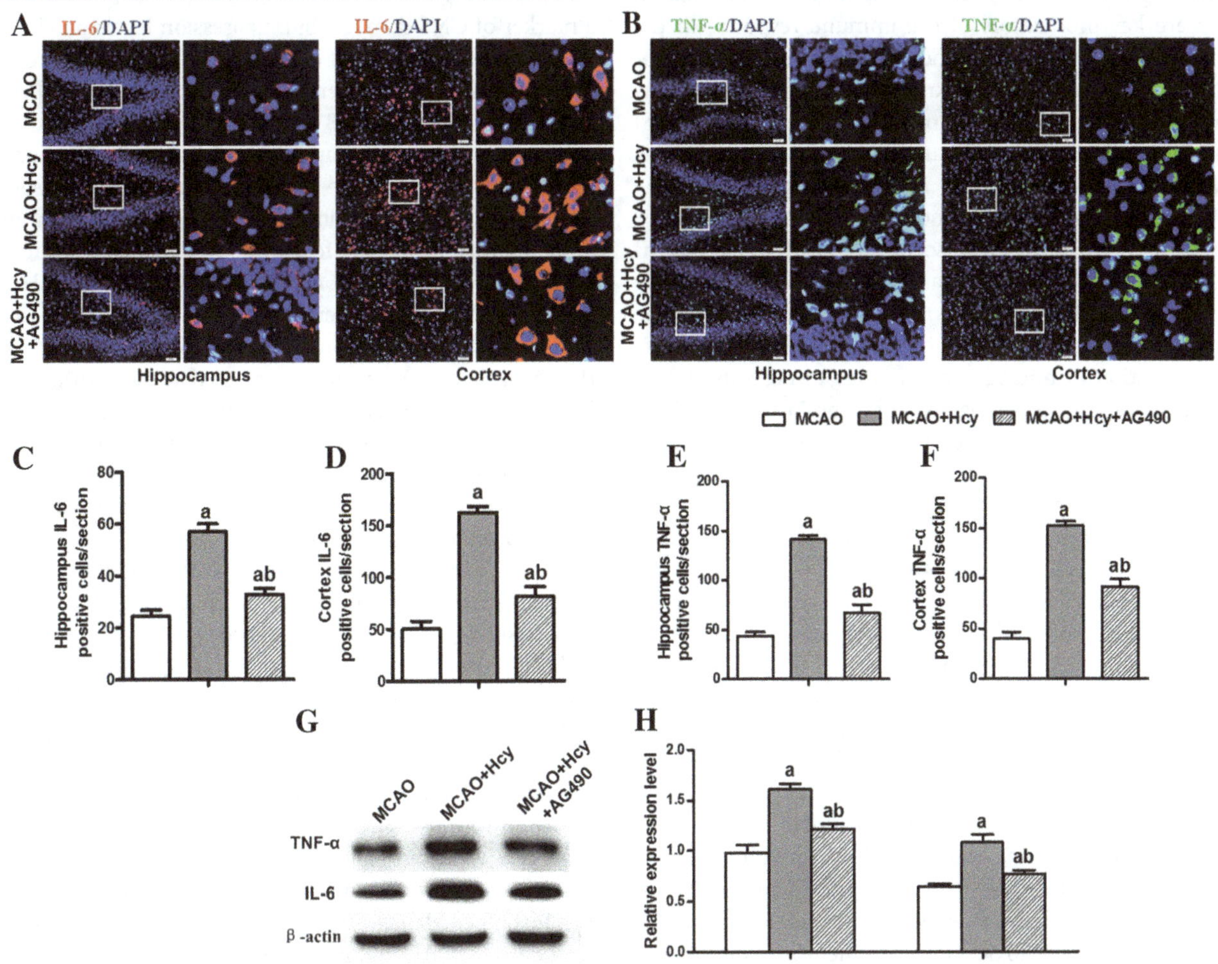

Fig. 6 The effects of AG490 on TNF-α and IL-6 production induced by Hcy. **a, b** TNF-α (green) and IL-6 (red) immunoreactivity in the DG region of the rat hippocampus and the cerebral ischemic cortex after Hcy and AG490 treatment. The blue staining represents DAPI. Scale bar = 50 μm. **c-f** Graph showing the mean fluorescence intensity for TNF-α and IL-6 (n = 6, 10 fields/brain). **g** Representative bands of TNF-α and IL-6 by western blot analysis. β-actin protein was used here as an internal control. **h** Bar graphs show semiquantitative levels of TNF-α and IL-6 as determined by band density analysis. The data are presented as the mean ± SD from four independent experiments. $^{a}p < 0.05$ vs. the SHAM group, $^{b}p < 0.05$ vs. the MCAO group

The previous studies demonstrated that the main cell types of the central nervous system involve Hcy neurotoxicity. High level of Hcy can cause the toxic effect, leading to neuron and neural cell death [23, 24] while low dose can promote glial cell proliferation [25]. In addition, some studies suggest that the neurotoxicity of Hcy may involve negative regulation of neural stem cell (NSC) proliferation [26]. Several reports have also found that Hcy promotes proliferation and activation of microglia through induction of NAD(P)H oxidase in vitro [25, 27]. Low-dose Hcy not only induced Bv2 cell proliferation but also activated these cells in a dose- and time-dependent manner. In our study, Hcy induced microglia activation in ischemic brain. This result is in line with in vitro study. Meanwhile, since Hcy affected the activities of several main brain cells, complex pathogenetic mechanisms may be involved in brain injury caused by Hcy after cerebral ischemia.

Microglia represent 5–20% of the total glial population and are key modulators of the immune response in the brain [28, 29]. Similar to the role of peripheral macrophages, Microglia are now known as the first line of immune defense against central nervous system (CNS) injuries and disorders. These highly plastic cells play dualistic roles in neuronal injury and recovery. Some studies have found that under physiologic conditions, resident microglia are quiescent and scattered throughout the CNS [30]. Occasionally microglia are moderately activated to play a classic role as "scavenger" for the maintenance and restoration of the CNS [31]. The moderate activation of microglia contributes to nervous system repair by engulfing pathogens within brain tissue and releasing neurotrophic factors. However, excessive and prolonged activation of microglial cells can lead to a variety of pathological damages in the central nervous system [3, 32]. Vehmas et al. [33] have confirmed that the amount of activated microglial cells is positively correlated with the progress of Alzheimer's disease. In our models, Hcy treatment activated microglial cells, markedly enlarged the infarct volume and induced cell injury, so the hyperactivation of microglial cells caused by Hcy appeared to be harmful for the ischemic brain. Thus, whether the activation of microglial cells is beneficial or detrimental appears to depend on the extent of cell activation.

In most cases, activated microglia initiate neuroinflammation by producing cytotoxic and inflammatory factors such as the cytokines IL-1β, TNF-α and IL-6, thereby aggravating brain damage [34]. High concentration of TNF-α has direct toxic effect on neurons and neural cells. TNF-α transgenic mice have severe inflammation and exhibit brain and neurodegenerative diseases [35]. Regarding IL-6, its high expression can accelerate the pathological processes of central nervous system disorders [36]. Meanwhile, there is increasing evidence that demonstrating inflammation not only immediately affects the infarcted tissue but also causes long-term damage in the ischemic penumbra after cerebral ischemia. The present study confirms that Hcy treatment induced activation of microglia and a significant up-regulation of the inflammatory factors TNF-α and IL-6 in the cortex and hippocampus of ischemic brains. Moreover, based on results of TTC staining and morphological assays, Hcy may exert a neurotoxic effect by microglia-mediated neuroinflammation injury.

To explore the potential mechanisms of the microglia-inflammatory enhancing effect of Hcy, we focused on investigating JAK2/STAT3 pathway. JAK2/STAT3, as critical immunological signaling molecules, are normally expressed in the brain and play a vital role in regulating microglial activation and inflammatory response [37, 38]. STAT3, an important downstream regulatory molecule of the JAK/STAT pathway, is a well-established regulator of inflammatory gene expression and a marker of CNS damage [39]. Expression levels of STAT3 have been shown to be enhanced in reactive microglia cells when the brain suffers focal ischemic injury [40] Aberrantly activated STAT3 has also been reported to involved in the neuroinflammatory injury after ischemic stroke. To investigate the potential function of the JAK2-STAT3 pathway in Hcy-induced microglia activation and inflammatory response following MCAO, we examine whether the JAK2 inhibitor AG490 could affect Hcy-induced pSTAT3, the microglia specific markers Iba-1and OX-42, and the proinflammatory mediators TNF-α and IL-6 expression. Our results revealed that the activation of STAT3 in microglia and secretion of TNF-α and IL-6 were significantly upregulated in Hcy-treated ischemic brains and this effect was reversed by AG490. These data provide further evidence that that the STAT3 expression raised by Hcy treatment might be involved in microglial activation and the neuroinflammatory injury in MCAO rats.

Focal ischemia-induced STAT3 phosphorylation was previously reported to be localized in various cell types including microglia/macrophages, astrocytes and neurons [39, 41, 42]. Activated microglia/macrophages (ED1 and OX42/Cd11b positive, microglia/macrophage markers) were observed to be the predominant cell type that showed pSTAT3 immunostaining at 24 and 72 h after brain ischemia/reperfusion injury [12]. Moreover, it has been reported that pSTAT3 immunoreactivity was also present in different brain regions following stroke. For instance, Planas et al. [39] showed that a transient episode of MCAO induced a strong microglial response. This was accompanied by increased expression of STAT3 in the ipsilateral cortex and striatum. However, little is known about changes in activation of microglial STAT3 in rat hippocampus after brain ischemia, despite the finding that hippocampus is one of the most vulnerable brain regions to ischemic damages. The present study demonstrated that a strong induction of microglial STAT3 occurred in rat hippocampus after cerebral ischemia by immunohistochemistry. In future study, two points will still need to be clarified: whether the activation of STAT3 in neurons, reactive astrocytes and microglia would play different roles in ischemia-induced injury and whether STAT3 activation in different brain regions may serve different functions.

Conclusions

Hcy further enhanced MCAO-induced microglial activation and inflammatory cytokine secretion including TNF-α and IL-6 production. AG490, a JAK inhibitor, diminished Hcy-enhanced phosphorylation of STAT3, significantly reduced Hcy-induced microglia cell activation and TNF-α and IL-6 production, indicating that Hcy triggered brain injury possibly through the JAK2/STAT3 signaling pathway. Our data provide significant new information regarding the molecular mechanisms underlying Hcy-induced microglial inflammation, and such knowledge will assist in the better understanding of the pathogenesis of brain disease.

Abbreviations

AG490: α-cyano-(3,4-dihydroxy)- N-benzylcin-namide; BCA: Bicinchoninic acid; CNS: Central nervous system; DAPI: 4,6-diaminido-2-phenylindole; DG: Dentate gyrus; Hcy: Homocysteine; HE: Hematoxylin-eosin staining; IL-6: Interleukin 6; JAK2: The Janus family of tyrosine kinase 2; MCAO: Middle cerebral artery occlusion reperfusion group; ROS: Reactive oxygen species; SHAM: Sham operation control group; STAT3: Signal transducer and activator of transcription 3; TBST: Tris buffered saline with Tween 20; TNF-α: Tumor necrosis factor α; TTC: 2,3,5-triphenyltetrazolium chloride

Acknowledgements

We specially thank Youming Wang (Tianjin Medical University) for excellent technical assistance with respect to rat tail vein injection and the establishment of MCAO model.

Funding

This work was supported by the grant from the National Natural Science Foundation of China (81373003).

Authors' contributions

SC performed the experimental design and most experiments and drafted the manuscript. ZD performed the immunohistochemical experiments and data analysis. MC performed some of the Western Blot analyses. YZ participated in establishing MCAO model. MW carried out HE staining. NS participated in TTC staining. XW performed the data analysis and manuscript revision. HL helped to draft the manuscript. GH participated in the design of the study. XZ conceive d of the study and participated in its design and coordination, did the general supervision of the research group, and helped to draft the manuscript. All authors read and approved the final manuscript.

Consent for publication

Not applicable.

Competing interests

The authors declare that they have no competing interests.

References

1. Lakhan SE, Kirchgessner A, Hofer M. Inflammatory mechanisms in ischemic stroke: therapeutic approaches. J Transl Med. 2009;7:97.
2. Yi JH, Park SW, Kapadia R, Vemuganti R. Role of transcription factors in mediating post-ischemic cerebral inflammation and brain damage. Neurochem Int. 2007;50:1014–27.
3. Patel AR, Ritzel R, McCullough LD, Liu F. Microglia and ischemic stroke: a double-edged sword. Int J Physiol Pathophysiol Pharmacol. 2013;5:73–90.
4. Shin JA, Lim SM, Jeong SI, Kang JL, Park EM. Noggin improves ischemic brain tissue repair and promotes alternative activation of microglia in mice. Brain Behav Immun. 2014;40:143–54.
5. Lucas SM, Rothwell NJ, Gibson RM. The role of inflammation in CNS injury and disease. Br J Pharmacol. 2006;147(Suppl 1):S232–40.
6. Obeid R, Herrmann W. Mechanisms of homocysteine neurotoxicity in neurodegenerative diseases with special reference to dementia. FEBS Lett. 2006;580:2994–3005.
7. Lehotsky J, Tothova B, Kovalska M, Dobrota D, Benova A, Kalenska D, Kaplan P. Role of homocysteine in the ischemic stroke and development of ischemic tolerance. Front Neurosci. 2016;10:538.
8. Wan L, Sun Y, Zhang F, Ren Y. Low-dose homocystine enhances proliferation and migration of Bv2 microglia cells. Cell Mol Neurobiol. 2016;36:1279–89.
9. Raible DJ, Frey LC, Brooks-Kayal AR. Effects of JAK2-STAT3 signaling after cerebral insults. JAKSTAT. 2014;3:e29510.
10. Liang Z, Wu G, Fan C, Xu J, Jiang S, Yan X, Di S, Ma Z, Hu W, Yang Y. The emerging role of signal transducer and activator of transcription 3 in cerebral ischemic and hemorrhagic stroke. Prog Neurobiol. 2016;137:1–16.
11. Zhu H, Zou L, Tian J, Du G, Gao Y. SMND-309, a novel derivative of salvianolic acid B, protects rat brains ischemia and reperfusion injury by targeting the JAK2/STAT3 pathway. Eur J Pharmacol. 2013;714:23–31.
12. Satriotomo I, Bowen KK, Vemuganti R. JAK2 and STAT3 activation contributes to neuronal damage following transient focal cerebral ischemia. J Neurochem. 2006;98:1353–68.
13. Longa EZ, Weinstein PR, Carlson S, Cummins R. Reversible middle cerebral artery occlusion without craniectomy in rats. Stroke. 1989;20:84–91.
14. Yu L, Chen C, Wang LF, Kuang X, Liu K, Zhang H, Du JR. Neuroprotective effect of kaempferol glycosides against brain injury and neuroinflammation by inhibiting the activation of NF-kappaB and STAT3 in transient focal stroke. PLoS One. 2013;8:e55839.
15. Yi J, He G, Yang J, Luo Z, Yang X, Luo X. Heat acclimation regulates the autophagy-lysosome function to protect against heat stroke-induced brain injury in mice. Cell Physiol Biochem. 2017;41:101–14.
16. Liu B, Hong JS. Role of microglia in inflammation-mediated neurodegenerative diseases: mechanisms and strategies for therapeutic intervention. J Pharmacol Exp Ther. 2003;304:1–7.
17. Sriram K, Miller DB, O'Callaghan JP. Minocycline attenuates microglial activation but fails to mitigate striatal dopaminergic neurotoxicity: role of tumor necrosis factor-alpha. J Neurochem. 2006;96:706–18.
18. Block ML, Zecca L, Hong JS. Microglia-mediated neurotoxicity: uncovering the molecular mechanisms. Nat Rev Neurosci. 2007;8:57–69.
19. Xuan YT, Guo Y, Han H, Zhu Y, Bolli R. An essential role of the JAK-STAT pathway in ischemic preconditioning. Proc Natl Acad Sci U S A. 2001;98: 9050_5.
20. Jung JE, Kim GS, Narasimhan P, Song YS, Chan PH. Regulation of Mn-SOD activity and neuroprotection by STAT3 in mice after cerebral ischemia. J Neurosci. 2009;29:7003–14.
21. Terwecoren A, Steen E, Benoit D, Boon P, Hemelsoet D. Ischemic stroke and hyperhomocysteinemia: truth or myth? Acta Neurol Belg. 2009;109:181–8.
22. van Beynum IM, Smeitink JA, den Heijer M, te Poele Pothoff MT, Blom HJ. Hyperhomocysteinemia: a risk factor for ischemic stroke in children. Circulation. 1999;99:2070–2.
23. Li XA, Ho YS, Chen L, Hsiao WL. The protective effects of icariin against the homocysteine-linduced neurotoxicity in the primary embryonic cultures of rat cortical neurons. Molecules. 2016;21
24. Lipton SA, Kim WK, Choi YB, Kumar S, D'Emilia DM, Rayudu PV, Arnelle DR, Stamler JS. Neurotoxicity associated with dual actions of homocysteine at the N-methyl-D-aspartate receptor. Proc Natl Acad Sci U S A. 1997;94:5923–8.

25. Zou CG, Zhao YS, Gao SY, Li SD, Cao XZ, Zhang M, Zhang KQ. Homocysteine promotes proliferation and activation of microglia. Neurobiol Aging. 2010;31:2069–79.
26. Yan H, Zhang X, Luo S, Liu H, Wang X, Gao Y, Wilson JX, Huang G. Effects of homocysteine on ERK signaling and cell proliferation in fetal neural stem cells in vitro. Cell Biochem Biophys. 2013;66:131–7.
27. Manolescu BN, Oprea E, Farcasanu IC, Berteanu M, Cercasov C. Homocysteine and vitamin therapy in stroke prevention and treatment: a review. Acta Biochim Pol. 2010;57:467–77.
28. Zhang Z, Chopp M, Powers C. Temporal profile of microglial response following transient (2 h) middle cerebral artery occlusion. Brain Res. 1997;744:189–98.
29. Schubert P, Morino T, Miyazaki H, Ogata T, Nakamura Y, Marchini C, Ferroni S. Cascading glia reactions: a common pathomechanism and its differentiated control by cyclic nucleotide signaling. Ann N Y Acad Sci. 2000;903:24–33.
30. Thomas WE. Brain macrophages: evaluation of microglia and their functions. Brain Res Brain Res Rev. 1992;17:61–74.
31. Nakamura Y. Regulating factors for microglial activation. Biol Pharm Bull. 2002;25:945–53.
32. Walter L, Neumann H. Role of microglia in neuronal degeneration and regeneration. Semin Immunopathol. 2009;31:513–25.
33. Vehmas AK, Kawas CH, Stewart WF, Troncoso JC. Immune reactive cells in senile plaques and cognitive decline in Alzheimer's disease. Neurobiol Aging. 2003;24:321–31.
34. Kraft AD, Harry GJ. Features of microglia and neuroinflammation relevant to environmental exposure and neurotoxicity. Int J Environ Res Public Health. 2011;8:2980–3018.
35. Probert L, Akassoglou K, Pasparakis M, Kontogeorgos G, Kollias G. Spontaneous inflammatory demyelinating disease in transgenic mice showing central nervous system-specific expression of tumor necrosis factor alpha. Proc Natl Acad Sci U S A. 1995;92:11294–8.
36. Gruol DL, Nelson TE. Physiological and pathological roles of interleukin-6 in the central nervous system. Mol Neurobiol. 1997;15:307–39.
37. Huang C, Ma R, Sun S, Wei G, Fang Y, Liu R, Li G. JAK2-STAT3 signaling pathway mediates thrombin-induced proinflammatory actions of microglia in vitro. J Neuroimmunol. 2008;204:118–25.
38. Dinapoli VA, Benkovic SA, Li X, Kelly KA, Miller DB, Rosen CL, Huber JD, O'Callaghan JP. Age exaggerates proinflammatory cytokine signaling and truncates signal transducers and activators of transcription 3 signaling following ischemic stroke in the rat. Neuroscience. 2010;170:633–44.
39. Planas AM, Soriano MA, Berruezo M, Justicia C, Estrada A, Pitarch S, Ferrer I. Induction of Stat3, a signal transducer and transcription factor, in reactive microglia following transient focal cerebral ischaemia. Eur J Neurosci. 1996;8:2612–8.
40. Schabitz WR, Kollmar R, Schwaninger M, Juettler E, Bardutzky J, Scholzke MN, Sommer C, Schwab S. Neuroprotective effect of granulocyte colony-stimulating factor after focal cerebral ischemia. Stroke. 2003;34:745–51.
41. Justicia C, Gabriel C, Planas AM. Activation of the JAK/STAT pathway following transient focal cerebral ischemia: signaling through Jak1 and Stat3 in astrocytes. Glia. 2000;30:253–70.
42. Suzuki S, Tanaka K, Nogawa S, Dembo T, Kosakai A, Fukuuchi Y. Phosphorylation of signal transducer and activator of transcription-3 (Stat3) after focal cerebral ischemia in rats. Exp Neurol. 2001;170:63–71.

4

Sulfosuccinimidyl oleate sodium is neuroprotective and alleviates stroke-induced neuroinflammation

Hiramani Dhungana, Mikko T. Huuskonen, Merja Jaronen, Sighild Lemarchant, Humair Ali, Velta Keksa-Goldsteine, Gundars Goldsteins, Katja M. Kanninen, Jari Koistinaho* and Tarja Malm*

Abstract

Background: Ischemic stroke is one of the main causes of death and disability worldwide. It is caused by the cessation of cerebral blood flow resulting in the insufficient delivery of glucose and oxygen to the neural tissue. The inflammatory response initiated by ischemic stroke in order to restore tissue homeostasis in the acute phase of stroke contributes to delayed brain damage.

Methods: By using in vitro models of neuroinflammation and in vivo model of permanent middle cerebral artery occlusion, we demonstrate the neuroprotective and anti-inflammatory effects of sulfosuccinimidyl oleate sodium (SSO).

Results: SSO significantly reduced the lipopolysaccharide/interferon-γ-induced production of nitric oxide, interleukin-6 and tumor necrosis factor-α, and the protein levels of inflammatory enzymes including nitric oxide synthase 2, cyclooxygenase-2 (COX-2), and p38 mitogen-activated protein kinase (MAPK) in microglia, without causing cell toxicity. Although SSO failed to directly alleviate glutamate-induced excitotoxicity in murine cortical neurons, it prevented inflammation-induced neuronal death in microglia-neuron co-cultures. Importantly, oral administration of SSO in Balb/c mice subjected to permanent occlusion of the middle cerebral artery reduced microglial activation in the peri-ischemic area and attenuated brain damage. This in vivo neuroprotective effect of SSO was associated with a reduction in the COX-2 and heme oxygenase-1 immunoreactivities.

Conclusions: Our results suggest that SSO is an anti-inflammatory and a possible therapeutic candidate in diseases such as stroke where inflammation is a central hallmark.

Keywords: Stroke, CD36, SSO, Inflammation, Microglia, Neuroprotection

Background

Ischemic damage following cerebral infarction is accompanied by a series of complex pathophysiological events including excitotoxicity, oxidative stress, inflammation, and apoptosis [1]. The post-ischemic inflammatory response in stroke is largely detrimental and contributes to the development of delayed brain damage [2]. Brain inflammation is mediated by microglia, astrocytes, and infiltrating peripheral leukocytes, primarily neutrophils and monocytes [3]. These inflammatory cells produce a variety of cytotoxic molecules, including pro-inflammatory cytokines, and reactive oxygen, and nitrogen species [4]. Microglia, in particular, are rapidly activated upon ischemia within hours of damage. Endogenous ligands including purines, peroxiredoxins, heat shock proteins, and high mobility group box-1 released from dying cells during ischemia bind to microglial surface receptors like cluster of differentiation 36 (CD36) and Toll-like receptors (TLRs) [5]. Intracellular signaling that follows the ligand-receptor interaction releases pro-inflammatory mediators like interleukin (IL)-1, IL-6, tumor necrosis factor-α (TNFα), cyclooxygenase-2 (COX-2), and nitric oxide synthase 1 (NOS1) that can damage the brain by further promoting inflammation and apoptosis. In contrast, anti-inflammatory cytokines like IL-10 and transforming growth factor-β

* Correspondence: jari.koistinaho@uef.fi; tarja.malm@uef.fi
A.I. Virtanen Institute for Molecular Sciences, University of Eastern Finland, P.O. box 1727, FI-70211 Kuopio, Finland

(TGF-β) are involved in the resolution of inflammation [2]. Drugs, such as curcumin [6] and minocycline [7, 8], that alleviate inflammatory reactions have been shown to reduce ischemic damage and aid in functional recovery in preclinical models of stroke. Despite the lack of translational success and efficacy of anti-inflammatory agents thus far in human stroke [9, 10], modulation of microglial activation still holds promise in the treatment of stroke.

Sulfosuccinimidyl oleate sodium (SSO) is a long chain fatty acid that inhibits fatty acid transport into cells. SSO is known to bind the CD36 receptor on the surface of microglia. CD36 activation is involved in many inflammatory pathways and contributes to cell or tissue damage through production of free radicals, cytokines, and chemokines [11–14]. However, the role of SSO in inhibiting inflammation either directly or independently of CD36 in ischemic stroke has not been reported. We thus aimed to investigate whether SSO is able to attenuate stroke-related neuroinflammation in vitro and in vivo and provide benefit in a mouse model of ischemic stroke. We demonstrate for the first time that SSO inhibits key inflammatory mediators both in vitro and in vivo and that this anti-inflammatory effect is mediated by inhibition of phosphorylated p38 mitogen-associated protein kinase. Our data show that SSO provides neuroprotection against ischemic insult and can be a candidate molecule for further drug development.

Methods

BV2 cell culture

The mouse BV2 microglial cell line was kindly provided by professor Rosario Donato (University of Perugia, Italy). Cells were maintained in a humidified chamber with 5% CO2 and 37 °C in RPMI-1620 medium (Invitrogen, CA, USA) supplemented with 10% heat-inactivated fetal bovine serum (FBS, Invitrogen) and 0.6 μg/ml gentamicin (Sigma-Aldrich, MO, USA). Cells were seeded at a density of 1.5×10^5 cells/ml for both protein and RNA extraction. Culture media was replaced by serum-free RPMI media 24 h after seeding. On the next day, the cells were stimulated with 100 ng/ml lipopolysaccharide (LPS, Sigma-Aldrich) and 5 ng/ml interferon-γ (IFN-γ, Peprotech, NJ, USA) and co-treated with SSO (TRC, Toronto, Canada) for a further 24 h.

Primary cortical neuron cultures

Primary neuronal cultures were prepared as described previously [15]. Briefly, cortical tissue from E15 C57BL/6J embryos was dissected out after carefully removing the meninges. The dissected cortices were transferred to Krebs buffer (0.126 M NaCl, 2.5 mM KCl, 25 mM $NaHCO_3$, 1.2 mM NaH_2PO_4, 1.2 mM $MgCl_2$, 2.5 mM $CaCl_2$, pH 7.4) containing 0.025% trypsin and incubated at 37 °C for 15 min. Then, the reaction was stopped by using trypsin inhibitor containing DNase (Sigma-Aldrich). Neurons were dissociated, counted, and plated in poly-L-lysine (Sigma-Aldrich)-coated 48-well plates at a density of 1.25×10^5 cells/well in neurobasal media (Gibco, NY, USA) supplemented with 2% B27 (Thermo Fisher Scientific, MA, USA), 500 μM L-glutamine (Thermo Fisher Scientific), and 1% penicillin-streptomycin (P/S, Thermo Fisher Scientific). Fifty percent of the media was changed 5 days after seeding. At day 6, the neurons were exposed to 50 μM of SSO for 2 h and then 400 μM of glutamate in the presence of 50 μM SSO for 24 h.

Primary microglia cultures

Primary microglia cultures were prepared as described previously [15]. Briefly, P0-P2 C57BL/6J mouse brains were dissected and rinsed in phosphate buffer solution (PBS) containing 1 g/l glucose. Brains were mechanically dissociated and digested using 0.5% trypsin-EDTA for 20 min at 37 °C. The tissue homogenate was suspended in DMEM/F12 (Gibco) containing 10% heat-inactivated FBS and 1% P/S (Thermo Fisher Scientific) and plated on 150-mm cell culture dishes for 3 weeks. After reaching confluency, astrocytes were removed using 0.25% trypsin in Hank's Balanced Salt Solution (HBSS, Gibco) in 1:4 dilution in serum-free DMEM/F12. After careful washes with PBS, the microglia attached on the bottom of the plates were isolated by using 0.25% trypsin in PBS. Fresh culture medium containing FBS was added to neutralize the effect of trypsin. Cells were then centrifuged and plated for co-culture studies.

Neuron-BV2 co-culture and neuron-primary microglia co-cultures

For primary neuron-BV2 co-culture, cortical neurons were plated onto a 48-well plate at a density of 1.25×10^5 cells/well in neurobasal media as described previously. At day 5, BV2 cells were plated on top of neurons at a density of 1:5 (25,000 BV2 cells for 125,000 neurons) for 2 h. Cells were pre-treated with SSO for 2 h and then exposed to 100 ng/ml LPS and 5 ng/ml IFNγ for 48 h. The co-cultures were rinsed with PBS, fixed with 4% PFA for 20 min, and washed again with PBS. Neuronal viability in the co-cultures was evaluated as described previously [16]. The co-cultures were stained with microtubule-associated protein 2 (MAP-2) peroxidase labeling, and the ABTS peroxidase substrate kit (Vector) was used to develop the color for the analysis according to the manufacturer's instructions. The green-colored product was formed after incubation for 30 min with ABTS kit in the dark. One hundred fifty microliter of the substrate solution was transferred to a 96-well plate, and the absorbance was measured using a microtiter plate reader Victor 2.0 (Perkin Elmer, MA, USA) at 405 nm. For primary neuron-microglia co-culture, cortical neurons were similarly plated onto 48-well plates at a density of 1.25×10^5 cells/well. At day 5, primary microglia were plated on top of neurons in neurobasal media at a density of 1:2 (62,500 microglia for 125,000 neurons). On the next day, the cells were pre-treated with SSO for 2 h and then exposed to 100 ng/ml LPS and 30 ng/ml IFN-γ for 48 h. The cells were then rinsed with PBS, fixed with 4% PFA, and the neuronal viability assessed by ABTS peroxidase substrate kit as described above.

Measurement of nitric oxide production and cell viability assay

Nitric oxide (NO) production was assessed in the culture media by using Griess assay 24 h after LPS/IFNγ stimulation and SSO treatment. Fifty microliter of culture supernatant was incubated with an equal volume of Griess reagent for 10 min at room temperature (RT), and the optical density was measured at 544 nm using Victor 2.0 plate reader.

Cell viability was measured using resazurin assay 24 h after exposure. Briefly, cells were incubated with 10 μM resazurin (Sigma-Aldrich) diluted in culture media for 2 h at 37 °C. The absorbance was then quantified at 485 nm using Victor 2.0 plate reader.

CBA assay

Culture supernatants obtained 24 h after SSO treatment were used to determine the levels of interleukin-6 (IL-6), IL-10, monocyte chemoattractant protein 1 (MCP-1), TNF-α, IFN-γ, and IL-12p70 using a mouse anti-inflammatory cytometric bead array (CBA) kit (BD Biosciences, CA, USA). After staining, the samples were run on a FACS Calibur flow cytometer (BD Biosciences). The results were analyzed using FCAP array software (Soft Flow Hungary Ltd., Pecs, Hungary).

Western blot

Twenty-four hours after SSO treatment, BV2 cells were washed with PBS and collected in SDS sample buffer (0.0625 M TRIS-HCl, 2.3% SDS, 5% β-mercaptoethanol, 10% glycerol, bromophenol blue). For analyzing the nuclear localization of NFκB, BV2 cells were treated as described above and subcellular fractions were generated with Cell Fractionation kit (Cell Signaling) according to the manufacturer's protocol. Ten micrograms of protein were loaded and run on 10% SDS-PAGE gels. The proteins were transferred onto PVDF-hybond membranes for 1 h at 4 °C. The membranes were then blocked in 5% milk in 0.2% PBS-tween (PBST) for 30 min. Primary antibodies for total cell lysates (nitric oxide synthase 2 (NOS2), 1:2000 dilution, EMD Millipore, MA, USA; COX-2, 1:1000 dilution, BD Biosciences; heme oxygenase-1 (HO-1), 1:1000 dilution, ENZO Lifesciences, NY, USA; P-p38, 1:1000 dilution, Cell Signaling Technology, MA, USA) and for nuclear fractions (NFκB p65, 1:1000 dilution, Santa Cruz, TX, USA) in 5% BSA in PBS and 0.02% NaN3 were incubated with the membranes overnight at 4 °C. After washing with PBST, appropriate secondary antibodies were incubated for 2 h at RT diluted at 1:2000 in a blocking solution (anti-mouse ECL-HRP; GE healthcare life science, Uppsala, Sweden, or anti-rabbit IgG HRP Conjugate, Bio-Rad, CA, USA). The membranes were washed again with PBST, and the protein bands were visualized using an ECL-plus kit (Thermo Fisher Scientific) under Storm 860 scanner (Molecular dynamics, Caesarea, Israel). β-actin (1:2000 dilution, Sigma-Aldrich) and histone-3 (H3) (1:1000 dilution, Abcam, Cambridge, UK) antibodies were used as loading controls for total cell lysates and nuclear fractions, respectively. Their immunoreactivities were detected with Cy3-conjugated anti-rabbit secondary antibody (Jackson ImmunoResearch Laboratories, PA, USA) and scanned with G:BOX imaging system (Syngene, Cambridge, UK). Densitometric analysis was performed using ImageQuant TL software (GE healthcare life science).

Quantitative real-time PCR

The relative expression levels of IL-6, NOS2, nuclear factor erythroid 2-related factor-2 (Nrf2), and HO-1were measured in BV2 cells exposed to LPS/IFNγ and SSO using quantitative PCR (qPCR). Total RNAs were isolated using the RNeasy mini kit (Qiagen, CA, USA) according to the manufacturer's instructions. The concentration and purity of RNA samples were determined using a NanoDrop 2000 (Thermo Fisher Scientific). Complementary DNA (cDNA) was synthesized by using 500 ng of total RNA, Maxima Reverse Transcriptase, dNTP, and random hexamer primers (Life Technologies, CA, USA). The final concentration of cDNA was 2.5 ng/μl. qPCR was run using the StepOne Plus Real-Time PCR system (Applied Bioscience, CA, USA). Gene expression analysis was carried out using comparative C_t method ($\Delta\Delta C_T$) where the threshold cycle of the target genes was normalized to glyceraldehyde 3-phosphate dehydrogenase (GAPDH) and ribosomal RNA internal housekeeping gene controls (ΔC_T). The mRNA expression is presented as a fold change.

Animals

A total of 21 4-month-old male BALB/cABom mice (Taconic, Köln, Germany) obtained by breeding in-house were used in this study. The mice were housed under a 12-h light/dark cycle and allowed for food and water ad libitum. All the animal experiments were approved by the National Animal Experiment Board of Finland and followed the Council of Europe Legislation and Regulation for Animal Protection. The animals were randomized and divided into two groups, SSO treated ($n = 10$) and control ($n = 11$) using GraphPad QuickCalcs software (GraphPad Software, Inc. La Jolla, CA, USA).

Ischemia surgery and treatment with SSO

All animals underwent distal permanent occlusion of the middle cerebral artery (MCA) (pMCAo) as described previously [17]. Briefly, mice were anesthetized with 5% isoflurane for induction and 2% isoflurane for maintenance (70% N_2O/30% O_2). The temperature of the mice was maintained at 36-5 ± 0.5 °C using a thermostatically controlled heating blanket connected to a rectal probe (PanLab, Harvard Apparatus, Barcelona, Spain). The temporalis muscle was retracted to expose the skull in between the ear and the eye, and a small hole of approximately 1 mm was drilled at the site of the MCA. The dura was carefully removed to expose the MCA. The artery was then gently lifted up and cauterized using a thermocoagulator (Bovie Medical Corporation, Clearwater, FL, USA). After the procedure, the muscle was lifted back and the skin wound was sutured. The animals were then placed back to their home cages. SSO was emulsified in 0.5% methyl cellulose and administered once by single oral gavage at the dose of 50 mg/kg immediately after the surgery, when the mice had retained their consciousness. The administration routes for SSO in vivo have been described previously [18, 19]. In addition, we performed a dose-response study and found that SSO at 50 mg/kg was suitable to see a beneficial effect after stroke. There was no mortality in this study.

Magnetic resonance imaging

Infarct size was imaged by magnetic resonance imaging (MRI) at 3 days post-injury using a vertical 9.4T Oxford NMR 400 magnet (Oxford Instrument PLC, Abingdon, UK). Mice were anesthetized and maintained at 1.5% isoflurane during the imaging. A quadrature volume radiofrequency coil was used for transmission and reception. Multislice T2-weighted images (repetition time 3000 ms, echo time 40 ms, matrix size 128 × 256, field of view 19.2 × 19.2 mm^2, slice thickness 0.8 mm, and number of slices 12) were taken with double spin-echo sequences with adiabatic refocusing pulses. Lesion volume was outlined manually on T2-weighted images using an in-house software (Aedes) under MATLAB (Math-works, Natick, MA, USA) environment. The total lesion volume and the volume of the left and right hemispheres were calculated by multiplying the number of pixels with the pixel size and slice thickness. The relative percentage of the infarction volume was calculated as described previously: infarction volume = (volume of left hemisphere − (volume of right hemisphere − measured infarct volume))/volume of left hemisphere [20]. The analysis was performed blinded to the study groups.

Perfusion, blood sampling, and immunohistochemistry

All mice were sacrificed immediately after MRI imaging at 3 days post-injury. The mice were anesthetized using 250 mg/kg of avertin and transcardially perfused with heparinized saline (2500 IU/l). The brains were removed and post-fixed in 4% paraformaldehyde (PFA) for 24 h followed by cryoprotection in 30% sucrose for 48 h. The brains were snap frozen in liquid nitrogen and cut into 20-µm-thick serial coronal sections at the start of the lesion using a cryostat (Leica Microsystems GmbH, Wetzlar, Germany).

For the detection of microglia, astrocytes, COX-2, and HO-1 immunoreactivity, a set of six consecutive sections at 400 µM intervals starting from the beginning of the lesion were used. The sections were incubated against primary antibody ionized calcium binding adapter molecule 1(Iba-1, 1:250 dilution, Wako Chemical GmbH, Neuss, Germany), CD45 (1:100 dilution, BioRad, Hercules, CA, USA), NeuN (1:200 dilution, EMD Millipore, Temecula, CA, USA), glial fibrillary acidic protein (GFAP, 1:500 dilution; DAKO; Glostrup, Denmark or 1:200 dilution; EMD Millipore), COX-2 (1:500 dilution; Cayman Chemicals, Ann Arbor, MI, USA), and HO-1 (1:1000, ENZO) overnight at RT. The sections were then incubated with biotinylated secondary antibody (1:200 dilution, Vector, Burlingame, CA, USA) for 2 h and then avidin-biotin complex reagent (Vector) according to the manufacturer's instructions. Alternatively, Alexa 568-conjugated secondary antibody (1:200 dilution; Invitrogen, Eugene, OR, USA) was used. Immunoreactivities were visualized by the development with nickel-enhanced 3, 3′-diaminodenzidine.

Immunoreactivities in the peri-ischemic area adjacent to the infarct border were imaged at ×10 magnification using AX70 microscope (Olympus Corporation, Tokyo, Japan) with an attached digital camera (Color View 12 of F-view, Soft Imaging System, Munster, Germany) and a computer running analysis software (Soft imaging system). The intensity of the immunoreactivities was quantified from an area of 718 × 532 µm adjacent to the infarct border using ImagePro Software (Media Cybernetics, Silver Spring, MD, USA) blinded to the study groups. A total of seven to ten mice per group were analyzed.

Statistical analysis and exclusion criteria

Statistical analysis was performed using GraphPad Prism (GraphPad Software Inc., CA, USA) by running one-way ANOVA with Tukey's post hoc test or student t test where appropriate. Statistical outliers were excluded from the data set after performing Grubb's test using GraphPad Prism QuickCalcs. All the data are expressed as mean ± SEM and $P < 0.05$ was used for the determination of statistical significance.

Results

SSO maintains the viability of BV2 microglia upon inflammatory stimuli

The ability of SSO to alter cell viability was first assessed with naïve BV2 cells or BV2 cells stimulated with 100 ng/ml LPS and 5 ng/ml IFNγ. Two concentrations of SSO (20 μM and 50 μM) were used. SSO alone did not alter the cellular viability as measured by the resazurin assay (Fig. 1a). Exposure to 100 ng/ml LPS + 5 ng/ml IFNγ modestly, yet significantly reduced the viability of the BV2 cells. Co-treatment with SSO prevented the LPS + IFNγ-induced reduction in the cell viability (Fig. 1a). In addition, LPS + IFNγ exposure induced a massive NO production in BV2 cells which was blocked by co-treatment with SSO at both concentrations (Fig. 1b).

SSO downregulates LPS/IFNγ-induced inflammatory mediators in BV2 cells

Since 50 μM dose of SSO did not exert any toxicity, we chose to use SSO at the 50 μM concentration for further experiments. Next analyses focused on analyzing whether SSO exhibits anti-inflammatory properties in vitro in LPS + IFNγ-stimulated BV2 cells. Of the various cytokines analyzed, LPS + IFNγ promoted a massive increase in the secretion of IL-6 and TNF-α, which were significantly reduced by co-treatment with SSO (Fig. 2a, b). The levels of IL-10 were unaltered in all treatment groups (Fig. 2c).

We next analyzed whether SSO influences the expression of genes involved in the inflammation and redox signaling. As expected, LPS + IFNγ significantly increased the mRNA expression of *IL-6* (Fig. 3a) and *NOS2* (Fig. 3b). Co-treatment with SSO blocked the increase in the expression levels of both *IL-6* and *NOS2*. Interestingly, LPS + IFNγ reduced the expression levels of *Nrf2* which was returned to basal levels by co-treatment with SSO (Fig. 3c). In contrast, SSO treatment alone or in combination with LPS + IFNγ did not affect the levels of heme oxygenase 1 (*HO-1*), one of the well-known targets genes of *Nrf2*(Fig. 3d).

To further establish the anti-inflammatory properties of SSO, we measured the protein levels of COX-2 and NOS2, which are responsible for the production of NO and pro-inflammatory mediators. Figure 4a shows a representative Western blot analysis which revealed that SSO co-treatment significantly reduced the LPS + IFNγ-induced expression of NOS2 and COX-2 in BV2 cells (Fig. 4b, c). Furthermore, SSO alone increased the basal protein levels of HO-1 but did not alter the LPS + IFNγ-induced levels of HO-1 (Fig 4d). Since both LPS and IFNγ are known to increase the production of NOS2 through activation of MAPK pathway, we analyzed the protein expression levels of the activated p38. Western blot analysis revealed a significant LPS/IFNγ-induced upregulation in the phosphorylated form of the p38, which was prevented by co-treatment with SSO (Fig. 4e). We observed no changes in the levels of phosphorylated JNK and ERK between treated and untreated groups (data not shown).

Furthermore, p38 MAPK signaling pathway is known to increase nuclear translocation of NFκB p65, whereas inhibition of CD36, especially by SSO, is known to block this translocation especially after ceramide stimulation in pancreatic beta cells [21]. This was confirmed in our in vitro model, where we were able to demonstrate a robust nuclear translocation of NFκB p65 upon LPS/IFNγ exposure, which was significantly alleviated by SSO treatment (Fig. 4f, g).

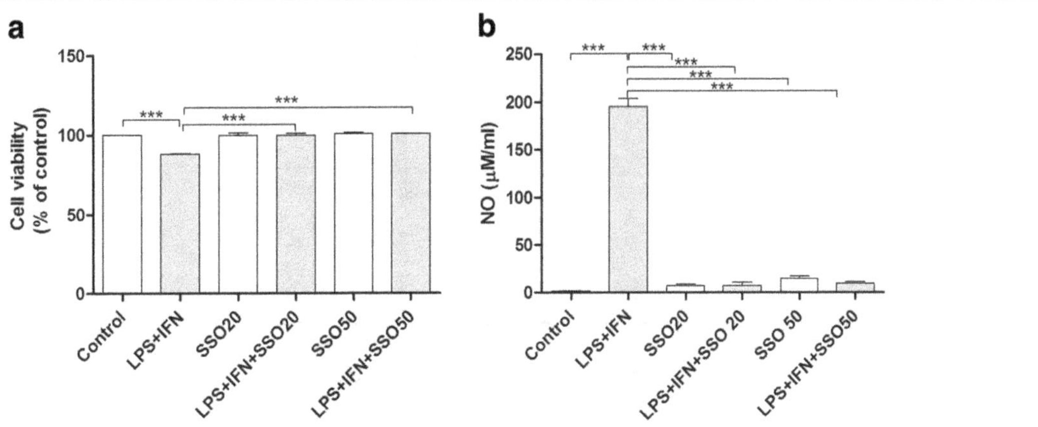

Fig. 1 SSO prevented inflammation-induced cell viability alteration and NO release. SSO alone did not alter the viability of BV2 cells. Exposure of BV2 cells to 100 ng/ml LPS and 5 ng/ml IFNγ significantly reduced the viability of BV2 cells while simultaneous treatment with SSO prevented it as revealed by resazurin assay (**a**). The values are normalized to control. In addition, LPS/IFNγ treatment induced a massive NO production in BV2 cells which was blocked by co-treatment with SSO at both concentrations as measured by Griess reaction (**b**). The results were analyzed with one-way ANOVA followed by Tukey's post hoc test. Data are expressed as mean ± SEM. $n = 3$ per group from three independent experiments. $^{*}p < 0.01$, $^{**}p < 0.01$ and $^{***}p < 0.001$

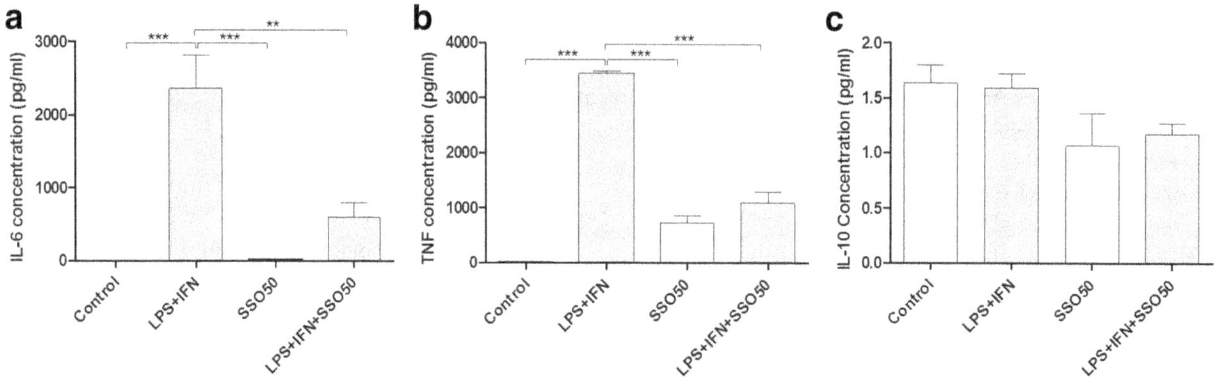

Fig. 2 SSO reduced the concentration of IL-6 and TNF-α secreted into the culture media in LPS + IFNγ-stimulated BV2 cells. Culture media were collected from BV2 cells stimulated with LPS + IFNγ for 24 h in the presence or absence of SSO. The collected media were analyzed for secreted levels of IL-6 (**a**), TNF-α (**b**), and IL-10 (**c**) using the CBA. The results were analyzed with one-way ANOVA followed by Tukey's post hoc test. Data are expressed as mean ± SEM. $n = 3$–4 per group derived from independent experiments. *$p < 0.01$, **$p < 0.01$, and ***$p < 0.001$

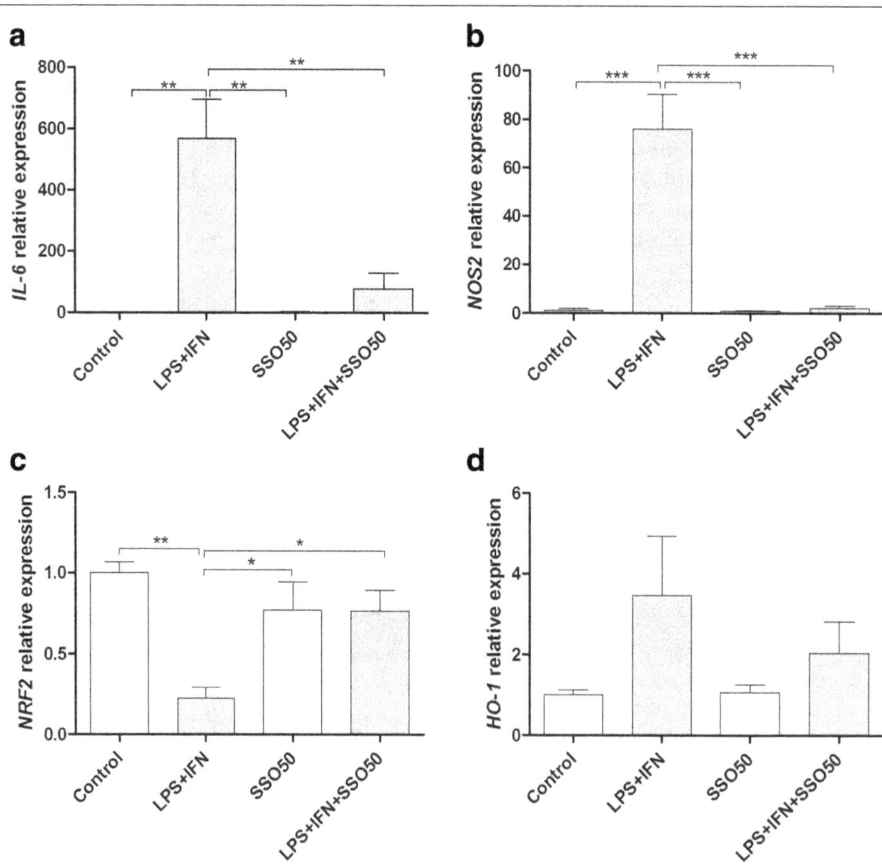

Fig. 3 SSO reduced the LPS + IFN-induced pro-inflammatory mediators *IL-6* and *NOS2* while increasing *Nrf2*, the main regulator of the antioxidant response. BV2 cells were exposed to LPS + IFNγ in the presence or absence of SSO for 24 h. The mRNA expression levels of *IL-6* (**a**), *NOS2* (**b**), *Nrf2* (**c**), and *HO-1* (**d**) were analyzed by qRT-PCR. Results are expressed as mean ± SEM. The results were analyzed with one-way ANOVA followed by Tukey's post hoc test. Data are expressed as mean ± SEM. $n = 3$ per group from three independent experiments, and the values were normalized to controls. *$p < 0.01$, **$p < 0.01$, and ***$p < 0.001$

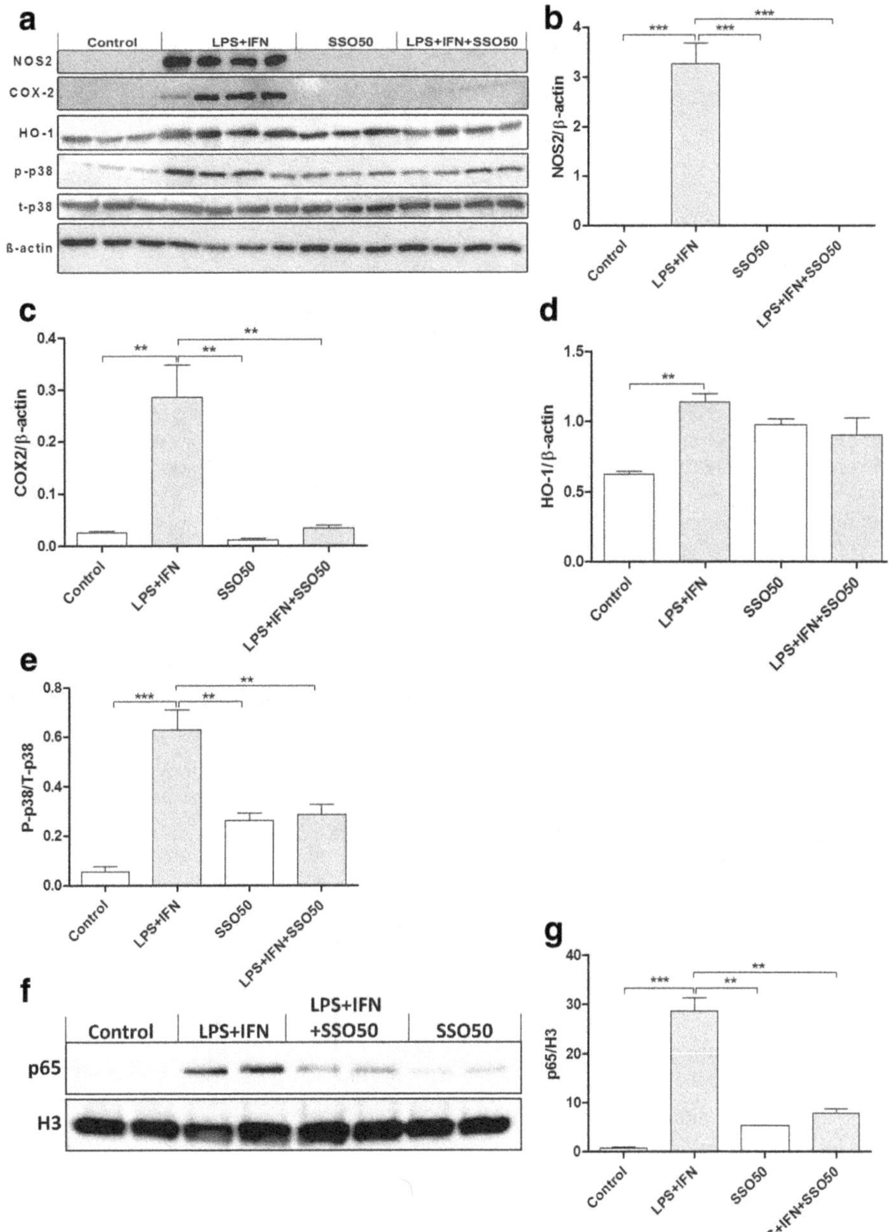

Fig. 4 SSO reduces the protein levels of activated p38, iNOS, and COX-2 in vitro. BV2 cells were exposed to 100 ng/ml of LPS and 5 ng/ml of IFNγ in the presence or absence of 50 μM SSO. Figure (**a**) shows the representative images of Western blots probed for NOS2, COX-2, HO-1, p-p38, t-p38, and β-actin as control. Stimulation of BV2 cells with LPS/IFNγ for 24 h drastically increased the levels of NOS2 (**b**), COX-2 (**c**), HO-1 (**d**), and P-p38/T-p38 (**e**). Representative image of nuclear NFκB p65 translocation after nuclear fractionation. Nuclear-specific marker H3 was used to normalize p65 translocation (**f**). LPS/IFNγ stimulation resulted in robust nuclear translocation of NFκB p65, which was significantly prevented by SSO co-treatment (**g**). The results were analyzed with one-way ANOVA followed by Tukey's post hoc test. Data are expressed as mean ± SEM. $n = 3$-4 per group from independent experiments. *$p < 0.01$, **$p < 0.01$, and ***$p < 0.001$

SSO rescues neurons from inflammation-induced death

We next assessed whether SSO is directly neuroprotective in cultured primary neurons exposed to glutamate-mediated excitotoxicity. Primary neurons were pre-treated with 50 μM SSO for 2 h followed by the exposure to 400 μM glutamate and 50 μM SSO for 24 h. SSO alone was not toxic to the neurons, yet it was unable to prevent glutamate-induced neuronal death (Fig. 5a). Since SSO was not able to rescue neuronal viability in pure neuronal cultures but has anti-inflammatory properties, we assessed whether SSO can prevent inflammation-induced neuronal death using primary neuron-BV2 co-cultures. The co-

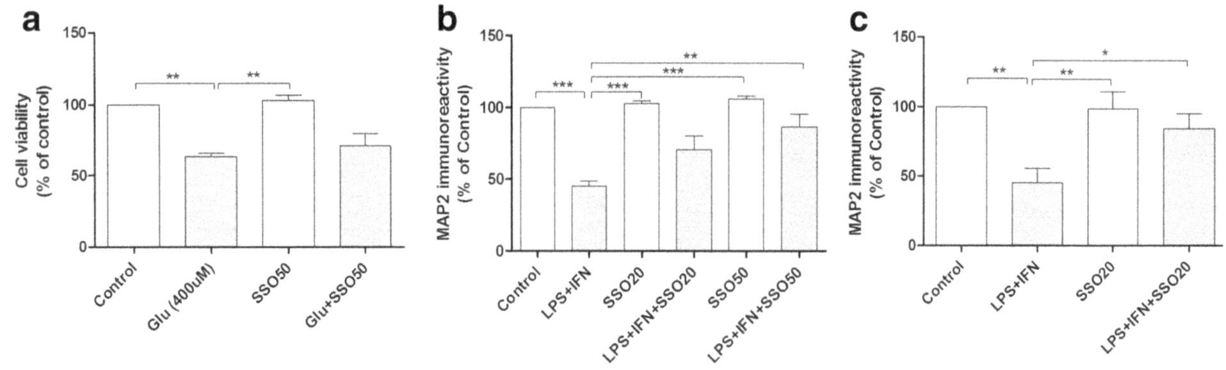

Fig. 5 SSO prevented inflammation-induced neuronal death in microglia/neuron co-culture. SSO was not directly protective against glutamate-mediated neurotoxicity. Primary neurons were pre-exposed to 50 μM SSO for 2 h followed by subsequent exposure to 400 μM glutamate and 50 μM SSO for 24 h. Cell viability was assayed using the MTT assay (**a**). SSO prevented inflammation-induced neuronal death in neuron-glial co-cultures. The co-cultures were pre-treated with two concentrations of SSO (20 μM and 50 μM) for 2 h followed by the exposure to LPS + IFNγ in the presence or absence of SSO. MAP-2 immunoreactivity was measured to determine neuronal viability using peroxidase-ABTS kit. SSO prevented the LPS + IFNγ-induced neuronal death in neuron/BV2 co-cultures (**b**) and neuron/primary microglia co-cultures (**c**). Data are expressed in mean ± SEM and statistical analysis carried out using one-way ANOVA followed by Tukey's post hoc test. $n = 3$ per group from three independent experiments, and the values are normalized to controls. *$p < 0.01$, **$p < 0.01$, and ***$p < 0.001$

cultures were pre-treated with two concentrations of SSO (20 μM and 50 μM) followed by the exposure to 100 ng/ml LPS and 5 ng/ml IFNγ. Measurement of neuronal viability using peroxidase-ABTS kit showed that SSO alone was not causing any loss of MAP-2 immunoreactivity. Moreover, SSO dose-dependently prevented the LPS/IFNγ-induced neuronal death (Fig. 5b). To confirm these findings on primary microglia, we exposed a primary neuron-primary microglia co-culture model to 20 μM SSO, and similarly, 2-h SSO pre-treatment significantly prevented LPS + IFNγ-induced neuron death (Fig. 5c).

SSO treatment attenuates brain damage following ischemia

Based on our in vitro data, we then tested the therapeutic effect of SSO in a mouse model of pMCAo. We chose the dose of 50 mg/kg of SSO, which caused no adverse effect to the mice. The mice underwent MRI imaging at 3 days post-injury. Quantification of the lesion volumes revealed that orally administered SSO significantly reduced the cortical ischemic infarct size compared to vehicle-treated controls (Fig. 6).

Peri-ischemic microgliosis but not astrogliosis was significantly reduced in SSO-treated mice

Ischemia-induced brain microgliosis was analyzed by immunohistochemical staining against Iba-1. As expected, we detected a significant upregulation of microgliosis in the peri-ischemic area of both the SSO-treated and control mice when compared to the corresponding area in the contralateral side at 3 days post-stroke (Fig. 7a). However, the extent of Iba-1 immunoreactivity in the peri-ischemic area of SSO-treated mice was significantly reduced compared to their vehicle-treated counterparts (Fig. 7a). Ischemia induced significant upregulation of GFAP immunoreactivity in the peri-ischemic area compared to the contralateral side, yet SSO failed to reduce stroke-induced increased GFAP immunoreactivity (Fig. 7b).

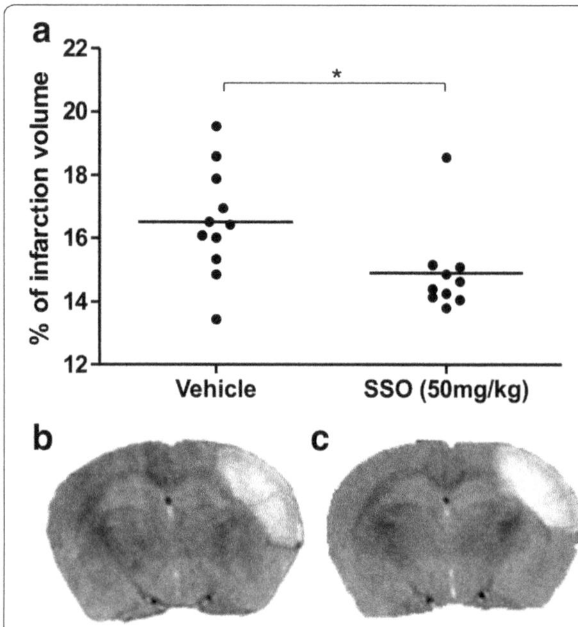

Fig. 6 SSO-treated mice show attenuated infarct size. Quantification of MRI images taken at 3 days post-injury revealed that oral administration of SSO reduced brain damage following ischemia (**a**). Data are expressed as mean ± SEM. Vehicle-treated mice ($n = 11$) and SSO-treated mice ($n = 10$). *$p < 0.05$. Figure (**b, c**) represents the typical T2 weighted image of vehicle- (**b**) and SSO-treated mice (**c**)

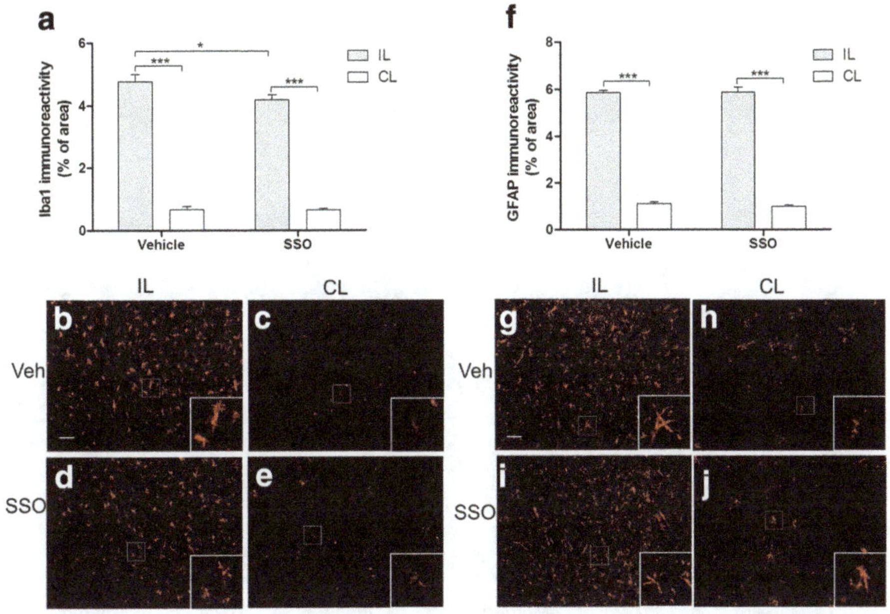

Fig. 7 Brain microgliosis is reduced upon treatment with SSO. GFAP and Iba-1 immunoreactivities were quantified at 3 days post-injury. Quantification of Iba-1 immunoreactivity (**a**) and representative images of Iba-1 staining in the peri-ischemic area of the ipsilateral (**b**) and contralateral hemisphere (**c**) of vehicle-treated mouse. The lower panels (**d**, **e**) represent the corresponding areas in SSO-treated mouse. Quantification of GFAP immunoreactivity (**f**) and the representative images from the peri-ischemic area of the ipsilateral (**g**) and contralateral (**h**) hemisphere in vehicle-treated mouse. Panels **i** and **j** represent corresponding areas in the SSO-treated mouse. High magnification insets show GFAP and Iba-1 positive cell morphologies. Data are expressed as mean ± SEM. GFAP immunoreactivity was quantified from vehicle-treated ($n = 10$) and SSO-treated ($n = 9$) mice. Iba- 1 immunoreactivity was quantified from vehicle-treated ($n = 10$) and SSO-treated ($n = 10$) mice. *$p < 0.05$ and ***$p < 0.001$. *IL* ipsilateral, *CL* contralateral

SSO-treated mice showed reduced expression of COX-2 and increased expression of HO-1 in the peri-ischemic area

Due to the ability of SSO to reduce the expression of COX-2 in vitro, we analyzed the extent of COX-2 immunoreactivity in the peri-ischemic area of the stroked animals at 3 days post-stroke. pMCAo induced a significant upregulation in COX-2 immunoreactivity in the peri-ischemic area (Fig. 8a). SSO-treated animals showed a reduced extent of COX-2 expression compared to vehicle-treated controls (Fig. 8a). To evaluate the cell types expressing COX-2, we carried out immunohistological double stainings with COX-2 and microglial/macrophage marker CD45, neuronal marker NeuN, and astrocytic marker GFAP. The double stainings revealed that COX-2 immunoreactivity was mainly localized in microglia/macrophages and neurons but not in astrocytes (Fig. 8f). To evaluate the impact of SSO to induce antioxidant response, we carried out a staining against HO-1 and detected a significant upregulation in HO-1 in the peri-ischemic area in the SSO-treated animals when compared to vehicle-treated controls (Fig. 8g). Double stainings of HO-1 with CD45, NeuN, and GFAP revealed colocalization similar to COX-2, HO-1 was mainly expressed in microglia/macrophages and neurons, but not in astrocytes (Fig. 8l).

Discussion

Here, we show for the first time that oral administration of SSO is neuroprotective in a mouse model of ischemic stroke. SSO-induced neuroprotection was associated to decreased levels of pro-inflammatory mediators and increased levels of the antioxidant HO-1. The neuroprotective effect of SSO was related to its anti-inflammatory activity, since SSO failed to directly prevent glutamate-induced neuronal death, yet it preserved microglia viability; attenuated the production of inflammatory mediators NO, IL-6, and TNF-α upon the exposure to LPS + IFNγ; and prevented inflammation-induced neuronal death in vitro.

Inflammation plays a pivotal role in many cerebral injuries and diseases including stroke. Stroke induces rapid microglial activation and promotes the secretion of a variety of inflammatory mediators including IL-1β, TNF-α, and IL-6 [22]. In addition, inflammatory enzymes like NOS, COX-2, and MAP kinases are rapidly upregulated, further exaggerate the inflammatory response and induce neuronal death. The pro-inflammatory events occurring in the ischemic brain can be modeled in vitro by exposing microglia to LPS. LPS binds to Toll-like receptors (TLRs), such as TLR4, and initiates the activation of the p38 MAPK and NFκB pathway resulting in the production of NOS2, NO, and various

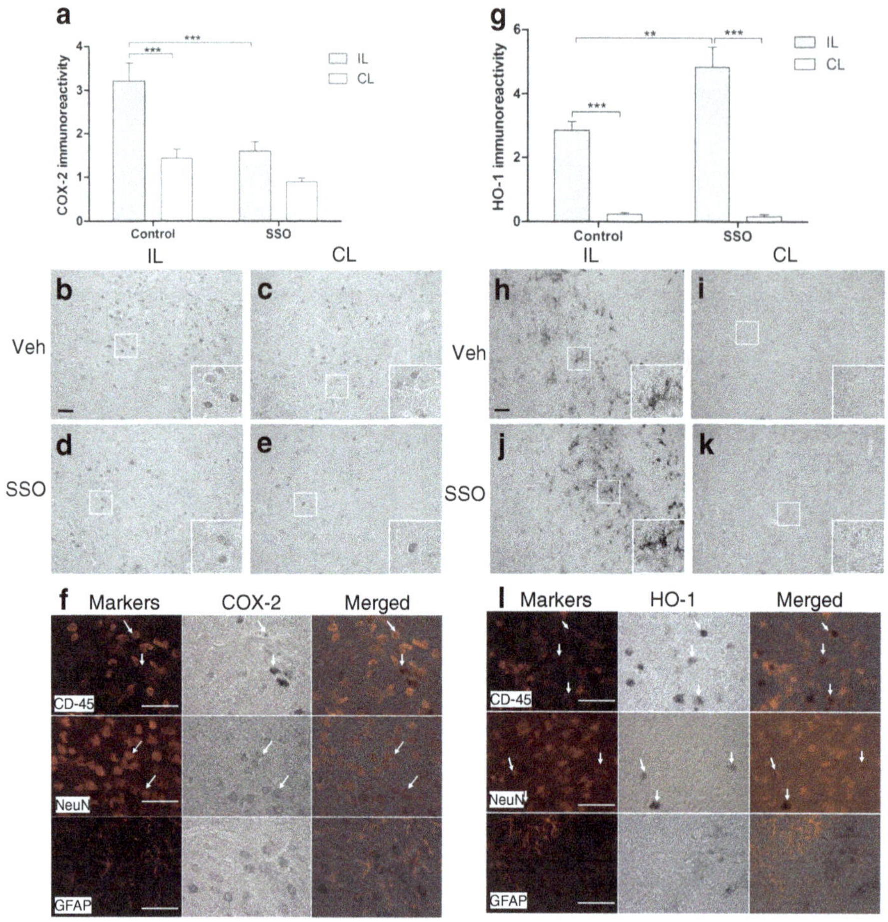

Fig. 8 COX-2 immunoreactivity was decreased while HO-1 immunoreactivity was increased in SSO-treated mice at 3 days post-stroke. pMCAo induced a significant increase in the levels of COX-2 immunoreactivity. COX-2 immunoreactivity was significantly reduced in SSO-treated mice compared to vehicle-treated mice (**a**). Representative images of COX-2 immunoreactivity in the peri-ischemic area of the ipsilateral (**b**) and contralateral side (**c**) of vehicle-treated mouse. Panels (**d** and **e**) represent the corresponding areas for the SSO treated mouse. HO-1 immunoreactivity was increased in SSO-treated mice when compared to vehicle-treated mice (**g**). Panels **h** and **i** show representative images of HO-1 immunoreactivities in the peri-ischemic ipsilateral and contralateral side of the vehicle-treated mouse, respectively. Panels **j** and **k** represent the corresponding areas in the SSO-treated mice, respectively. High magnification insets show the cellular morphology of the staining. Panels **f** and **l** show double staining of COX-2 (**f**) and HO-1 (**l**) together with markers of microglia/macrophage (CD45), neurons (NeuN), and astrocytes (GFAP) to confirm the cell types expressing these inflammatory mediators. Scale bar = 50 μm. Data are expressed as mean ± SEM. Immunoreactivities were quantified from the total of seven to ten mice per group. $^{**}p < 0.01$ and $^{***}p < 0.001$. *IL* ipsilateral, *CL* contralateral

pro-inflammatory cytokines, including IL-6 and TNF-α [23–25]. NO, IL-6, and TNF-α are classical TLR4-regulated pro-inflammatory mediators known to be induced in ischemic stroke and propagate apoptosis and the secondary ischemic damage mediated by [26, 27]. TLR4 deficiency reduces the levels of NO, IL-6, TNF-α and protects against ischemic-induced neuronal damage [9, 26, 28]. In accordance, inhibition of p38 MAPK pathway has been reported to be protective in both transient and permanent focal cerebral ischemia [29–31]. Similarly, preventing the activation of the NFκB pathway is protective in both permanent and transient cerebral ischemia [32, 33]. Neuroprotective agents modulating inflammation such as curcumin [6], hydroxysafflor yellow A [34], and minocycline [7, 8] inhibit microgliosis and the activation of NFκB and p38 pathways. Thus, it is not surprising that the neuroprotective and anti-inflammatory effects of SSO were associated with diminished activation of these pathways. Moreover, NO is the key mediator of neuronal death in neuron-microglia co-culture model used in this study [16], and SSO inhibited the secretion of NO, together with IL-6 and TNF-α upon the exposure to LPS + IFNγ and microgliosis in vivo, thus supporting the potent anti-inflammatory capacity of SSO.

SSO has been shown to act as an inhibitor of CD36 in vitro [35–37]. CD36 is a scavenger receptor involved in pathogen recognition and phagocytosis and is abundantly expressed in microglia/macrophages. CD36 is bound by a wide variety of ligands to promote downstream signaling resulting in pro-inflammatory activation [5, 38] including the activation of the NFκB pathway [39, 40]. Indeed, CD36 signaling is induced after cerebral stroke and plays a pivotal role in stroke-induced inflammation [41]. Thus, it is not surprising that CD36-deficient mice show reduced levels of NFκB activation and oxidative stress which alleviates brain damage [39]. Cao et al. [42] have shown that CD36 participates in LPS-induced inflammation in goat mammary epithelial cells by regulating NFκB and JNK activation but not p38-MAPK pathway. It is therefore plausible that SSO binds to the active site of CD36 to exert neuroprotection. However, reduced p38 activation by SSO in the current study suggests that also other mechanisms may underlie the neuroprotective effect of SSO. In fact, the impact of CD36 downstream signaling may be model- and context-dependent. This hypothesis is supported by a study demonstrating an increase in the extent of injury in mice lacking CD36 after acute neonatal stroke [43] and on the other hand by a study in which genetic deletion of CD36 provided benefit in a transient model of ischemic stroke [13]. Moreover, Kim et al. reported that a specific tetrapeptide inhibitor for CD36, SS-31, or genetic deletion of CD36 is protective only in transient but not permanent MCAo [44]. Noteworthy is that the dose of SS-31 used by Kim et al. and SSO used in the current study cannot be compared also due to different administration routes and time points. Likewise, the permanent stroke model used in the current study (distal pMCAo) is different from that used by Kim et al., possibly explaining the differences in the outcome.

Our in vitro data are well in line with our in vivo data showing the ability of SSO to reduce microglial activation and the expression of COX-2. COX-2, an enzyme upregulated following cerebral ischemia, contributes to the ischemic brain injury [45]. CD36 deficiency has been shown to be associated with downregulation of COX-2 in a rodent model of age-related macular degeneration [46], and CD36 activation has been proposed to increase the expression of COX-2 [47]. In line with these data, we found an upregulation of COX-2 immunoreactivity in the peri-ischemic area after stroke which was attenuated in SSO-treated mice. COX-2 immunoreactivity was mainly co-localized in neurons and microglia/macrophages. In addition, our in vitro data also show a reduction in the protein levels of COX-2 in SSO-treated microglia following the exposure to LPS + IFNγ. CD36 activation has been shown to contribute to the generation of pro-inflammatory eicosanoids in vitro [48]. Thus, the reduction in COX-2 activity by SSO might restrict the formation of pro-inflammatory eicosanoids by binding to CD36 and hence reduced brain damage which is likely to be reflected as decreased COX-2 expression also in affected neurons.

HO-1 induction has been reported to be beneficial in cerebral stroke in many models. HO-1 is an endogenous antioxidant enzyme upregulated in cerebral ischemia and catalyzes the conversion of heme to carbon monoxide and biliverdin. HO-1 expression is controlled and driven by Nrf2 [49]. Antioxidant agents driving the upregulation of HO-1, such as dimethyl fumarate [50], gastrodin [51], and thioredoxin [52], have been reported beneficial in models of stroke and also reduce microglial activation and stroke-related neuroinflammation. Moreover, similar to our study, upregulation in HO-1 has been shown to be associated with reduced expression in COX-2 and NOS2 [53] and silencing HO-1 expression promotes LPS-induced pro-inflammatory response [54]. In the current study, HO-1 was expressed in both microglia/macrophages and neurons, and SSO was able to reverse LPS + IFNγ-induced downregulation of Nrf2 expression in microglia cultures. In fact, stimulation of the Nrf2 pathway has been shown to inhibit microglial activation [55, 56] supporting the anti-inflammatory capacity of Nrf2 pathway upregulation, our observations of the increased HO-1 expression in both microglia/macrophages and neurons, and reduced microgliosis and neuronal damage in SSO-treated ischemic mice. The fact that we did not observe an increase in HO-1 in SSO-treated BV2 cells may be related to the fact that in ischemic brains, crosstalk between microglia and neurons is likely to take place and both neurons and microglia contribute to the increased levels of HO-1. This indeed was evident by co-staining of HO-1 with NeuN and CD45 showing that both cell types express HO-1.

Conclusions

Microglia play a prominent role in regulating stroke-induced inflammation. Microglia have been discussed to exacerbate brain damage following cerebral ischemia through the production of reactive nitrogen and oxygen species [4, 57, 58] but also secrete anti-inflammatory cytokines and aid in the process of inflammation resolution [27]. We have here shown for the first time that SSO is able to reduce the harmful microglial activation, promote the anti-oxidative response, and importantly reduce ischemic brain damage. Our in vitro data show that this is likely to be related to the inhibition of the p38 MAPK and NFκB pathways. Further studies are needed to determine the exact mechanism involved in SSO neuroprotection following ischemic stroke.

Abbreviations

NFκB: Nuclear factor kappa-B; CBA: Cytokine bead array; COX-2: Cyclooxygenase-2; H3: Histone-3; HBSS: Hank's Balanced Salt Solution; HO-1: Heme oxygenase-1; IFN-γ: Interferon-gamma; IL-1: Interleukin-1; IL-6: Interleukin-6; LPS: Lipopolysaccharide; MAPK: Mitogen-activated protein kinase; MCA: Middle cerebral artery; MCP-1: Monocyte chemoattractant protein-1; MRI: Magnetic resonance imaging; NO: Nitric oxide; Nrf2: Nuclear factor (erythroid-derived 2)-like 2; PBS: Phosphate buffer solution; PFA: Paraformaldehyde; pMCAo: Distal permanent occlusion of the MCA; SSO: Sulfosuccinimidyl oleate sodium; TLR: Toll-like receptor; TNF-α: Tumor necrosis factor-α

Acknowledgements
We thank Ms. Mirka Tikkanen for the technical assistance.

Funding
This study was supported by funding from EU FP7, Academy of Finland and Emil Aaltonen foundation.

Authors' contributions
HD, KMK, JK, and TM contributed to the study conception and design. HD, GG, VK-G, MJ, SL, HA, MH, and TM contributed to the acquisition of data. HD, MH, MJ, and TM contributed to the analysis and interpretation of data. HD and TM contributed to the drafting of the manuscript. HD, TM, KMK, JK, and MJ contributed to the critical revision of the manuscript. All authors read and approved the final manuscript.

Consent for publication
Not applicable.

Competing interests
The authors declare that they have no competing interests.

References
1. Dirnagl U, Iadecola C, Moskowitz MA. Pathobiology of ischaemic stroke: an integrated view. Trends Neurosci. 1999;22:391–7.
2. Vidale S, Consoli A, Arnaboldi M, Consoli D. Postischemic inflammation in acute stroke. J Clin Neurol (Seoul, Korea), 13. 2017:1–9.
3. Wang Q, Tang XN, Yenari MA. The inflammatory response in stroke. J Neuroimmunol. 2007;184:53–68.
4. Jin R, Yang G, Li G. Inflammatory mechanisms in ischemic stroke: role of inflammatory cells. J Leukoc Biol. 2010;87:779–89.
5. Iadecola C, Anrather J. The immunology of stroke: from mechanisms to translation. Nat Med. 2011;17:796–808.
6. Dong HJ, Shang CZ, Peng DW, Xu J, PX X, Zhan L, Wang P. Curcumin attenuates ischemia-like injury induced IL-1beta elevation in brain microvascular endothelial cells via inhibiting MAPK pathways and nuclear factor-kappaB activation. Neurol Sci. 2014;35:1387–92.
7. Tikka TM, Koistinaho JE. Minocycline provides neuroprotection against N-methyl-D-aspartate neurotoxicity by inhibiting microglia. J Immunol. 2001; 166:7527–33.
8. Yrjanheikki J, Keinanen R, Pellikka M, Hokfelt T, Koistinaho J. Tetracyclines inhibit microglial activation and are neuroprotective in global brain ischemia. Proc Natl Acad Sci U S A. 1998;95:15769–74.
9. Caso JR, Pradillo JM, Hurtado O, Lorenzo P, Moro MA, Lizasoain I. Toll-like receptor 4 is involved in brain damage and inflammation after experimental stroke. Circulation. 2007;115:1599–608.
10. Minnerup J, Sutherland BA, Buchan AM, Kleinschnitz C. Neuroprotection for stroke: current status and future perspectives. Int J Mol Sci. 2012;13:11753–72.
11. Abe T, Shimamura M, Jackman K, Kurinami H, Anrather J, Zhou P, Iadecola C. Key role of CD36 in Toll-like receptor 2 signaling in cerebral ischemia. Stroke. 2010;41:898–904.
12. Cho S. CD36 as a therapeutic target for endothelial dysfunction in stroke. Curr Pharm Des. 2012;18:3721–30.
13. Cho S, Park EM, Febbraio M, Anrather J, Park L, Racchumi G, Silverstein RL, Iadecola C. The class B scavenger receptor CD36 mediates free radical production and tissue injury in cerebral ischemia. J Neurosci. 2005;25:2504–12.
14. Simantov R, Silverstein RL. CD36: a critical anti-angiogenic receptor. Front Biosci. 2003;8:s874–82.
15. Malm T, Mariani M, Donovan LJ, Neilson L, Landreth GE. Activation of the nuclear receptor PPARδ is neuroprotective in a transgenic mouse model of Alzheimer's disease through inhibition of inflammation. J Neuroinflammation. 2015;12:7.
16. Gresa-Arribas N, Viéitez C, Dentesano G, Serratosa J, Saura J, Solà C. Modelling neuroinflammation in vitro: a tool to test the potential neuroprotective effect of anti-inflammatory agents. Plos One. 2012;7:e45227.
17. Dhungana H, Rolova T, Savchenko E, Wojciechowski S, Savolainen K, Ruotsalainen A-K, Sullivan P, Koistinaho J, Malm T. Western-type diet modulates inflammatory responses and impairs functional outcome following permanent middle cerebral artery occlusion in aged mice expressing the human apolipoprotein E4 allele. J Neuroinflammation. 2013;10:102.
18. Hrometz SL, Ebert JA, Grice KE, Nowinski SM, Mills EM, Myers BJ, Sprague JE. Potentiation of Ecstasy-induced hyperthermia and FAT/CD36 expression in chronically exercised animals. Temperature. 2016;3:557–66.
19. Liu H, Xu W, Yu Q, Yang Q. 4,4'-diaponeurosporene-producing Bacillus subtilis increased mouse resistance against S. Typhimurium infection in a CD36 dependent manner. Front Immunol. 2017;8
20. Shuaib A, Xu Wang C, Yang T, Noor R. Effects of nonpeptide V(1) vasopressin receptor antagonist SR-49059 on infarction volume and recovery of function in a focal embolic stroke model. Stroke. 2002;33:3033–7.
21. Karunakaran U, Moon JS, Lee HW, Won KC. CD36 initiated signaling mediates ceramide-induced TXNIP expression in pancreatic beta-cells. Biochim Biophys Acta (BBA) - Mol Basis Dis. 2015;1852:2414–22.
22. Kim JY, Kawabori M, Yenari MA. Innate inflammatory responses in stroke: mechanisms and potential therapeutic targets. Curr Med Chem. 2014;21: 2076–97.
23. Chan ED, Riches DWH. IFN-γ + LPS induction of iNOS is modulated by ERK, JNK/SAPK, and p38^{<em>mapk</em>} in a mouse macrophage cell line. Am J Physiol Cell Physiol. 2001;280:C441–50.
24. Jung YS, Park JH, Kim H, Kim SY, Hwang JY, Hong KW, Bae SS, Choi BT, Lee S-W, Shin HK. Probucol inhibits LPS-induced microglia activation and ameliorates brain ischemic injury in normal and hyperlipidemic mice. Acta Pharmacol Sin. 2016;37:1031–44.
25. W-J O, Jung U, Eom H-S, Shin H-J, Park H-R. Inhibition of lipopolysaccharide-induced proinflammatory responses by Buddleja officinalis extract in BV-2 microglial cells via negative regulation of NF-kB and ERK1/2 signaling. Molecules. 2013;18:9195.
26. Kilic U, Kilic E, Matter CM, Bassetti CL, Hermann DM. TLR-4 deficiency protects against focal cerebral ischemia and axotomy-induced neurodegeneration. Neurobiol Dis. 2008;31:33–40.
27. Zhao S-C, Ma L-S, Chu Z-H, Xu H, Wu W-Q, Liu F. Regulation of microglial activation in stroke. Acta Pharmacol Sin. 2017;38:445–58.
28. Cao CX, Yang QW, Lv FL, Cui J, Fu HB, Wang JZ. Reduced cerebral ischemia-reperfusion injury in Toll-like receptor 4 deficient mice. Biochem Biophys Res Commun. 2007;353:509–14.
29. Barone FC, Irving EA, Ray AM, Lee JC, Kassis S, Kumar S, Badger AM, White RF, McVey MJ, Legos JJ, et al. SB 239063, a second-generation p38 mitogen-activated protein kinase inhibitor, reduces brain injury and neurological deficits in cerebral focal ischemia. J Pharmacol Exp Ther. 2001;296:312–21.
30. Legos JJ, Erhardt JA, White RF, Lenhard SC, Chandra S, Parsons AA, Tuma RF, Barone FC. SB 239063, a novel p38 inhibitor, attenuates early neuronal injury following ischemia. Brain Res. 2001;892:70–7.
31. Piao CS, Kim JB, Han PL, Lee JK. Administration of the p38 MAPK inhibitor SB203580 affords brain protection with a wide therapeutic window against focal ischemic insult. J Neurosci Res. 2003;73:537–44.
32. Nurmi A, Lindsberg PJ, Koistinaho M, Zhang W, Juettler E, Karjalainen-Lindsberg ML, Weih F, Frank N, Schwaninger M, Koistinaho J. Nuclear factor-kappaB contributes to infarction after permanent focal ischemia. Stroke. 2004;35:987–91.
33. Schneider A, Martin-Villalba A, Weih F, Vogel J, Wirth T, Schwaninger M. NF-kappaB is activated and promotes cell death in focal cerebral ischemia. Nat Med. 1999;5:554–9.

34. Lv Y, Qian Y, Ou-Yang A, Fu L. Hydroxysafflor yellow A attenuates neuron damage by suppressing the lipopolysaccharide-induced TLR4 pathway in activated microglial cells. Cell Mol Neurobiol. 2016;36:1241–56.
35. Coort SLM, Willems J, Coumans WA, van der Vusse GJ, Bonen A, Glatz JFC, Luiken JJFP. Sulfo-N-succinimidyl esters of long chain fatty acids specifically inhibit fatty acid translocase (FAT/CD36)-mediated cellular fatty acid uptake. Mol Cell Biochem. 2002;239:213–9.
36. Kuda O, Pietka TA, Demianova Z, Kudova E, Cvacka J, Kopecky J, Abumrad NA. Sulfo-N-succinimidyl oleate (SSO) inhibits fatty acid uptake and signaling for intracellular calcium via binding CD36 lysine 164: SSO also inhibits oxidized low density lipoprotein uptake by macrophages. J Biol Chem. 2013;288:15547–55.
37. Pohl J, Ring A, Korkmaz U, Ehehalt R, Stremmel W. FAT/CD36-mediated long-chain fatty acid uptake in adipocytes requires plasma membrane rafts. Mol Biol Cell. 2005;16:24–31.
38. Cho S, Kim E. CD36: a multi-modal target for acute stroke therapy. J Neurochem. 2009;109:126–32.
39. Kunz A, Abe T, Hochrainer K, Shimamura M, Anrather J, Racchumi G, Zhou P, Iadecola C. Nuclear factor-kappaB activation and postischemic inflammation are suppressed in CD36-null mice after middle cerebral artery occlusion. J Neurosci. 2008;28:1649–58.
40. Triantafilou M, Gamper FG, Haston RM, Mouratis MA, Morath S, Hartung T, Triantafilou K. Membrane sorting of Toll-like receptor (TLR)-2/6 and TLR2/1 heterodimers at the cell surface determines heterotypic associations with CD36 and intracellular targeting. J Biol Chem. 2006;281:31002–11.
41. Cho S, Febbraio M. CD36: an inflammatory mediator in acute brain injury. In: Chen J, Hu X, Stenzel-Poore M, Zhang JH, editors. Immunological mechanisms and therapies in brain injuries and stroke. New York, NY: Springer New York; 2014. p. 321–47.
42. Woo MS, Wang X, Faustino JV, Derugin N, Wendland MF, Zhou P, Iadecola C, Vexler ZS. Genetic deletion of CD36 enhances injury after acute neonatal stroke. Ann Neurol. 2012;72:961–70.
43. Cao D, Luo J, Chen D, Xu H, Shi H, Jing X, Zang W. CD36 regulates lipopolysaccharide-induced signaling pathways and mediates the internalization of Escherichia coli in cooperation with TLR4 in goat mammary gland epithelial cells. Sci Rep. 2016;6:23132.
44. Kim E, Tolhurst AT, Szeto HH, Cho S. Targeting CD36-mediated inflammation reduces acute brain injury in transient, but not permanent, ischemic stroke. CNS Neurosci Therapeut. 2015;21:385–91.
45. Iadecola C, Gorelick PB. The janus face of cyclooxygenase-2 in ischemic stroke: shifting toward downstream targets. Stroke. 2005;36:182–5.
46. Houssier M, Raoul W, Lavalette S, Keller N, Guillonneau X, Baragatti B, Jonet L, Jeanny JC, Behar-Cohen F, Coceani F, et al. CD36 deficiency leads to choroidal involution via COX2 down-regulation in rodents. PLoS Med. 2008;5:e39.
47. Bujold K, Rhainds D, Jossart C, Febbraio M, Marleau S, Ong H. CD36-mediated cholesterol efflux is associated with PPARγ activation via a MAPK-dependent COX-2 pathway in macrophages. Cardiovasc Res. 2009;83:457–64.
48. Kuda O, Jenkins CM, Skinner JR, Moon SH, Su X, Gross RW, Abumrad NA. CD36 protein is involved in store-operated calcium flux, phospholipase A2 activation, and production of prostaglandin E2. J Biol Chem. 2011;286:17785–95.
49. Loboda A, Damulewicz M, Pyza E, Jozkowicz A, Dulak J. Role of Nrf2/HO-1 system in development, oxidative stress response and diseases: an evolutionarily conserved mechanism. Cell Mol Life Sci. 2016;73:3221–47.
50. Yao Y, Miao W, Liu Z, Han W, Shi K, Shen Y, Li H, Liu Q, Fu Y, Huang D, Shi F-D. Dimethyl fumarate and monomethyl fumarate promote post-ischemic recovery in mice. Transl Stroke Res. 2016;7:535–47.
51. Peng Z, Wang S, Chen G, Cai M, Liu R, Deng J, Liu J, Zhang T, Tan Q, Hai C. Gastrodin alleviates cerebral ischemic damage in mice by improving anti-oxidant and anti-inflammation activities and inhibiting apoptosis pathway. Neurochem Res. 2015;40:661–73.
52. Wang B, Tian S, Wang J, Han F, Zhao L, Wang R, Ning W, Chen W, Qu Y. Intraperitoneal administration of thioredoxin decreases brain damage from ischemic stroke. Brain Res. 2015;30:89–97.
53. Suh SJ, Chung TW, Son MJ, Kim SH, Moon TC, Son KH, Kim HP, Chang HW, Kim CH. The naturally occurring biflavonoid, ochnaflavone, inhibits LPS-induced iNOS expression, which is mediated by ERK1/2 via NF-kappaB regulation, in RAW264.7 cells. Arch Biochem Biophys. 2006;447:136–46.
54. Rushworth SA, MacEwan DJ, O'Connell MA. Lipopolysaccharide-induced expression of NAD(P)H:quinone oxidoreductase 1 and heme oxygenase-1 protects against excessive inflammatory responses in human monocytes. J Immunol (Baltimore, Md : 1950). 2008;181:6730–7.
55. Kwon Y-W, Cheon SY, Park SY, Song J, Lee J-H. Tryptanthrin suppresses the activation of the LPS-treated BV2 microglial cell line via Nrf2/HO-1 antioxidant signaling. Front Cell Neurosci. 2017;11:18.
56. Min KJ, Kim JH, Jou I, Joe EH. Adenosine induces hemeoxygenase-1 expression in microglia through the activation of phosphatidylinositol 3-kinase and nuclear factor E2-related factor 2. Glia. 2008;56:1028–37.
57. del Zoppo GJ, Milner R, Mabuchi T, Hung S, Wang X, Berg GI, Koziol JA. Microglial activation and matrix protease generation during focal cerebral ischemia. Stroke. 2007;38:646–51.
58. Pun PBL, Lu J, Moochhala S. Involvement of ROS in BBB dysfunction. Free Radic Res. 2009;43:348–64.

5

Infiltration and persistence of lymphocytes during late-stage cerebral ischemia in middle cerebral artery occlusion and photothrombotic stroke models

Yan Feng[1,2†], Shiwei Liao[1†], Changjuan Wei[1], Dongmei Jia[1], Kristofer Wood[3], Qiang Liu[1,3], Xiaoying Wang[4], Fu-Dong Shi[1,2,3] and Wei-Na Jin[1,2,3*]

Abstract

Background: Evidence suggests that brain infiltration of lymphocytes contributes to acute neural injury after cerebral ischemia. However, the spatio-temporal dynamics of brain-infiltrating lymphocytes during the late stage after cerebral ischemia remains unclear.

Methods: C57BL/6 (B6) mice were subjected to sham, photothrombosis, or 60-min transient middle cerebral artery occlusion (MCAO) procedures. Infarct volume, neurodeficits, production of reactive oxygen species (ROS) and inflammatory factors, brain-infiltrating lymphocytes, and their activation as well as pro-inflammatory cytokine IFN-γ production were assessed. Brain-infiltrating lymphocytes were also measured in tissue sections from post-mortem patients after ischemic stroke by immunostaining.

Results: In mice subjected to transient MCAO or photothrombotic stroke, we found that lymphocyte infiltration persists in the ischemic brain until at least day 14 after surgery, during which brain infarct volume significantly diminished. These brain-infiltrating lymphocytes express activation marker CD69 and produce proinflammatory cytokines such as IFN-γ, accompanied with a sustained increase of reactive oxygen species (ROS) and inflammatory cytokines release in the brain. In addition, brain-infiltrating lymphocytes were observed in post-mortem brain sections from patients during the late stage of ischemic stroke.

Conclusion: Our results demonstrate that brain-infiltration of lymphocytes persists after the acute stage of cerebral ischemia, facilitating future advanced studies to reveal the precise role of lymphocytes during late stage of stroke.

Keywords: Inflammation, Lymphocytes, Ischemic stroke, Photothrombosis, Transient middle cerebral artery occlusion

Background

Peripheral lymphocytes infiltrating ischemic brain regions orchestrate inflammatory responses, catalyze neuronal death, and worsen clinical outcomes of acute ischemic stroke (AIS) [1–3]. Previous studies have focused on the dynamics and function of brain-infiltrating lymphocytes during the acute stage of brain ischemia, i.e., from hours to days after onset [4–10]. In acute ischemic stroke, the majority of infiltrating lymphocyte subsets can damage neural structures and exacerbate stroke outcome [11–15]. For example, γδ T, $CD8^+$ T, and NK cells contribute to acute brain injury after stroke onset [16, 17], while regulatory T and B cells are reported to be protective [18]. However, little is known about the presence and functional status of brain-infiltrating lymphocytes during the late stage of cerebral ischemia.

Transient middle cerebral artery occlusion (MCAO) and photothrombotic ischemia are two commonly used murine models to study neuroinflammation in stroke.

* Correspondence: Weina.Jin@DignityHealth.org
†Equal contributors
1Department of Neurology, Tianjin Neurological Institute, Tianjin Medical University General Hospital, Tianjin 300052, China
2Center for Neuroinflammation, Beijing TianTan Hospital, Beijing 100070, China
Full list of author information is available at the end of the article

Although the post-ischemic inflammation and injury have been well documented during the early stage of ischemia in these two models, the features of cellular immune responses have not been adequately studied during the late stage.

In this study, we determined the dynamics, activation, and cytokine production profiles of brain-infiltrating lymphocytes up to 14 days after photothrombotic and MCAO in mice during which brain infarct volume has significantly diminished, in conjunction with post-mortem human brain tissues from patients with ischemic stroke. Our results suggest that lymphocyte responses can persist in the brain at least for weeks after cerebral ischemia.

Methods

Mice

Male C57BL/6 (B6, $H2^b$) mice and $Rag2^{-/-}\gamma c^{-/-}$mice ($H2^b$) were purchased from Taconic (Oxnard, CA, USA). Mutant mice were backcrossed to the B6 background for at least 12 generations. Mice were maintained under specific pathogen-free conditions, and used at 10–12 weeks of age. They were housed with no more than five animals per cage under standardized light-dark cycle conditions with ad libitum access to food and water. For all experiments, age-matched male littermates were used. All animal experiments were performed in accordance with the ARRIVE (Animal Research: Reporting in vivo Experiments) guidelines. All procedures were approved by Animal Care and Use Committees of the Barrow Neurological Institute and Tianjin Neurological Institute.

Transient middle cerebral artery occlusion procedure

Adult male 10- to 12-week-old mice were subjected to 60 min focal cerebral ischemia produced by transient intraluminal occlusion of the middle cerebral artery (MCAO) as described previously [19–23]. MCAO was performed under anesthesia induced by inhalation of 3.5% isoflurane and maintained by inhalation of 1.0–2.0% isoflurane in 70% N_2O and 30% O_2. Body temperature was monitored throughout surgery with a rectal probe and maintained at 37.0 ± 0.5 °C using a heating pad (Sunbeam, Neosho, MO, USA). Cerebral blood flow was monitored for 5 min both before and after MCAO, and immediately before and after reperfusion with a laser Doppler probe (model P10, Moor Instruments, Wilmington, DE, USA). A monofilament made of 6–0 nylon with rounded tip was used to induce focal cerebral ischemia for 60 min by occlusion of the right middle cerebral artery. After 60 min of MCAO, the occluding filament was withdrawn gently back into the common carotid artery to allow reperfusion. Mice were excluded upon death or non-satisfactory cerebral blood flow (CBF) during occlusion or 10 min after reperfusion. Mice that had a residual CBF < 20% of pre-ischemic levels throughout the ischemic period and CBF recovery > 80% within 10 min of reperfusion were used in the study. Sham-operated mice were subjected to the same surgical procedure, but the filament was not advanced far enough to occlude the middle cerebral artery. 7T-MRI was used to determine infarct volume 1–14 days after MCAO [19]. In the MCAO model, the mortality rate was 13.4% (13 of total 97) and exclusion rate was 18.5% (13 of total 97 for inadequate reperfusion, 5 of total 97 for criteria limitations set for the mNSS scoring system).

Photothrombotic stroke procedure

Photothrombotic occlusion was performed as previously reported [24]. Mice subjected to photothrombotic surgery were anesthetized by inhalation of 3.5% isoflurane and maintained by inhalation of 1.0–2.0% isoflurane in 70% N_2O and 30% O_2. Mice were injected intraperitoneally with rose Bengal at a dose of 150 mg/kg (Sigma Aldrich, St. Louis, MO, USA) 5 min prior to illumination. After receiving Rose Bengal, mice were placed into a stereotaxic apparatus (Stoelting Co, Wood Dale, IL, USA). The bregma was identified and the end of a fiber optic cable with a diameter of 4 mm was placed over the top of the skull rostrocaudally centered on and approximately 2 mm lateral to the bregma. Five minutes after injection of the Rose Bengal solution, a cold light source (Schott KL 1600 LED, Elmsford, NY, USA) with a green bandpass filter (Thor Labs, Newton, NJ, USA) was turned on and the skull was illuminated for 20 min. Once the region had been illuminated for 20 min, the mouse was removed from the stereotaxic apparatus and the incision was sutured and sterilized. Sham-operated mice were subjected to the same surgical procedure without Rose Bengal injection. Mice were excluded upon death or non-satisfactory modified Neurological Severity Score [mNSS score < 6 or above a score of 13 at 24 h after photothrombosis (prior to treatment) were excluded]. In the photothrombotic stroke model, the mortality rate was 6% (5 of total 84) and exclusion rate was 8.3% (7 of total 84 non-satisfactory mNSS score).

Behavior assessment

Behavioral tests were performed at days 1, 3, 7, and 14 after ischemic stroke as we previously described and published reports [19, 20, 25–28]. The modified Neurological Severity Score (mNSS) test consisted of motor, sensory, reflex, and balance assessments. The rating scale was as follows: A score of 13–18 indicates severe injury, 7–12 indicates moderate injury, and 1–6 indicates mild injury. Following surgery, each mouse was assessed on a scale from 0 to 18 after recovery from the stroke procedure. Mice with score < 6 or above a score of 13 at 24 h post surgery (prior to treatment) were not included in the study. In all experiments, 12 mice were excluded due to criteria limitations set for the mNSS scoring system.

For the adhesive removal test, an adhesive patch (0.35 × 0.45 cm) was applied to the forelimb contralateral to the ischemic hemisphere [29]. The mouse was then put into a cage. Time taken to contact and remove adhesive tape was recorded with 120 s being the time limit. The Corner turning test was used to assess sensorimotor and postural asymmetries [30]. All mice tested were allowed to enter a corner with an angle of 30° which required the subject to turn either to the left or the right to exit the corner. This was repeated and recorded ten times, with at least 30 s between trials, and the percentage of right turns out of total turns was calculated. The ability of a mouse to respond to a vibrissae-elicited excitation by forward movement of its forelimb was evaluated with the forelimb placing test, as previously described [22]. Briefly, animals held by their trunk were positioned parallel to a table top and slowly moved up and down, allowing the vibrissae on one side of the head to brush along the table surface. Refractory placements of the impaired (left) forelimb were evaluated and a score was calculated as number of successful forelimb placements out of ten consecutive trials. The rotarod test was performed as previously reported [31]. Mice from sham or stroke groups were placed on an accelerating rotating rod. The speed was increased from 4 to 40 rpm (the acceleration rate to 20 rpm/min) within 5 min. Mice were tested three times daily with a break of at least 5 min between tests. The latency to fall off the rotating rod was recorded by a blinded investigator [31].

Neuroimaging

Infarct size of both ischemic stroke models was assessed with a 7T small animal MRI (Bruker Daltonics Inc., Billerica, MA, USA) with a 72 mm linear transmitter coil and a mouse surface receiver coil for mouse brain imaging, as we previously described [19, 32]. Mice were under anesthesia by inhalation of 3.5% isoflurane and maintained by inhalation of 1.0–2.0% isoflurane in 70% N_2O and 30% O_2 by a face mask. During MRI scanning (10 min per mouse), the animal's respiration was continually monitored by a small animal monitoring and gating system (SA Instruments, Stoney Brook, NY, USA) via a pillow sensor positioned under the abdomen. Mice were placed on a heated circulating water blanket (Bruker, Billerica, MA) to maintain normal body temperature (36–37 °C). Axial 2D multi-slice T2-weighted images of brain with fat-suppressed Rapid Acquisition with Relaxation Enhancement (RARE) sequence (TR = 4000 ms, effective TE = 60 ms, number of average = 4, FOV = 19.2 mm × 19.2 mm, matrix size = 192 × 192). The ten gradient echoes were acquired for T2*-mapping by using a Multi-slice Gradient Echo sequence (MGE, TR = 120 ms, echo time = 3.0, 6.0, 9.0, 12.0, 15.0, 18.0, 21.0, 24.0, 27.0, 30.0 ms, field of view = 35.0 × 35.0 mm, matrix = 128 × 128, slice thickness = 1.0 mm, flip angle 80°). The MRI data were analyzed using ImageJ software (National Institutes of Health, Bethesda MD, USA).

The live bioluminescence images were captured to detect reactive oxygen species (ROS) generation in the brain, using the Xenogen IVIS200 imager (Caliper LifeSciences, Hopkinton, MA, USA) [19, 32, 33]. ROS production was assessed using luminol as we and others previously described [22, 23, 26, 33]. Briefly, mice were injected i.p. with 200 mg/kg luminol (Invitrogen, Carlsbad, CA, USA). At 10 min after luminol injection, bioluminescence images were captured. A region of interest tool was used to define and measure the chemiluminescent intensity within the brain. Data were collected as photons per second per cm^2 using Living Image software (Caliper Life Sciences, Hopkinton, MA, USA).

Cell isolation, labeling, and passive transfer

Splenocytes of C57BL/6 mice were isolated using red cell lysis buffer (BD Biosciences) as we previously described [19, 34]. For the SPIO-Molday ION Rhodamine-B (MIRB) labeling assay, lymphocytes were sorted using flow cytometry, and cultured with MIRB (BioPhysics Assay Laboratory, Inc., Worcester, MA, USA) at a concentration of 25 μg/ml, in RPMI culture medium with 10% FBS (Invitrogen, Grand Island, NY, USA), L-glutamine (2 mM), IL-2 (10 μg/ml), penicillin (100 U/ml), and streptomycin (0.1 mg/ml) at 5% CO_2/37 °C, as we previously described [20]. After MIRB incubation for 24 h, cells were centrifuged (400 g for 5 min) and washed twice with PBS to remove extracellular MIRB. Further, 2×10^7 MIRB-labeled lymphocytes in 200 μl PBS were then injected via the tail vein into $Rag2^{-/-}\gamma c^{-/-}$ recipient mice. Immediately after transfer, the $Rag2^{-/-}\gamma c^{-/-}$ recipients were subjected to sham, 60 min MCAO, or photothrombosis surgeries.

Flow cytometry

The lymphocytes for FACS assessment were isolated from spleens or brains as we previously described [19, 32, 34]. In brief, splenocytes were isolated using red cell lysis buffer (BD Biosciences). For brain mononuclear cells isolation, after perfusion with cold PBS, the whole brain was dissected, cut into small pieces, and digested in 1 mg/ml Collagenase IV in DMEM at 37 °C for 30 min to obtain the single cells. Single cells were resuspended in 70% percoll and transferred into 15 ml tubes, then overlaid with 37% percoll. The mononuclear cells were harvested after centrifuging at 1800 rpm for 20 min at RT (without brake). Antibodies were labeled with one of the following fluorescent tags: fluorescein isothiocyanate (FITC), phycoerythrin (PE), PerCP-Cy5.5, allophycocyanin (APC), PE-

Cy7, or APC-Cy7. The following antibodies were used in this study: CD3 (145-2C11, 553066, BD Biosciences, San Jose, CA, USA), CD4 (RM4-5, 552775, BD Biosciences, San Jose, CA, USA), CD8 (53-6.7, 557654, BD Biosciences, San Jose, CA, USA), NK1.1 (PK136, 551114, BD Biosciences, San Jose, CA, USA), B220 (RA3-6B2, 553093, BD Biosciences, San Jose, CA, USA), IFN-γ (XMG1.2, 505814, Biolegend, San Diego, CA, USA), CD69 (H1.2F3, 104508, Biolegend, San Diego, CA, USA). Flow cytometric measurements were performed on a FACSAria (BD Biosciences, San Jose, CA, USA) and analyzed using FACSDiva and Flowjo 7.6 software (Informer Technologies, Ashland, OR, USA).

Immunostaining

The immunostaining was performed as we previously described [19, 25, 26, 32, 35, 36]. Briefly, mice were euthanized and whole brain tissue was removed after perfusion, fixed in 4% paraformaldehyde, and then dehydrated with 15 and 30% sucrose. Whole brains were embedded in OCT for preparation of frozen sections. The frozen slices of 30 μm thickness were blocked in 5% goat or donkey serum for 1 h at room temperature. Tissue sections were incubated with primary antibodies against mouse CD4 (MT310, sc-19,641; Santa Cruz Biotechnology, Dallas, Texas, USA), CD8 (ab4055, Abcam, Cambridge, MA, USA), NKp46 (MAB2225, R&D systems, Minneapolis, MN, USA) at 4 °C overnight, and then incubated with appropriate fluorochrome-conjugated secondary antibodies. Nuclei were co-stained with 4′,6-diamidino-2-phenylindole (DAPI; Abcam, Cambridge, MA, USA). For human brain tissue staining, primary antibodies against human CD4 (MAB379-100, R&D systems, Minneapolis, MN, USA), CD8 (MAB1509, R&D systems, Minneapolis, MN, USA), and NKp46 (MAB1850, R&D systems, Minneapolis, MN, USA) were used. Images were acquired on a fluorescence microscope (Olympus, model BX-61, Center Valley, PA, USA) [19, 32, 34]. After immunostaining, positive cell numbers were counted in the every tenth tissue section through the entire tissue block. The number of positive cells in brain sections was expressed as a percentage of immunolabeled cells relative to the total number of cells assessed by DAPI [20, 37]. Image analysis was performed using ImageJ software (National Institutes of Health).

ELISA

Cytokines in brain homogenates were measured using a customized ELISA kit (SA Biosciences, Valencia, CA, USA). Protein homogenates were extracted from mouse brain using the Halt Protease Inhibitor Cocktail kit (Thermo Fisher Scientific, Fremont, CA, USA) and centrifuged at 13,000 rpm for 20 min at 4 °C, and supernatants were collected. Cytokine levels were detected at 1:20 dilutions according to the manufacturer's instructions, and reactions analyzed at a wavelength of 450 nm using a 96-well microplate reader (Model 680; Bio-Rad Laboratories, Hercules, CA, USA).

Human brain tissue

Paraffin-embedded brain tissue sections of stroke patients were obtained from the Sun Health Research Institute (Sun City, AZ) and Department of Pathology, Ohio State University (Columbus, OH). Among the ten human samples used in this study, five tissues were obtained from patients who died within 7–14 days after stroke onset (male, 2; female, 3). The locations of stroke lesions were within the cortical areas supplied by the middle cerebral artery. The tissue was collected from the middle cerebral artery field of perfusion. Five control sections were from patients who died from nonneurological diseases (trauma, 1; kidney failure, 1; gastric cancer, 1; liver cancer, 2) (male, 2; female, 3), and the location of selected tissue sections was matched with stroke patients. All included patients have no acute myocardial infarction, heart failure, autoimmune disease, hematological system disease, or any infection before stroke at the time of death. Patients with ischemic stroke and controls did not differ significantly for mean age at death (stroke patients, 76.2 ± 7 years; controls, 79.5 ± 9.2 years, mean ± SEM; $p > 0.05$, Student's t test). Brain tissues were collected within 4 h after death.

Statistical analyses

Power analysis and sample size calculations were performed using SAS 9.1 software (SAS Institute Inc. Cary, NC, USA). The experimental design was based on previous publications with similar mechanistic studies [19, 32, 34, 38, 39]. The exclusion criteria are described in the individual method section. Randomization was based on the random number generator function in Microsoft Excel software. All results were analyzed by investigators blinded to different groups. Data are presented as the means ± s.e.m. Statistical significance was determined by the two-tailed unpaired Student's t test for two groups, one-way analysis of variance (ANOVA) followed by Tukey post-hoc test for three or more groups, or two-way ANOVA accompanied by Bonferroni post hoc test for multiple comparisons. Values of $p < 0.05$ were considered significant. All statistical analyses were performed using Prism 6.0 software (GraphPad, San Diego, CA, USA).

Results

Evaluation of ischemic damages over time in photothrombotic stroke and MCAO model

7T-MRI T2-w imaging was used to measure the infarct lesion over time (day 1, 3, 7, and 14) after ischemic stroke. The ischemic lesion was evident at 1–3 days both in photothrombosis and MCAO, featured by heterogeneous hyperintense signals on T2-w images (Photothrombosis vs. sham, $n = 10$ per group, $p < 0.01$; MCAO vs. sham, $n = 10$ per group, $p < 0.01$; Fig. 1a, b). Decline of hyperintense signals was found after day 7 on T2-w images both in MCAO and photothrombosis mice. Since day 7 after photothrombosis, a hypointense signal was observed surrounding lesion area in photothrombosis mice, suggesting the formation of glia scar in photothrombosis mice which was also identified by immunostaining (Fig. 2). The MRI T2-w signal at 14 days after surgery can still be observed in photothrombosis model but hardly observed in MCAO model (Fig. 1**a**, **b**). However in both models, Iba-1 expressing microglia were accumulated around the infarct lesion at day 14 after surgery with functional marker CD68 expression, prompting a functional activation status of microglia after 14 days ischemia (Fig. 2, see Additional file 1).

To determine neurodeficits in photothrombosis and MCAO model, a battery of behavioral tests on sensory-motor function were conducted, including mNSS score, the forelimb placing test, the adhesive-removing test, corner turning test, and rotarod test. As shown in Fig. 1c, the behavioral tests demonstrated that the greatest neurodeficits occurred from day 1 to day 3 in both photothrombosis and MCAO mice. Functional recovery started from day 7 post-stroke. Both photothrombosis and MCAO mice gradually and spontaneously recovered thereafter, but still exhibited neurodeficits up to 14 days after stroke as compared to sham control (Photothrombosis vs. sham, $n = 10$ per group, $p < 0.01$; MCAO vs. sham, $n = 10$ per group, $p < 0.01$; Fig. 1c). This result indicates that the impaired behavioral outcomes last up to 14 days after brain ischemia.

Brain inflammation persists in photothrombosis and MCAO model during late-phase of brain ischemia

To date, brain inflammation has been studied in many experimental models and human specimens during the acute phase of ischemic stroke. But the long-term features of inflammatory cells are still obscure. So we next investigated the inflammation status in CNS at late phase of brain ischemia in photothrombotic stroke model as well as MCAO model. As shown in Fig. 3, at 14 days after brain ischemia, a significantly higher level of reactive oxygen species (ROS; as one of the inflammatory parameters) was noted in photothrombosis mice and a slightly higher level of ROS was detected in MCAO mice as compared to sham mice (Photothrombosis vs. sham, $n = 6$ per group, $p < 0.01$; MCAO vs. sham, $n = 6$ per group, $p > 0.05$; Fig. 3a, b).

Using a customized mouse cytokine ELISA panel, we assessed the expression of pro-inflammatory cytokines in the brain homogenates of photothrombosis and MCAO mice 14 days after surgery. We found that both photothrombosis and MCAO for 14 days showed upregulation of pro-inflammatory cytokines release including IL-1α, IL-1β, IFN-γ, IL-6, TNF-α, and CD69 compared with sham control (Photothrombosis vs. sham, $n = 4$ per group, IL-1α, IL-1β, IFN-γ,

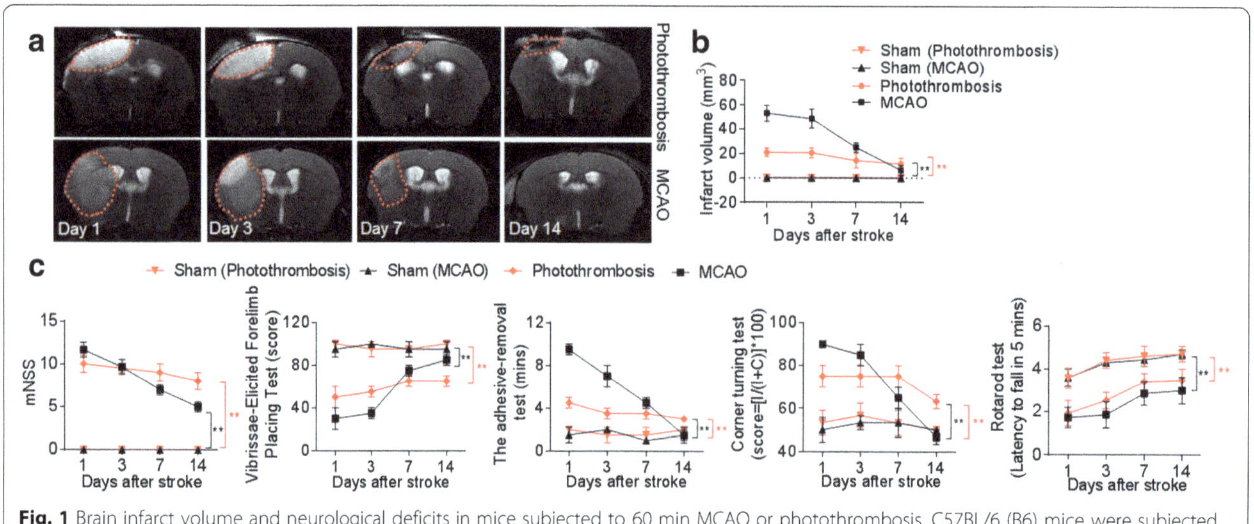

Fig. 1 Brain infarct volume and neurological deficits in mice subjected to 60 min MCAO or photothrombosis. C57BL/6 (B6) mice were subjected to sham, photothrombosis, or 60 min MCAO operation. At day 1, 3, 7, or 14 after surgery, mice were subjected to MR imaging and neurological assessment. **a** Representative MRI images show time course of infarct volume (outlined in red) in mice subjected to sham, photothrombosis, or MCAO. **b** Line graphs show the quantification of infarct volume of photothrombosis and MCAO mice at indicated time points after surgery. **c** Cumulative data illustrate the indicated neurological assessments (including mNSS score, the forelimb placing test, adhesive-removing test, corner turning test, and rotarod test) of photothrombosis and MCAO mice from day 1 to day 14 after surgery. $n = 10$ mice per group. Error bars represent s.e.m.; $^{**}p < 0.01$, sham vs. stroke group (photothrombosis/MCAO) by two-way ANOVA

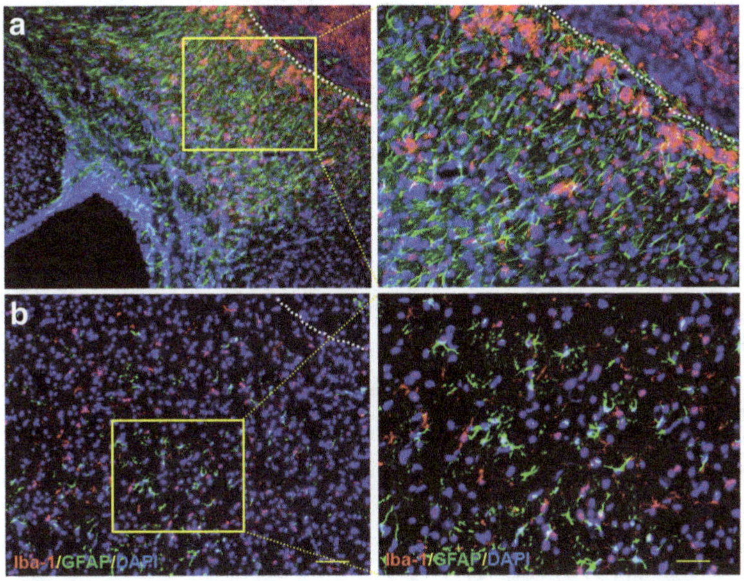

Fig. 2 Stroke lesion diminished at day 14 after brain ischemia in mice. Immunostaining of brain sections showing the lesion in the middle of infarction and perilesional area (separated by dashed line) at 14 day after photothrombotic stroke (**a**) and MCAO (**b**). Scale bars: 100 μm (left), 40 μm (right)

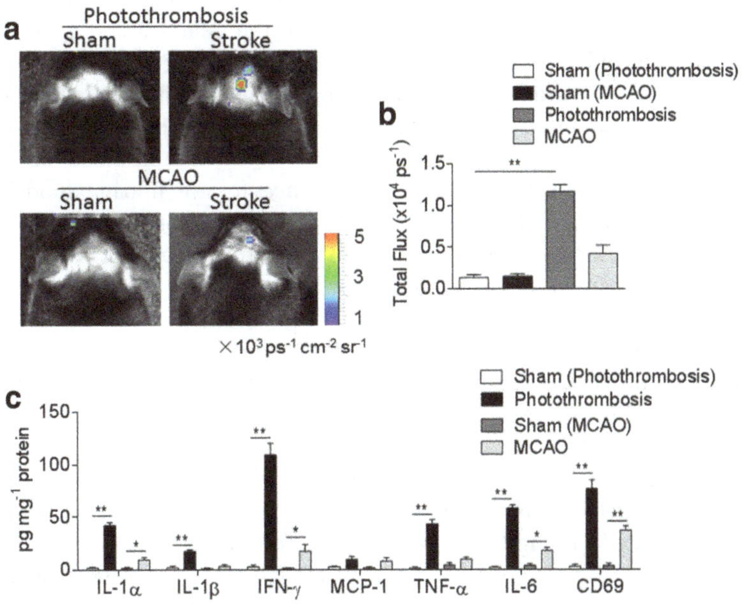

Fig. 3 Production of ROS and inflammatory factors in the ischemic brain at day 14 after onset in mice. C57BL/6 (B6) mice were subjected to sham operation, photothrombosis, or 60 mins MCAO for 14 days. **a** At day 14 after surgery, bioluminescence images show ROS generation in photothrombosis and MCAO mice. **b** Quantification analysis showed ROS generation in photothrombosis and MCAO mice 14 days after ischemia. $n = 6$ mice per group. **c** At 14 days after ischemia, brain tissues were obtained from photothrombosis and MCAO mice. Brain tissues from sham-operated mice were used as control. Brain homogenates were prepared, and cytokine concentrations were measured by a customized Mouse Cytokines ELISA kit, including IL-1α, IL-1β, IFN-γ, MCP-1, IL-6, TNF-α, and CD69. Results shown are from three independent experiments with a pool of 4 mice per group. Error bars represent s.e.m.; $*p < 0.05$; $**p < 0.01$, sham vs. stroke group (photothrombosis/MCAO) by one-way ANOVA

IL-6, TNF-α, and CD69, $p < 0.01$; MCAO vs. sham, $n = 4$ per group, IL-1α, IFN-γ, IL-6, $p < 0.05$; CD69, $p < 0.01$), suggesting the brain inflammation persists until 14 days after brain ischemia (Fig. 3c).

Lymphocytes infiltration and activation persist in late phase of brain ischemia in photothrombosis and MCAO mice

As lymphocyte infiltration prominently contributes to brain inflammation during the delayed phase of ischemia, we further compared the brain lymphocyte infiltration in photothrombosis and MCAO mice at 14 days after brain ischemia. We used Molday ION Rhodamine B (MIRB), which is an ultra-small, super paramagnetic iron oxide particle (USPIO) of 35 nm that is not toxic for immune cells and can be visualized by MRI [20]. Lymphocytes were obtained from wild-type mice, labeled with MIRB in vitro, and then passively transferred into $Rag2^{-/-}\gamma c^{-/-}$ recipient mice (lacking T, B, NK, and NKT cells). Using 7T-MRI, we non-invasively tracked inflammatory infiltration until 7 days after MCAO. We found that MIRB-labeled lymphocytes (visualized as hypointensive dots on MRI) could be tracked 7 days after surgery in both models, but with significantly stronger signal intensity in photothrombosis mice, indicating inflammatory infiltration of lymphocytes into the brain 7 days after stroke (Photothrombosis vs. sham, $n = 8$ per group, $p < 0.01$; MCAO vs. sham, $n = 8$ per group, $p > 0.05$; Fig. 4a, b).

Brain-infiltrating $CD4^+$ T, $CD8^+$ T, NK, and B cells can be observed both in photothrombosis and MCAO mice at 14 days after surgery. We found significantly increased $CD4^+$ T, $CD8^+$ T, NK cells in stroke models compared with sham mice. Comparing the two models, there are more $CD4^+$ T, $CD8^+$ T, NK cells in photothrombosis model than MCAO model, while no difference in B cell populations was observed between the two models (Photothrombosis vs. sham, $n = 8$ per group, $CD4^+$ T, $CD8^+$ T, NK, and B cells, $p < 0.01$; MCAO vs. sham, $n = 8$ per group, $CD4^+$ T, $CD8^+$ T, NK cells, $p < 0.05$; B cells, $p < 0.01$; Fig. 4c, d; Photothrombosis vs. sham, $n = 5$ per group, $CD4^+$ T, $CD8^+$ T, NK, $p < 0.01$; MCAO vs. sham, $n = 5$ per group, $CD4^+$ T and NK cells, $p < 0.05$; Fig. 4e, f). This result suggested the lymphocyte infiltration can be observed in the delayed phase of brain ischemia, which might be implicated in long-term post-stroke injury.

Next, to further study the possible role of increased $CD4^+$ T, $CD8^+$ T, and NK cell infiltration in ischemic brain during the late phase, we compared the activation of these cells in brains of photothrombosis and MCAO mice with sham controls. We found that the activating lymphocyte marker CD69 and IFN-γ were over-expressed in both stroke models compared with sham mice, but more in photothrombosis mice as compared to MCAO mice at 14 days after surgery. Of note, in photothrombosis mice, IFN-γ expression was significantly increased in $CD4^+$ T cells, which was not dramatic in $CD8^+$ T or NK cells (IFN-γ: Photothrombosis vs. sham, $n = 8$ per group, $CD4^+$ T cells, $p < 0.01$, $CD8^+$ T and NK cells, $p < 0.05$; MCAO vs. sham, $n = 8$ per group, $CD4^+$ T cells, $p < 0.05$; CD69: Photothrombosis vs. sham, $n = 8$ per group, $CD4^+$ T, $CD8^+$ T, and NK cells, $p < 0.01$; MCAO vs. sham, $n = 8$ per group, $CD4^+$ T cells, $p < 0.05$; Fig. 5a–c). As IFN-γ is a critical cytokine in the mediation of Th1 responses that have been indicated as a key player to promote ischemic brain injury, these results indicate that the activation of infiltrated lymphocytes, especially IFN-γ-expressing $CD4^+$ T cells, may be involved in the late phase of ischemic stroke. However, there is no significant difference in splenic and circulating lymphocyte populations between the sham and ischemic groups in the two models (Fig. 6).

Rodent models mimic the inflammatory brain infiltration in ischemia stroke patients during delayed stage

Ischemic stroke in human is a heterogeneous disorder with a complex pathophysiology at different stages, so it is not feasible to mimic all aspects of human stroke in one animal model. Here we examined brain infiltration of $CD4^+$ T, $CD8^+$ T, and NK cells in post-mortem brain sections from ischemic stroke patients who died within 7–14 days after stroke onset. Patients with ischemic stroke exhibited marked increase of T cells and NK cells around the infarct lesion area (Stroke vs. control, $n = 15$ sections, $p < 0.01$; Fig. 7). This result is paralleled with the lymphocyte infiltration in mice model, suggesting the persistence of inflammatory infiltration in both stroke patients and mice models, which provide the evidence to use murine models for mirroring the ischemic stroke patients, and for investigating immuno-inflammatory features at delayed stage of cerebral ischemia.

Discussion

In this study, we demonstrate that lymphocyte infiltration persists during late stage of cerebral ischemia when brain infarcts become significantly decreased in two experimental stroke models. Together with the activation of infiltrating lymphocytes, we noted the increased ROS production, inflammatory factors release, and IFN-γ and CD69 upregulation in brain-infiltrated lymphocytes, suggesting that lymphocytes may retain their capability to impact the inflammatory microenvironment in the brain during the late stage of ischemia.

Infiltrating immune cells orchestrate the brain inflammatory environment by producing various effector molecules or inflammatory mediators [40]. In this study, we found that brain inflammation last to 14 days after brain

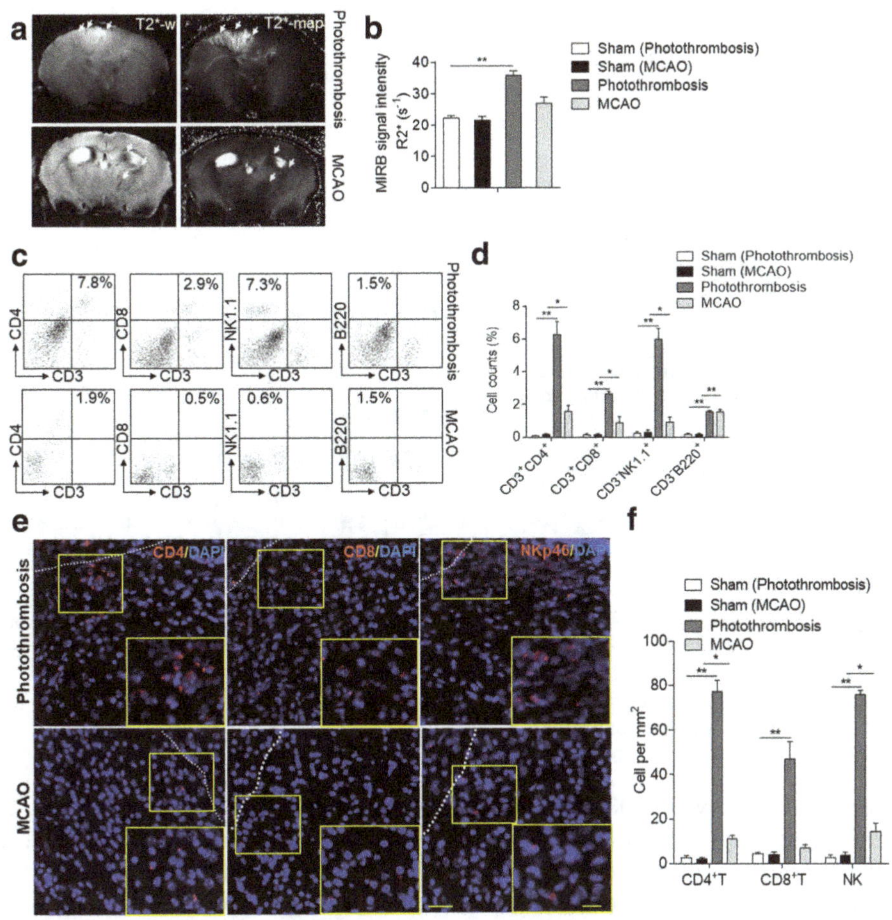

Fig. 4 Lymphocyte infiltration persists in the ischemic brain at day 14 after onset in mice. **a** Lymphocytes were isolated from spleens of C57BL/6 (B6) mice and co-cultured with MIRB. 2×10^7 MIRB-labeled cells were then adoptively transferred into $Rag2^{-/-}\gamma c^{-/-}$ mice followed by sham or stroke procedures. MRI images show hypointensive dots that indicate MIRB-labeled lymphocytes in the ischemic brains of $Rag2^{-/-}\gamma c^{-/-}$ mice. **b** Summarized results show signal of MIRB-labeled lymphocytes in mice receiving either sham or MCAO operations. $n = 8$ mice per group. **c** Dot plots of flow cytometry assay show $CD4^+$ T, $CD8^+$ T, NK, and B cells in single cell suspension from brains of photothrombosis- or MCAO-operated mice at 14 days after stroke. **d** Bar graphs summarize the cumulative data for quantifying $CD4^+$ T, $CD8^+$ T, NK, and B cell population from brains of photothrombosis- or MCAO-operated mice at 14 days after stroke. $n = 8$ mice per group. **e** At 14 day after surgery, representative immunostaining images show infiltrated $CD4^+$ T, $CD8^+$ T, and NK cells around ischemic lesion area in photothrombosis and MCAO mice. Red: CD4, CD8 or NKp46; blue: DAPI. Scale bars: 40 μm, 20 μm (inset). **f** Quantification analysis shows the infiltrated $CD4^+$ T, $CD8^+$ T, and NK cell counts from ipsilateral brain in photothrombosis and MCAO mice 14 days after ischemia. $n = 5$ mice per group. Error bars represent s.e.m.; $^*p < 0.05$; $^{**}p < 0.01$, sham vs. stroke group (photothrombosis/MCAO) by one-way ANOVA

ischemia in both models, and the photothrombotic mice elicited higher levels of inflammatory cytokines/chemokines in the brain and more lymphocyte infiltration from the periphery than MCAO mice during the late phase of stroke. This result may due to the different features of these two models: photothrombosis produces a permanent and persistent injury resulting from the production of free radicals and thrombus production in small vessels. In contrast, transient MCAO with an intraluminal occlusion produces a temporary occlusion of a main vessel that is resolved by reperfusion and collateral vessel perfusion. Furthermore, there is significant disruption of the blood-brain barrier surrounding photothrombotic regions for at least 7 and up to 14 days after injury [41], whereas the blood-brain barrier disruption is resolved within 4 days in MCAO [42], which indicates a more intact blood-brain barrier in MCAO mice by 14 days after injury. This factor may account for the differences observed in lymphocyte infiltration. Another possibility is the coagulation of peripheral blood during photothrombosis. In order to offset the possible confounding peripheral blood in the lesion, we also set up ET-1 focal stroke model with ET-1/L-NAME injection. We observed lymphocytes infiltration at day 14 after brain ischemia in ET-1 model, which supports our finding that inflammatory infiltration at late stage of brain ischemia (see Additional file 2). We further performed experiments to test how the coagulated blood within the

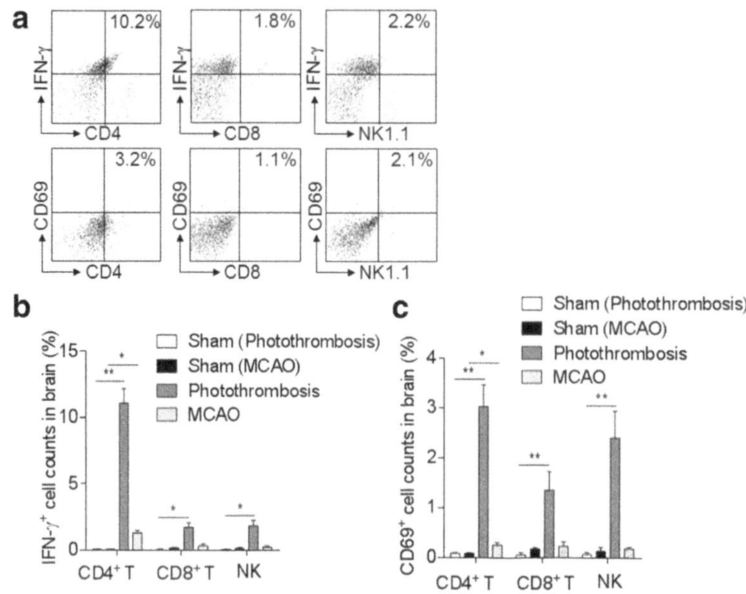

Fig. 5 Brain-infiltrating lymphocytes express CD69 and IFN-γ at day 14 after brain ischemia in mice. **a** Flow cytometry dot plots show IFN-γ and CD69 expression in $CD4^+$ T, $CD8^+$ T, and NK cells in single cell suspension from brains of photothrombosis- or MCAO-operated mice at 14 days after stroke. **b**, **c** Bar graphs summarize the cumulative data for quantifying IFN-γ (**b**) and CD69 (**c**) expression in $CD4^+$ T, $CD8^+$ T, and NK cells from brains of photothrombosis- or MCAO-operated mice at 14 days after stroke. $n = 8$ mice per group. Error bars represent s.e.m.; $^{**}p < 0.01$, sham vs. stroke group (photothrombosis/MCAO) by one-way ANOVA

cerebral vasculature affect observed ROS production and MIRB-labeled cell signal in photothrombosis model, by injecting lymphocytes before or immediately after photothrombosis procedure. As compared to the pre-stroke cell transfer, post-stroke transferred mice exhibit slightly reduced ROS production and MIRB signal but with no significance. This data indicates coagulation may produce artificial signal in the infarct region, but it may not significantly affect the lymphocyte infiltration-induced inflammation after brain ischemia (see Additional file 3). Our study suggests that lymphocytes may retain their capability to impact the inflammatory micro-environment in the brain during the late stage of ischemia. Cotrina ML et al. reported an enhanced inflammatory response and increased periphery infiltration within 7 days after photothrombotic stroke compared with MCAO, but did not study the long-term stroke outcome comparing the two models [43]. Our study also evaluated post-stroke neurological outcome, showing that in both models, neurodeficits still persist at late phase after brain ischemia. Vandeputte C et al. characterized the inflammatory response in photothrombotic

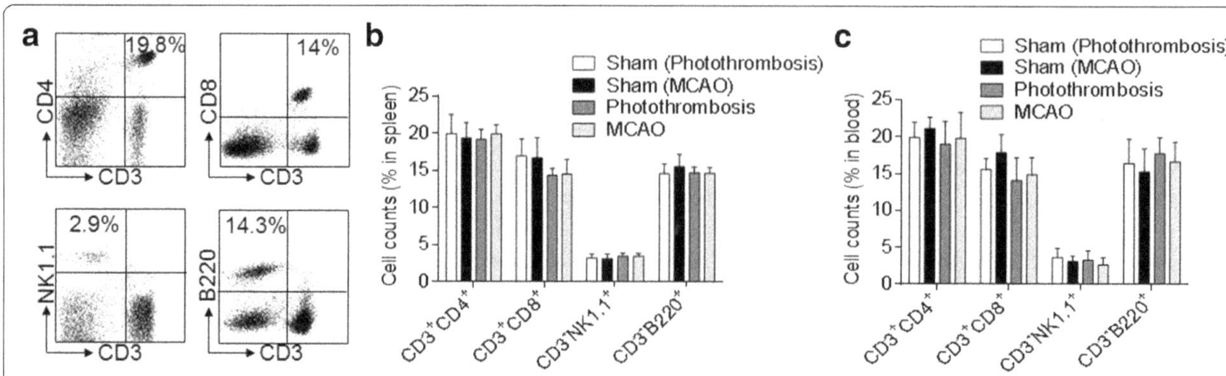

Fig. 6 Assessment of peripheral lymphocyte subsets at day 14 after brain ischemia in mice. **a** Dot plots of flow cytometry show gating strategy of $CD4^+$ T, $CD8^+$ T, NK, and B cells in single cell suspension from spleens of photothrombosis- or MCAO-operated mice at 14 days after stroke. **b** Bar graphs summarize the cumulative data for $CD4^+$ T, $CD8^+$ T, NK, and B cell counts from spleens of photothrombosis- or MCAO-operated mice at 14 days after stroke. **c** Bar graphs summarize the cumulative data for $CD4^+$ T, $CD8^+$ T, NK, and B cell counts from blood of photothrombosis- or MCAO-operated mice at 14 days after stroke. $n = 8$ mice per group. Error bars represent s.e.m

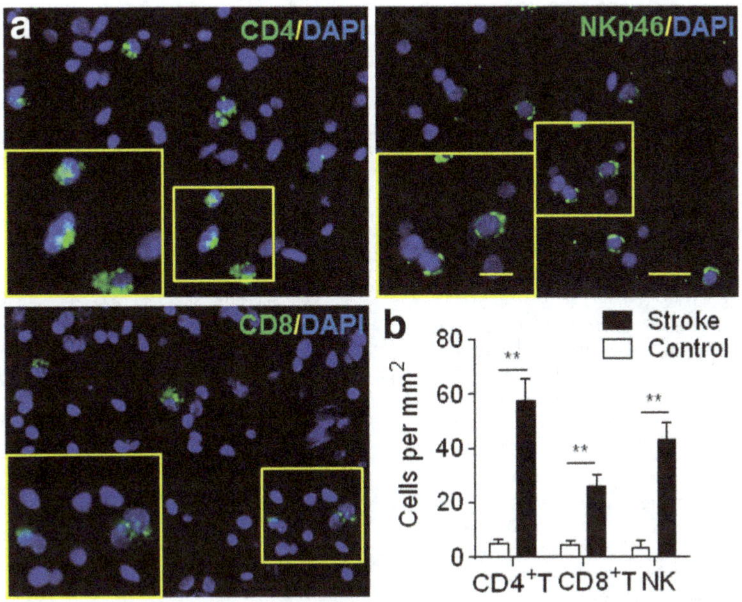

Fig. 7 Lymphocyte infiltration persists in the brain of patients with ischemic stroke during delayed stage after onset. **a** Representative immunostaining images show CD4$^+$ T, CD8$^+$ T, and NK cells in brain perilesional area in an ischemic stroke patient. **b** Bar graph shows the quantification of CD4$^+$ T, CD8$^+$ T, and NK cells in controls and patients with ischemic stroke during later phases. $n = 15$ sections from five patients with ischemic stroke; $n = 15$ sections from five controls with non-neurological disease. Scale bars: 20 μm, 10 μm (inset). Error bars represent s.e.m.; $^{**}p < 0.01$ sham vs. stroke patients by two-tailed unpaired Student's t test

stroke model by MRI [44], which is in line with our MRI results.

Early detrimental roles of lymphocytes such as T cells have been reported in ischemic stroke [16, 17]. Evidence suggests that CD4$^+$ T and CD8$^+$ T lymphocytes, but not B lymphocytes, contribute to the inflammatory thrombosis, brain injury, and neurological deficit in experimental stroke models [16, 17]. In an effort to identify the fate of brain-infiltrating lymphocytes, we measured the presence, activation, and functional status of these cells during the resolution phase of ischemic brain injury. The expression of the activation marker CD69 and cytokines such as IFN-γ by these lymphocytes suggest their competence to tune the inflammatory environment in the brain. Of interest, we found higher expression of IFN-γ in stroke mice, especially by CD4$^+$ T cells. This finding suggests that T cells may be potentially involved in the process of tissue remodeling and impact disease outcome during the resolution phase of ischemic stroke. However, still unclear are how lymphocyte subsets such as T cells impact on brain ischemia-induced brain injury, what chronic factors and which neuro-immune pathways may be responsible. These aspects will certainly need to be investigated in future studies.

Although the precise temporal and spatial dynamics of lymphocyte response in human stroke may not entirely match that found in experimental stroke models because the overall disease time course is usually significantly longer in human stroke, it is notable that the persisted infiltration of lymphocytes were also seen in the brain sections from stroke patients during the delayed stage of ischemia. Comparing the two mice models with stroke patients, MCAO model is more similar in the vessel occluded and the reperfusion style expected in clinical cases, so better mirrors the ischemic stroke patient. While because of the lasting and distinct inflammatory infiltration, photothrombosis might be a useful animal model to study the brain inflammation during late phase of brain injury. This finding presents a need for further investigation to better understand the role of infiltrating lymphocytes during the late stage of cerebral ischemia.

Conclusions

In summary, we demonstrate that lymphocyte infiltration persists during late-stage cerebral ischemia. The activation and expression of effector molecules in these cells suggests their potential involvement in the resolution phase of ischemic brain injury. These findings may provide a better knowledge base for future advanced studies to reveal the precise role of lymphocyte responses during late stage of stroke.

Additional files

Additional file 1: Microglial phenotype at day 14 after photothrombosis and MCAO. C57BL/6 (B6) mice were subjected to sham operation, photothrombosis, or 60 mins MCAO for 14 days. At day 14 after surgery, mice were subjected to flow cytometry assessment. **(A)** Dot plots of flow cytometry assay show the gating strategy for microglia and CD68-expression. (**B**) Bar graphs summarize the cumulative data for quantifying microglia population and CD68-expression from brains of photothrombosis- or MCAO-operated mice at 14 days after stroke. $n = 4$ mice per group. $^{*}P < 0.05$; $^{**}P < 0.01$, sham vs. stroke (photothrombosis/MCAO) by one-way ANOVA.

Additional file 2: Lymphocytes infiltration at day 14 after brain ischemia in ET-1 model. (**A**) ET-1 model induction. ET-1 and L-NAME were dissolved in sterile saline, and were delivered into the cortex by stereotaxic injection (AP +1.0, ML +1.0, DV -1.0, ET-1 at 1 μg and L-NAME at 2.7 μg). The ipsilateral common carotid artery were permanently occluded just prior to the ET-1 injection. (**B**) Lymphocyte infiltration at late stage of brain ischemia in mice subjected to ET-1 model. Dot plots of flow cytometry assay show $CD4^{+}$ T, $CD8^{+}$ T, NK, and B cells in single cell suspension from brains of sham (PBS injection) or ET-1/L-NAME injected mice at 14 days after procedures. (**C**) Bar graphs summarize the cumulative data for quantifying $CD4^{+}$ T, $CD8^{+}$ T, NK, and B cell counts from brains of ET-1 model at 14 days after stroke. $n = 8$ mice per group. Error bars represent s.e.m.; $^{*}P < 0.05$; $^{**}P < 0.01$, sham vs. ET-1 model by two-tailed unpaired Student's *t* test.

Additional file 3: ROS generation and lymphocytes infiltration in photothrombosis model with lymphocytes pre- or post-stroke transfer. Lymphocytes were isolated from spleens of C57BL/6 mice. 2×10^{7} isolated cells were then adoptively transferred into $Rag2^{-/-}\gamma c^{-/-}$ mice followed by sham or photothrombosis procedures, or transferred immediately after procedure. (**A**) Imaging ROS activity in vivo. Bioluminescent images were captured for 1 min using the cooled IVIS imaging system (Xenogen IVIS-200) after luminol i.p. injection, to monitor the ROS generation in $Rag2^{-/-}\gamma c^{-/-}$ photothrombosis brains. (**B**) Quantification and statistical analysis of the images. As compared to the pre-stroke cell transfer, post-stroke transferred mice exhibit slightly fewer ROS signal but with no significance. $n = 3$ mice per group. (**C**) Lymphocytes were isolated from spleens of C57BL/6 (B6) mice and co-cultured with MIRB. 2×10^{7} MIRB-labeled cells were then adoptively transferred into $Rag2^{-/-}\gamma c^{-/-}$ mice followed by sham or stroke procedures, or transferred immediately after procedure. MRI was used to track MIRB-labeled lymphocytes in the ischemic brains of $Rag2^{-/-}\gamma c^{-/-}$ mice. Bar graph shows MIRB signal in mice receiving either sham or photothrombosis model. MIRB signals can be observed in the ischemic brain of post-stroke transferred mice, with comparable intensity to the pre-transferred group. Error bars represent s.e.m.; $^{*}P < 0.05$; $^{**}P < 0.01$, sham vs. stroke by one-way ANOVA.

Acknowledgements
Not applicable.

Funding
This study was supported in part by the US National Institutes of Health grant (R01NS092713); American Heart Association grant (16SDG27250236); National Multiple Sclerosis Society grant (RG-1507-05318); National Science Foundation of China grant (81771274, 91642205, 81471220, 81471535), Ministry of Human Resources and Social Security of China grant 2016.

Authors' contributions
YF, SL, CW, and DJ acquired, analyzed and interpreted the data. KS acquired, interpreted the data, and edited the language of manuscript. QL designed the study, drafted the manuscript, and acquired funding for the study. XW drafted the manuscript and interpreted the data. FDS formulated the study concept, designed the study, drafted the manuscript, and acquired funding for the study. W-NJ designed the study, acquired, analyzed and interpreted the data, drafted the manuscript, and acquired funding for the study. All authors read and approved the final manuscript.

Consent for publication
Not applicable.

Competing interests
The authors declare that they have no competing interests.

Author details
[1]Department of Neurology, Tianjin Neurological Institute, Tianjin Medical University General Hospital, Tianjin 300052, China. [2]Center for Neuroinflammation, Beijing TianTan Hospital, Beijing 100070, China. [3]Department of Neurology, Barrow Neurological Institute, St. Joseph's Hospital and Medical Center, Phoenix 85013, AZ, USA. [4]Neuroprotection Research Laboratory, Departments of Radiology and Neurology, Massachusetts General Hospital, Harvard Medical School, Boston 02129, MA, USA.

References
1. Schroeter M, Jander S, Witte OW, Stoll G. Local immune responses in the rat cerebral cortex after middle cerebral artery occlusion. J Neuroimmunol. 1994;55:195–203.
2. Jander S, Kraemer M, Schroeter M, Witte OW, Stoll G. Lymphocytic infiltration and expression of intercellular adhesion molecule-1 in photochemically induced ischemia of the rat cortex. J Cereb Blood Flow Metab. 1995;15:42–51.
3. Benakis C, Garcia-Bonilla L, Iadecola C, Anrather J. The role of microglia and myeloid immune cells in acute cerebral ischemia. Front Cell Neurosci. 2014;8:461.
4. Hurn PD, Subramanian S, Parker SM, Afentoulis ME, Kaler LJ, Vandenbark AA, Offner H. T- and B-cell-deficient mice with experimental stroke have reduced lesion size and inflammation. J Cereb Blood Flow Metab. 2007; 27:1798–805.
5. Urra X, Cervera A, Villamor N, Planas AM, Chamorro A. Harms and benefits of lymphocyte subpopulations in patients with acute stroke. Neuroscience. 2009;158:1174–83.
6. Sun JC, Lanier LL. NK cell development, homeostasis and function: parallels with CD8(+) T cells. Nat Rev Immunol. 2011;11:645–57.
7. Sun JC, Beilke JN, Bezman NA, Lanier LL. Homeostatic proliferation generates long-lived natural killer cells that respond against viral infection. J Exp Med. 2011;208:357–68.
8. Jaeger BN, Donadieu J, Cognet C, Bernat C, Ordonez-Rueda D, Barlogis V, Mahlaoui N, Fenis A, Narni-Mancinelli E, Beaupain B, et al. Neutrophil depletion impairs natural killer cell maturation, function, and homeostasis. J Exp Med. 2012;209:565–80.
9. Sun JC, Beilke JN, Lanier LL. Adaptive immune features of natural killer cells. Nature. 2009;457:557–61.
10. Yokoyama WM, Kim S, French AR. The dynamic life of natural killer cells. Annu Rev Immunol. 2004;22:405–29.
11. Ransohoff RM, Brown MA. Innate immunity in the central nervous system. J Clin Invest. 2012;122:1164–71.
12. Gadani SP, Walsh JT, Lukens JR, Kipnis J. Dealing with danger in the CNS: the response of the immune system to injury. Neuron. 2015;87:47–62.
13. Chamorro A, Meisel A, Planas AM, Urra X, van de Beek D, Veltkamp R. The immunology of acute stroke. Nat Rev Neurol. 2012;8:401–10.
14. Fu Y, Liu Q, Anrather J, Shi FD. Immune interventions in stroke. Nat Rev Neurol. 2015;11:524–35.
15. Iadecola C, Anrather J. The immunology of stroke: from mechanisms to translation. Nat Med. 2011;17:796–808.
16. Yilmaz G, Arumugam TV, Stokes KY, Granger DN. Role of T lymphocytes and interferon-gamma in ischemic stroke. Circulation. 2006;113:2105–12.
17. Kleinschnitz C, Schwab N, Kraft P, Hagedorn I, Dreykluft A, Schwarz T, Austinat M, Nieswandt B, Wiendl H, Stoll G. Early detrimental T-cell effects in experimental cerebral ischemia are neither related to adaptive immunity nor thrombus formation. Blood. 2010;115:3835–42.
18. Liesz A, Suri-Payer E, Veltkamp C, Doerr H, Sommer C, Rivest S, Giese T, Veltkamp R. Regulatory T cells are key cerebroprotective immunomodulators in acute experimental stroke. Nat Med. 2009;15:192–9.
19. Gan Y, Liu Q, Wu W, Yin JX, Bai XF, Shen R, Wang Y, Chen J, La Cava A, Poursine-Laurent J, et al. Ischemic neurons recruit natural killer cells that accelerate brain infarction. Proc Natl Acad Sci U S A. 2014;111:2704–9.
20. Jin WN, Yang X, Li Z, Li M, Shi SX, Wood K, Liu Q, Fu Y, Han W, Xu Y, et al. Non-invasive tracking of CD4+ T cells with a paramagnetic and fluorescent nanoparticle in brain ischemia. J Cereb Blood Flow Metab. 2016;36:1464–76.
21. Yan T, Chopp M, Chen J. Experimental animal models and inflammatory cellular changes in cerebral ischemic and hemorrhagic stroke. Neurosci Bull. 2015;31:717–34.
22. Jin WN, Li Z, Li M, Wood K, Gonzales R, Liu Q. Depletion of microglia exacerbates postischemic inflammation and brain injury. J Cereb Blood Flow Metab. 2017;37:2224-36.

23. Liu Q, Jin WN, Liu Y, Shi K, Sun H, Zhang F, Zhang C, Gonzales R, Sheth KN,La Cava A, Shi FD. Brain ischemia suppresses immunity in the periphery and brain via different neurogenic innervations. Immunity. 2017;46(3):474-87.
24. Li H, Zhang N, Lin HY, Yu Y, Cai QY, Ma L, Ding S. Histological, cellular and behavioral assessments of stroke outcomes after photothrombosis-induced ischemia in adult mice. BMC Neurosci. 2014;15:58.
25. Liu Q, Tang Z, Gan Y, Wu W, Kousari A, La Cava A, Shi FD. Genetic deficiency of beta2-containing nicotinic receptors attenuates brain injury in ischemic stroke. Neuroscience. 2014;256:170–7.
26. Tang Z, Gan Y, Liu Q, Yin JX, Shi J, Shi FD. CX3CR1 deficiency suppresses activation and neurotoxicity of microglia/macrophage in experimental ischemic stroke. J Neuroinflammation. 2014;11:26.
27. Balkaya M, Krober J, Gertz K, Peruzzaro S, Endres M. Characterization of long-term functional outcome in a murine model of mild brain ischemia. J Neurosci Methods. 2013;213:179–87.
28. Mirza MA, Ritzel R, Xu Y, McCullough LD, Liu F. Sexually dimorphic outcomes and inflammatory responses in hypoxic-ischemic encephalopathy. J Neuroinflammation. 2015;12:32.
29. Bouet V, Boulouard M, Toutain J, Divoux D, Bernaudin M, Schumann-Bard P, Freret T. The adhesive removal test: a sensitive method to assess sensorimotor deficits in mice. Nat Protoc. 2009;4:1560–4.
30. Schaar KL, Brenneman MM, Savitz SI. Functional assessments in the rodent stroke model. Exp Transl Stroke Med. 2010;2:13.
31. Liu X, Liu J, Zhao S, Zhang H, Cai W, Cai M, Ji X, Leak RK, Gao Y, Chen J, Hu X. Interleukin-4 is essential for microglia/macrophage M2 polarization and long-term recovery after cerebral ischemia. Stroke. 2016;47:498–504.
32. Hao J, Liu R, Piao W, Zhou Q, Vollmer TL, Campagnolo DI, Xiang R, La Cava A, Van Kaer L, Shi FD. Central nervous system (CNS)-resident natural killer cells suppress Th17 responses and CNS autoimmune pathology. J Exp Med. 2010;207:1907–21.
33. Khan P, Idrees D, Moxley MA, Corbett JA, Ahmad F, von Figura G, Sly WS, Waheed A, Hassan MI. Luminol-based chemiluminescent signals: clinical and non-clinical application and future uses. Appl Biochem Biotechnol. 2014;173:333–55.
34. Liu Q, Sanai N, Jin WN, La Cava A, Van Kaer L, Shi FD. Neural stem cells sustain natural killer cells that dictate recovery from brain inflammation. Nat Neurosci. 2016;19:243–52.
35. Shi FD, Van Kaer L. Reciprocal regulation between natural killer cells and autoreactive T cells. Nat Rev Immunol. 2006;6:751–60.
36. Liu Q, Xie X, Lukas RJ, St John PA, Wu J. A novel nicotinic mechanism underlies beta-amyloid-induced neuronal hyperexcitation. J Neurosci. 2013; 33:7253–63.
37. Schmitt C, Strazielle N, Ghersi-Egea JF. Brain leukocyte infiltration initiated by peripheral inflammation or experimental autoimmune encephalomyelitis occurs through pathways connected to the CSF-filled compartments of the forebrain and midbrain. J Neuroinflammation. 2012;9:187.
38. Prass K, Meisel C, Hoflich C, Braun J, Halle E, Wolf T, Ruscher K, Victorov IV, Priller J, Dirnagl U, et al. Stroke-induced immunodeficiency promotes spontaneous bacterial infections and is mediated by sympathetic activation reversal by poststroke T helper cell type 1-like immunostimulation. J Exp Med. 2003;198:725–36.
39. Offner H, Subramanian S, Parker SM, Wang C, Afentoulis ME, Lewis A, Vandenbark AA, Hurn PD. Splenic atrophy in experimental stroke is accompanied by increased regulatory T cells and circulating macrophages. J Immunol. 2006;176:6523–31.
40. Seifert HA, Pennypacker KR. Molecular and cellular immune responses to ischemic brain injury. Transl Stroke Res. 2014;5:543–53.
41. Liu NW, Ke CC, Zhao Y, Chen YA, Chan KC, Tan DT, Lee JS, Chen YY, Hsu TW, Hsieh YJ, et al. Evolutional characterization of Photochemically induced stroke in rats: a multimodality imaging and molecular biological study. Transl Stroke Res. 2017;8:244–56.
42. Garrigue P, Giacomino L, Bucci C, Muzio V, Filannino MA, Sabatier F, Dignat-George F, Pisano P, Guillet B. Single photon emission computed tomography imaging of cerebral blood flow, blood-brain barrier disruption, and apoptosis time course after focal cerebral ischemia in rats. Int J Stroke. 2016;11:117–26.
43. Cotrina ML, Lou N, Tome-Garcia J, Goldman J, Nedergaard M. Direct comparison of microglial dynamics and inflammatory profile in photothrombotic and arterial occlusion evoked stroke. Neuroscience. 2017;343:483–94.
44. Vandeputte C, Thomas D, Dresselaers T, Crabbe A, Verfaillie C, Baekelandt V, Van Laere K, Himmelreich U. Characterization of the inflammatory response in a photothrombotic stroke model by MRI: implications for stem cell transplantation. Mol Imaging Biol. 2011;13:663–71.

Heparanase promotes neuroinflammatory response during subarachnoid hemorrhage in rats

Benjarat Changyaleket[1†], Zhao Zhong Chong[1], Randal O. Dull[1], Danop Nanegrungsunk[1] and Haoliang Xu[2*†]

Abstract

Background: Heparanase, a mammalian endo-β-D-glucoronidase that specifically degrades heparan sulfate, has been implicated in inflammation and ischemic stroke. However, the role of heparanase in neuroinflammatory response in subarachnoid hemorrhage (SAH) has not yet been investigated. This study was designed to examine the association between heparanase expression and neuroinflammation during subarachnoid hemorrhage.

Methods: Rats were subjected to SAH by endovascular perforation, and the expression of heparanase was determined by Western blot analysis and immunofluorescence in the ipsilateral brain cortex at 24 h post-SAH. Pial venule leukocyte trafficking was monitored by using intravital microscopy through cranial window.

Results: Our results indicated that, compared to their sham-surgical controls, the rats subjected to SAH showed marked elevation of heparanase expression in the ipsilateral brain cortex. The SAH-induced elevation of heparanase was accompanied by increased leukocyte trafficking in pial venules and significant neurological deficiency. Intracerebroventricular application of a selective heparanase inhibitor, OGT2115, which was initiated at 3 h after SAH, significantly suppressed the leukocyte trafficking and improved the neurological function.

Conclusions: Our findings indicate that heparanase plays an important role in mediating the neuroinflammatory response after SAH and contributes to SAH-related neurological deficits and early brain injury following SAH.

Keywords: Heparanase, Inflammation, Subarachnoid hemorrhage, Neurological function

Background

Subarachnoid hemorrhage (SAH) is a devastating disease. Although it accounts for only a small percentage (5%) of overall stroke, SAH is associated with a high mortality rate that reaches up to 50% [1]. In addition, those who survive the initial bleeding may experience permanent, severe neurological deficits, excluding them from the workforce [1]. Since approximate 50% of SAH occurs in patients younger than 55 years of age, the disease poses a great economic burden in society. As a result, identifying therapeutic strategies to treat SAH and its complications is of extreme importance.

Neuroinflammation is believed to play a key role in the poor outcome of SAH [2], but its exact mechanisms are not well defined. Delayed cerebral ischemia (DCI) is a major complication of SAH characterized by inflammation, cerebral edema, and microthrombosis, collectively leading to brain infarction and neurological deficits, typically appearing 3 days after SAH [3]. Cerebral vasospasm was considered to be a major mechanism of DCI [2, 4] with inflammation as a key factor contributing to the induction of vasospasm following SAH [5]. For example, proinflammatory cytokine levels in the brain 4–6 days following SAH correlates with the severity of radiographically proven vasospasm [6]. By contrast, inhibitors of these cytokines attenuate the SAH-induced vasospasm [7–11]. In addition, general anti-inflammatory treatment using corticosteroids has been shown to reduce vasospasm, attenuate delayed cerebral ischemia, and improve outcomes in both experimental and clinical SAH [12–15].

Heparanase is emerging as a potential candidate that regulates neuroinflammation. Heparanase is a heparan

* Correspondence: hlxu@uic.edu
†Equal contributors
[2]Department of Pathology, University of Illinois at Chicago, 840 South Wood Street, Chicago, IL 60612, USA
Full list of author information is available at the end of the article

sulfate degrading enzyme that cleaves heparan sulfate (HS) on the HS proteoglycans (HSPG) and has been implicated in tumor metastasis and inflammation [16]. Heparanase is extensively expressed in many cells, including neurons, astrocytes, endothelial cells, and macrophages [17–21]. Heparanase is synthesized and secreted as a latent 65 kDa precursor and is retained at pericellular sites binding to cell surface HS components [22, 23]. Acidic environments as observed in tumor or inflammatory conditions are optimal for the enzymatic activity [24–26]. In contrast, heparanase expressed on the surface of cells do not enzymatically degrade HS in tissues with normal physiologic conditions [27]. HSPG is a major component of the extracellular matrix (ECM). Thus, the cleavage of HSPG may regulate the remodeling of the ECM and allow for tissue invasion of circulating cells and/or leukocyte trafficking across the endothelium, a critical process in inflammation. Inhibition of heparanase was shown to be effective in reducing inflammation [28–31].

The information concerning the role of heparanase in neuroinflammation during different types of strokes is limited. A few reports have demonstrated that heparanase is upregulated in the rat brain after ischemic stroke [16, 19, 32]. No data is available regarding the association between heparanase and SAH. Our current study examined heparanase expression in the rat cerebral cortex in the early phase of brain injury post SAH. We also examined the effect of inhibiting heparanase function on neurological outcome and leukocyte trafficking in rats. Our findings illustrate that heparanase expression is increased after SAH and inhibition of heparanase attenuates SAH-induced neurovascular inflammation and improves neurological function after SAH.

Methods

Animal preparation and procedures

The protocol was approved by the University of Illinois Institutional Animal Care and Use Committee. Male Sprague-Dawley rats, weighing 250–300 g (Charles River, Wilmington, MA), were randomly assigned to undergo sham surgery (group 1), SAH surgery (group 2), SAH surgery + vehicle (group 3), or SAH surgery + heparanase inhibitor (group 4). In groups 1 and 2, we examined the effect of SAH on heparanase expression and determined its localization to specific cell types in the brain via western blot analysis ($n = 4$) and immunofluorescence stain ($n = 6$). These animal groups were sacrificed at 24 h post sham/SAH surgeries. In groups 3 and 4, we tested the hypothesis that inhibiting endogenous heparanase activity, using heparanase inhibitor, OGT2115, prevents post-SAH neuroinflammation ($n = 4$–6) and improves neurologic outcome ($n = 6$). Three hours after SAH induction, animals in these two groups received either a vehicle treatment or OGT2115 via the osmotic pump. Neurological scores were assessed at 48 h post-SAH, followed by pial venule intravascular leukocyte adhesion (PVLA) evaluation via a cranial window-intravital microscopy system. An additional sham surgical group that is identical to group 1 ($n = 6$) was added to this study for better comparison.

Subarachnoid hemorrhage (SAH) model

The details of SAH endovascular perforation model were previously described [33]. Briefly, rats weighing 250–300 g were anesthetized with 70% N_2O/30% O_2/2% isoflurane using a rodent ventilator. The tail artery was cannulated to monitor arterial pressure. Blood pressure, blood gases, and body temperature were recorded and kept within normal ranges by adjusting ventilating rate and using a servo-controlled heating pad. Regional cerebral blood flow (rCBF) over the middle cerebral artery (MCA) territory was continuously monitored before, during, and 30 min after SAH via laser-Doppler flowmetry (LDF).

To induce SAH, the right external carotid artery (ECA), common carotid artery (CCA), and internal carotid artery (ICA) were exposed. After the CCA were temporarily occluded, a polytetrafluoroethylene tube was inserted into the ICA via the ECA until resistance was felt. SAH was induced by a 2-mm protrusion of a tungsten wire inside tube, puncturing the proximal anterior cerebral artery. After retracting the wire and tubing, the CCA was reopened to allow reperfusion via the ICA. The arterial catheter was removed, the wounds were closed, and anesthesia was discontinued. When spontaneous breathing was reestablished, the rats were extubated and returned to their cages. This modified SAH model has shown high reproducibility. However, maintaining blood gas and blood pressure among all experimental groups, as well as puncturing the appropriate intracranial vascular site, is important to minimize the variation of intracranial hemorrhage. At the end of the experiment, the presence of SAH was confirmed by direct observation of blood accumulation around the proximal anterior cerebral artery where the perforation occurred. Based on our previous findings, successful SAH showed remarkable blood accumulation within the first 24 h that would then decrease in size. In most cases, blood accumulation could no longer be detected after 72 h post-SAH (data not shown).

Alzet osmotic pump installation

Three hours after SAH/sham surgeries, the Alzet osmotic pumps (Model 1003D, Alzet, Cupertino, CA) were installed subcutaneously in the neck region to provide the animals either vehicle or heparanase inhibitor, OGT2115

(MW: 495.3, Tocris Bioscience, Cat. #2710). The method has been described previously in details [34]. Briefly, rats were placed in a stereotactic frame under isoflurane anesthesia. The skull was exposed and a small hole over the right lateral ventricle (8 mm caudal to bregma, 1.5 mm lateral to midline, and 4 mm beneath the skull surface) was made to allow intracerebroventricular drug delivery. An initial loading dose of OGT2115 [0.05 μg in 5 μl artificial cerebrospinal fluid (aCSF)] or 5 μl vehicle (aCSF) was injected slowly into the lateral ventricle, followed by implantation of an infusion cannula with attached osmotic pump. This provided a continuous drug delivery at a rate of 1 μL/h to maintain CSF concentration of OGT2115 at approximate 0.4 μM, which is its IC50 for heparanase inhibition [35]. The OGT2115 was administered continuously until animals were sacrificed at 48 h.

Cranial window and intravital microscopy

To assess leukocyte trafficking, the cranial windows were installed at 48 h after SAH as previously described [36]. Briefly, the animals were intubated and mechanically supported under 70% N_2O/30%O_2/2% isoflurane. Femoral artery and vein were cannulated for monitoring arterial blood pressure and for obtaining samples for arterial blood gases. Body temperature was kept at 37 °C. A 10-mm craniotomy was performed midline over the skull. After removing the dura, a 11-mm diameter glass window equipped with three ports (inflow, outflow, and intracranial pressure monitoring) was glued to the skull with cyanoacrylate. The intracranial pressure (ICP) under the cranial window was monitored and maintained within 7 to 11 mmHg range, by adjusting the height of the outflow port, throughout the experiment. After completion of the surgery, the anesthesia with isoflurane was switched to fentanyl infusion for monitoring of rhodamine-6G (R6G)-labeled leukocyte. This semi-quantitative method of in vivo assessment of leukocyte trafficking has been described in details in our previous publications [33, 37]. Briefly, loading dose of R6G (0.2 mg) was applied intravenously, followed by 0.2 mg/h maintenance dose. Pial venules (approximate 40 to 60 μm in diameter) were randomly selected for study. Images of R6G-labeled leukocytes were captured using a digital camera (CoolSnap ES, Photometrics, Tucson, AZ, USA) mounted on a fluorescence microscope (Nikon, Melville, NY, USA) and analyzed using MetaMorph software (Molecular Devices, Downingtown, PA, USA). Leukocyte adhesion was reported as the percentage of adherent leukocytes (this includes both tightly adhered and slow-rolling leukocytes) occupying the viewed venular area in the microscopic field and was used as a surrogate marker of neuroinflammation [37].

Western blots

Brain cortical homogenate was centrifuged and the supernatant collected for protein determination (Bradford method). Western blot analysis of protein expression changes of heparanase was performed according to a protocol previously described [38]. Briefly, the blots were hybridized with rabbit anti-heparanase polyclonal antibody (1:1000, MyBioSource, Inc., San Diego, CA) and subsequently incubated with donkey anti-rabbit IgG secondary antibody conjugated with infrared fluorescent dye (IRDye 800 from LI-COR technology, Lincoln, NE) diluted 1:10,000 in 0.5× Odyssey blocking buffer and 0.1% Tween 20. β-actin was used as a loading control (anti β-actin rabbit monoclonal, 1:1000, Cell Signaling Technology Inc., Boston, MA). Blot membranes were then scanned using the LI-COR Odyssey Infrared Imaging System (LI-COR Biosciences, Lincoln, NE). The protein level of heparanase in each brain sample ($n = 4$ in each group) was expressed as the ratio of the optical densities of heparanase and β-actin bands.

Immunohistochemistry

Twenty-four hours after surgery, rats were sacrificed and transcardially perfused with cold phosphate-buffered saline (PBS) followed by 20 ml paraformaldehyde (4%). Brains were harvested and paraffin-embedded. Coronal sections (8 μm) were obtained and prepared for immunofluorescence staining. The primary antibodies were used at the following dilution: 1:200 for rabbit polyclonal anti-heparanase (MyBiosource, San Diego, CA) and 1:100 for mouse monoclonal anti-NeuN (EMD Millipore, CA). After overnight incubation, sections were washed and incubated for 1 h at 37 °C with the secondary antibodies which were donkey anti-rabbit rhodamine red-X and donkey anti-mouse conjugated with FITC. Nuclei were stained with 400 ng/ml DAPI. Image acquisition was obtained on a Zeiss Axioplan2 fluorescence microscope quipped with an Axiocam MRm digital camera and Axiovision 4.5 imaging software. Images were taken from sections of ipsilateral parietal cortex stained simultaneously and exposed to identical conditions and amount of time, allowing the comparison of fluorescence intensity among regions of interest. Acquisition settings were calibrated for the most optimal signal to noise ratio, and subsequent images were taken under identical settings.

Neurological assessments

Neurological assessments were performed in animals at 48 h post-SAH by a blinded observer. The assessments were based on a 21-point scale as previously described [33]. The ratings were taken from a sum of scores from seven categories: (i) spontaneous activity, (normal = 3, akinesia = 0); (ii) side stroking (bilateral brisk response =

3, no response = 0); (iii) vibrissae touch (bilateral brisk response = 3, no response = 0); (iv) limb symmetry (forelimb and hindlimb extended = 3, contralateral forelimb and hindlimb completely flexed = 0); (v) lateral turning (bilateral turning ≥ 45° = 3, no turning = 0); (vi) forelimb walking (briskly walks forward in symmetry = 3, cannot move on forelimbs = 0); and (vii) slope climbing (climbs to the top of slope with prompting and strong grip = 3, weak grips and falls off = 0).

Statistics

Results were presented as means ± SEM. A $p < 0.05$ was considered as statistically significant. Several statistical analyses were used. Protein expression and leukocyte adhesion were analyzed using one-way analysis of variance (ANOVA) combined with a post hoc Tukey's analysis. Non-parametric neurological behavioral data were analyzed using Mann–Whitney rank sum test. The result was expressed as medians and ranges (boxplot design).

Results

Physiological variables

Physiologic parameters including mean arterial pressure (MAP), temperature, and arterial blood gases were maintained within normal physiologic range. In the SAH animals, there was a transient drop in MAP of ~30 mmHg at the initiation of MCA perforation which resolved within 5 min. rCBF also decreased abruptly to 10–20% of the initial baseline at the time of perforation, followed by a gradual recovery to 60% of baseline values within 20 min (Table 1). SAH was also confirmed by post-mortem inspection of the presence of blood accumulation around the proximal anterior cerebral artery where the perforation occurred [37]. No significant differences were observed when comparing temperature, $PaCO_2$, pH, and MABP values at equivalent experimental time points among all experimental groups. The mortality rate was 33% in the SAH groups. All animals died within the first 24 h after SAH initiation. No animals died in the sham group.

Table 1 Subarachnoid hemorrhage (SAH)-induced cerebral blood flow changes in rats

Subgroup	Number of animals	CBF changes (% of the initial values)	
		1 min post-SAH	20 min post-SAH
Sham surgery (group 1)	16	90.3 ± 7.7	103.2 ± 6.1
SAH surgery (group 2)	10	14.6 ± 3.5*	64.2 ± 5.9*
SAH surgery + vehicle (group 3)	6	16.9 ± 5.2*	62.3 ± 9.0*
SAH surgery + heparanase inhibitor (group 4)	6	15.3 ± 5.7*	58.2 ± 4.6*

Cerebral blood flow (CBF) changes were measured throughout SAH surgical procedure. CBF changes were calculated for 30 min post-SAH and expressed as percentage of initial CBF values. SAH was accompanied with an abrupt CBF drop, followed by a gradual recovery toward its initial value and reached a plateau after 20 min. Three hours post-SAH, animals in groups 3 and 4 received intracerebroventricular treatment of either vehicle (aCSF) or heparanase inhibitor (OGT2115) via Alzet osmotic pump installation. Values are mean ± SE

*$p < 0.05$ vs the sham surgical controls

The expression of brain heparanase after SAH

To investigate the expression of heparanase in the brain after SAH, Western blot was performed for heparanase in the protein extract of ipsilateral cortex in rats at 24 h following SAH (Fig. 1). SAH was accompanied by a significant elevation of heparanase expression, compared to their matched sham controls (SAH: 9.96 ± 4.1 vs Sham: 3.42 ± 2.0, $p < 0.05$; values were expressed as the ratio of the optical densities of heparanase and β-actin). The result was confirmed by immunofluorescence stain for heparanase, which showed a substantial increase of heparanase expression in the SAH-ipsilateral brain cortex when compared to the sham surgical controls (representative pictures are shown in Fig. 2).

Heparanase inhibition attenuates pial venular leukocyte trafficking induced by SAH

To investigate the inflammatory response to SAH, PVLA was observed through an intravital microscope. PVLA was expressed as the percentage of the pial venular area

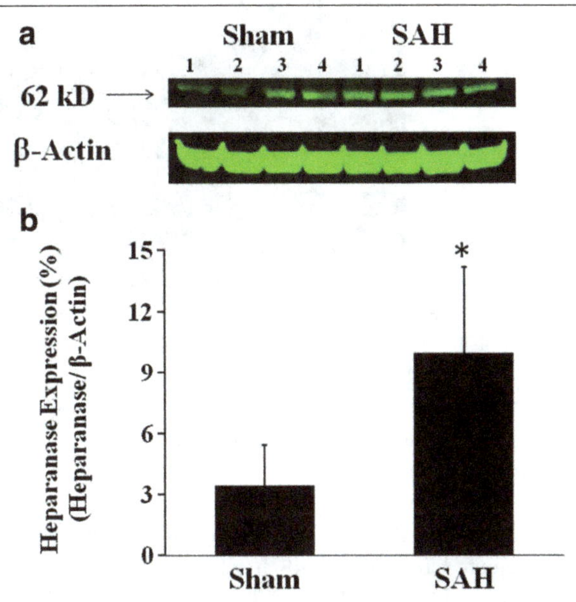

Fig. 1 The expression of heparanase increases in cerebral cortex after subarachnoid hemorrhage (SAH) in rats. Western blot was performed for heparanase in the ipsilateral cerebral cortex at 24 h following SAH. **a** Representative images showing the expression of heparanase to be increased at 24 h after SAH. **b** The quantitative results demonstrated that the expression ratio of heparanase/β-actin in density was significantly increased at 24 h after SAH. In **b**, values are mean ± SEM, $n = 4$, *$p < 0.05$ *vs* sham

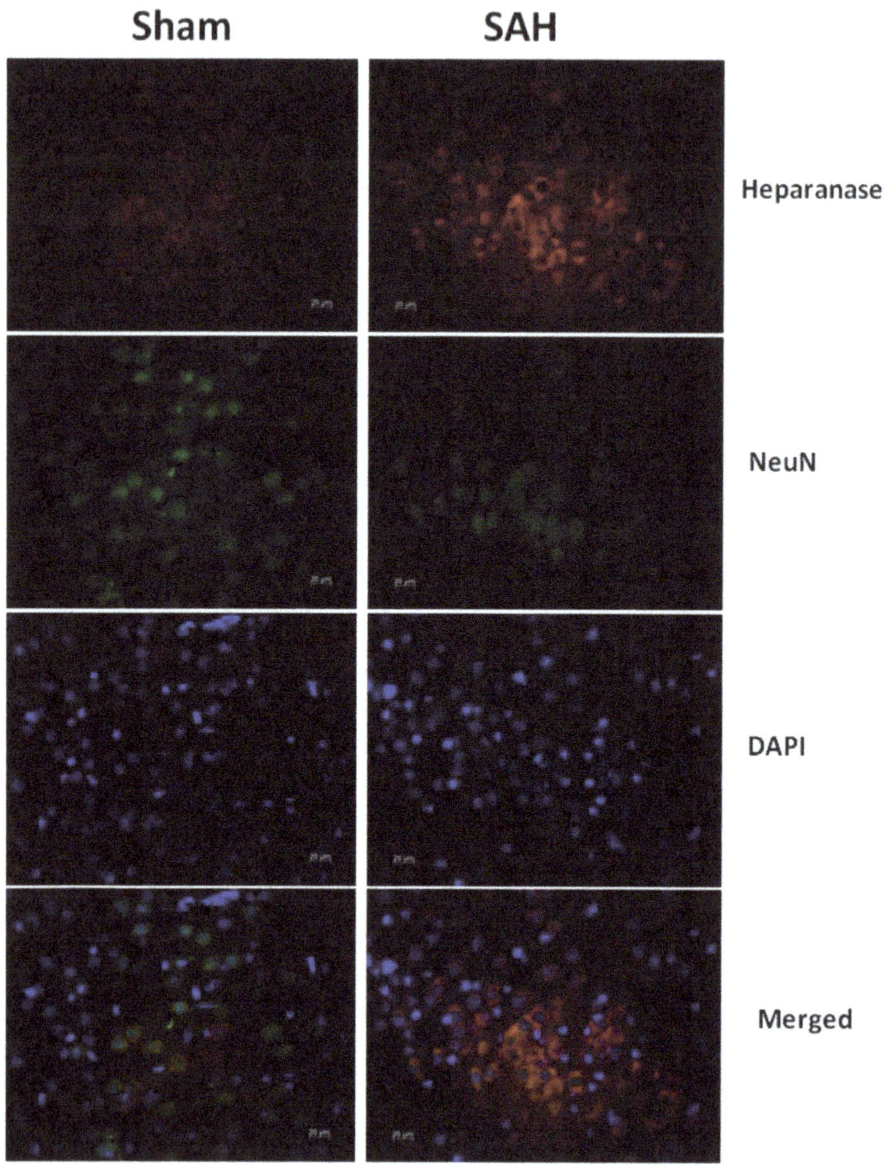

Fig. 2 Representative pictures show upregulation of heparanase expression induced by subarachnoid hemorrhage (SAH) in rats from the SAH group compared to their sham controls. Tri-color staining for heparanase (*red*), DAPI (*blue*), and NeuN (*green*) were performed in coronal sections of rat ipsilateral cortex at 24 h post-SAH

occupied by adherent R6G-labeled leukocytes at 48 h post-SAH. The representative images and quantitative results were shown in Fig. 3a, b, respectively. A markedly increase in PVLA was observed in vehicle-treated rats subjected to SAH at 48 h when compared to the sham surgical group (12.8 ± 4.3% *vs* 1.4 ± 1.2%). Treatment with heparanase inhibitor OGT2115 significantly reduced PVLA levels relative to vehicle (2.2 ± 1.2%).

Heparanase inhibition improves neurologic scores after SAH

The neurologic outcome scores for the sham, SAH, SAH + vehicle, or SAH + OGT2115 group are summarized in Fig. 4. Neurologic assessments were performed using the scoring system described in the "Methods" section. The maximum achievable score was 21, which translates to no functional deficit. The nonparametric data are presented as a boxplot, with median values for each group. Since both SAH group and SAH + vehicle group showed virtually no significant difference, the data of these two groups were pooled. Neurologic deficit scores of the sham surgical group were tightly distributed, ranging from 20 to 21. All the SAH-exposed rats displayed median neurologic scores that were significantly lower than in the sham group. However, a significant improvement of neurologic function was noted when the SAH + OGT2115 control

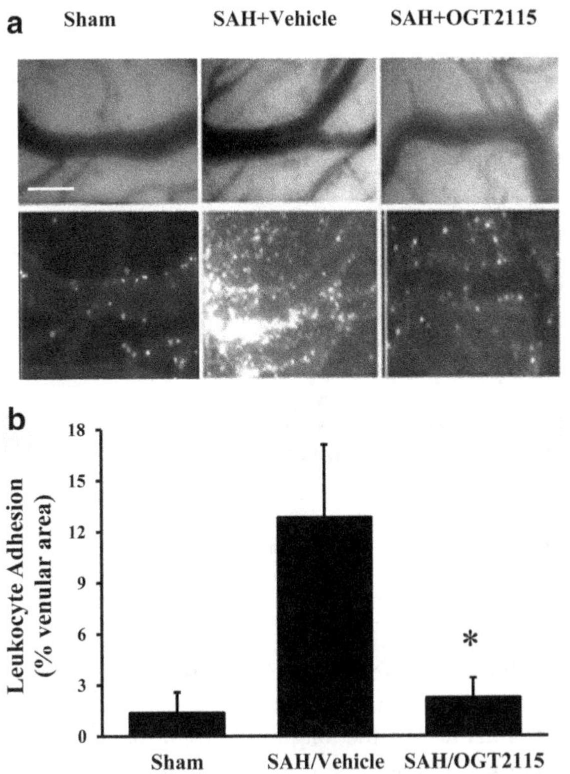

Fig. 3 Inhibition of heparanase attenuates leukocyte adhesion in pial venules induced by subarachnoid hemorrhage (SAH). **a** Representative images showed the effect of heparanase inhibition (via OGT2115) on SAH-associated pial venular leukocyte trafficking at 48 h post-SAH. The contour of the pial venules was observed under the bright field (upper panels). The leukocyte adhesion was expressed as the bright area occupied by Rhodamine-6G-labeled leukocytes (lower panels). Scale = 50 μm. **b** Quantitative results of the effects of heparanase inhibitor (OGT2115) on SAH associated pial venular leukocyte adhesion in SAH. Leukocyte adhesion is expressed as the percentage of the viewed venular area occupied by rhodamined-6G-labeled leukocytes. In **b**, values are mean ± SEM, n = 4–6 per group

group was compared with the SAH + vehicle group (11 ± 3 vs 15 ± 3; p <0.05) (Fig. 4).

Discussion

In the present study, SAH in rat is produced via an endovascular perforation method that has been employed by many laboratories [39, 40]. This method has been characterized as one of the best models for investigating subarachnoid hemorrhage, since it mimics the rupture of human cerebral aneurysm and closely matches its clinical manifestation in terms of morbidity, mortality, and severity [41].

We observed that heparanase expression was increased during early brain injury following SAH and that heparanase was detected exclusively in neurons at 24 h post SAH. Moreover, inhibiting heparanase activity abolished SAH-induced leukocyte adhesion in pial venules. Heparanase upregulation has been considered as one of the mechanisms underlying the induction of angiogenesis during repeated hypoxic exposures and tumor metastasis [19, 42–46]. Navarro and colleagues showed that upregulation of both heparanase and vascular endothelial growth factor (VEGF) under repeated hypoxic conditions promoted angiogenesis [19]. Angiogenesis under pathological condition may represent a compensatory mechanism to promote blood flow to the ischemic, or injured, area of the brain. In particular, increased angiogenesis in the penumbra area attenuates ischemic neuronal cell death [44]. The higher density of blood vessels seems to correlate with better functional recovery, longer survival, and increased cerebral blood flow to areas surrounding the brain infarcts in stroke patients [47–49]. However, the role of heparanase in SAH-associated neuropathy is still unknown. Our current study is the first report to investigate the association between the upregulation of heparanase, cerebrovascular inflammation, and neurological impairment in SAH.

In the current study, we found that SAH induced significant leukocyte migration through the pial venule, indicating an inflammatory response following SAH. Interestingly, inhibition of heparanase (by OGT2115) significantly reduced leukocyte trafficking at 48 h post-SAH, suggesting that heparanase activation is involved in SAH-associated inflammatory reaction. It has been well known that heparanase cleaves heparan sulfate on HSPG, a major constituent of ECM that functions as a storage depot of numerous enzymes and cytokines [50], leading to ECM degradation, tissue invasion, and angiogenesis. As such, heparanase-induced impairment of the structural integrity of the ECM may lead to inflammation as represented by the promotion of leukocyte migration across the endothelium. This has been linked to a compensatory angiogenesis, which is considered beneficial in reperfusion post stroke. However, it may inadvertently lead to an inflammatory response and tissue injury in the brain. Sasaki and colleagues reported that heparanase expression on the cell surface of macrophages was essential for its leukocyte extravasation through the basement membrane [21]. In a recent study, Level et al. also found that heparanase augmented the adhesion of neutrophils and mononuclear cells to vascular endothelial cells in a concentration-dependent manner [51]. Heparanase exists as a 65-kDa inactive precursor form and a 50-kDa active form. Both forms can mediate cell adhesion via a β1-integrin-dependent mechanisms that is unrelated to their enzymatic activity [52]. However, enzymatic activity of heparanase, or at least the ability to be processed to an enzymatically active form, is still essential for its proinflammatory activity in vivo [51]. Consistent with this finding, our preliminary experimental results showed an elevation of active form

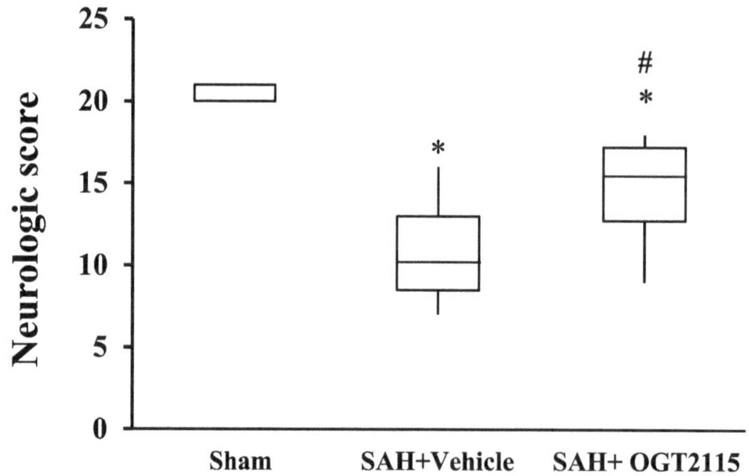

Fig. 4 Inhibition of heparanase improves neurological score after subarachnoid hemorrhage (SAH). The data, presented in boxplot form, represents neurological scores obtained at 48 h of post-SAH, where the *upper* and *lower box* edges represent the 25th and 75th percentiles, and the whiskers represent the 95% confidence intervals. The median values are depicted by the *horizontal lines within the boxes*. Significant decrease in neurological score was observed in SAH rats. In contrast, application of heparanase inhibitor OGT2115 is associated with significantly increased neurological score. Values are mean ± SEM, *$p < 0.05$ *vs* sham, #$p < 0.05$ vs SAH+ vehicle control, $n = 6$ per group

of heparanase expression in the ipsilateral cortex at 24 h after SAH (data not shown), which is suggestive of the contributory role of heparanase in SAH-induced cerebrovascular inflammation. This issue needs further investigation.

We further investigated the role of heparanase in SAH-related early neurological dysfunction. Based on our previous experience, the neurological function cannot be assessed accurately within 24 h post-surgery due to the stress and residual influence from either anesthesia and/or surgical procedure. Stable and more reliable neurological scores can only be obtained at 48 h, which was our earliest evaluation time point during this study. Nevertheless, we found that inhibition of heparanase by OGT2115 within the first 24 h post-SAH prevented SAH-associated neurological deficits at 48 h post-SAH, suggesting an important role of heparanase in mediating early brain injury following SAH.

Our previous findings indicate that blocking SAH-induced leukocyte adhesion and transmigration into the brain parenchyma improves neurological outcome [37]. In SAH, the initial insult induces an inflammatory state characterized by early recruitment of leukocytes and increased production of cytokines and chemokines [1, 53]. This immune response correlates with SAH severity and has been linked to neural cell injury, BBB dysfunction, and delayed cerebral ischemia [54–57]. Therefore, the enhanced leukocyte trafficking may be an important prerequisite in promoting neuropathology that are likely to be an effective treatment target to prevent SAH-associated neurological impairment.

There are limitations of the present study. First, in this study, early application of heparanase inhibitor resulted in significant suppression of SAH-associated cerebrovascular inflammation and improvement of neurological function. However, the long-term prognosis of this intervention was not addressed. Considering that heparanase promotes angiogenesis and that angiogenesis provides neuroprotection against ischemic brain damage, a delayed complication of SAH, it is of great importance to assess the efficacy of heparanase inhibition over the late phase of SAH. As such, an extended observation window is needed. Another limitation of this study is that the localization (i.e., the cellular and/or compartmental specificity) of heparanase expression needs to be emphasized. Navarro et al. reported [19] that, after ischemic stroke, the upregulation of heparanase expression was localized predominately in neurons and not in astrocytes, microglia, or endothelium. Another study, however, identified that heparanase expression was confined to the endothelial cells at 7 days, but then shifted to astrocytes at 14 days post ischemia [16]. Takahashi et al. also detected heparanase expression only in astrocytes after the subacute phase (3–7 days) post brain ischemia. Apparently, expression of heparanase correlates temporally and spatially in different cell types in the brain in different stroke models [16, 19, 32].Consistent with these findings, in our current study, a significant population of heparanase-positive cells in the SAH brain sections were not positive for NeuN staining, indicating SAH-associated heparanase expression in cells other than neurons (Fig. 2.). Nevertheless, our experiments focused on the early phase of SAH within 24 h; further investigation is warranted to investigate other time points both in the early and delayed phases of SAH to delineate the regulation of heparanase expression.

Conclusions

Taken together, the present findings show a significant elevation of SAH-associated heparanase expression that is linked to post-SAH leukocyte trafficking. Selective blocking heparanase by OGT2115 attenuates cerebrovascular inflammation and prevents SAH-induced neurological impairment, suggesting an involvement of heparanase in SAH-associated neuropathy.

Abbreviations

aCSF: Artificial Cerebrospinal fluid; ANOVA: Analysis of variance; CCA: Common carotid artery; DCI: Delayed cerebral ischemia; ECA: External carotid arteries; HS: Heparan sulfate; HSPG: HS proteoglycans; ICA: Internal carotid artery; ICP: Intracranial pressure; LDF: Laser doppler flowmetry; MAP: Mean arterial pressure; MCA: Middle cerebral artery; PVLA: Pial venule intravascular leukocyte adhesion; R6G: Rhodamine-6G; rCBF: Regional cerebral blood flow; SAH: Subarachnoid hemorrhage

Acknowledgements

The authors dedicate this manuscript to the memory of Professor Dale Pelligrino who was a dedicated neuroscientist and encouraging mentor.

Funding

Not applicable.

Authors' contributions

BC and HLX were involved in the design of the study, carried out the majority of the experiment, and participated in the data analysis and manuscript preparation. ROD and ZZC participated in the manuscript preparation. DN participated in immunochemistry stain for the study. All authors read and approved the final manuscript.

Consent for publication

Not applicable.

Competing interests

The authors declare that they have no competing interests.

Author details

[1]Department of Anesthesiology, University of Illinois at Chicago, Chicago, IL, USA. [2]Department of Pathology, University of Illinois at Chicago, 840 South Wood Street, Chicago, IL 60612, USA.

References

1. Kooijman E, Nijboer CH, van Velthoven CT, Mol W, Dijkhuizen RM, et al. Long-term functional consequences and ongoing cerebral inflammation after subarachnoid hemorrhage in the rat. PLoS One. 2014;9:e90584.
2. Ayer R, Zhang J. Connecting the early brain injury of aneurysmal subarachnoid hemorrhage to clinical practice. Turk Neurosurg. 2010;20:159–66.
3. Rowland MJ, Hadjipavlou G, Kelly M, Westbrook J, Pattinson KT. Delayed cerebral ischaemia after subarachnoid haemorrhage: looking beyond vasospasm. Br J Anaesth. 2012;109:315–29.
4. Prunell GF, Svendgaard NA, Alkass K, Mathiesen T. Delayed cell death related to acute cerebral blood flow changes following subarachnoid hemorrhage in the rat brain. J Neurosurg. 2005;102:1046–54.
5. Vecchione C, Frati A, Di Pardo A, Cifelli G, Carnevale D, et al. Tumor necrosis factor-alpha mediates hemolysis-induced vasoconstriction and the cerebral vasospasm evoked by subarachnoid hemorrhage. Hypertension. 2009;54: 150–6.
6. Hanafy KA, Stuart RM, Khandji AG, Connolly ES, Badjatia N, et al. Relationship between brain interstitial fluid tumor necrosis factor-alpha and cerebral vasospasm after aneurysmal subarachnoid hemorrhage. J Clin Neurosci. 2010;17:853–6.
7. Jiang Y, Liu DW, Han XY, Dong YN, Gao J, et al. Neuroprotective effects of anti-tumor necrosis factor-alpha antibody on apoptosis following subarachnoid hemorrhage in a rat model. J Clin Neurosci. 2012;19:866–72.
8. Lin CL, Dumont AS, Calisaneller T, Kwan AL, Hwong SL, et al. Monoclonal antibody against E selectin attenuates subarachnoid hemorrhage-induced cerebral vasospasm. Surg Neurol. 2005;64:201–5. discussion 205-206.
9. Clatterbuck RE, Gailloud P, Ogata L, Gebremariam A, Dietsch GN, et al. Prevention of cerebral vasospasm by a humanized anti-CD11/CD18 monoclonal antibody administered after experimental subarachnoid hemorrhage in nonhuman primates. J Neurosurg. 2003;99:376–82.
10. Bowman G, Bonneau RH, Chinchilli VM, Tracey KJ, Cockroft KM. A novel inhibitor of inflammatory cytokine production (CNI-1493) reduces rodent post-hemorrhagic vasospasm. Neurocrit Care. 2006;5:222–9.
11. Nishino A, Umegaki M, Fujinaka T, Yoshimine T. Cilostazol attenuates cerebral vasospasm after experimental subarachnoid hemorrhage. Neurol Res. 2010;32:873–8.
12. Chyatte D, Sundt Jr TM. Response of chronic experimental cerebral vasospasm to methylprednisolone and dexamethasone. J Neurosurg. 1984; 60:923–6.
13. Yoneko M, Katayama Y, Moro N, Kamei J, Kojima J. Inhibitory effect of hydrocortisone on cerebral salt wasting after subarachnoid hemorrhage in rats. Methods Find Exp Clin Pharmacol. 2010;32:727–31.
14. Katayama Y, Haraoka J, Hirabayashi H, Kawamata T, Kawamoto K, et al. A randomized controlled trial of hydrocortisone against hyponatremia in patients with aneurysmal subarachnoid hemorrhage. Stroke. 2007;38:2373–5.
15. Chyatte D, Fode NC, Nichols DA, Sundt Jr TM. Preliminary report: effects of high dose methylprednisolone on delayed cerebral ischemia in patients at high risk for vasospasm after aneurysmal subarachnoid hemorrhage. Neurosurgery. 1987;21:157–60.
16. Li J, Li JP, Zhang X, Lu Z, Yu SP, et al. Expression of heparanase in vascular cells and astrocytes of the mouse brain after focal cerebral ischemia. Brain Res. 2012;1433:137–44.
17. Gingis-Velitski S, Zetser A, Flugelman MY, Vlodavsky I, Ilan N. Heparanase induces endothelial cell migration via protein kinase B/Akt activation. J Biol Chem. 2004;279:23536–41.
18. Marchetti D, Li J, Shen R. Astrocytes contribute to the brain-metastatic specificity of melanoma cells by producing heparanase. Cancer Res. 2000;60: 4767–70.
19. Navarro FP, Fares RP, Sanchez PE, Nadam J, Georges B, et al. Brain heparanase expression is up-regulated during postnatal development and hypoxia-induced neovascularization in adult rats. J Neurochem. 2008;105: 34–45.
20. Parish CR, Freeman C, Hulett MD. Heparanase: a key enzyme involved in cell invasion. Biochim Biophys Acta. 2001;1471:M99–108.
21. Sasaki N, Higashi N, Taka T, Nakajima M, Irimura T. Cell surface localization of heparanase on macrophages regulates degradation of extracellular matrix heparan sulfate. J Immunol. 2004;172:3830–5.
22. Goldshmidt O, Zcharia E, Aingorn H, Guatta-Rangini Z, Atzmon R, et al. Expression pattern and secretion of human and chicken heparanase are determined by their signal peptide sequence. J Biol Chem. 2001;276:29178–87.
23. Gingis-Velitski S, Zetser A, Kaplan V, Ben-Zaken O, Cohen E, et al. Heparanase uptake is mediated by cell membrane heparan sulfate proteoglycans. J Biol Chem. 2004;279:44084–92.
24. Gilat D, Hershkoviz R, Goldkorn I, Cahalon L, Korner G, et al. Molecular behavior adapts to context: heparanase functions as an extracellular matrix-degrading enzyme or as a T cell adhesion molecule, depending on the local pH. J Exp Med. 1995;181:1929–34.
25. Toyoshima M, Nakajima M. Human heparanase. Purification, characterization, cloning, and expression. J Biol Chem. 1999;274:24153–60.

26. Vlodavsky I, Friedmann Y. Molecular properties and involvement of heparanase in cancer metastasis and angiogenesis. J Clin Invest. 2001;108: 341–7.
27. Goldshmidt O, Zcharia E, Cohen M, Aingorn H, Cohen I, et al. Heparanase mediates cell adhesion independent of its enzymatic activity. FASEB J. 2003; 17:1015–25.
28. Zhao H, Liu H, Chen Y, Xin X, Li J, et al. Oligomannurarate sulfate, a novel heparanase inhibitor simultaneously targeting basic fibroblast growth factor, combats tumor angiogenesis and metastasis. Cancer Res. 2006;66:8779–87.
29. Parish CR, Freeman C, Brown KJ, Francis DJ, Cowden WB. Identification of sulfated oligosaccharide-based inhibitors of tumor growth and metastasis using novel in vitro assays for angiogenesis and heparanase activity. Cancer Res. 1999;59:3433–41.
30. Uno F, Fujiwara T, Takata Y, Ohtani S, Katsuda K, et al. Antisense-mediated suppression of human heparanase gene expression inhibits pleural dissemination of human cancer cells. Cancer Res. 2001;61:7855–60.
31. Gao J, Su L, Qin R, Chang Q, Huang T, et al. Transfection of antisense oligodeoxynucleotide inhibits heparanase gene expression and invasive ability of human pancreatic cancer cell in vitro. J Huazhong Univ Sci Technolog Med Sci. 2006;26:72–4.
32. Takahashi H, Matsumoto H, Kumon Y, Ohnishi T, Freeman C, et al. Expression of heparanase in nestin-positive reactive astrocytes in ischemic lesions of rat brain after transient middle cerebral artery occlusion. Neurosci Lett. 2007;417:250–4.
33. Xu HL, Garcia M, Testai F, Vetri F, Barabanova A, et al. Pharmacologic blockade of vascular adhesion protein-1 lessens neurologic dysfunction in rats subjected to subarachnoid hemorrhage. Brain Res. 2014;1586:83–9.
34. Changyaleket B, Xu H, Vetri F, Valyi-Nagy T, Paisansathan C, et al. Intracerebroventricular application of S100B selectively impairs pial arteriolar dilating function in rats. Brain Res. 2016;1634:171–8.
35. Courtney SM, Hay PA, Buck RT, Colville CS, Phillips DJ, et al. Furanyl-1,3-thiazol-2-yl and benzoxazol-5-yl acetic acid derivatives: novel classes of heparanase inhibitor. Bioorg Med Chem Lett. 2005;15:2295–9.
36. Xu HL, Salter-Cid L, Linnik MD, Wang EY, Paisansathan C, et al. Vascular adhesion protein-1 plays an important role in postischemic inflammation and neuropathology in diabetic, estrogen-treated ovariectomized female rats subjected to transient forebrain ischemia. J Pharmacol Exp Ther. 2006; 317:19–29.
37. Xu HL, Pelligrino DA, Paisansathan C, Testai FD. Protective role of fingolimod (FTY720) in rats subjected to subarachnoid hemorrhage. J Neuroinflammation. 2015;12:16.
38. Xu HL, Vetri F, Lee HK, Ye S, Paisansathan C, et al. Estrogen replacement therapy in diabetic ovariectomized female rats potentiates postischemic leukocyte adhesion in cerebral venules via a RAGE-related process. Am J Physiol Heart Circ Physiol. 2009;297:H2059–67.
39. Sugawara T, Ayer R, Jadhav V, Zhang JH. A new grading system evaluating bleeding scale in filament perforation subarachnoid hemorrhage rat model. J Neurosci Methods. 2008;167:327–34.
40. Ostrowski RP, Tang J, Zhang JH. Hyperbaric oxygen suppresses NADPH oxidase in a rat subarachnoid hemorrhage model. Stroke. 2006;37:1314–8.
41. Cahill JZJ. Monofilament perforation: subarachnoid hemorrhage model. USA: Humana Press; 2009.
42. Bernaudin M, Nedelec AS, Divoux D, MacKenzie ET, Petit E, et al. Normobaric hypoxia induces tolerance to focal permanent cerebral ischemia in association with an increased expression of hypoxia-inducible factor-1 and its target genes, erythropoietin and VEGF, in the adult mouse brain. J Cereb Blood Flow Metab. 2002;22:393–403.
43. Chavez JC, Agani F, Pichiule P, LaManna JC. Expression of hypoxia-inducible factor-1alpha in the brain of rats during chronic hypoxia. J Appl Physiol. 2000;89:1937–42.
44. Greenberg DA, Jin K. From angiogenesis to neuropathology. Nature. 2005; 438:954–9.
45. Plate KH. Mechanisms of angiogenesis in the brain. J Neuropathol Exp Neurol. 1999;58:313–20.
46. Plate KH, Breier G, Weich HA, Risau W. Vascular endothelial growth factor is a potential tumour angiogenesis factor in human gliomas in vivo. Nature. 1992;359:845–8.
47. Krupinski J, Kaluza J, Kumar P, Kumar S, Wang JM. Role of angiogenesis in patients with cerebral ischemic stroke. Stroke. 1994;25:1794–8.
48. Cramer SC, Nelles G, Benson RR, Kaplan JD, Parker RA, et al. A functional MRI study of subjects recovered from hemiparetic stroke. Stroke. 1997;28:2518–27.
49. Weiller C, Ramsay SC, Wise RJ, Friston KJ, Frackowiak RS. Individual patterns of functional reorganization in the human cerebral cortex after capsular infarction. Ann Neurol. 1993;33:181–9.
50. Beckouche N, Bignon M, Lelarge V, Mathivet T, Pichol-Thievend C, et al. The interaction of heparan sulfate proteoglycans with endothelial transglutaminase-2 limits VEGF165-induced angiogenesis. Sci Signal. 2015;8:ra70.
51. Lever R, Rose MJ, McKenzie EA, Page CP. Heparanase induces inflammatory cell recruitment in vivo by promoting adhesion to vascular endothelium. Am J Physiol Cell Physiol. 2014;306:C1184–90.
52. Sotnikov I, Hershkoviz R, Grabovsky V, Ilan N, Cahalon L, et al. Enzymatically quiescent heparanase augments T cell interactions with VCAM-1 and extracellular matrix components under versatile dynamic contexts. J Immunol. 2004;172:5185–93.
53. Lad SP, Hegen H, Gupta G, Deisenhammer F, Steinberg GK. Proteomic biomarker discovery in cerebrospinal fluid for cerebral vasospasm following subarachnoid hemorrhage. J Stroke Cerebrovasc Dis. 2012;21:30–41.
54. Kubota T, Handa Y, Tsuchida A, Kaneko M, Kobayashi H, et al. The kinetics of lymphocyte subsets and macrophages in subarachnoid space after subarachnoid hemorrhage in rats. Stroke. 1993;24:1993–2000. discussion 2000-1991.
55. Kooijman E, Nijboer CH, van Velthoven CT, Kavelaars A, Kesecioglu J, et al. The rodent endovascular puncture model of subarachnoid hemorrhage: mechanisms of brain damage and therapeutic strategies. J Neuroinflammation. 2014;11:2.
56. Kasius KM, Frijns CJ, Algra A, Rinkel GJ. Association of platelet and leukocyte counts with delayed cerebral ischemia in aneurysmal subarachnoid hemorrhage. Cerebrovasc Dis. 2010;29:576–83.
57. McMahon CJ, Hopkins S, Vail A, King AT, Smith D, et al. Inflammation as a predictor for delayed cerebral ischemia after aneurysmal subarachnoid haemorrhage. J Neurointerv Surg. 2013;5:512–7.

7

Recombinant CTRP9 administration attenuates neuroinflammation via activating adiponectin receptor 1 after intracerebral hemorrhage in mice

Lianhua Zhao[1,2], Shengpan Chen[2,3], Prativa Sherchan[2], Yan Ding[2], Wei Zhao[1], Zaiyu Guo[1], Jing Yu[2], Jiping Tang[2*] and John H. Zhang[2*]

Abstract

Background: Neuroinflammation is a crucial factor contributing to neurological injuries after intracerebral hemorrhage (ICH). C1q/TNF-related protein 9 (CTRP9), an agonist of adiponectin receptor 1 (AdipoR1), has recently been shown to reduce inflammatory responses in systemic diseases. The objective of this study was to investigate the protective role of CTRP9 against neuroinflammation after ICH in a mouse model and to explore the contribution of adenosine monophosphate-activated protein kinase (AMPK)/nuclear factor kappa B (NFκB) pathway in AdipoR1-mediated protection.

Methods: Adult male CD1 mice ($n = 218$) were randomly assigned to different groups for the study. ICH was induced via intrastriatal injection of bacterial collagenase. Recombinant CTRP9 (rCTRP9) was administered intranasally at 1 h after ICH. To elucidate the underlying mechanism, AdipoR1 small interfering ribonucleic acid (siRNA) and selective phosphorylated AMPK inhibitor Dorsomorphin were administered prior to rCTRP9 treatment. Brain edema, short- and long-term neurobehavior evaluation, blood glucose level, western blot, and immunofluorescence staining were performed.

Results: Endogenous CTRP9 and AdipoR1 expression was increased and peaked at 24 h after ICH. AdipoR1 was expressed by microglia, neurons, and astrocytes. Administration of rCTRP9 reduced brain edema, improved short- and long-term neurological function, enhanced the expression of AdipoR1 and p-AMPK, and decreased the expression of phosphorylated NFκB and inflammatory cytokines after ICH. The protective effects of rCTRP9 were abolished by administration of AdipoR1 siRNA and Dorsomorphin.

Conclusions: Our findings demonstrated that administration of rCTRP9 attenuated neuroinflammation through AdipoR1/AMPK/NFκB signaling pathway after ICH in mice, thereby reducing brain edema and improving neurological function after experimental ICH in mice. Therefore, CTRP9 may provide a potential therapeutic strategy to alleviate neuroinflammation in ICH patients.

Keywords: C1q/TNF-related protein 9, Adiponectin receptor 1, Intracerebral hemorrhage, Neuroinflammation, Adenosine monophosphate-activated protein kinase

* Correspondence: jtang@llu.edu; johnzhang3910@yahoo.com
[2]Department of Physiology and Pharmacology, Loma Linda University, 11041 Campus St, Loma Linda, CA 92354, USA
Full list of author information is available at the end of the article

Background

Spontaneous intracerebral hemorrhage (ICH) is a severe type of stroke with high morbidity and mortality, accounting for about 15% of all stroke patients [1]. Intracerebral hematoma oppresses surrounding brain tissue is considered primary brain injury. Then, red blood cell debris and blood components breakdown can initiate the secondary brain injury and persist for several days to weeks in the perihematoma area [2]. Increasing evidence indicates that inflammatory response that occurs in the early stage after ICH is a key factor leading to secondary brain injury induced by ICH. Treatment to inhibit neuroinflammation after the onset of ICH can provide critical therapeutic strategy to improve outcomes after ICH.

Adiponectin is a major adipocyte-derived hormone that exerts its beneficial physiological effects such as regulation of metabolism, anti-atherosclerosis, and anti-inflammatory effects by activating its receptors [3–5]. Adiponectin receptor 1 (AdipoR1) is the main isoform of adiponectin receptors. Activation of AdipoR1 has been shown to have anti-inflammatory effects in the brain [6]. The C1q/TNF-related protein (CTRP) family is a novel analog of adiponectin, among which the globular C1q domain of CTRP9 has the highest degree of amino acid sequence homology with adiponectin. Studies have shown that CTRP9 has a protective effect against inflammation after cardiac ischemia [7, 8]. However, its role in stroke has not been investigated.

Adenosine monophosphate-activated protein kinase (AMPK) signaling system plays a key role in cellular and organismal survival by its ability to maintain metabolic homeostasis. Activation of AMPK has been shown to inhibit inflammatory response in various injury models while suppression of AMPK activity was associated with increased inflammation [9, 10]. Furthermore, the nuclear factor kappa B (NFκB) signaling system is one of the primary pathways involved in pro-inflammatory responses. Previous studies have shown that activation of AMPK signaling can downregulate the function of NFκB system [11–13]. To date, the anti-inflammatory role of CTRP9 in the brain has not been studied.

In the present study, we hypothesized the following three points: (1) rCTRP9 administration by intranasal route improves neurological deficits and brain edema after ICH; (2) rCTRP9 administration attenuates the production of inflammatory mediators following ICH; (3) the anti-inflammatory effect of rCTRP9 is mediated through the AdipoR1/AMPK/NFκB pathway after ICH.

Methods

Animals

Eight-week-old male CD1 mice (weight 30–40 g, Charles River, Wilmington, MA) were housed in a 12-h light/dark cycle at a controlled temperature and humidity with unlimited access to food and water. All experimental procedures were performed following the study protocol approved by the Institutional Animal Care and Use Committee (IACUC) at Loma Linda University in accordance with the National Institutes of Health Guide for the Care and Use of Laboratory Animals.

Experimental design

In the present study, all mice were randomly assigned to the following experiments. The following five separate experiments are shown in the timeline of experimental design (Additional file 1: Figure S1). The summary of experimental groups, animal numbers, and mortality rate in the study are listed in a table (Additional file 2: Table S1).

Experiment 1

To evaluate time course expression of endogenous CTRP9 and AdipoR1 after ICH, 36 mice were randomly divided into 6 groups for western blot: sham, ICH after 3, 6, 12, 24, and 72 h ($n = 6$/group). Additional two mice were used for immunofluorescence staining at 24 h post-ICH. Western blot was used to detect the expression of CTRP9 and AdipoR1 in the ipsilateral (right) hemisphere. Immunofluorescence staining was performed to localize AdipoR1 on neurons, astrocytes, and microglia.

Experiment 2

To determine the best treatment dosage for rCTRP9, 30 mice were randomly divided into 5 groups, $n = 6$/group: sham, ICH + vehicle (PBS), ICH + rCTRP9 (0.03 μg/g), ICH + rCTRP9 (0.1 μg/g), ICH+ rCTRP9 (0.3 μg/g). rCTRP9 was administered intranasally at 1 h post-ICH. Neurobehavioral tests and brain water content (BWC) were assessed at 24 h post-ICH. Blood glucose level was measured starting 1, 2, 3, 6, and 24 h after ICH.

Experiment 3

To determine the presence of rCTRP9 in the brain after intranasal administration, mice ($n = 24$) were divided into 4 groups, $n = 6$/group: naive, naïve+rCTRP9 (0.1 μg/g), ICH, ICH + rCTRP9 (0.1 μg/g). Based on results from experiment 2, medium dosage (0.1 μg/g) of rCTRP9 was chosen for the study. Neurobehavioral tests and western blot to measure rCTRP9 expression in ipsilateral (right) hemisphere were performed at 24 h post-ICH. Next, for the effects of the drug at 72 h after ICH, 18 mice were divided into 3 groups, $n = 6$/group: sham, ICH + vehicle (PBS), ICH + rCTRP9 (0.1 μg/g). Neurobehavioral tests and BWC were evaluated at 72 h post-ICH.

Experiment 4

To assess long-term neurobehavioral function, 24 mice were divided into 3 groups: sham, ICH + vehicle (PBS), ICH + rCTRP9 (0.1 μg/g), $n = 8$/group. The foot fault test and rotarod test were performed on days 7, 14, and 21 post-ICH. Morris water maze test was conducted on days 21–25 post-ICH.

Experiment 5

To verify the efficacy of AdiporR1 siRNA to knockdown the expression of AdipoR1, 24 mice were divided into 4 groups, $n = 6$/group: naive, naïve+AdipoR1 small interfering ribonucleic acid (siRNA), ICH, ICH + AdipoR1 siRNA. Next, to verify the anti-inflammatory mechanism of rCTRP9, mice ($n = 42$) were divided into seven groups: sham, ICH + vehicle (PBS), ICH + rCTRP9 (0.1 μg/g), ICH + rCTRP9 + AdipoR1 siRNA, ICH + rCTRP9 + scramble siRNA (Scr siRNA), ICH + rCTRP9 + Dorsomorphin, ICH + rCTRP9 + DMSO (5 μl of 5% dimethyl sulfoxide in PBS), $n = 6$/group. Neurobehavioral tests and western blot were performed at 24 h post-ICH.

ICH model

ICH was induced by intrastriatal injection of bacterial collagenase into the right basal ganglia as previously described [14]. Briefly, mice were anesthetized with ketamine (100 mg/kg) and xylazine (10 mg/kg) (2:1 vol/vol, intraperitoneal injection) and positioned prone in a stereotaxic head frame. Bacterial collagenase (0.075 units, type VII-S; Sigma-Aldrich, St. Louis, MO) was dissolved in 0.5 μL PBS and infused into the right basal ganglia at a rate of 0.1667 μL/min, using an infusion pump (Stoelting, IL). The needle was left for an additional 5 min to prevent possible leakage of the collagenase solution, and withdrawn slowly at a rate of 1 mm/min. After removal of the needle, the cranial burr hole was sealed with bone wax, the incision was sutured, and 0.4 mL of normal saline was injected subcutaneously, and the mice were allowed to recover. The sham operation was performed with PBS only. All ICH animals with hematoma and neurological deficits were included. Animals that died before experimental endpoints reached were replaced with new animals. Animals with no hematoma were excluded.

Drug administration

Recombinant CTRP9 (rCTRP9) (Novus, CO) dissolved in PBS was administered intranasally at 1 h post-ICH as previously reported [15]. Briefly, rCTRP9 was diluted in PBS, and three different doses of rCTRP9 (0.03, 0.1, and 0.3 μg/g) were treated. Nasal administration of rCTRP9 was performed at 1 h after ICH induction. A total volume 20 μL of rCTRP9 was administered intranasally. Mice, still under anesthesia, were placed in a supine position, and rCTRP9 was administered alternating drops (5 μL/drop) every 2 min between the left and right nares over a period of 20 min. The ICH + vehicle group received an equal volume of phosphate-buffered saline (PBS).

Intracerebroventricular injection

AdipoR1 siRNA and scramble siRNA (scr siRNA) (Life Technologies, NY) were delivered via intracerebroventricular (ICV) injection 48 h before ICH as previously described [16]. Briefly, AdipoR1 SiRNA or scr siRNA (100 pmol/mouse) was dissolved in sterile RNAs free resuspension buffer according to the manufacturer's instructions (Life Technologies, NY). The ICV injections into the left ventricle were performed using the following coordinates relative to bregma (0.22 mm posterior, 1.0 mm lateral, and 2.25 mm deep) at a rate of 0.667 μL/min at 48 h prior to surgery. After waiting for 5 min, the needle was removed over a period of 3 min. The burr hole was sealed with bone wax. Dorsomorphin (5 μg/mouse, Sigma, MO) was dissolved in DMSO and given by ICV injection into left ventricle as described above at 30 min before ICH surgery.

Short-term neurobehavior assessment

Short-term neurobehavioral tests were performed with modified Garcia score test, forelimb placement test, and corner turn test by an experienced investigator who was blinded to the experimental groups at 24 and 72 h post-ICH, as previously reported [17]. Garcia score assessment with a 21-point score evaluating spontaneous activity, axial sensation, vibrissae proprioception, symmetry of limb movement, lateral turning, forelimb walking, climbing, and grabbing was conducted. The forelimb placement test was used to investigate the animals' responsiveness to vibrissae stimulation; the placement of the left and right forelimbs was investigated for 10 consecutive trials. Then, left forelimb placement was calculated as left forelimb placement/(left forelimb placement + right forelimb placement) × 100%. For the corner turn test, animals were allowed to advance into a 30° corner and exit by turning either to the left or right. Choice of turning was recorded for a total of 10 trials, and a score was calculated as number of left turns/all trials × 100.

Brain water content measurement

The brain water content (BWC) was measured as previously reported using the wet/dry method [17]. Mice were euthanized under deep anesthesia and the brains were removed immediately and divided into five parts: ipsilateral and contralateral cortex, ipsilateral and contralateral basal ganglia, and cerebellum. All brain samples were weighed on analytical microbalance (APX-60 Denver Instrument, NY) to obtain the wet weight (WW). Then the samples were dried at 100 °C for 48 h to obtain the dry weight (DW). Brain water content (%) was calculated using the following formula: (WW – DW)/WW*100%.

Blood glucose measurement

Plasma glucose level was measured by blood glucose meter (Ascensia Diabetes Care US Inc., NJ) in the blood collected from tail vein before ICH and at 1, 2, 3, 6, and 24 h after ICH in each group.

Long-term neurobehavior assessment

Foot-fault and rotarod test were performed at the first, second, and third weeks post-ICH to assess sensorimotor function, coordination, and balance as previously described [18]. Water maze tests, including swim distance and escape latency, were performed at days 21 to 25 post-ICH to evaluate memory and spatial learning as previously described [19]. Morris water maze test probe quadrant duration was evaluated on day 25 post-ICH.

Western blot analysis

Western blotting was performed as described previously [20]. Briefly, the brain protein samples were prepared using Ripa Lysis buffer (Bio-Rad, CA), and equal amounts of protein were run on an SDS-PAGE gel. After being electrophoresed and transferred to a nitrocellulose membrane, the membrane was blocked and incubated with primary antibody overnight at 4 °C. The following primary antibodies were used: AdipoR1 (1:1000, ab126611), p-AMPKα (1:1000, ab133448), AMPKα (1:1000, ab32047), p-NFκB (1:1000, ab86299), NFκB (1:2000, ab16502), tumor necrosis factorα (TNFα) (1:1000, ab6671), interleukin-6 (IL-6) (1:1000, ab6672) (all from Abcam, MA), CTRP9 (1:500, NBP2–46834, Novus, CO), and adaptor protein, phosphotyrosine interacting with PH domain and leucine zipper 1 (APPL1) (1:1000, sc-271,901, Santa Cruz Biotechnology, CA). β-actin was used as an internal loading control. The respective secondary antibodies were incubated for 1 h at room temperature. The bands were probed with an ECL Plus chemiluminescence reagent Kit (Amersham Biosciences, Arlington Heights, PA) and visualized with the image system (Bio-Rad, Versa Doc, model 4000). Relative density of the protein immunoblot images were analyzed by ImageJ software (ImageJ 1.4, NIH, USA).

Immunofluorescence staining

At 24 h following ICH, mice were perfused under deep anesthesia with cold PBS (pH 7.4). Mice were then infused with 10% formalin. Brains were then removed and fixed in formalin at 4 °C for a minimum of 3 days. Samples were then dehydrated with 30% sucrose in PBS (pH 7.4). The frozen coronal slices (8 μm thick) were sectioned in cryostat (CM3050S; Leica Microsystems). Double immunofluorescence staining was performed as previously described [20]. The primary antibodies included anti-AdipoR1 (1:200, ab126611), anti-Iba-1 (1:200, ab178847), anti-NeuN (1:200, ab177487), and anti-GFAP (1:200, ab16997) (all from Abcam, MA).

Statistical analysis

All animals were randomly assigned to different groups. All the experimental tests were blinded to the surgeons and researchers who did the experiments and analyzed the research data. All tests for exploratory studies were performed two-sided. All data were expressed as the mean and standard deviation (mean ± SD). Statistical analysis was performed with GraphPad Prism (Graph Pad Software, San Diego, CA). One-way analysis of variance (ANOVA) is followed by multiple comparisons between groups using Tukey's post hoc test. Two-way repeated measures ANOVA was used to analyze the long-term neurobehavioral functions over time. Statistical significance was set at $p < 0.05$.

Results

Animal mortality rate

A total of 218 mice were used of which 56 were sham and 162 mice underwent ICH induction. None of the sham mice died, and the mortality rate in ICH group was 9.2% (15/162). Three mice were excluded from the study because of no hemorrhage. An additional file shows this in more details (Additional file 2: Table S1).

Endogenous CTRP9 and AdipoR1 expression were increased after ICH

The expression of endogenous CTRP9 and AdipoR1 was increased after ICH with a peak at 24 h compared to sham group and then decreased at 72 h after ICH ($p <$ 0.05, Fig. 1a, b). Immunofluorescence staining showed that AdipoR1 was expressed in microglia (Iba-1), neurons (NeuN), and astrocytes (GFAP) at 24 h post-ICH (Fig. 1c).

rCTRP9 attenuated neurobehavioral deficits and reduced brain edema at 24 h after ICH

The neurobehavioral score was significantly decreased in vehicle group compared with the sham group at 24 h post-ICH. Administration of medium dose and high dose of rCTRP9 significantly improved neurological function and decreased BWC in the right basal ganglia and cortex compared with ICH + vehicle group ($p < 0.05$, Fig. 2a–d).

rCTRP9 did not change blood glucose level after ICH

Blood glucose level increased significantly at 1 h post-surgery in all groups compared to baseline before surgery ($p < 0.05$), then continued to decline and reached nadir at 24 h post-ICH (Fig. 2e). There was no significant difference in blood glucose levels between experimental groups when compared at the same time point ($p > 0.05$). Based on above results, medium dosage rCTRP9 was used in the following experiments.

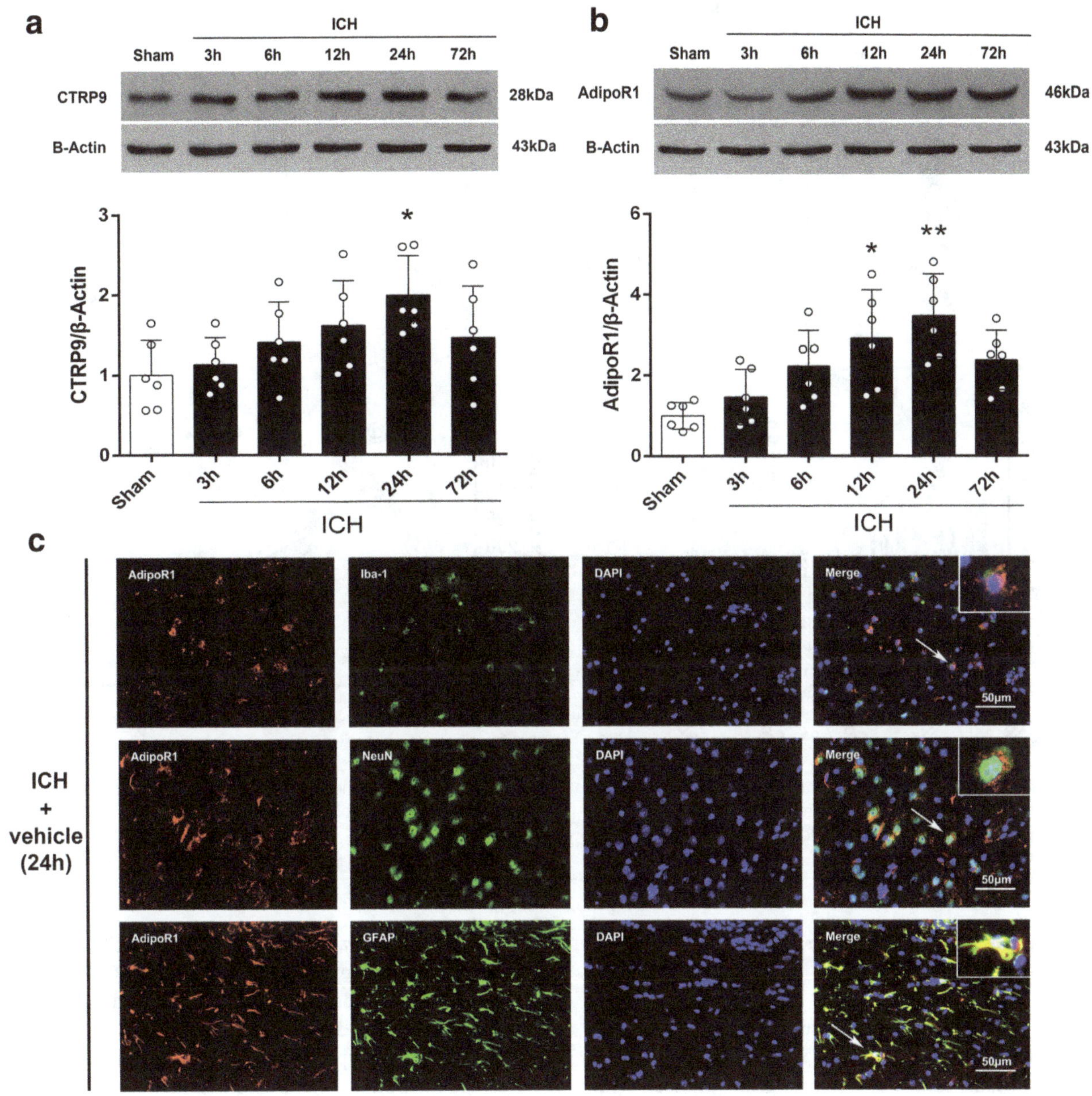

Fig. 1 Expression of C1q/TNF-related protein 9 (CTRP9) and adiponectin receptor 1 (AdipoR1) after intracerebral hemorrhage (ICH). **a** Representative western blot images and quantitative analyses of CTRP9 time course after ICH. **b** Representative western blot images and quantitative analyses of AdipoR1 time course after ICH. Values are expressed as mean ± SD. $*p < 0.05$, $**p < 0.01$ vs. sham group. $N = 6$. **c** Double immunofluorescence staining for AdipoR1 (red) in microglia (Iba-1, green), neurons (NeuN, green), and astrocytes (GFAP, green) in right basal cortex 24 h after ICH. Scale bar = 50 μm. $N = 2$. DAPI, 4′,6-diamidino-2-phenylindole; Iba-1, ionized calcium binding adaptor molecule-1; NeuN, neuronal nuclear; GFAP, glial fibrillary acidic protein

Nasal rCTRP9 administration increased the brain expression level of CTRP9 in naïve and ICH mice

At 24 h after nasal administration of rCTRP9, the expression of CTRP9 in naïve+CTRP9 group was significantly increased compared with naïve group. The expression level of CTRP9 was significantly increased in ICH + rCTRP9 group compared to ICH group at 24 h after ICH ($p < 0.05$, Fig. 3a). The neurobehavioral score in the ICH + rCTRP9 group was significantly improved compared with ICH group ($p < 0.05$, Fig. 3b–d).

rCTRP9 attenuated neurobehavioral deficits and reduced brain edema at 72 h after ICH

The neurobehavioral score was significantly improved, and brain edema in the right basal ganglia and cortex was reduced with rCTRP9 treatment

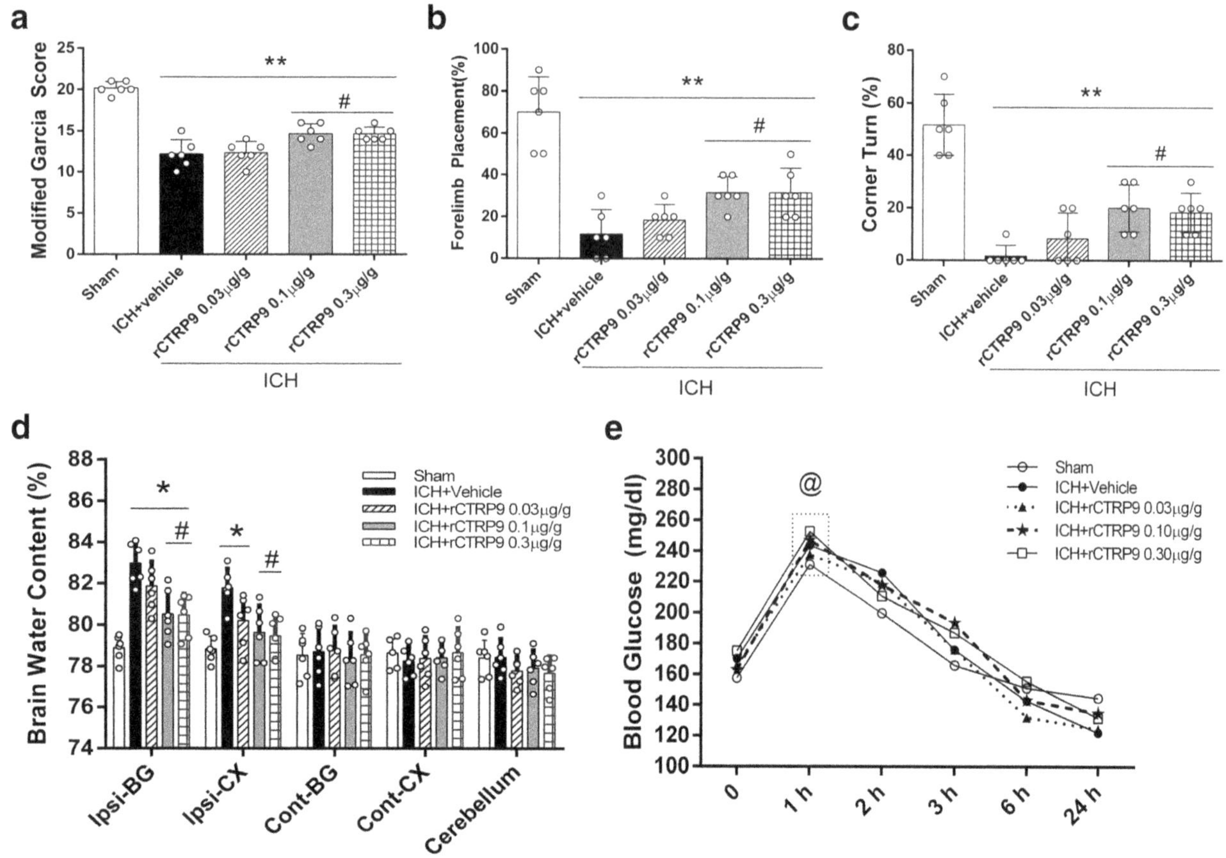

Fig. 2 The effects of different doses of rCTRP9 on neurobehavior tests, brain water content (BWC), and blood glucose at 24 h post-ICH. **a** Modified Garcia test, **b** forelimb placement test, **c** corner turn test, and **d** BWC at 24 h post-ICH. **e** Blood glucose levels measured at 0, 1, 2, 3, 6, and 24 h post-ICH. Values are expressed as mean ± SD. *$p < 0.05$, **$p < 0.01$ vs. sham group; #$p < 0.05$ vs. ICH + vehicle group; @$p < 0.05$ vs. before ICH (0 h); $N = 6$

compared with ICH + vehicle group at 72 h after ICH ($p < 0.05$, Fig. 4a–d).

rCTRP9 improved long-term neurobehavioral outcomes after ICH

In the foot fault test, ICH + vehicle group showed significantly increased foot faults compared to sham group and in the rotarod test, ICH + vehicle group had shorter latency to fall compared to sham group at 1, 2, and 3 weeks after ICH. Animals with rCTRP9 treatment showed significant improvement in both tests ($p < 0.05$; Fig. 5a, b).

In the water maze test, ICH + vehicle group showed significantly longer swim distance and escape latency. The rCTRP9 treatment group had significantly improved performance on days 3 to 5 of testing ($p < 0.05$; Fig. 5c, d). In the probe trial, the ICH + vehicle group spent less time in the target quadrant compared with sham group, while rCTRP9 treatment markedly increased the time spent in the probe quadrant ($p < 0.05$, Fig. 5e).

AdipoR1 siRNA aggravated neurological deficits and decreased AdipoR1 expression in naïve and ICH mice

AdipoR1 siRNA administration significantly decreased the expression of AdipoR1 and reduced neurobehavioral score in naïve+AdipoR1 siRNA group compared with naïve group. Similarly, the expression level of AdipoR1 was significantly decreased, and neurobehavior score was reduced in ICH + AdipoR1 siRNA group compared with ICH group ($p < 0.05$, Fig. 6a–d).

AdipoR1 siRNA and Dorsomorphin abolished the anti-inflammatory effects of rCTRP9

AdipoR1 siRNA but not scramble siRNA reversed neurobehavioral improvement observed in ICH + rCTRP9 mice at 24 h post-ICH. Likewise, Dorsomorphin significantly decreased neurobehavioral score compared with ICH + rCTRP9 + DMSO group ($p < 0.05$, Fig. 7a–c).

The expression of CTRP9 was significantly increased in all ICH groups that received rCTPR9 via intranasal administration compared to sham and ICH + vehicle groups. The expression of AdipoR1, APPL1, and p-AMPK increased

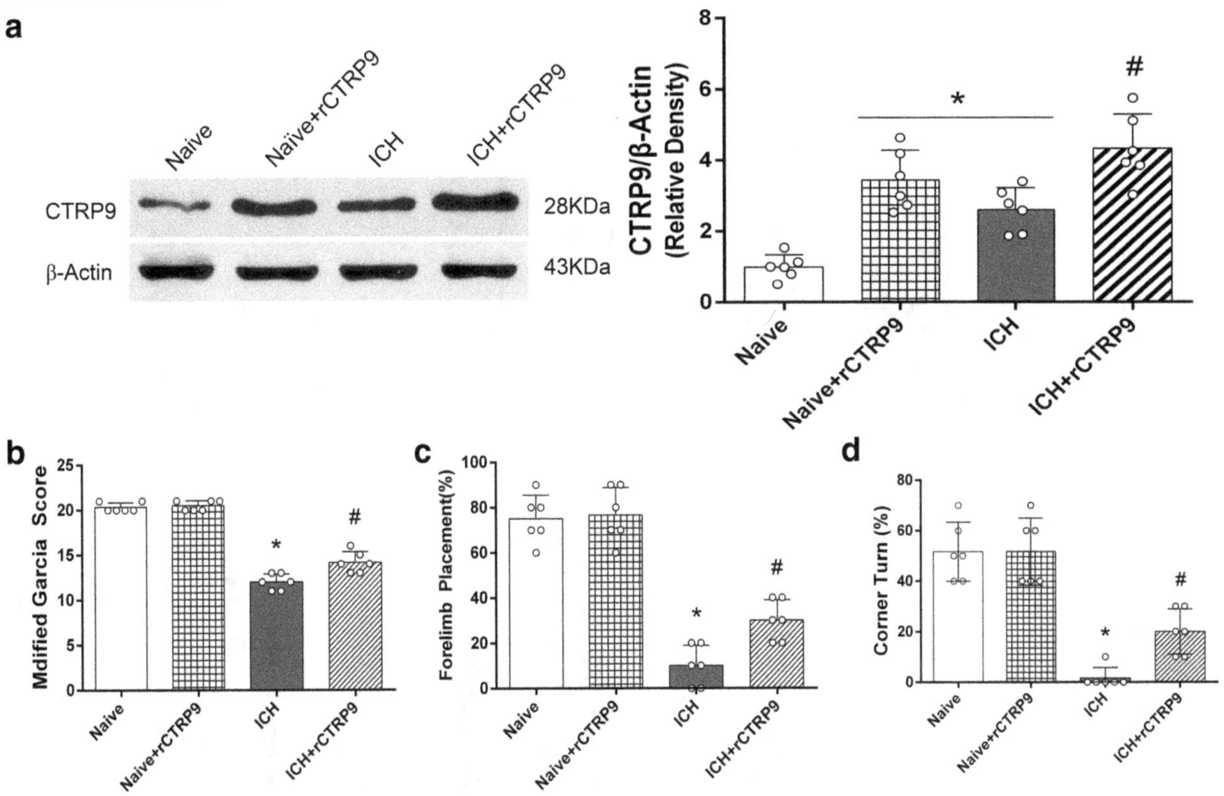

Fig. 3 Brain expression of CTRP9 and neurological function evaluation after nasal administration of rCTRP9 at 24 h post-ICH. **a** Representative western blot images and quantitative analyses of CTRP9. Nasal administration of rCTRP9 increased the expression level of CTRP9 in naïve mice and ICH mice at 24 h post-ICH. **b** Modified Garcia test, **c** forelimb placement test, and **d** corner turn test showed that nasal administration of rCTRP9 improved neurological function at 24 h post-ICH. Values are expressed as mean ± SD. *$p < 0.05$ vs. naive group; #$p < 0.05$ vs. ICH group; $N = 6$

after rCTRP9 administration in ICH + rCTRP9 group compared to ICH + vehicle group. AdipoR1 siRNA significantly decreased the expression of AdipoR1, APPL1, and p-AMPK, while increasing the expression of p-NFκB, TNFα, and IL-6 when compared with ICH + rCTRP9 + Scr siRNA group. In addition, Dorsomorphin intervention significantly suppressed p-AMPK expression, while increasing p-NFκB, TNFα, and IL-6 expression when compared with ICH + rCTRP9 + DMSO group ($p < 0.05$; Fig. 7d).

Discussion

In the present study, we first showed that the expression of CTRP9 and AdipoR1 increased in the brain at 24 h after ICH. Moreover, we found that rCTRP9 administration improved both short- and long-term neurobehavioral outcomes, alleviated brain edema, and attenuated neuroinflammation after ICH, which were accompanied by an increase in AdipoR1 and p-AMPK expression and a decrease in pro-inflammatory factors TNFα and IL-6 expression. Additionally, we determined that AdipoR1/AMPK/NFκB signaling pathway was involved in the anti-inflammatory effects of rCTRP9 after ICH. These findings suggest that rCTRP9 administration possibly improved outcomes after ICH at least in part by attenuating neuroinflammation through AdipoR1/AMPK/NFκB signaling pathway. The schematic mechanism was shown in a figure (Additional file 3: Figure S2).

Adiponectin is a biologically active polypeptide secreted by adipocytes and plays important roles in the regulation of energy homeostasis and insulin sensitivity. However, adiponectin knockout mice showed a relatively modest phenotype in the absence of diet or metabolic stress [21]. These findings suggested that there was a potential effective compensatory mechanism involved. CTRP9 shares the highest degree of sequence identity with adiponectin at the presumed functional globular domain, and has similar biochemical properties to adiponectin [22]. Existing research shows that CTRP9 has a variety of beneficial functions such as relaxing blood vessels, protecting the vascular endothelium, regulating metabolism, and reducing the expression of inflammatory factors [23, 24]. In addition, CTRP9 has also been shown to decrease myocardial infarct size by inhibiting the inflammatory response [25]. However, its role in the brain has never been studied.

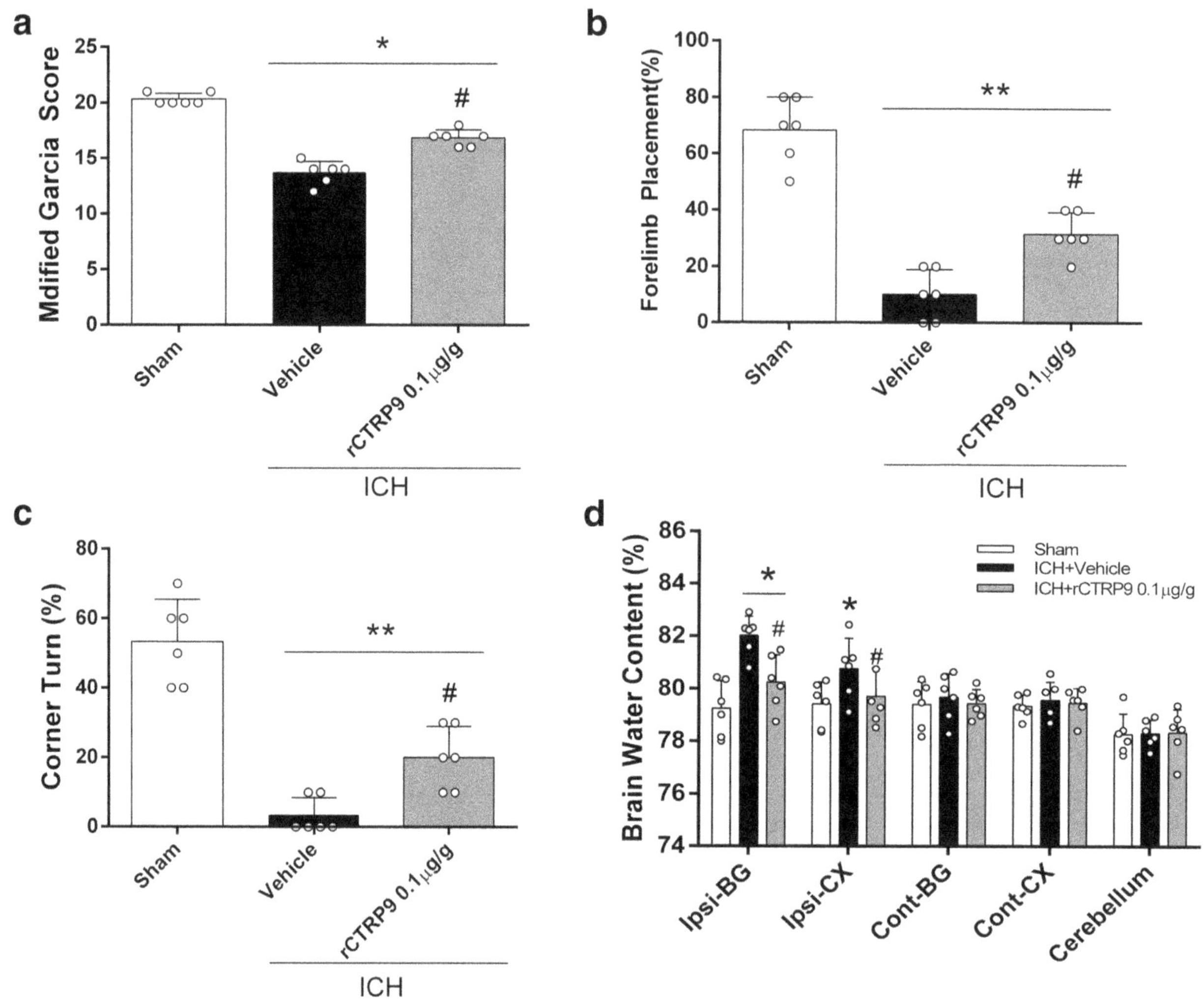

Fig. 4 rCTRP9 improved neurological deficits and decreased brain water content (BWC) at 72 h post-ICH. **a** Modified Garcia test, **b** forelimb placement test, **c** corner turn test, and **d** BWC at 72 h post-ICH. Values are expressed as mean ± SD. *$p < 0.05$, **$p < 0.01$ vs. sham group; #$p < 0.05$ vs. ICH + vehicle group; $N = 6$

In the present study, we demonstrated for the first time that CTRP9 has anti-inflammatory effects in ICH mouse model. The outcomes that we measured in this study have been utilized as standard outcome measurement in previously published ICH rodent model studies in which thrombin inhibition, microglia inactivation, and iron chelation were shown to have similar beneficial effects as observed in our study [26–28]. We evaluated the temporal expression of endogenous CTRP9 for 3 days after ICH. The results indicated that CTRP9 expression increased after ICH and reached the highest level at 24 h post-ICH. It has been reported that physiological levels of adiponectin in both human and mouse serum were elevated in response to inflammatory stimuli [29–32]. Our findings are consistent with a previous study that showed endogenous adiponectin expression significantly increased in cerebral ischemic areas after middle cerebral artery occlusion (MCAO) [33]. Acute injury or stress has been proposed to increase plasma concentration of elastase, which promotes the generation of globular adiponectin from full-length adiponectin [22, 34]. The acute stress following ICH injury may therefore contribute to increase endogenous CTRP9 expression after ICH. In addition, we observed that nasal administration of rCTRP9 increased the brain expression of CTRP9 and improved neurobehavioral deficits and brain edema after ICH. Even though the endogenous expression of CTRP9 was increased after ICH, it may not be sufficient to significantly reduce the massive neuroinflammatory insult after ICH. Exogenous administration of rCTRP9 further potentiates potential protective pathways against neuroinflammation after ICH.

Previous studies report that CTRP9 increased insulin sensitivity and lowered blood sugar levels in the hyperglycemia model [22]. Thus, we tested blood glucose changes during the first 24 h after rCTRP9 administration. We

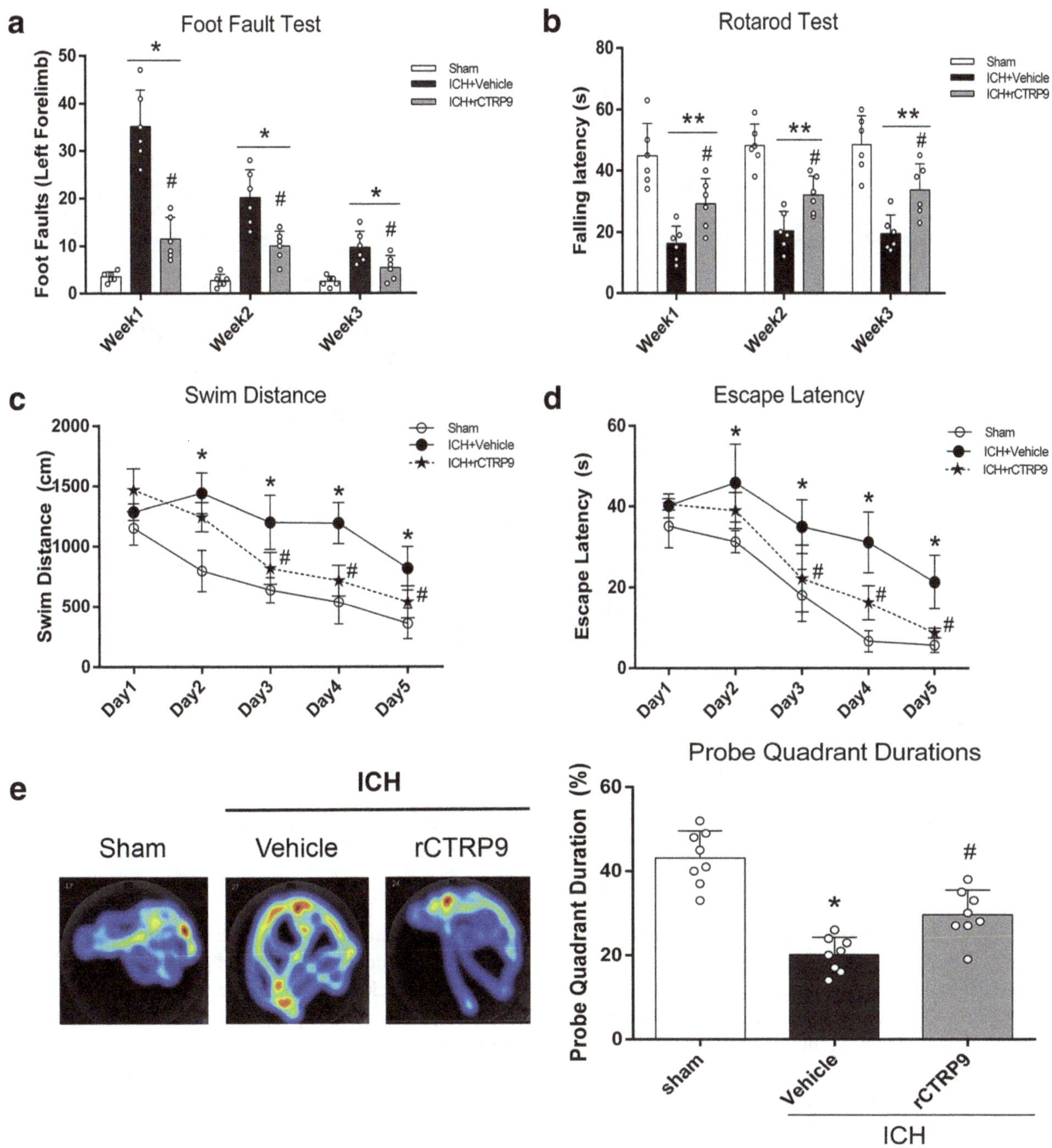

Fig. 5 rCTRP9 improved long-term neurobehavioral function after ICH. **a** Foot fault test and rotarod test on days 7, 14, and 21 after ICH. **b** Morris water maze indicated by swim distance and escape latency on 21–25 days after ICH. **c** Morris water maze test probe quadrant duration on day 25 post-ICH. Values are expressed as mean ± SD. *$p < 0.05$, **$p < 0.01$ vs. sham group; #$p < 0.05$ vs. ICH + vehicle group. $N = 8$

observed that intranasal administration of rCTRP9 did not affect blood glucose levels. Blood glucose in all the groups, including vehicle or rCTRP9 groups, reached highest levels at 1 h post-surgery, possibly a response to surgery-related stress. Additionally, subsequent blood glucose levels continued to decline in all groups, reaching the lowest levels at 24 h after ICH. These findings can possibly be attributed to surgery-induced stress and hematoma that increases energy expenditure as well as reduce food intake capacity of the animals. Since there were no difference observed in blood glucose levels between groups after intranasal rCTRP9 administration, it is reasonable to consider that rCTRP9 did not cause hypoglycemia in our ICH model.

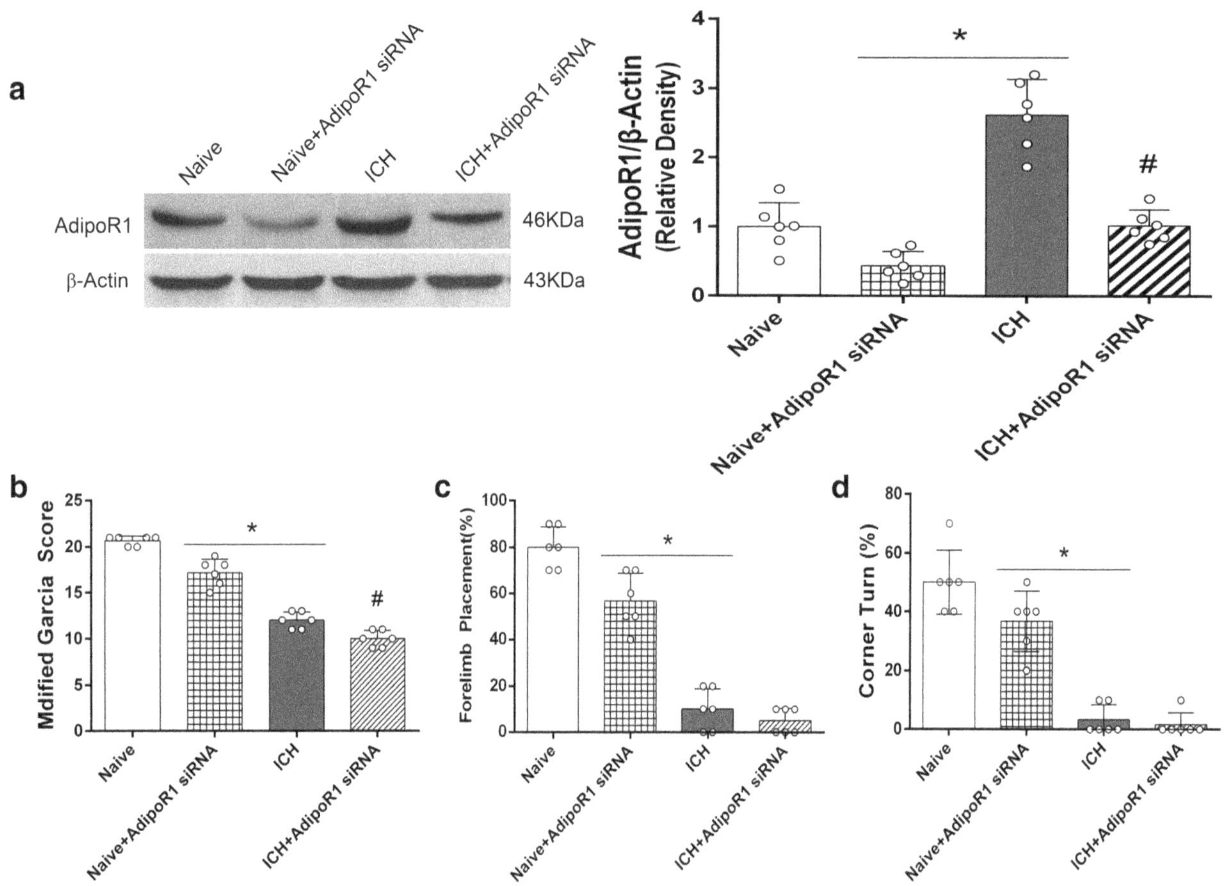

Fig. 6 AdipoR1 expression and neurological function evaluation after AdipoR1 siRNA administration in naïve and ICH mice. **a** Representative western blot images and quantitative analyses of AdipoR1 expression. AdipoR1 siRNA decreased the expression of AdipoR1 in naïve mice and ICH mice at 24 h post-ICH. **b** Modified Garcia test, **b** forelimb placement test, and **c** corner turn test showed that AdipoR1 siRNA aggravated neurological deficits in naïve mice and ICH mice at 24 h post-ICH. Values are expressed as mean ± SD. *$p < 0.05$ vs. naive group; #$p < 0.05$ vs. ICH group; $N = 6$

We found that AdipoR1 was expressed not only in microglia but also in neurons and astrocytes by immunofluorescence staining. These results are consistent with previous reports. Although adiponectin receptors have been shown to exist abundantly in the brain, its exact role in brain diseases remains unclear. Currently, two adiponectin receptors have been identified, AdipoR1 and AdipoR2. The expression of AdipoR1 has been reported to be more pronounced than AdipoR2 in the brain [35]. In addition, AdipoR1 and AdipoR2 have differential binding affinities to various adiponectin multimers. AdipoR1 binds to globular adiponectin (gAd) with high affinity, while AdipoR2 has an intermediate affinity with both gAd and full-length adiponectin [36]. In addition, AdipoR1 predominantly binds to adiponectin and suppresses NFκB activation and subsequently reduces the expression of pro-inflammatory cytokine, while AdipoR2 does not mediate the effects of adiponectin on microglial cells [6]. In this study, we observed that intracerebroventricular injection of AdipR1 siRNA decreased the expression of AdipoR1 and worsened neurological function in naïve and ICH mice. These results indicated a beneficial role of AdipR1 as well as demonstrated the knockdown efficacy AdipoR1.

The expression of AdipoR1 is regulated by many factors; obesity, alcohol, and insulin resistance can lower while exercise, stress, and cerebral ischemic conditions can increase the levels of AdipoR1. Our findings showed that AdipoR1 expression temporarily increased after ICH and reached peak levels at 24 h post-ICH. The receptor AdipoR1 is a high-affinity receptor for globular adiponectin. An increase in AdipoR1 expression may be necessary to perform its function given the increase in expression of globular domain of CTRP9 after ICH injury. This may be a possible explanation for the increase in AdipoR1 expression after ICH. Additionally, our results showed that AdipoR1 was modulated in a similar manner to CTRP9 levels after ICH, which indicates that rCTRP9 may exert its function through AdipoR1. Furthermore, rCTRP9 administration increased the expression of AdipoR1. The results were consistent with previous study which showed that adiponectin increased

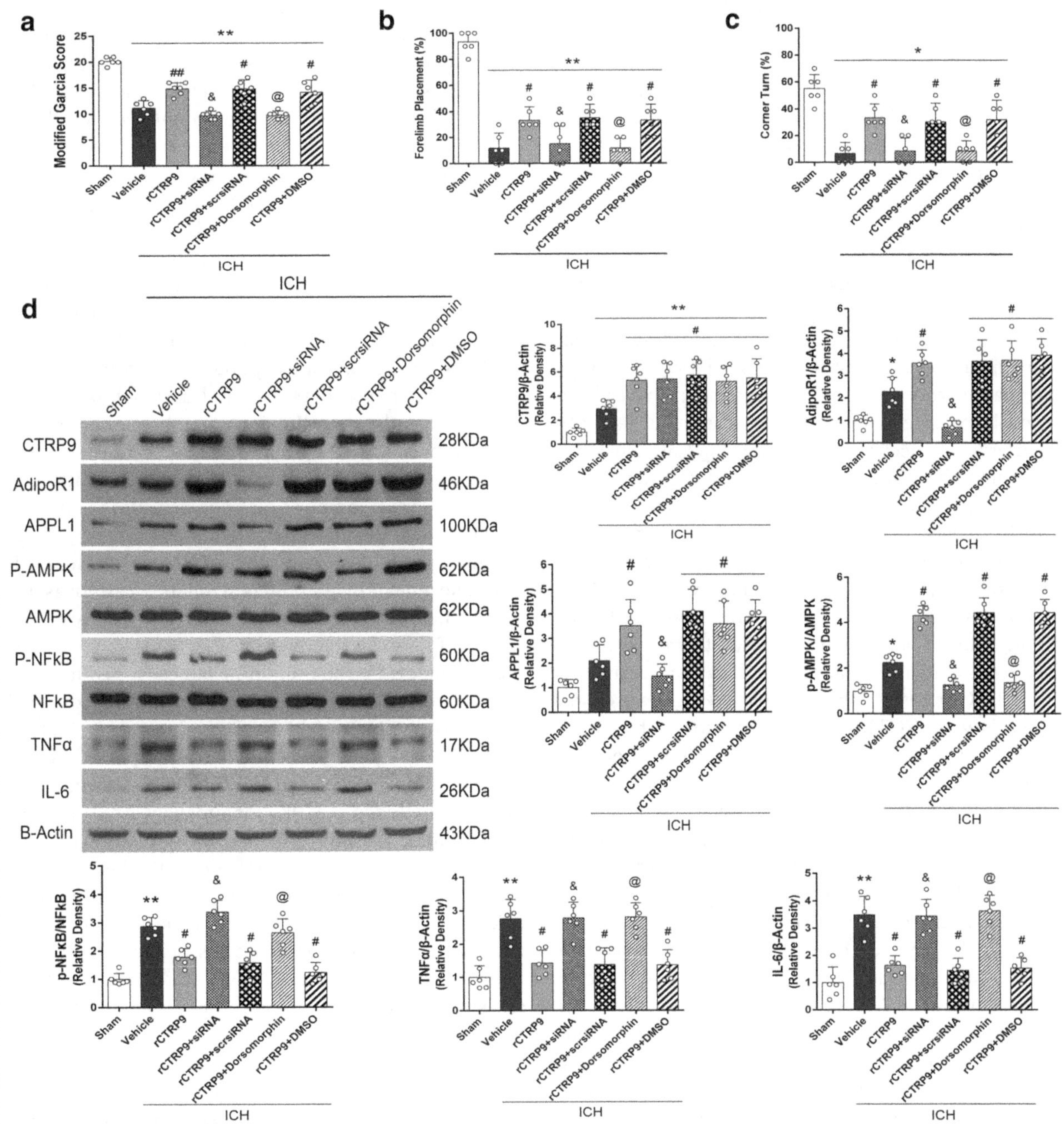

Fig. 7 Knockdown of AdipoR1 and p-AMPK abolished improvement in neurological function and anti-inflammatory effects of rCTRP9 at 24 h post-ICH. **a** Modified Garcia test, **b** forelimb placement test, **c** corner turn test, and **d** representative western blot images and quantitative analyses of CTRP9, AdipoR1, APPL1, p-AMPK/AMPK, p-NFκB/NFκB, TNF-α, and IL-6 at 24 h post-ICH. Values are expressed as mean ± SD. *$p < 0.05$, **$p < 0.01$ vs. sham group; #$p < 0.05$, ##$p < 0.01$ vs. ICH + vehicle group; &$p < 0.05$ vs. rCTRP9 + Scr siRNA, and @$p < 0.05$ vs. rCTRP9 + DMSO group. Scr, scramble; siRNA, small interfering RNA. $N = 6$

the expression of AdipoR1 and protected the brain against cerebral ischemic stroke [37]. We speculate that acute ICH injury may initially activate the inflammasome pathway and then trigger the stress reaction of adiponectin AdipoR1 signaling to reduce local inflammation. This is supported by the findings of our study which demonstrated that CTRP9/AdipoR1 showed anti-inflammatory effects in the ICH model, which is consistent with a previous study in which adiponectin was protective against cerebral ischemic stroke [38]. We measured inflammatory cytokines expression in the brain after ICH and with rCTRP9 administration. Local immune cells such as microglia and peripheral immune cells have been implicated in contributing to neuroinflammation after ICH. Since we administered rCTRP9 via intranasal administration which allows direct delivery of the agent to the brain, we measured changes in cytokine expression in the brain and levels of circulating cytokines were not measured in this study. Furthermore, to demonstrate the role of AdipoR1 in the anti-inflammatory mechanism of rCTRP9, AdipoR1 siRNA was administered by intracerebroventricular injection at 48 h before ICH with rCTRP9 treatment. The results showed that knockdown of AdipoR1 abolished the protective effects of rCTRP9 and reversed the expression of downstream proteins, suggesting that AdipoR1 played an essential role in the activating the downstream anti-inflammatory pathway by rCTRP9.

Neuroinflammation is a key process leading to secondary neurological damage after ICH [39]. Although anti-inflammatory effects of adiponectin have been previously reported in many disease models [40–42], the underlying mechanism remains unclear. Next, we investigated the downstream signaling pathway mediated via AdipoR1 activation. APPL1 is the only adiponectin receptor (AdipoR)-interacting protein that has been identified. The NH2-terminal intracellular region of AdipoR directly interacts with the PTB domain of APPL1. APPL1 was required for AdipoR-induced activation of downstream pathways to exert its anti-inflammatory and cytoprotective effects [43]. Our results showed that APPL1 expression increased with rCTRP9 administration after ICH. AMPK is a major downstream signaling molecule activated by APPL1 and has been demonstrated by studies on adiponectin-dependent AMPK signaling. A recent study suggested that bakkenolide B inhibited lipopolysaccharide-induced pro-inflammatory cytokines via AMPK activation in microglia [44]. In our study, administration of rCTRP9 markedly increased the expression of p-AMPK. This finding was consistent with a previous study in which CTRP9 protected against acute cardiac injury following ischemia-reperfusion via AMPK-dependent mechanism [45]. Due to its role in inducing the expression of proinflammatory cytokines, the nuclear factor NFκB pathway has long been considered as a typical proinflammatory signaling pathway. Prior published studies showed that the anti-inflammatory effects of adiponectin may be mediated via AMPK/NFκB signaling pathway [46]. In this study, we observed that rCTRP9 treatment upregulated the expression of AdipoR1, APPL1, and p-AMPK, and downregulated the pro-inflammatory p-NFκB after ICH. Furthermore, AdipoR1 siRNA and Dorsomorphin reversed the anti-inflammatory effects by rCTRP9. Overall, our results indicated that rCTRP9 treatment exerted anti-inflammatory effects through AdipoR1/AMPK/NFκB pathway in ICH model.

There are some limitations in the present study. First, AdipoR1 is expressed in astrocytes and may play a role in blood-brain barrier protective effects of rCTRP9, which may also contribute to the beneficial effects of rCTRP9 after ICH. Second, the pathophysiology of neuroinflammation after ICH is a complex network. Other downstream factors such as CAMKKβ and PPARα may be modulated by rCTRP9 administration after ICH which was not explored in this study. In the current study, we focused on APPL1/AMPK signaling anti-inflammatory mechanisms. Further studies need to be conducted to explore other potential signaling pathways contributed by rCTRP9 and AdipoR1 activation. Third, we did not evaluate the effects of CTRP9 in different age groups or in ICH with systemic co-morbidities. ICH tends to occur in older population with hypertension, vascular disorders, cerebral amyloid angiopathy, or anticoagulation. Previous publications indicate that adiponectin may have effect on hypertension and aging. Clinical studies have shown a relationship between serum adiponectin concentrations and the activity of renin-angiotensin-aldosterone system (RAAS), leading to changes in blood pressure [47, 48]. The effect of adiponectin on the cardiovascular system has been demonstrated partly by activation of the AMPK and cyclooxygenase-2 (COX-2) pathways, relaxation of vascular endothelial cells, reduction of endothelial cell apoptosis, and promotion of nitric oxide production [49, 50]. The lifespan of AdipoR1 or AdipoR2 knockout mice was reported to be shorter than that of control mice, the mechanisms involved included AMPK, mammalian target of rapamycin (mTOR) and SIRT, which are known to be key longevity molecules [51]. Overall, these findings indicate a need to study the relationship between adiponectin and CTRP9 with hypertension, aging, and systemic co-morbidities associated with ICH. Fourth, in this study, we did not evaluate sex-specific differences in the effects of CTRP9 in ICH. Estrogen has been reported to have neuroprotective effects, and it reduced neurological impairment after ICH and subarachnoid hemorrhage in rats [52, 53]. We therefore, used 8-week-old male adult CD1 mice for this study in order to eliminate the interference due to the effects of female sex hormones in the study outcomes.

Conclusions

In summary, we first showed that rCTRP9 administration improved neurological function, reduced brain edema, and alleviated inflammation through AdipoR1/AMPK/NFκB pathway after ICH. CTRP9, the closest analogue of adiponectin, may be a potential therapeutic target against neuroinflammation after ICH.

Additional files

Additional file 1: Figure S1. Experimental design and animal groups. ICH, intracerebral hemorrhage; rCTRP9, recombinant C1q/TNF-related protein 9; WB, western blot; IHC, immunohistochemistry; BS, blood sugar; siRNA, small interfering ribonucleic acid.

Additional file 2: Table S1. Summary of experimental groups and mortality rate in the study.

Additional file 3: Figure S2. Schematic mechanism of the effects of rCTRP9 on anti-neuroinflammation after ICH. rCTRP9, recombinant C1q/TNF-related protein 9; AdipoR1, adiponectin receptor 1; APPL1, adaptor protein, phosphotyrosine interacting with PH domain and leucine zipper 1; p-AMPK, phosphorylated-adenosine monophosphate-activated protein kinase; p-NFκB, phosphorylated-nuclear factor kappa B; TNFα, tumor necrosis factor α; IL-6, interleukin-6.

Abbreviations

AdipoR1: Adiponectin receptor 1; AMPK: Adenosine monophosphate-activated protein kinase; APPL1: Adaptor protein, phosphotyrosine interacting with PH domain and leucine zipper 1; BWC: Brain water content; CTRP9: C1q/TNF-related protein 9; DMSO: Dimethyl sulfoxide; GFAP: Glial fibrillary acidic protein; Iba-1: Ionized calcium binding adaptor molecule-1; ICH: intracerebral hemorrhage; IL-6: Interleukin-6; NeuN: Neuronal nuclear; p-AMPK: Phosphorylated-AMPK; PBS: Phosphate-buffered saline; p-NFκB: Phosphorylated-nuclear factor kappa B; Scr siRNA: Scramble siRNA; siRNA: Small interfering ribonucleic acid; TNFα: Tumor necrosis factor

Funding

This study is supported partially by grants from National Institutes of Health (NS091042 and NS082184) to Dr. J. H. Zhang.

Authors' contributions

JHZ, LHZ, and PS conceived and designed the study. LHZ, SPC, and JPT conducted the experiments, analyzed the data, and drafted the manuscript. PS and YD worked on the manuscript revision. SPC and JPT participated in the experimental design, data analysis and interpretation, and manuscript preparation. All authors read and approved the final manuscript.

Consent for publication

Not applicable.

Competing interests

The authors declare that they have no conflicts of interest.

Author details

[1]Department of Neurology, Tianjin TEDA Hospital, Tianjin, China. [2]Department of Physiology and Pharmacology, Loma Linda University, 11041 Campus St, Loma Linda, CA 92354, USA. [3]Department of Neurosurgery, Affiliated Haikou Hospital, Xiangya School of Medicine, Central South University, Haikou, China.

References

1. Keep RF, Hua Y, Xi G. Intracerebral haemorrhage: mechanisms of injury and therapeutic targets. Lancet Neurol. 2012;11:720–31.
2. Wilkinson DA, Pandey AS, Thompson BG, Keep RF, Hua Y, Xi G. Injury mechansims in acute intracerebral hemorrhage. Neuropharmacology. 2018; 134:240–8.
3. Okamoto Y, Kihara S, Ouchi N, Nishida M, Arita Y, Kumada M, Ohashi K, Sakai N, Shimomura I, Kobayashi H, et al. Adiponectin reduces atherosclerosis in apolipoprotein E-deficient mice. Circulation. 2002;106: 2767–70.
4. Whitehead JP, Richards AA, Hickman IJ, Macdonald GA, Prins JB. Adiponectin--a key adipokine in the metabolic syndrome. Diabetes Obes Metab. 2006;8:264–80.
5. Kang KH, Higashino A, Kim HS, Lee YT, Kageyama T. Molecular cloning, gene expression, and tissue distribution of adiponectin and its receptors in the Japanese monkey, Macaca fuscata. J Med Primatol. 2009;38:77–85.
6. Nicolas S, Cazareth J, Zarif H, Guyon A, Heurteaux C, Chabry J, Petit-Paitel A. Globular adiponectin limits microglia pro-inflammatory phenotype through an AdipoR1/NF-kappaB signaling pathway. Front Cell Neurosci. 2017;11:352.
7. Bai S, Cheng L, Yang Y, Fan C, Zhao D, Qin Z, Feng X, Zhao L, Ma J, Wang X, et al. C1q/TNF-related protein 9 protects diabetic rat heart against ischemia reperfusion injury: role of endoplasmic reticulum stress. Oxidative Med Cell Longev. 2016;2016:1902025.
8. Sun Y, Yi W, Yuan Y, Lau WB, Yi D, Wang X, Wang Y, Su H, Wang X, Gao E, et al. C1q/tumor necrosis factor-related protein-9, a novel adipocyte-derived cytokine, attenuates adverse remodeling in the ischemic mouse heart via protein kinase A activation. Circulation. 2013;128:S113–20.
9. Myerburg MM, King JD Jr, Oyster NM, Fitch AC, Magill A, Baty CJ, Watkins SC, Kolls JK, Pilewski JM, Hallows KR. AMPK agonists ameliorate sodium and fluid transport and inflammation in cystic fibrosis airway epithelial cells. Am J Respir Cell Mol Biol. 2010;42:676–84.
10. Wang Y, Huang Y, Xu Y, Ruan W, Wang H, Zhang Y, Saavedra JM, Zhang L, Huang Z, Pang T. A dual AMPK/Nrf2 activator reduces brain inflammation after stroke by enhancing microglia M2 polarization. Antioxid Redox Signal. 2018;28:141–63.
11. Hattori Y, Suzuki K, Hattori S, Kasai K. Metformin inhibits cytokine-induced nuclear factor kappaB activation via AMP-activated protein kinase activation in vascular endothelial cells. Hypertension. 2006;47:1183–8.
12. Yang Z, Kahn BB, Shi H, Xue BZ. Macrophage alpha1 AMP-activated protein kinase (alpha1AMPK) antagonizes fatty acid-induced inflammation through SIRT1. J Biol Chem. 2010;285:19051–9.
13. Mancini SJ, White AD, Bijland S, Rutherford C, Graham D, Richter EA, Viollet B, Touyz RM, Palmer TM, Salt IP. Activation of AMP-activated protein kinase rapidly suppresses multiple pro-inflammatory pathways in adipocytes including IL-1 receptor-associated kinase-4 phosphorylation. Mol Cell Endocrinol. 2017;440:44–56.
14. Ma Q, Huang B, Khatibi N, Rolland W 2nd, Suzuki H, Zhang JH, Tang J. PDGFR-alpha inhibition preserves blood-brain barrier after intracerebral hemorrhage. Ann Neurol. 2011;70:920–31.
15. Zhang Y, Chen Y, Wu J, Manaenko A, Yang P, Tang J, Fu W, Zhang JH. Activation of dopamine D2 receptor suppresses Neuroinflammation through alphaB-crystalline by inhibition of NF-kappaB nuclear translocation in experimental ICH mice model. Stroke. 2015;46:2637–46.
16. Yu L, Lu Z, Burchell S, Nowrangi D, Manaenko A, Li X, Xu Y, Xu N, Tang J, Dai H, Zhang JH. Adropin preserves the blood-brain barrier through a Notch1/Hes1 pathway after intracerebral hemorrhage in mice. J Neurochem. 2017;143:750–60.
17. Krafft PR, Caner B, Klebe D, Rolland WB, Tang J, Zhang JH. PHA-543613 preserves blood-brain barrier integrity after intracerebral hemorrhage in mice. Stroke. 2013;44:1743–7.
18. Lekic T, Hartman R, Rojas H, Manaenko A, Chen W, Ayer R, Tang J, Zhang JH. Protective effect of melatonin upon neuropathology, striatal function, and memory ability after intracerebral hemorrhage in rats. J Neurotrauma. 2010;27:627–37.
19. Sherchan P, Lekic T, Suzuki H, Hasegawa Y, Rolland W, Duris K, Zhan Y, Tang J, Zhang JH. Minocycline improves functional outcomes, memory deficits, and histopathology after endovascular perforation-induced subarachnoid hemorrhage in rats. J Neurotrauma. 2011;28:2503–12.
20. Chen Y, Zhang Y, Tang J, Liu F, Hu Q, Luo C, Tang J, Feng H, Zhang JH. Norrin protected blood-brain barrier via frizzled-4/beta-catenin pathway after subarachnoid hemorrhage in rats. Stroke. 2015;46:529–36.
21. Ma K, Cabrero A, Saha PK, Kojima H, Li L, Chang BH, Paul A, Chan L. Increased beta-oxidation but no insulin resistance or glucose intolerance in mice lacking adiponectin. J Biol Chem. 2002;277:34658–61.
22. Wong GW, Krawczyk SA, Kitidis-Mitrokostas C, Ge G, Spooner E, Hug C, Gimeno R, Lodish HF. Identification and characterization of CTRP9, a novel secreted glycoprotein, from adipose tissue that reduces serum glucose in mice and forms heterotrimers with adiponectin. FASEB J. 2009;23:241–58.
23. Zheng Q, Yuan Y, Yi W, Lau WB, Wang Y, Wang X, Sun Y, Lopez BL, Christopher TA, Peterson JM, et al. C1q/TNF-related proteins, a family of

novel adipokines, induce vascular relaxation through the adiponectin receptor-1/AMPK/eNOS/nitric oxide signaling pathway. Arterioscler Thromb Vasc Biol. 2011;31:2616–23.

24. Li J, Zhang P, Li T, Liu Y, Zhu Q, Chen T, Liu T, Huang C, Zhang J, Zhang Y, Guo Y. CTRP9 enhances carotid plaque stability by reducing pro-inflammatory cytokines in macrophages. Biochem Biophys Res Commun. 2015;458:890–5.
25. Kambara T, Shibata R, Ohashi K, Matsuo K, Hiramatsu-Ito M, Enomoto T, Yuasa D, Ito M, Hayakawa S, Ogawa H, et al. C1q/tumor necrosis factor-related protein 9 protects against acute myocardial injury through an adiponectin receptor I-AMPK-dependent mechanism. Mol Cell Biol. 2015;35:2173–85.
26. Wu CH, Shyue SK, Hung TH, Wen S, Lin CC, Chang CF, Chen SF. Genetic deletion or pharmacological inhibition of soluble epoxide hydrolase reduces brain damage and attenuates neuroinflammation after intracerebral hemorrhage. J Neuroinflammation. 2017;14:230.
27. Yang Z, Zhao T, Zou Y, Zhang JH, Feng H. Curcumin inhibits microglia inflammation and confers neuroprotection in intracerebral hemorrhage. Immunol Lett. 2014;160:89–95.
28. Ma B, Day JP, Phillips H, Slootsky B, Tolosano E, Dore S. Deletion of the hemopexin or heme oxygenase-2 gene aggravates brain injury following stroma-free hemoglobin-induced intracerebral hemorrhage. J Neuroinflammation. 2016;13:26.
29. Toussirot E, Streit G, Nguyen NU, Dumoulin G, Le Huede G, Saas P, Wendling D. Adipose tissue, serum adipokines, and ghrelin in patients with ankylosing spondylitis. Metabolism. 2007;56:1383–9.
30. Brochu-Gaudreau K, Rehfeldt C, Blouin R, Bordignon V, Murphy BD, Palin MF. Adiponectin action from head to toe. Endocrine. 2010;37:11–32.
31. Yang Q, Fu C, Xiao J, Ye Z. Uric acid upregulates the adiponectinadiponectin receptor 1 pathway in renal proximal tubule epithelial cells. Mol Med Rep. 2018;17:3545–54.
32. Delaigle AM, Jonas JC, Bauche IB, Cornu O, Brichard SM. Induction of adiponectin in skeletal muscle by inflammatory cytokines: in vivo and in vitro studies. Endocrinology. 2004;145:5589–97.
33. Shen L, Miao J, Yuan F, Zhao Y, Tang Y, Wang Y, Zhao Y, Yang GY. Overexpression of adiponectin promotes focal angiogenesis in the mouse brain following middle cerebral artery occlusion. Gene Ther. 2013;20:93–101.
34. Huang H, Iida KT, Sone H, Ajisaka R. The regulation of adiponectin receptors expression by acute exercise in mice. Exp Clin Endocrinol Diabetes. 2007; 115:417–22.
35. Guillod-Maximin E, Roy AF, Vacher CM, Aubourg A, Bailleux V, Lorsignol A, Penicaud L, Parquet M, Taouis M. Adiponectin receptors are expressed in hypothalamus and colocalized with proopiomelanocortin and neuropeptide Y in rodent arcuate neurons. J Endocrinol. 2009;200:93–105.
36. Yamauchi T, Kamon J, Ito Y, Tsuchida A, Yokomizo T, Kita S, Sugiyama T, Miyagishi M, Hara K, Tsunoda M, et al. Cloning of adiponectin receptors that mediate antidiabetic metabolic effects. Nature. 2003;423:762–9.
37. Guo F, Jiang T, Song W, Wei H, Wang F, Liu L, Ma L, Yin H, Wang Q, Xiong L. Electroacupuncture attenuates cerebral ischemia-reperfusion injury in diabetic mice through adiponectin receptor 1-mediated phosphorylation of GSK-3beta. Mol Neurobiol. 2015;51:685–95.
38. Nishimura M, Izumiya Y, Higuchi A, Shibata R, Qiu J, Kudo C, Shin HK, Moskowitz MA, Ouchi N. Adiponectin prevents cerebral ischemic injury through endothelial nitric oxide synthase dependent mechanisms. Circulation. 2008;117:216–23.
39. Wang J, Dore S. Inflammation after intracerebral hemorrhage. J Cereb Blood Flow Metab. 2007;27:894–908.
40. Ohashi K, Shibata R, Murohara T, Ouchi N. Role of anti-inflammatory adipokines in obesity-related diseases. Trends Endocrinol Metab. 2014; 25:348–55.
41. Yang Y, Hu W, Jiang S, Wang B, Li Y, Fan C, Di S, Ma Z, Lau WB, Qu Y. The emerging role of adiponectin in cerebrovascular and neurodegenerative diseases. Biochim Biophys Acta. 2015;1852:1887–94.
42. Wang Y, Zhou M, Lam KS, Xu A. Protective roles of adiponectin in obesity-related fatty liver diseases: mechanisms and therapeutic implications. Arq Bras Endocrinol Metabol. 2009;53:201–12.
43. Deepa SS, Dong LQ. APPL1: role in adiponectin signaling and beyond. Am J Physiol Endocrinol Metab. 2009;296:E22–36.
44. Park SY, Choi MH, Park G, Choi YW. Petasites japonicus bakkenolide B inhibits lipopolysaccharideinduced proinflammatory cytokines via AMPK/Nrf2 induction in microglia. Int J Mol Med. 2018;41:1683–92.
45. Kambara T, Ohashi K, Shibata R, Ogura Y, Maruyama S, Enomoto T, Uemura Y, Shimizu Y, Yuasa D, Matsuo K, et al. CTRP9 protein protects against myocardial injury following ischemia-reperfusion through AMP-activated protein kinase (AMPK)-dependent mechanism. J Biol Chem. 2012;287:18965–73.
46. Devaraj S, Torok N, Dasu MR, Samols D, Jialal I. Adiponectin decreases C-reactive protein synthesis and secretion from endothelial cells: evidence for an adipose tissue-vascular loop. Arterioscler Thromb Vasc Biol. 2008;28:1368–74.
47. Yilmaz MI, Sonmez A, Kilic S, Celik T, Bingol N, Pinar M, Mumcuoglu T, Ozata M. The association of plasma adiponectin levels with hypertensive retinopathy. Eur J Endocrinol. 2005;152:233–40.
48. Nowak L, Adamczak M, Wiecek A. Blockade of sympathetic nervous system activity by rilmenidine increases plasma adiponectin concentration in patients with essential hypertension. Am J Hypertens. 2005;18:1470–5.
49. Wang ZV, Scherer PE. Adiponectin, cardiovascular function, and hypertension. Hypertension. 2008;51:8–14.
50. Ouedraogo R, Gong Y, Berzins B, Wu X, Mahadev K, Hough K, Chan L, Goldstein BJ, Scalia R. Adiponectin deficiency increases leukocyte-endothelium interactions via upregulation of endothelial cell adhesion molecules in vivo. J Clin Invest. 2007;117:1718–26.
51. Okada-Iwabu M, Yamauchi T, Iwabu M, Honma T, Hamagami K, Matsuda K, Yamaguchi M, Tanabe H, Kimura-Someya T, Shirouzu M, et al. A small-molecule AdipoR agonist for type 2 diabetes and short life in obesity. Nature. 2013;503:493–9.
52. Nakamura T, Hua Y, Keep RF, Park JW, Xi G, Hoff JT. Estrogen therapy for experimental intracerebral hemorrhage in rats. J Neurosurg. 2005;103:97–103.
53. Shih HC, Lin CL, Lee TY, Lee WS, Hsu C. 17beta-estradiol inhibits subarachnoid hemorrhage-induced inducible nitric oxide synthase gene expression by interfering with the nuclear factor kappa B transactivation. Stroke. 2006;37:3025–31.

8

Dimethylarginines in patients with intracerebral hemorrhage: association with outcome, hematoma enlargement, and edema

Hans Worthmann[1*†], Na Li[1,2†], Jens Martens-Lobenhoffer[3], Meike Dirks[1], Ramona Schuppner[1], Ralf Lichtinghagen[4], Jan T. Kielstein[5,6], Peter Raab[7], Heinrich Lanfermann[7], Stefanie M. Bode-Böger[3†] and Karin Weissenborn[1†]

Abstract

Background: Asymmetric dimethylarginine (ADMA)--the most potent endogenous NO-synthase inhibitor, has been regarded as mediator of endothelial dysfunction and oxidative stress. Considering experimental data, levels of ADMA and its structural isomer symmetric dimethylarginine (SDMA) might be elevated after intracerebral hemorrhage (ICH) and associated with clinical outcome and secondary brain injury.

Methods: Blood samples from 20 patients with acute ICH were taken at ≤ 24 h and 3 and 7 days after the event. Nine patients had favorable (modified Rankin Scale (mRS) at 90 days 0–2) outcome, and 11 patients unfavorable outcome (mRS 3–6). Patients' serum ADMA, SDMA, and L-arginine levels were determined by high-performance liquid chromatography–tandem mass spectrometry. Levels were compared to those of 30 control subjects without ICH. For further analysis, patients were grouped according to outcome, hematoma and perihematomal edema volumes, occurrence of hematoma enlargement, and cytotoxic edema as measured by computed tomography and serial magnetic resonance imaging.

Results: Levels of ADMA--but not SDMA and L-arginine--were elevated in ICH patients compared to controls (binary logistic regression analysis: ADMA ≤ 24 h, $p = 0.003$; 3 days $p = 0.005$; 7 days $p = 0.004$). If patients were grouped according to outcome, dimethylarginines were increased in patients with unfavorable outcome. The binary logistic regression analysis confirmed an association of SDMA levels ≤ 24 h ($p = 0.048$) and at 3 days ($p = 0.028$) with unfavorable outcome. ADMA ≤ 24 h was increased in patients with hematoma enlargement ($p = 0.003$), while SDMA ≤ 24 h was increased in patients with large hematoma ($p = 0.029$) and perihematomal edema volume ($p = 0.023$).

Conclusions: Our data demonstrate an association between dimethylarginines and outcome of ICH. However, further studies are needed to confirm this relationship and elucidate the mechanisms behind.

Keywords: ADMA, SDMA, Intracerebral hemorrhage, Outcome, Hematoma enlargement, Edema

* Correspondence: worthmann.hans@mh-hannover.de
†Equal contributors
[1]Department of Neurology, Hannover Medical School, 30623 Hannover, Germany
Full list of author information is available at the end of the article

Background

Intracerebal hemorrhage (ICH) is a detrimental disease with high morbidity and mortality [1]. Deterioration by secondary hematoma enlargement and perihematomal edema occurs frequently during the first days leading to a high rate of poor outcome underlining the need for effective therapy. Knowledge about molecular mechanisms being involved in these important complications that could facilitate therapeutic approaches is still sparse.

After ICH, thrombin and hemin, a hemoglobin metabolite, enter the brain parenchyma. Experimental data from cell culture models of microglia and cortical astrocytes indicate that these components lead to overexpression of inducible nitric oxide synthase (iNOS) and increased production of superoxide [2, 3]. Importantly, in ICH patients, levels of NO or NO metabolites were correlated with outcome. Chiang et al. showed an association of increased NO levels in cerebrospinal fluid with poor outcome at 6 months [4]. In contrast to this, Rashid et al. detected lower serum levels of NO metabolites in patients with poor outcome at discharge [5]. NO levels are differently influenced by dimetyhlarginines asymmetric dimetyhlarginine (ADMA) and its structural isomer symmetric dimethylarginine (SDMA).

Mono and dimethylarginines L-NG-monomethylarginine (N-NMMA), ADMA, and SDMA are generated by proteolysis from proteins with methylated arginine residues as catalyzed by protein arginine methyltransferases (PRMTs) [6, 7]. The structure of ADMA resembles L-arginine, which acts as the substrate of NOS to synthesize NO. For this reason, ADMA represents the most potent endogenous NOS inhibitor as it competes with L-arginine for NOS binding [8]. In acute ischemic stroke, it has been regarded as mediator of oxidative stress by inhibition and uncoupling of NO-synthases (for a review see [9]). Its structural isomer symmetric dimethylarginine (SDMA) inhibits production of NO levels differently through impairment of intracellular L-arginine uptake since L-arginine acts as the substrate of NOS [10]. SDMA increases the production of reactive oxygen species (ROS) as shown in monocytes [11].

By these mechanisms, dimethylarginines and L-arginine may contribute to the NO metabolism and oxidative stress also after ICH and might be involved in clinical outcome and secondary complications such as hematoma enlargement or perihematomal edema.

So far, dimethylarginine levels have been measured in only one study of ICH patients ($n = 22$) and did not differ from levels in control subjects [12]. However, the study by Wanby and colleagues leaves several questions unanswered since neither the time point of blood sampling has been specified nor have any clinical or radiological outcomes been analyzed in the study. Dimethylarginine levels may vary during the first days after ICH––similar to patients with ischemic stroke [13]. We expected a delayed increase in ADMA levels in ICH patients comparable to the findings in subarachnoid hemorrhage (SAH) patients [14, 15].

We aimed to investigate the temporal pattern of ADMA, SDMA, and L-arginine after ICH in regard to clinical outcome. In addition, we intended to examine the association of dimethylarginines with hematoma and perihematomal volumes and occurrence of hematoma enlargement and cytotoxic edema.

Methods

Study population

Twenty patients with primary ICH who presented within 24 h of symptom onset and were treated either at the stroke unit or the intensive care unit in the Department of Neurology at Hannover Medical School were enrolled. The patient cohort derived from a cohort of a former study [16]. Intracerebral hemorrhage was diagnosed by computed tomography (CT) scan or magnetic resonance tomography (MRI). Exclusion criteria were surgical ICH procedures, contraindication to MRI or refusal of participation. Thirty healthy subjects adjusted for sex and age served as controls. Patients and controls were assessed for age, sex, arterial hypertension, diabetes mellitus, estimated glomerular filtration rate (evaluated by CKD-EPI equation), hyperlipidemia, status of smoking, and treatment with anticoagulants and antiplatelets. In addition, in patients, baseline stroke severity (according to National Institutes of Health Stroke Scale Score (NIHSS) on admission) and clinical outcome (modified Rankin Scale (mRS) at 90 days) were obtained (favorable outcome mRS 0–2, unfavorable outcome mRS 3–6). For the definition of outcome groups, moderately and severely disabled patients as used in other studies [17] were combined in the unfavorable outcome group since in our patient cohort, the most severely disabled patients could not be included due to surgical procedures and impossibility of performance of serial MRI investigation.

The study was approved by the ethics committee of Hannover Medical School. Patients or a relative gave written informed consent.

Blood collection and measurement of ADMA, SDMA, and L-arginine

Venous blood samples were taken at ≤ 24 h (median 12 h) and 3 and 7 days after the event. Serum was stored at −80 °C until assayed. Serum ADMA, SDMA, and L-arginine were assessed blindly without knowledge of any of the clinical information using high-performance liquid chromatography–tandem mass spectrometry (HPLC–MS–MS) [18]. The lower limits of quantification for ADMA were 0.15 μmol/l, for SDMA were 0.20 μmol/l, and for L-arginine were 7.5 μmol/l. The inter-assay precision was 3.77%, and the intra-assay precision was 2.12% for

ADMA, 3.86, and 2.83% for SDMA and 4.01 and 0.82% for L-arginine.

Imaging protocol and analysis

On admission, CT was performed for clinical diagnosis. Magnetic resonance imaging (MRI) was conducted at ≤ 24 h ($n = 18$), 3 days ($n = 18$), and 7 days ($n = 16$) after the event, as feasible. For detection of hematoma and perihematomal edema volume by manual segmentation on 3D-fluid-attenuated-inversion recovery-data, ITK-SNAP analysis software was used. Cytotoxic edema was defined by area of elevated diffusion-weighted imaging (DWI)-b1000-signal and decreased apparent diffusion coefficient (ADC) value (by > 10% compared with mirror region of interest (ROI)) outside of hematoma on T2*- and DWIb0-sequences. The manually outlined area was confirmed by 3D-multiplanar localization using the image analysis software. Patients were grouped according to median hematoma volume considering the initial MRI. In two patients, no MRI was conducted at ≤ 24 h due to a severe clinical deficit on admission. In these patients, MRI at 3 days was used for categorization of hematoma volume. Hematoma enlargement was defined by increase of hematoma volume > 33% or 6.0 ml calculated from first imaging (CT or MRI) to follow-up MRIs. When hematoma volumes from CT and MRI were compared, MRI volumes were adapted as proposed by Burgess et al. (CT volume = 0.8* MRI volume) [19]. Patients without MRI at 3 or 7 days ($n = 2$) were excluded from this analysis. For analysis of patient groups according to perihematomal edema volume, the maximum values from MRI (≤ 24 h and 3 or 7 days) were used. In addition, patients were grouped for occurrence of cytotoxic edema as detected by MRI (≤ 24 h and 3 or 7 days).

Statistical analysis

Statistical analysis was performed with the IBM SPSS Statistics 23. The data are presented as numbers and portion for categorical variables and median with interquartile range for continuous variables. The data were tested for statistically significant differences between patients and controls by Mann-Whitney *U* test for continuous data and Pearson chi-square for categorical data. The binary logistic regression analysis included ADMA levels and adjusted for co-variables age and estimated glomerular filtration rate (eGFR) using the method of backward stepwise. Within group comparisons of ADMA, SDMA and L-arginine levels at different time points were analyzed by Wilcoxon test. For the outcome analysis, patients were grouped into those with favorable and unfavorable outcome. In addition, Spearman rank correlation was performed between molecular marker levels and mRS at 90 days. To analyze the association of ADMA, SDMA, and L-arginine with imaging outcomes, patients were grouped according to hematoma and perihematomal edema volume and occurrence of hematoma enlargement and cytotoxic edema. For the analysis of clinical and imaging outcomes, the data were tested for statistically significant differences between patient groups by Mann-Whitney *U* test for continuous data and Pearson chi-square for categorical data. The binary logistic regression analysis tested ADMA and SDMA levels for association with clinical outcome including age and eGFR as co-variables (method of backward stepwise). A p value < 0.05 was considered to indicate statistical significance.

Results

The study population consisted of 20 patients with ICH with a median age of 77 years (interquartile range 72–84). Clinical and demographical characteristics in patients and controls are shown in Table 1. Patients and controls did not significantly differ in regard to these parameters.

Temporal pattern of dimethylarginines after acute ICH

In controls ADMA levels were 0.438 μmol/L (interquartile range 0.389–0.476), SDMA levels were 0.551 μmol/L (interquartile range 0.465–0.631), and L-arginine levels

Table 1 Clinical characteristics of patients and controls

	ICH ($n = 20$)	Controls ($n = 30$)	*P*
Female	11 (55.0)	17 (56.7)	0.907
Male	9 (45.0)	13 (43.3)	
Age (years)	77 (72; 84)	71 (63; 76)	0.106
Hypertension	15 (75.0)	24 (80.0)	0.676
Smoker	1 (5.0)	4 (13.3)	0.336
Hyperlipoproteinemia	6 (30.0)	15 (50.0)	0.160
Diabetes mellitus	1 (5.0)	4 (13.3)	0.336
History of CVD	0 (0.0)	3 (10.0)	0.145
History of CHD	1 (5.0)	5 (16.7)	0.214
History of antiplatelets	4 (20.0)	9 (30.0)	0.430
History of anticoagulants	1 (5.0)	0 (0.0)	0.216
eGFR (ml/min per 1.73 m^2)	86.9 (65.4; 98.2)	70.7 (61.7; 86.6)	0.104
NIHSS on admission	9 (6; 15)	n.a.	–
mRS 90 days	3 (2; 4)	n.a.	–
Deep location of ICH	15 (75.0)	n.a.	–
IVH extension	2 (10.0)	n.a.	–
Hematoma volume (ml)	10.3 (3.1; 24.4)	n.a.	–
Hematoma enlargement	5 (25.0)	n.a.	–
Perihematomal edema (ml)	23.0 (11.9; 61.5)	n.a.	–
Cytotoxic edema	9 (45.0)	n.a.	–

Data are presented as numbers (percentages) or median (interquartile range). $P < 0.05$ was considered statistically significant

CHD coronary heart disease, *CVD* cerebrovascular disease, *eGFR* estimated glomerular filtration rate, *IVH* intraventricular hematoma, *mRS* modified Rankin Scale, *NIHSS* National Institutes of Health Stroke Scale

were 74.65 μmol/L (interquartile range 63.70–91.43). Levels of ADMA, SDMA, and L-arginine with interquartile range for ICH patients are shown in Fig. 1a–c. ADMA levels were significantly increased at any time point in ICH patients compared to controls (≤ 24 h, $p < 0.001$; 3 days $p = 0.001$; 7 days, $p > 0.001$), while SDMA and L-arginine levels were not (Fig. 1a–c). However, L-arginine showed a trend for lower levels at ≤ 24 h ($p = 0.060$) and 3 days ($p = 0.063$).

The binary logistic regression analysis with co-variables age, and eGFR showed a significant elevation of ADMA levels at days 1, 3, and 7 in ICH patients compared to levels in controls (ADMA ≤ 24 h, $p = 0.003$; ADMA 3 days, $p = 0.005$; ADMA 7 days $p = 0.004$).

ADMA levels increased after the initial time point (≤ 24 h) until day 7 ($p = 0.030$) (Fig. 1a). SDMA levels decreased between the initial time point (≤ 24 h) and day 3 ($p = 0.029$) (Fig. 1b). No significant differences were seen for L-arginine levels in regard to the temporal evolution (Fig. 1c).

Dimethylarginines in relation to outcome

Patients were grouped according to mRS at 90 days as favorable (mRS 0–2) and unfavorable (mRS 3–6) outcome. Nine patients had favorable outcome, and 11 patients had unfavorable outcome. Outcome groups did not differ in regard to baseline characteristics and cardiovascular risk factors.

ADMA levels ≤ 24 h were significantly higher in patients with unfavorable than in patients with favorable outcome ($p = 0.031$) (Fig. 2a). SDMA levels at any time point were significantly elevated in patients with unfavorable outcome compared to those with favorable outcome (SDMA ≤ 24 h, $p = 0.016$; SDMA at 3 days, $p = 0.004$; SDMA at 7 days, $p = 0.031$) (Fig. 2b). For L-arginine, no significant differences were detected in regard to outcome groups (Fig. 2c).

The binary logistic regression analysis did not confirm increased ADMA levels ≤ 24 h in patients with unfavorable outcome ($p = 0.059$). Increased SDMA levels ≤ 24 h ($p = 0.048$) and at 3 days ($p = 0.028$) but not at 7 days ($p = 0.122$) remained significantly associated with unfavorable outcome.

Correlation analysis revealed a significant correlation of SDMA levels at ≤ 24 h and 3 days with mRS at 90 days, whereas SDMA at 7 days and ADMA levels ≤ 24 h only tended to correlate with mRS at 90 days (ADMA ≤ 24 h, $p = 0.088$; SDMA ≤ 24 h, $p = 0.029$; SDMA at 3 days, $p = 0.005$; SDMA at 7 days, $p = 0.081$) (Fig. 3a, b). At other time points, no association between ADMA, SDMA, or L-arginine and mRS at 90 days was detected.

Dimethylarginines in relation to secondary brain injury in ICH

Hematoma enlargement occurred in five patients and cytotoxic edema in nine patients (Table 1). To test the hypothesis that early levels of dimethylarginines (≤ 24 h) are associated with secondary brain injury, patients were grouped according to the median of hematoma and perihematomal edema volume as well as according to the occurrence of hematoma enlargement and cytotoxic

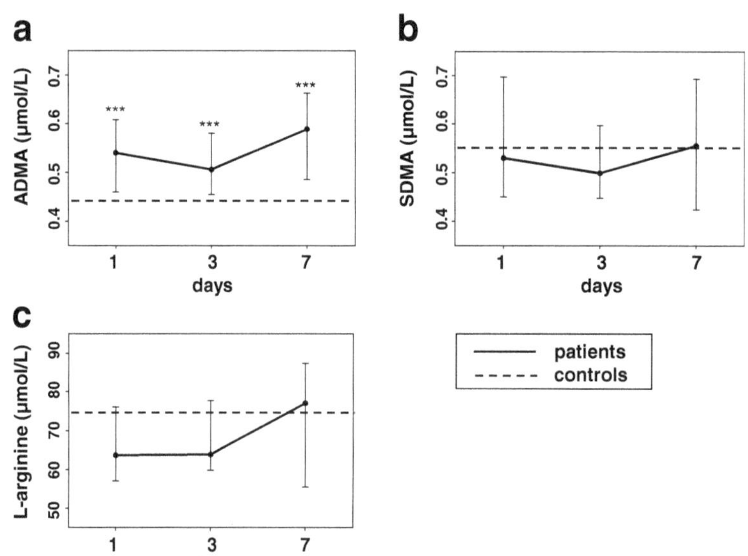

Fig. 1 a–c Time courses of ADMA, SDMA, and L-arginine in acute ICH. Data are presented as median (interquartile range). Values in controls are presented by dashed line. Differences between patients and controls: *** $p \leq 0.001$. Within group comparisons of marker levels between initial (≤ 24 h) and follow-up time points: significant differences were detected for ADMA (≤ 24 h versus 7 days; $p = 0.030$) and SDMA (≤ 24 h versus 3 days; $p = 0.029$)

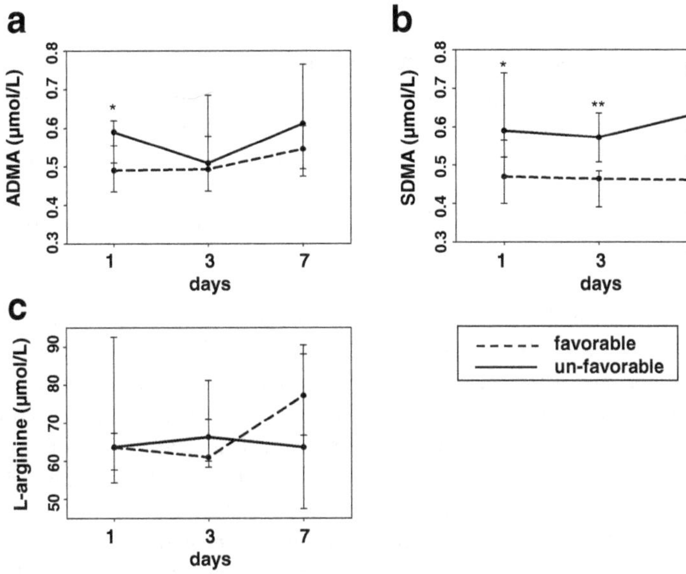

Fig. 2 a–c Comparison of time courses of ADMA, SDMA, and L-arginine after acute ICH in patients with favorable and unfavorable outcome. The data are presented as median (interquartile range). Differences between outcome groups: *$p \leq 0.05$; **$p \leq 0.01$

edema. Of note, these outcome groups did not differ in regard to baseline characteristics and cardiovascular risk factors.

In patients with higher hematoma volume (> median; $n = 10$), SDMA levels but not ADMA levels (≤ 24 h) were significantly higher compared to those with smaller hematoma volume (< median; $n = 10$) ($p = 0.029$). ADMA levels (≤ 24 h) were significantly higher in patients developing hematoma enlargement ($n = 5$) compared to patients without hematoma enlargement ($n = 13$) ($p = 0.003$). SDMA levels (≤ 24 h) were significantly higher in patients with larger perihematomal edema volume (> median; $n = 10$) compared to those with smaller perihematomal edema volume (< median; $n = 10$) ($p = 0.023$), while perihematomal edema mostly consists of vasogenic edema, in part of the patients cytotoxic edema, could be detected. In patients with occurrence of cytotoxic edema ($n = 9$), ADMA and SDMA levels (≤ 24 h) did not differ from those in patients without cytotoxic edema ($n = 11$).

Discussion

Our data show that (i) levels of ADMA are increased after acute ICH, (ii) higher levels of SDMA are associated with poor functional outcome, (iii) ADMA is associated with the occurrence of hematoma enlargement, and (iv) SDMA is associated with large hematoma and perihematomal edema volumes.

After ICH, inflammation, cellular damage, and proteolysis cause oxidative stress, which is known to increase protein arginine methyltransferase (PRMT) activity and decrease dimethylarginine dimethylaminohydrolase (DDAH) activity leading to elevated ADMA levels [20, 21]. In our study, ADMA levels but not SDMA levels were increased at each time point in ICH patients compared to controls. Of note,

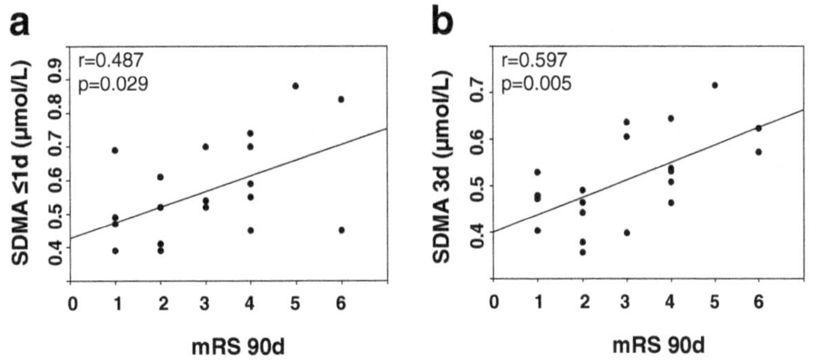

Fig. 3 a, b Correlation of SDMA ≤ 1 and 3 days with mRS at 90 days

Wanby et al. reported no increase of ADMA levels in 22 ICH patients [12]. But the design of both studies seems barely comparable. Wanby and colleagues took only one blood sample at an undefined time point during the first days after admission. However, in our study, ADMA levels were increased at each of the specified time points during the first week after the event. Therefore, differences in study results might not be related to the blood sampling schedule but to the patient cohort. We demonstrated an increase of ADMA in patients with poor outcome in the univariate analysis, while after adjustment for co-variables ADMA levels only tended to be associated with unfavorable outcome. Since Wanby et al. did not report clinical severity or outcome for their patients, it cannot be discussed if the difference between the study results might be due to differences in ICH severity. An association of ADMA levels with outcome might be explained by the larger extent of damage inducing more oxidative stress. Importantly, this hypothesis is supported by elevated ADMA levels in patients with hematoma enlargement. However, it remains unclear if ADMA is directly involved in the pathophysiology of hematoma enlargement. ADMA may trigger oxidative stress via uncoupling of endothelial NOS (eNOS) and iNOS resulting in production of the toxic compounds superoxide ($O_2\cdot^-$) and peroxynitrite ($ONOO\cdot^-$) [22, 23]. This may lead to further damage of the blood-brain barrier (BBB) facilitating hematoma enlargement. However, so far, direct evidence for ADMA-induced uncoupling of eNOS and iNOS is lacking for the cerebral circulation.

The continuous increase in ADMA levels between day 1 and day 7, as shown in our patient cohort, could possibly be explained by massive inflammation, proteolysis, and oxidative stress during the first days after ICH. Of note, follow-up data from a fraction of the patient cohort suggest that ADMA levels might be still elevated at day 90, although levels tended to decrease compared to those on day 7 (data not shown). However, so far, the length of and the reason for prolonged elevation of ADMA levels after ICH remain unclear.

Wanby et al. demonstrated lower levels of L-arginine in ICH patients than in controls [12]. In our study L-arginine--levels were also lower in the ICH patients than in the controls until day 3 after the event, but the level of significance was missed. Under conditions of L-arginine depletion, neuronal NOS (nNOS) synthesizes $O_2\cdot^-$ [24]. Therefore, it is suggested that lower levels of L-arginine in ICH patients result in increased $O_2\cdot^-$ production, potentially harming the zone of hypoperfusion surrounding the hematoma. Interestingly, addition of ADMA inhibited the nNOS-derived $O_2\cdot^-$ production [24]. This might indicate a beneficial effect of ADMA after ICH, potentially limiting the pathology of BBB damage. Another beneficial effect of ADMA might be reduction of perfusion by increase of vascular tone to lower the volume of bleeding. In healthy subjects, infusion of ADMA with 0.10 mg/kg/min significantly decreased cerebral blood flow [25].

These ADMA effects might be pronounced in patients with poor outcome and hematoma enlargement since in these patients, ADMA production following cellular damage and proteolysis is particularly high. However, since these secondary complications are particularly detrimental and cause poor outcome, obviously any discussed beneficial ADMA effect might not be sufficient.

After ICH, elevated ADMA levels might also affect systemic blood pressure. Experimental data in rats showed that microinjection of ADMA in the rostral ventrolateral medulla reduced NO synthesis and increased blood pressure [26]. Importantly, high blood pressure after ICH has been associated with poor clinical outcome and secondary complications such as hematoma enlargement [27]. In addition, high blood pressure variability is associated with unfavorable outcome, possibly due to secondary injury of hypoperfused tissue affected by perihematomal edema [28]. However, optimized clinical management such as early intensive blood pressure-lowering is still discussed [29]. In particular, any treatment directly influencing NO levels cannot be recommended due to insufficient evidence. Recently, a systematic review has investigated safety and efficacy of the NO donor transdermal glyceryl trinitrate when applied after stroke. Patients showed blood pressure lowering, but outcome was not ameliorated [30]. Of note, the analyzed studies included both ischemic and hemorrhagic stroke patients.

SDMA levels were not different between ICH patients and controls in the current study and in the study of Wanby and colleagues [12]. Importantly, the current study showed a significant association of SDMA levels with outcome at 90 days. Giving a hint that SDMA is involved in the pathophysiology after acute ICH, SDMA levels measured in blood samples from the first day after the event were significantly higher in patients with larger compared to those with smaller hematoma and perihematomal edema volume. However, studies explaining these associations are so far missing in acute ICH patients and only data from other pathologies can be discussed. Recently, Feliers et al. demonstrated in glomerular endothelial cells, that SDMA causes eNOS uncoupling [31], a mechanism resulting in increased ROS production. It remains unclear, whether SDMA leads to eNOS uncoupling also in acute ICH. In another study, SDMA triggered ROS synthesis of monocytes by modulation of store-operated calcium channels [11]. Another mechanism, by which SDMA may add to poor outcome after ICH could be via pro-inflammatory effects.

Inflammation during the acute stage of ICH is of particular importance. Recently, leukocyte counts and the neutrophil-to-lymphocyte ratio on admission have been shown to be associated with functional outcome in ICH patients potentially contributing to neurological deterioration via edema formation [32]. Interestingly, also in ischemic stroke patients who developed parenchymal hematoma or in patients with symptomatic ICH after thrombolytic treatment, the neutrophil-to-lymphocyte ratio is increased [33]. SDMA might be involved in increased inflammation after ICH since in monocytes, it triggers nuclear factor kappa-light-chain-enhancer of activated B cell (NF-kappaB) activation and tumor necrosis factor-alpha (TNF-alpha) and interleukin-6 (IL-6) expression [34]. However, to our knowledge the association between dimethylarginines and inflammation in ICH patients has not been studied so far.

Limitations

This study was the first to investigate the temporal pattern of dimethylarginine levels after ICH and their association with clinical outcomes. Due to the small number of patients included, it is necessary to confirm the results in a larger study. In addition, there is no evidence that the demonstrated association of dimethylarginines with functional and radiological outcome reflects a causative effect of these mediators in the pathophysiology of ICH. However, in the current study, elaborated serial MRI imaging provided detection of radiological outcome markers which cannot be achieved in routine clinical care. Thereby, the association of dimethylarginine levels with hematoma enlargement and perihematomal edema could be investigated. To confirm these data, a step from bedside to bench to elucidate the underlying mechanisms in experimental studies is warranted.

Conclusions

ADMA and SDMA levels are increased after the acute event of ICH in relation to outcome and might be--though differentially--involved in secondary brain injury such as hematoma enlargement and perihematomal edema. However, further studies are needed to elucidate the mechanisms behind to investigate if there is any causal relationship between dimethylarginine levels, inflammatory response to, and outcome of intracerebral hemorrhage.

Abbreviations

ADC: Apparent diffusion coefficient; ADMA: Asymmetric dimethylarginine; BBB: Blood-brain barrier; CHD: Coronary heart disease; CT: Computed tomography; CVD: Cerebrovascular disease; DDAH: Dimethylarginine dimethylaminohydrolase; DWI: Diffusion weighted imaging; eGFR: Estimated glomerular filtration rate; eNOS: Endothelial nitric oxide synthase; HE: Hematoma enlargement; HPLC-MS-MS: High-performance liquid chromatography-tandem mass spectrometry; ICH: Intracerebral hemorrhage; IL-6: Interleukin-6; iNOS: Inducible nitric oxide synthase; IVH: Intraventricular hematoma; MRI: Magnetic resonance imaging; mRS: Modified Rankin Scale; NF-kappaB: Nuclear factor kappa-light-chain-enhancer of activated B cells; NIHSS: National Institutes of Health Stroke Scale Score; nNOS: Neuronal nitric oxide synthase; NOS: Nitric oxide synthase inhibitor; $ONOO^-$: Peroxynitrite; $O_2^{.-}$: Superoxide; PRMT: Protein arginine methyltransferase; ROI: Region of interest; ROS: Reactive oxygen species; SAH: Subarachnoid hemorrhage; SDMA: Symmetric dimethylarginine; TNF-alpha: Tumor necrosis factor-alpha

Acknowledgements

The authors thank Frank Dsiosa, Klaus Burfeind, and Bernadette Lüns for excellent technical assistance.

Funding

None

Authors' contributions

HW contributed to the conception and design of the study, the data acquisition, analysis, and interpretation, and the drafting and revision of the manuscript. NL contributed to the conception and design of the study, the data acquisition, analysis, and interpretation, and the revision of the manuscript. JM, MD, RS, and RL contributed to the data acquisition, analysis and interpretation, and to the revision of the manuscript. JTK and HL contributed to the data analysis and interpretation and to the revision of the manuscript. PR and SMB contributed to the design of the study, the data acquisition, analysis and interpretation and to the revision of the manuscript. KW contributed to the conception and design of the study, the data analysis and interpretation, and the revision of the manuscript. All authors read and approved the final manuscript.

Consent for publication

Not applicable

Competing interests

The other authors declare that they have no competing interests.

Author details

[1]Department of Neurology, Hannover Medical School, 30623 Hannover, Germany. [2]Department of Neurology, Beijing Tiantan Hospital, Capital Medical University, Beijing, China. [3]Department of Clinical Pharmacology, Otto-von-Guericke-University of Magdeburg, University Hospital, Magdeburg, Germany. [4]Department of Clinical Chemistry, Hannover Medical School, Hannover, Germany. [5]Department of Nephrology and Hypertension, Hannover Medical School, Hannover, Germany. [6]Medical Clinic V, Academic Teaching Hospital Braunschweig, Braunschweig, Germany. [7]Institute of Diagnostic and Interventional Neuroradiology, Hannover Medical School, Hannover, Germany.

References

1. Van Asch CJ, Luitse MJ, Rinkel GJ, van der Tweel I, Algra A, Klijn CJ. Incidence, case fatality, and functional outcome of intracerebral haemorrhage over time, according to age, sex, and ethnic origin: a systematic review and meta-analysis. Lancet Neurol. 2010 Feb;9(2):167–76.
2. Ryu J, Pyo H, Jou I, Joe E. Thrombin induces NO release from cultured rat microglia via protein kinase C, mitogen-activated protein kinase, and NF-kappa B. J Biol Chem. 2000 Sep 29;275(39):29955–9.
3. Laird MD, Wakade C, Alleyne CH Jr, Dhandapani KM. Hemin-induced necroptosis involves glutathione depletion in mouse astrocytes. Free Radic Biol Med. 2008;45:1103–14.
4. Chiang MF, Chiu WT, Lin FJ, Thajeb P, Huang CJ, Tsai SH. Multiparametric analysis of cerebral substrates and nitric oxide delivery in cerebrospinal fluid

in patients with intracerebral haemorrhage: correlation with hemodynamics and outcome. Acta Neurochir. 2006;148:615–21.

5. Rashid PA, Whitehurst A, Lawson N, Bath PM. Plasma nitric oxide (nitrate/nitrite) levels in acute stroke and their relationship with severity and outcome. J Stroke Cerebrovasc Dis. 2003;12:82–7.
6. Nakajima T, Matsuoka Y, Kakimoto Y. Isolation and identification of N-G-monomethyl, N-G, N-G-dimethyl- and N-G, N' G-dimethylarginine from the hydrolysate of proteins of bovine brain. Biochim Biophys Acta. 1971 Feb 23; 230(2):212–22.
7. Lee DY, Teyssier C, Strahl BD, Stallcup MR. Role of protein methylation in regulation of transcription. Endocr Rev. 2005 Apr;26(2):147–70.
8. Vallance P, Leone A, Calver A, Collier J, Moncada S. Endogenous dimethylarginine as an inhibitor of nitric oxide synthesis. J Cardiovasc Pharmacol. 1992;20(Suppl 12):S60–2.
9. Chen S, Li N, Deb-Chatterji M, Dong Q, Kielstein JT, Weissenborn K, Worthmann H. Asymmetric dimethyarginine as marker and mediator in ischemic stroke. Int J Mol Sci 2012 Nov 28;13(12):15983-6004. Review.
10. Closs EI, Basha FZ, Habermeier A, Forstermann U. Interference of L-arginine analogues with L-arginine transport mediated by the y+ carrier hCAT-2B. Nitric Oxide. 1997;1:65–73.
11. Schepers E, Glorieux G, Dhondt A, Leybaert L, Vanholder R. Role of symmetric dimethylarginine in vascular damage by increasing ROS via store-operated calcium influx in monocytes. Nephrol Dial Transplant. 2009;24:1429–35.
12. Wanby P, Teerlink T, Brudin L, Brattstrom L, Nilsson I, Palmqvist P, et al. Asymmetric dimethylarginine (ADMA) as a risk marker for stroke and TIA in a Swedish population. Atherosclerosis. 2006;185:271–7.
13. Worthmann H, Chen S, Martens-Lobenhoffer J, Li N, Deb M, Tryc AB, Goldbecker A, Dong Q, Kielstein JT, Bode-Böger SM, Weissenborn K. High plasma dimethylarginine levels are associated with adverse clinical outcome after stroke. J Atheroscler Thromb. 2011;18(9):753–61.
14. Jung CS, Oldfield EH, Harvey-White J, Espey MG, Zimmermann M, Seifert V, et al. Association of an endogenous inhibitor of nitric oxide synthase with cerebral vasospasm in patients with aneurysmal subarachnoid hemorrhage. J Neurosurg. 2007;107:945–50.
15. Martens-Lobenhoffer J, Sulyok E, Czeiter E, Büki A, Kohl J, Firsching R, Tröger U, Bode-Böger SM. Determination of cerebrospinal fluid concentrations of arginine and dimethylarginines in patients with subarachnoid haemorrhage. J Neurosci Methods. 2007 Aug 15;164(1):155–60.
16. Li N, Worthmann H, Heeren M, Schuppner R, Deb M, Tryc AB, Bueltmann E, Lanfermann H, Donnerstag F, Weissenborn K, Raab P. Temporal pattern of cytotoxic edema in the perihematomal region after intracerebral hemorrhage: a serial magnetic resonance imaging study. Stroke. 2013 Apr;44(4):1144–6.
17. Phan TG, Chen J, Beare R, Ma H, Clissold B, Van Ly J, Srikanth V, VISTA-ICH Collaboration. Classification of different degrees of disability following intracerebral hemorrhage: a decision tree analysis from VISTA-ICH collaboration. Front Neurol. 2017 Feb 28;8:64.
18. Martens-Lobenhoffer J, Bode-Böger SM. Quantification of l-arginine, asymmetric dimethylarginine and symmetric dimethylarginine: a step improvement in precision by stable isotope dilution mass spectrometry. J Chromatogr B. 2012;904:140–3.
19. Burgess RE, Warach S, Schaewe TJ, Copenhaver BR, Alger JR, Vespa P, Martin N, Saver JL, Kidwell CS. Development and validation of a simple conversion model for comparison of intracerebral hemorrhage volumes measured on CT and gradient recalled echo MRI. Stroke. 2008 Jul;39(7):2017–20.
20. Leiper J, Murray-Rust J, McDonald N, Vallance P. S-nitrosylation of dimethylarginine dimethylaminohydrolase regulates enzyme activity: further interactions between nitric oxide synthase and dimethylarginine dimethylaminohydrolase. Proc Natl Acad Sci U S A. 2002 Oct 15;99(21):13527–32.
21. Sydow K, Münzel T. ADMA and oxidative stress. Atheroscler Suppl. 2003 Dec;4(4):41–51.
22. Wells SM, Holian A. Asymmetric dimethylarginine induces oxidative and nitrosative stress in murine lung epithelial cells. Am J Respir Cell Mol Biol. 2007 May;36(5):520–8.
23. Wadham C, Mangoni AA. Dimethylarginine dimethylaminohydrolase regulation: a novel therapeutic target in cardiovascular disease. Expert Opin Drug Metab Toxicol. 2009 Mar;5(3):303–19.
24. Cardounel AJ, Xia Y, Zweier JL. Endogenous methylarginines modulate superoxide as well as nitric oxide generation from neuronal nitric-oxide synthase: differences in the effects of monomethyl- and dimethylarginines in the presence and absence of tetrahydrobiopterin. J Biol Chem. 2005;280:7540–9.
25. Kielstein JT, Donnerstag F, Gasper S, Menne J, Kielstein A, Martens-Lobenhoffer J, Scalera F, Cooke JP, Fliser D, Bode-Böger SM. ADMA increases arterial stiffness and decreases cerebral blood flow in humans. Stroke. 2006 Aug;37(8):2024–9.
26. Tan X, Li JK, Sun JC, Jiao PL, Wang YK, Wu ZT, Liu B, Wang WZ. The asymmetric dimethylarginine-mediated inhibition of nitric oxide in the rostral ventrolateral medulla contributes to regulation of blood pressure in hypertensive rats. Nitric Oxide. 2017 Jul 1;67:58–67.
27. Rodriguez-Luna D, Piñeiro S, Rubiera M, Ribo M, Coscojuela P, Pagola J, Flores A, Muchada M, Ibarra B, Meler P, Sanjuan E, Hernandez-Guillamon M, Alvarez-Sabin J, Montaner J, Molina CA. Impact of blood pressure changes and course on hematoma growth in acute intracerebral hemorrhage. Eur J Neurol. 2013 Sep;20(9):1277–83.
28. Lattanzi S, Cagnetti C, Provinciali L, Silvestrini M. Blood pressure variability and clinical outcome in patients with acute Intracerebral hemorrhage. J Stroke Cerebrovasc Dis. 2015 Jul;24(7):1493–9.
29. Lattanzi S, Cagnetti C, Provinciali L, Silvestrini M. How should we lower blood pressure after cerebral hemorrhage? A systematic review and meta-analysis. Cerebrovasc Dis. 2017;43(5–6):207–13.
30. Bath PM, Krishnan K, Appleton JP. Nitric oxide donors (nitrates), L-arginine, or nitric oxide synthase inhibitors for acute stroke. Cochrane Database Syst Rev. 2017 Apr 21;4:CD000398.
31. Feliers D, Lee DY, Gorin Y, Kasinath BS. Symmetric dimethylarginine alters endothelial nitric oxide activity in glomerular endothelial cells. Cell Signal. 2015 Jan;27(1):1–5.
32. Lattanzi S, Cagnetti C, Provinciali L, Silvestrini M. Neutrophil-to-lymphocyte ratio predicts the outcome of acute intracerebral hemorrhage. Stroke. 2016 Jun;47(6):1654–7.
33. Guo Z, Yu S, Xiao L, Chen X, Ye R, Zheng P, Dai Q, Sun W, Zhou C, Wang S, Zhu W, Liu X. Dynamic change of neutrophil to lymphocyte ratio and hemorrhagic transformation after thrombolysis in stroke. J Neuroinflammation. 2016 Aug 26;13(1):199.
34. Schepers E, Barreto DV, Liabeuf S, Glorieux G, Eloot S, Barreto FC, Massy Z, Vanholder R, European Uremic Toxin Work Group (EUTox). Symmetric dimethylarginine as a proinflammatory agent in chronic kidney disease. Clin J Am Soc Nephrol. 2011 Oct;6(10):2374–83.

9

RAS modulation prevents progressive cognitive impairment after experimental stroke

Heba A. Ahmed[1], Tauheed Ishrat[2], Bindu Pillai[1], Abdelrahman Y. Fouda[1], Mohammed A. Sayed[1], Wael Eldahshan[1], Jennifer L. Waller[5], Adviye Ergul[1,3] and Susan C. Fagan[1,4*]

Abstract

Background: With the aging population, the prevalence and incidence of cerebrovascular disease will continue to rise, as well as the number of individuals with vascular cognitive impairment/dementia (VCID). No specific FDA-approved treatments for VCID exist. Although clinical evidence supports that angiotensin receptor blockers (ARBs) prevent cognitive decline in older adults, whether ARBs have a similar effect on VCID after stroke is unknown. Moreover, these agents reduce BP, which is undesirable in the acute stroke period, so we believe that giving C21 in this acute phase or delaying ARB administration would enable us to achieve the neurovascular benefits without the risk of unintended and potentially dangerous, acute BP lowering.

Methods: The aim of our study was to determine the impact of candesartan (ARB) or compound-21 (an angiotensin type 2 receptor-–AT2R-–agonist) on long-term cognitive function post-stroke, in spontaneously hypertensive rats (SHRs). We hypothesized that AT2R stimulation, either directly with C21, or indirectly by blocking the angiotensin type 1 receptor (AT1R) with candesartan, initiated after stroke, would reduce cognitive impairment. Animals were subjected to a 60-min transient middle cerebral artery occlusion and randomly assigned to either saline/C21 monotherapy, for the full study duration (30 days), or given sequential therapy starting with saline/C21 (7 days) followed by candesartan for the remainder of the study (21 days). Outcome measures included sensorimotor/cognitive-function, amyloid-β determination, and histopathologic analyses.

Results: Treatment with RAS modulators effectively preserved cognitive function, reduced cytotoxicity, and prevented chronic-reactive microgliosis in SHRs, post-stroke. These protective effects were apparent even when treatment was delayed up to 7 days post-stroke and were independent of blood pressure and β-amyloid accumulation.

Conclusion: Collectively, our findings demonstrate that RAS modulators effectively prevent cognitive impairment after stroke, even when treatment is delayed.

Keywords: Angiotensin modulators, Cognitive-impairment, Hypertension, Stroke

* Correspondence: sfagan@uga.edu
[1]Program in Clinical and Experimental Therapeutics, Charlie Norwood VA Medical Center and University of Georgia College of Pharmacy, HM Bldg., 1120 15th St, Augusta, GA 30912, USA
[4]Department of Neurology, Augusta University, Augusta, GA, USA
Full list of author information is available at the end of the article

Background

Vascular cognitive impairment/dementia (VCID), which defines alterations in cognition attributable to cerebrovascular causes regardless of pathogenesis or severity [1, 2], is an extremely common and debilitating, albeit understudied, long-term complication of stroke, impacting nearly 30–40% of all stroke survivors [3]. The severity of VCI can range from subtle cognitive deficits to overt dementia [4]. At a time when stroke mortality is going down, the rate of stroke-related dementia almost doubled between 1990 and 2000 [5]. Unlike sensorimotor deficits, which are often maximal in the hours following stroke and tend to gradually improve, cognitive deficits increase over time, in both patients [6] and experimental animal models [7]. Until recently, it was thought that vascular dementia develops in a step-wise fashion, due to repeated ischemic events, but recent data from a large, NIH-funded, epidemiologic trial proved that patients often experience a slowly progressive cognitive decline after a single-stroke lesion, in addition to an acute change [3, 5]. This continuous deterioration occurs even in the absence of any new stroke lesions [8].

Unfortunately, no FDA-approved treatments exist for VCID, increasing the urgency for treatment development in this area, as identifying drug therapies that target the pathological processes associated with progressive VCID continues to be a vital unmet need [9].

One of the most important risk factors for development and progression of cognitive impairment and dementia is hypertension [5, 10]. Hypertension, which is associated with vascular dysfunction, has been established to increase the risk of dementia both independently and by increasing the risk of stroke. In fact, hypertension alone can predict the development of dementia in nearly 60% of subjects with executive dysfunction [11].

Even with Alzheimer's disease (AD), vascular dysfunction may be of greater importance than amyloid accumulation in terms of influencing the disease course, especially in older individuals [5, 7]. Likewise, vascular brain injury is now considered a very early, and perhaps initial, pathogenic mechanism not only in VCID but also in AD [8].

Angiotensin II (Ang II), the major effector/ligand of the intrinsic brain renin angiotensin system (RAS), is a neuropeptide produced mostly by glial cells in the CNS [12] and targets the brain's two major receptor subtypes AT1R and AT2R, both primarily expressed in the vasculature [13]. Hyperactivation of brain AT1R is responsible for the damaging effects associated with RAS as it promotes vasoconstriction, reduces CBF, and increases oxidative stress and vulnerability to ischemia, in addition to promoting vascular and tissue inflammation and exacerbating neurodegeneration [12].

Our group has shown that ARBs, by indirectly stimulating brain AT2Rs, are both vascular and neuroprotective after ischemic stroke [14]. These agents also effectively preserved cognitive function and prevented the development/progression of VCID in aged animals with chronic cerebral hypoperfusion [15]. Stimulation of the AT2R has emerged as a novel therapeutic strategy in vascular and CNS diseases by virtue of its anti-inflammatory, neuroprotective, and tissue-regenerating properties [6, 8]. In our recent large, randomized preclinical trial of the AT2R agonist, compound 21, although neuroprotection was modest, we found a consistent benefit of C21 on cognition after stroke [16]. The purpose of this investigation was to determine the impact of RAS modulation on the development of cognitive impairment after stroke in hypertensive animals, as a proposed model of VCID.

Clinical trial evidence supports that ARBs, when used for the treatment of hypertension, prevent cognitive and functional decline in older adults and lower the risk of dementia and AD [2, 11, 17]. Unfortunately, these agents also reduce blood pressure (BP), an AT1R effect which is undesirable in the acute stroke period (first 7 days) [18]. This is because during the acute phase post-stroke, a fall in BP may lead to an excessive reduction in cerebral perfusion, and is especially true with long-standing hypertension, due to associated impairments in cerebrovascular autoregulation. Moreover, based on the findings of the large clinical (SCAST) study, significant acute reductions in BP with candesartan should be avoided, to allow perfusion through collateral vessels and optimize salvage of penumbral tissue post-stroke [18]. We hence decided to initiate treatment with candesartan, only after the first 7 days (replacing C21 or saline). This approach was taken in order to harness the neurovascular benefits of AT2 receptor stimulation with C21, in the acute phase, while avoiding the early antihypertensive effects of candesartan, and to model what could be an effective strategy in clinical practice.

Methods

Experimental design, animals, and treatment

As summarized in Fig. 1, this was a 2 × 2, randomized, double-blind (investigators and statistician), preclinical trial. In total, we used 41 young adult (4 months old), male SHRs, weighing 290–300 g, obtained from Charles River Laboratories. Of these animals, 33 were subjected to a 60-min temporary middle cerebral artery occlusion (tMCAO) and 8 animals were exposed to sham surgery. Animals were housed in a pathogen-free environment with free access to food and water on a 12-h light/dark cycle before and after surgery. All animals exposed to 60 min of temporary middle cerebral artery occlusion (tMCAO) were randomized, after reperfusion, using a random number generator, to one of 4 groups. Animals received either C21 (0.03 mg/kg/day) (VicorePharma, G teborg, Sweden) or saline, initiated IP 2 h after the

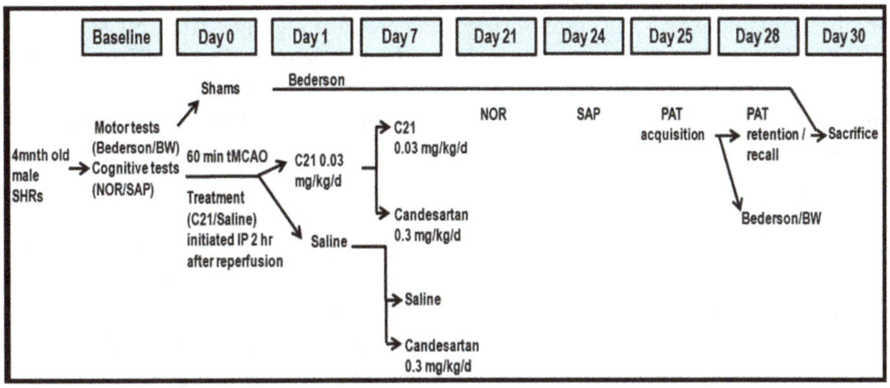

Fig. 1 Schematic time-line and description of the experimental design. This was a long-term 2 × 2, randomized, double-blind preclinical trial aimed to study the impact of RAS modulation, after stroke, on long-term cognitive function in spontaneously hypertensive rats (SHRs)

onset of reperfusion, and continued for a total of 7 days, after which the animals were either switched to a low dose of candesartan (0.3 mg/kg) IP or continued with their initial treatments (C21 or saline), daily for the remainder of the study. Treatments were prepared in identical syringes by an investigator not involved in the administration or assessment of the animals and unblinding only occurred after all data was collected and analyzed. The entire set of data was reported, and included in the final data analyses, for each and every animal that survived and completed all the necessary behavioral tests in the study, without exclusion of any animals/data points. Therefore, all the animals that started the study, with the exception of the 3 animals that did not complete any of the behavioral tests (one animal died at 24 h, the other 2 did not survive past 9 days post-stroke due to excessive weight loss) successfully completed the study and were included in the final analyses. Animal experiments were conducted and reported in accordance with the *Animal Research: Reporting of In Vivo Experiments (ARRIVE)*, *Stroke Therapy Academic Industry Roundtable* (*STAIR*), and Reporting Guidelines for Risk Models (RiGoR) guidelines [13–15].

Focal cerebral ischemia

The skin on the cervical region was incised to access the common carotid artery, under anesthesia maintained at 3% isoflurane mixed with 30% oxygen and 70% nitrogen. Ischemia/reperfusion injury was achieved by occluding the middle cerebral artery (MCA) using 4–0 silicon-coated nylon suture with rounded tip, which was inserted into external carotid artery and advanced through internal carotid artery until it blocked the origin of the MCA. Successful MCAO was confirmed by the presence of hemiparesis prior to reperfusion. After the 60-min occlusion, animals were re-anesthetized and sutures removed to allow reperfusion of ischemic brain areas. Animals were returned to their home cages after MCAO with easy access to food and water [14].

Assessment of functional outcome

Body weight

Weight monitoring gives an independent and unambiguous measure of an animal's overall health and welfare [19]. For our studies, animals were weighed before surgery and then daily after stroke until the day of sacrifice.

Blood pressure monitoring

To study the effect of different doses of C21 (0.1, 0.03, 0.06 mg/kg/day) and candesartan (0.3, 1 mg/kg/day) on BP, a separate set of animals (6 adult male SHRs) was monitored using continuous BP telemetry. Blood pressure was monitored before tMCAO, after occlusion and following reperfusion, using continuous BP telemetry with transmitters (Data Sciences International, St Paul, MN, USA). These were implanted in rats, under 3–5% isoflurane inhalation anesthesia, as reported previously according to the manufacturer's specifications [20]. In brief, a midline incision was performed to expose the abdominal aorta, which was shortly occluded to allow insertion of the transmitter catheter, which was secured in place using tissue glue. The incision was closed using non-absorbable suture (3–0). Rats were returned to their individual cages and allowed to recover from surgery for 10 days. By placing cages on top of the telemetry receivers, arterial pressure waveforms were continuously recorded throughout the study. These animals were later treated with increasing doses of C21 (0.01, 0.03, 0.06 mg/kg/day). Each dose was given for three consecutive days and followed up by a 24-h washout period before initiation of the next dosage increment. After the final washout, the animals were treated with two different doses of candesartan 0.3 and 1 mg/kg/day (separated by a 48-h washout period). The following week animals underwent a 60-min tMCAO and were given saline/C21

(0.03 mg/kg/d) for 7 days followed by candesartan (0.3 mg/kg/d) for the remainder of the monitoring period [20].

Neurobehavioral testing

All neurobehavioral tests were conducted, recorded, and analyzed in a blinded manner.

Sensorimotor testing

To assess sensorimotor function, animals underwent Bederson and beam walk tests at baseline and at day 1 and day 28 post-stroke.

Bederson score Animals were assigned a score from 0 to 3, given one point for each of the following: forelimb flexion, diminished resistance to lateral push, and contralateral circling with lower scores indicating better performance [21].

Beam walk Animals were placed on a horizontal beam (60 cm long, 4.5 cm wide) for 60 s and assigned a score from 0 to 6 as follows: balances on the beam with a steady posture = 0, grasps side of the beam = 1, hugs the beam with 1 limb falling = 2, hugs the beam with two limbs falling = 3, falls off the beam within 40–60 s = 4, falls off the beam within 20–40 s = 5, and falls off the beam in less than 20 s = 6 [14].

Memory, cognitive, and neurobehavioral testing

Cognitive tests were performed at baseline and prior to sacrifice at 30 days. In a subset of animals treated with either saline or C21, cognition (novel object recognition--NOR) was tested at 14 and 21 days. The NOR and spontaneous alternation performance (SAP) tests were performed to evaluate non-spatial and spatial working memories [22–25], respectively, while the passive avoidance test (PAT) assessed associative learning and reference memory [26, 27].

The novel object recognition (NOR) test

The NOR test was performed to evaluate non-spatial working memory related to frontal-subcortical circuits [22]. This test was based on the spontaneous tendency of animals to interact with a novel object more than a familiar one, and consisted of 2 trials separated by a retention period and preceded by a habituation phase. The habituation phase was conducted on 2 separate days, before the start of the test, to allow animals to acclimate to their arena, which consisted of placing them in an empty standard size box for 15 min. On the designated test day, animals were first subjected to an acquisition/sample trial, where the animal is presented with 2 identical (sample) objects and allowed to explore for 10 min [28, 29]. Following sample object exposure, the animal was returned to its home cage for a 1-h retention period. The 2nd preference trial/test session (5 min), which follows the retention period, was conducted in the same manner as the 1st trial, except that a new/novel object replaces one of the familiar/sample objects. The arena and objects were cleaned after each session with 70% ethanol. The time spent in exploring each object during the preference trial/test session was recorded and the discrimination index, which is the difference in exploration time for the objects divided by total time of exploration, was calculated. The discrimination index (DI) and the recognition index (RI), which is the time spent exploring the novel object relative to the total time of exploration, were taken as indicators of working memory [28, 30].

$$\text{Discrimination index (DI)} = (T_N - T_F)/(T_N + T_F)$$

$$\text{Recognition index (RI)} = T_N/(T_N + T_F)$$

- Time spent interacting with the familiar object ($\mathbf{T_F}$)
- Time spent interacting with the novel object ($\mathbf{T_N}$)

All animals passed the required exploratory criteria, exploring the objects for > 4 out of the 5 min. All the objects to be discriminated were unified between animals and chosen according to recommendations of Heyser and Chemero; they were symmetrical and transparent, and made of odorless, durable, and easy to clean plastic and glass [24].

The spontaneous alternation performance (SAP) test

The SAP test evaluates spatial working memory using a spontaneous alternation paradigm, which also takes advantage of rodents' natural preference for environmental novelty. Assessment was performed using a typical Y-maze apparatus, with 3 equidistant arms of similar size and dimensions (50 × 10 × 19 cm) each having acrylic walls adorned with specific motifs, serving as visual cues to aid in spatial navigation. After introduction to the center of the maze, the animal was allowed to freely explore all 3 arms. Over the course of multiple arm entries, the subject should show a tendency to enter the least recently visited arm and thus tend to alternate visits between the 3 arms. The number of arm entries and the number of triads are recorded in order to calculate the percentage of alternation. An entry occurs when all four limbs are within the arm. The SAP was assessed by scoring the pattern of entries into each arm during the 5-min test. Alternations were defined as successive entries into each of the 3 arms as on overlapping triplet sets (i.e., ABC, BCA). %SAP is defined as the ratio of actual (= total alternations) to possible (= total arm entries-2) number of alternations × 100 [23].

The passive avoidance test (PAT)

The inhibitory avoidance (IA) test (commonly referred to as passive avoidance test) was used to assess aversive associative learning and related reference memory. This test is designed to condition against an animal's urge to enter a dark chamber or explore a novel compartment, when exposed to an aversive stimulus [25]. The animal must therefore "actively inhibit" its desire and withhold the response, to re-enter a dark or novel compartment, after it has experienced an aversive stimulus in that location. For this test, one of the compartments of the Y-maze was equipped with a metal floor connected to an electric circuit box, adjusted to deliver brief, moderate intensity electric shocks (3 s duration, 0.6–1 mA). For the acquisition trial, the shock compartment/arm was blocked and the animal placed in one of the "safe" arms and allowed 10 min to explore the 2 open arms. Upon completion of 10 min, the door blocking the shock arm was opened allowing the animal to enter. Once the animal had fully entered the shock arm, its initial latency was recorded and it received a brief electric shock before being returned to its cage. After a 72-h retention period, the test trial was conducted. This was performed in a manner similar to that of the acquisition trial except that the foot shock was omitted and all 3 arms were accessible to the animal from the start. The difference, between training and test sessions, in latency for entering into the desired compartment (shock arm) was used as a measure of retention. This latency was recorded for up to 300 s, as the index of long-term aversive associative memory consolidation [20–22].

Animal sacrifice and tissue collection

At day 30, animals were anesthetized with IP ketamine/xylazine and transcardially perfused with 300 ml of ice cold PBS. Animals were decapitated, and their brains collected. Sections A and B, from brain matrix, were snap frozen and kept for ELISA. The remaining brain tissue was immersed in 10% formalin (Fischer Scientific, Waltham, MA, USA) for 48 h and then transferred to a 30% sucrose solution until taken for sectioning [14].

Immunofluorescent staining and confocal microscopy

Frozen brain sections (5 μm thick) were processed and stained following a standard technique as previously described [14]. Briefly, sections were heated in 10 mM sodium citrate buffer (pH 6) and then washed in TBS plus 0.025%/Triton X-100 with gentle agitation, blocked for 2 h in 10% normal goat serum/1% BSA, and incubated overnight at 4 °C with Alexa fluor 488 anti-amyloid-β1–16 (6E10; 1:1000; Biolegend) or anti-ionized calcium-binding adapter molecule-1 (Iba-1; 1:1000; Wako). After washing, slides were incubated with their appropriate fluorophore-conjugated goat secondary antibodies (1:1000; Abcam) for 1 h at room temperature and washed and cover-slipped with Vectashield mounting medium (Vector Laboratories, Burlingame, California, USA). Images were taken using Zeiss LSM 510 confocal microscope (Carl Zeiss).

Histopathologic analyses and quantification

The number of activated microglia, determined by Iba-1 staining, and degree of apoptotic cell death, determined by the ApopTag fluorescein in situ apoptosis detection kit [S7110, Chemicon (Millipore), Temecula, CA], in the ischemic borderzone region of the ipsilateral hemisphere for each brain section, was quantified using ImageJ software (NIH), in 3 different fields per section, digitized with a ×20 objective lens [14]. To quantitatively characterize microglia morphology, we used the particle measurement feature in ImageJ to automatically measure the 2D area, perimeter and Feret's diameter which is the greatest distance between any two points along the cell perimeter. This is a measure of cell length and serves partly as an indicator of microglial phenotype. We also evaluated other parameters including circularity and transformation index, [perimeter of cell (μm)]^2/4π [cell area(μm^2)], which reflect the degree of process extension and serve as established indicators categorizing microglial ramification status [23–25].

Protein expression

Quantitative determination of $A\beta_{1-42}$ concentrations in cortical and hippocampal lysates were carried out, using a rat specific sandwich amyloid-β ELISA kit (Wako, USA), according to manufacturer's protocol.

Endothelial cell culture and treatments

Amyloid-β ($A\beta_{1-42}$) preparation

Synthetic $A\beta_{1-42}$ was prepared to form soluble oligomeric peptides for endothelial cell culture studies, according to manufacturer's recommendations (AnaSpec, San Jose, CA, USA). The end product was a clear homogenous preparation, free from insoluble aggregates. Absence of aggregates or fibrils was confirmed under microscope.

Oxygen and glucose deprivation (OGD)

Human cerebral microvascular endothelial cells (hCMEC/D3), generously donated by Dr. J Zastre (University of Georgia), were cultured to confluence in normal oxygen/glucose, MCDB-131 complete medium (VEC Technologies, Rensselaer, NY). To mimic in vivo ischemia-reperfusion, these cells were subjected to 8 h OGD by incubation in glucose-free DMEM (GIBCO), at 37 °C in a hypoxia chamber (ProOx model C21; BioSpherix, Lacona, NY) with an

O_2 concentration of 1% and CO_2 of 5%, followed by 16 h of standard normoxic conditions (95% air, 5% CO_2) and replacing the glucose-free DMEM with serum-free Eagle's minimum essential medium (EMEM; American Type Culture Collection, Manassas, VA, USA), in the presence or absence of $A\beta_{1-42}$ (100 nM) with or without treatment, using angiogenic concentrations of C21 (100 nM, 1000 nM) [14] or candesartan (1 µg/ml, 10 µg/ml), before being subjected to the MTT cell viability assay [31].

Mitochondrial tetrazole test (MTT)

The extent of cell death was determined indirectly by the MTT cell viability assay. This test is based on the ability of living, metabolically active, cells to reduce a yellow tetrazole compound, 3-(4,5-dimethylthiazol-2-yl)-2,5-diphenyltetrazolium bromide, into an insoluble purple formazan product, with an absorbance maximum at 570 nm, measured using a microplate reader (Synergy HT, BioTek, VT, USA). Intensity of color formation/absorbance serves as a marker of cell viability [32].

Statistical analysis

All behavioral analysis was performed using SAS 9.4 by a blinded statistician, and statistical significance was assessed using an alpha level of 0.05, unless otherwise noted. Repeated measures mixed models were used to examine differences in outcomes between the five groups (SHAM, Stroke Saline, Stroke C21, Stroke Candesartan, and Stroke C21 + Candesartan) over days (0 and 21 days for NOR measures; 25 and 28 days for PAT). For each outcome, the mixed model contained fixed effects of group, day, and the two-factor interaction between group and day. Animal nested within group was considered a random effect. As there were only two measurement times, an unstructured correlation structure was used to model the correlation between days. The F-test for the two-factor interaction between group and day was the statistical test of interest and, if statistically significant, indicates that the changes in the outcomes over time are different in the five groups. Post hoc, pair-wise comparisons between groups over time were performed using a Bonferroni adjustment to the overall alpha level. To examine differences in weight over a 31-day period (from pre-surgery, 0 to 30 day following surgery) between Candesartan and C21 groups (Candesartan/C21, Candesartan/Saline, C21/Saline, Saline/Saline), a quadratic growth curve model was utilized. Fixed effects in the model included Candesartan and C21. Day was considered a continuous variable. Random effects included the intercept, linear day term, and the quadratic day^2 term. An unstructured variance co-variance structure provided the best model fit. The interaction between Candesartan, C21 and the quadratic day term and the interaction between Candesartan and the quadratic day term which were not statistically significant were removed from the model. Statistical significance for differences between groups for specific days (0, 1, 7, 10, 30) were examined using the estimated least squares means from a repeated measures mixed model and denoted by $^*P < 0.0001$, using a Bonferroni adjustment to the overall α-level for the number of post hoc pair-wise comparisons performed within group between measurement days and within days between groups was used to control for the number of tests performed. Differences between groups in immunostaining experiments were examined using ANOVA followed by Tukey test for post hoc analysis using GraphPad prism software (5.1). Exact power calculations were not performed in this study as the effect size could not be accurately estimated due to lack of previous studies utilizing these specific groups.

Results

Compound 21 had no effect on BP in SHRs before or after stroke

Stroke increased BP from baseline by over 30 mmHg in SHRs after a 60-min tMCAO. This was reduced slightly after reperfusion, but remained elevated for at least 24 h. This is similar to the trend we had previously observed after a 3-h tMCAO in both SHRs [20] and Wistar rats [14]. In SHRs, C21 treatment had no effect on BP compared to saline either before or after stroke (Fig. 2). Doses of 0.03 mg/kg/day C21 and 0.3 mg/kg/d candesartan were chosen based on our preliminary findings and previous publications [8, 33]. These doses were shown to have superior cognitive benefits than other doses when administered intraperitoneally, with little or no effect on BP. Moreover, C21 when administered daily, starting at 2 h after tMCAO and reperfusion, significantly ameliorated weight loss at day 7, compared to saline-treated controls (Additional file 1), with animals showing most rapid weight recovery, between days 7 and 30, when treatment was followed with candesartan.

All animals experienced complete motor recovery after transient ischemic stroke

Hypertensive animals subjected to a 60-min tMCAO showed visible sensorimotor deficits within the first few hours of stroke. These deficits, marked with high Bederson and beam walk scores (Fig. 3a), were pronounced at 24 h post-stroke, and all treatment groups showed similar recovery at 28 days post-stroke.

RAS modulation effectively prevented cognitive decline post-stroke

Sham animals did not demonstrate cognitive decline at 28 days. Despite complete recovery of sensorimotor function, the saline-treated animals demonstrated a

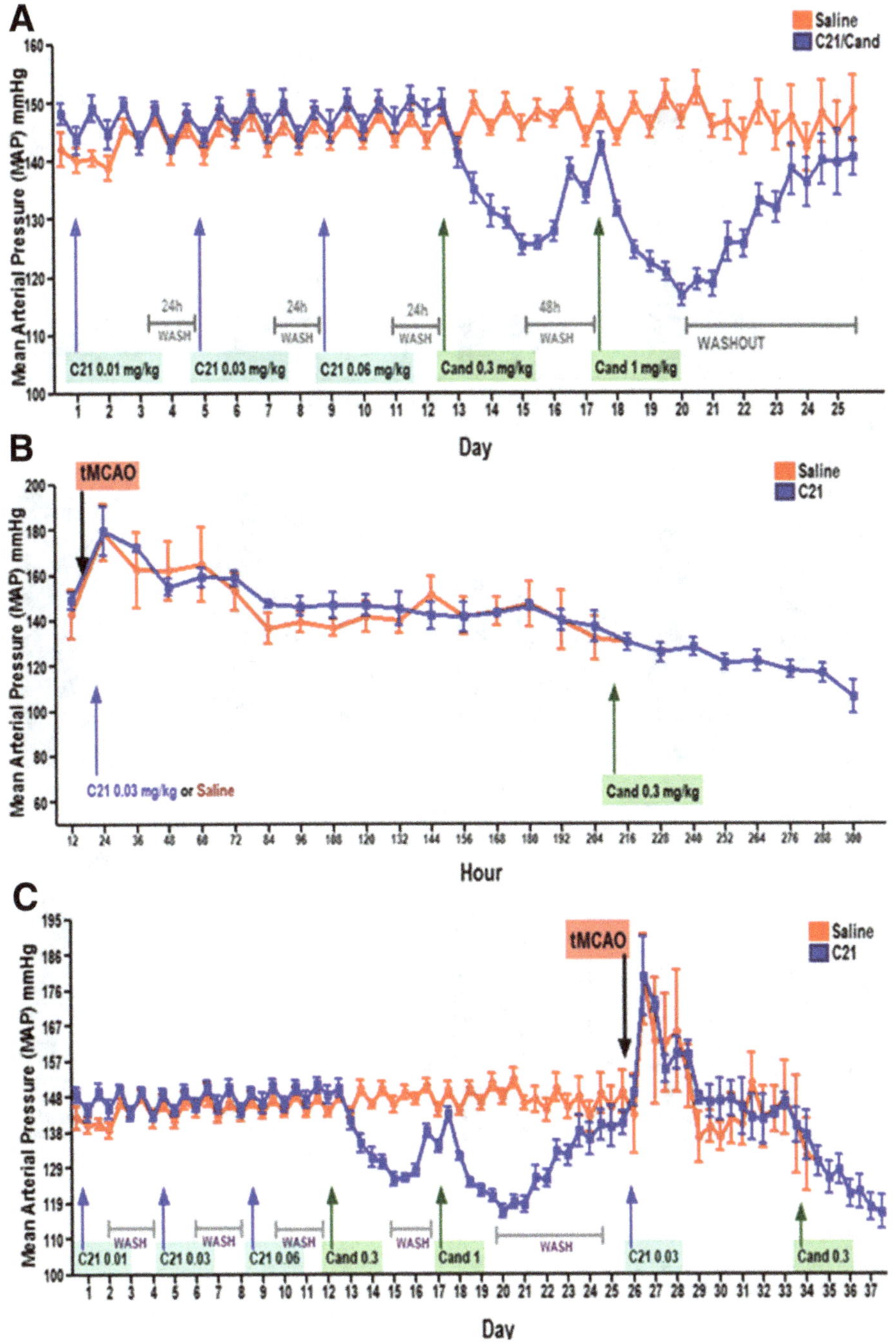

Fig. 2 Compound 21 had no effect on blood pressure in SHRs after a 60-min tMCAO. **a** Mean arterial pressure (MAP), as measured by telemetry, showed no effect of C21 on BP, in unstroked animals. **b** There was an increase in MAP from baseline after transient middle cerebral artery occlusion (tMCAO) and this was not affected by C21 administration 2 h after reperfusion, and the average BP trend was similar for both C21 and saline-treated animals. **c** Figure depicting complete MAP trend, before and after tMCAO, with the effect of treatments administered at different points in time

continuous decline in cognition from days 14 to 28 (Additional file 2). Chronic administration of C21, or candesartan, prevented this decline, even when treatment was initiated at 7 days after the ischemic insult. The groups treated with C21 and candesartan demonstrated superior performance on the NOR test, compared to saline-treated animals (Fig. 3b). In fact, most of the C21 and candesartan-treated animals showed discrimination and recognition indices that were not much different from their original baseline pre-stroke values. These animals also tended to display more efficient SAP, indicating better spatial working

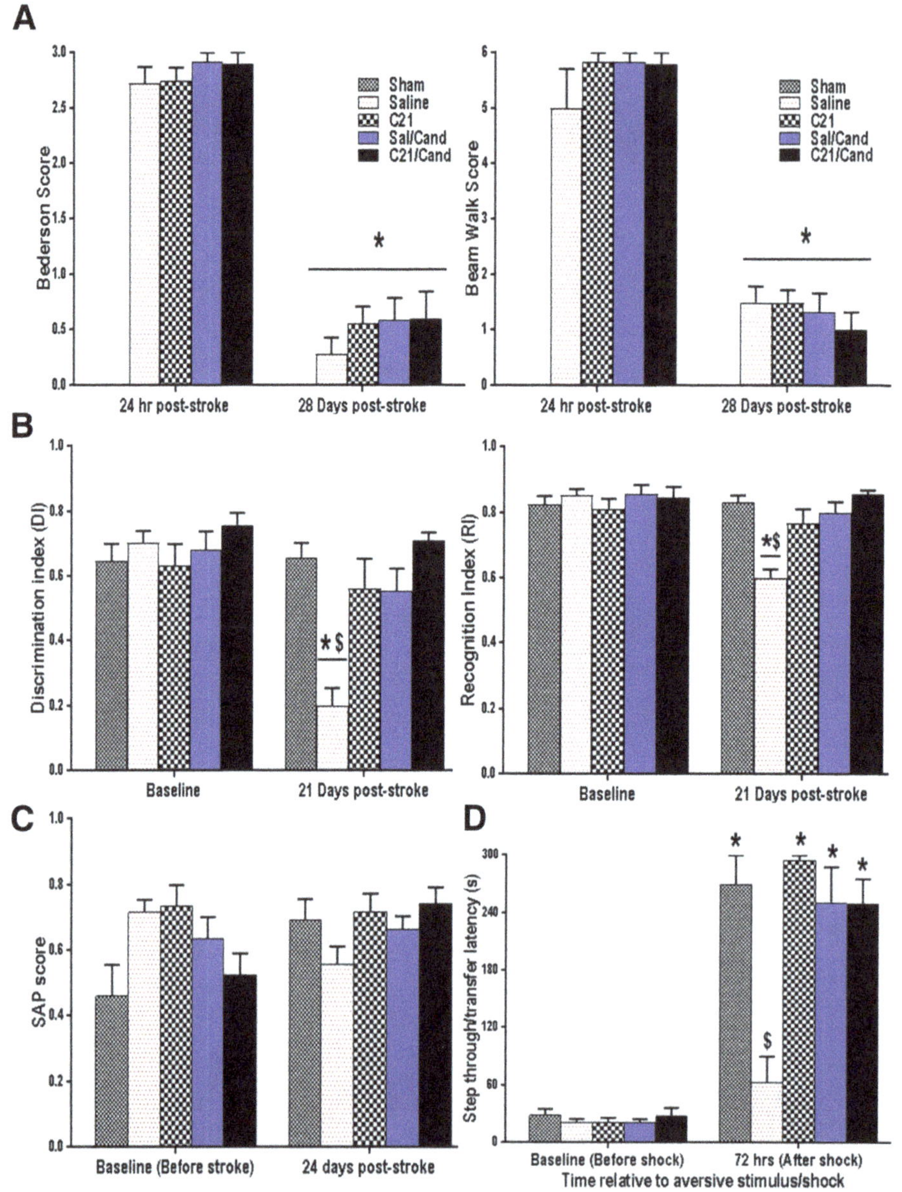

Fig. 3 RAS modulation improved learning and preserved spatial, non-spatial working, and long-term reference memories despite lack of effect on long-term motor recovery post-stroke. **a** All animals showed a significant recovery of sensorimotor function, as measured by Bederson (C21 × candesartan × time interaction $F_{(1,48)} = 0.22$, $P = 0.6384$) and Beam walk (C21 × candesartan × time interaction $F_{(1,31)} = 0.41$, $P = 0.5278$), at 28 days post-stroke, irrespective of their assigned treatment group. On the other hand, **b** for the novel object recognition (NOR) test, saline-treated animals showed a significant reduction in discrimination index (DI) and recognition index (RI), compared to their baseline values as well as to all other groups post-stroke, while sham and C21/candesartan-treated animals retained their ability to recognize the novel object during the preference trial indicating preserved non-spatial working memory (group × time interaction $F_{(1,30)} = 14.58$, $P < 0.0001$). **c** Spontaneous alternation performance (SAP) was also noticeably better for these animals with plots of the means from baseline to 24 days showing distinctive changes within each group, shams, and candesartan/C21-treated groups having either no change from baseline or an increased SAP, while the saline group showed a clear decrease in SAP from 0 to 24 days indicating worsened spatial working memory (C21 × candesartan × time interaction $F_{(1,17)} = 0.12$, $P = 0.7314$). **d** On the passive avoidance test (PAT), sham animals and those treated with C21/candesartan showed significantly enhanced step-through latency, indicating better memory retention and recall of the association between properties of the chamber and the foot shock, compared to their saline-treated counterparts. (group × time interaction $F_{(1,39)} = 19.00$, $P < 0.0001$). For all tests $n = 5$–10 animals/group, error bars indicate SEM. Statistical significance is denoted by *$P < 0.0001$ for post hoc pair-wise comparisons from baseline and **#**$P < 0.0001$ for post hoc pair-wise comparisons "between groups" post-stoke, using the Bonferroni-adjusted alpha

memory (Fig. 3c), and exhibited significantly higher transfer/step-through latencies on the PAT retention as compared to the acquisition trials (Fig. 3d). This not only indicates an intact reference memory, with retention of the aversive event, it also signifies effectual associative learning and recall of the connection between properties of the chamber and the foot shock. The saline-treated animals, however, exhibited compromised learning and memory as they failed to show any meaningful increase in transfer/step-through latency on the retention trial.

C21 prevented accumulation of $A\beta_{1-42}$ in the hippocampus of SHRs post-stroke

$A\beta$ accumulation was assessed using an $A\beta_{1-42}$ specific ELISA kit and confirmed visually by immunofluorescent staining, illustrating dense core plaques in the hippocampus (Fig. 4a). Animals treated with C21 for the first 7 days after ischemic stroke had markedly lower hippocampal concentrations of $A\beta_{1-42}$ at 30 days post-stroke than those treated with saline (Fig. 4b). Similar results were found in the cortical ischemic borderzone (Additional file 3). This finding, although novel, may not be responsible for the cognitive benefits associated with RAS modulators since animals that were switched to candesartan after having been treated with saline for 7 days also displayed preserved cognitive function, despite sustained elevations in hippocampal $A\beta_{1-42}$.

RAS modulation prevented $A\beta_{42}$-mediated cytotoxicity in HBECs subjected to OGD

Cell viability was significantly reduced in both neurons (Additional file 4) and HBECs incubated with $A\beta_{1-42}$ compared with untreated controls, under similar conditions. This $A\beta_{1-42}$-mediated cytotoxicity was prevented when cells were co-treated with candesartan. This was true with both the 1 and 10 μg/ml doses of candesartan and was apparent under both normoxic and hypoxic conditions. Although both doses of Candesartan (1 μg/ml, 10 μg/ml) were equally effective at preventing $A\beta_{1-42}$-associated endothelial cell death under hypoxic conditions, only the higher dose of C21 (1000 nM) was effective under normoxic conditions (Fig. 4c).

RAS modulation prevented chronic-reactive microgliosis in SHRs post-stroke

Representative immunofluorescent images of microglial morphology/ramification status changes are depicted in Fig. 5a. Hypertensive animals subjected to a 60-min tMCAO showed a significantly higher proportion of total (Fig. 5b) and reactive (Fig. 5c) microglia in the ischemic borderzone at 30 days post-stroke, relative to shams. These microglia displayed classic phenotypic features of an activated, amoeboid morphology, with relatively high circularity (Fig. 5d) and stubby or absent processes, in addition to a low Feret's maximum diameter (Fig. 5e) and transformation index (TI < 3) (Fig. 5f). This sustained activation (inflammatory), which was prevented in the C21 and candesartan-treated animals, was associated with delayed, albeit significant, cognitive decline. These agents, already established to possess potent anti-inflammatory and antioxidant properties [12], completely abolished chronic reactive microgliosis, known to be the chief source of cytokines and reactive oxygen species that drive progressive neuronal damage. Consistent with a transformation of amoeboid to healthy ramified microglia in these RAS-treated animals, the TI and Feret's maximum diameter was significantly higher and cell circularity was significantly lower than those of saline-treated animals, values that were not much different from sham animals.

RAS modulation reduced apoptotic cell death post-stroke

Animals subjected to tMCAO had significantly more TUNEL positive cells in their ischemic hemisphere than unstroked (sham) animals (Fig. 6a, b). Cell death was greatly reduced in animals treated long-term with C21/candesartan.

RAS modulation reduced infarct/cavitation size in SHRs post-stroke

Several weeks after ischemia/reperfusion injury, a focal infarction typically develops into a cavitation with a unilateral loss of tissue in the infarct region [34, 35]. Due to the long-term nature of our study, the infarct area was replaced with a discrete cavitation in the ipsilateral hemisphere. This is difficult to accurately quantify due to collapsing of the tissue upon collection. For the brains where it was possible, we provide the data, which was quantified using ImageJ software (NIH) and calculated as percent of contralesional hemisphere (Additional file 5), but we believe it may not accurately reflect the drug effects. We have hence chosen functional outcomes as our primary endpoint.

Discussion

The most important finding of our investigation was that chronic administration of RAS modulators, initiated after stroke, effectively prevented the development of cognitive impairment in hypertensive animals. This was true even when treatment was delayed to 7 days post-stroke and appeared to be independent of $A\beta$ accumulation and blood pressure effects. This was consistent across a series of blinded tests, assessing different aspects of cognitive function. The C21 and candesartan-treated animals showed preserved short-term working memory at 21 and 24 days post-stroke. These animals also displayed better associative learning and reference memory at 28 days

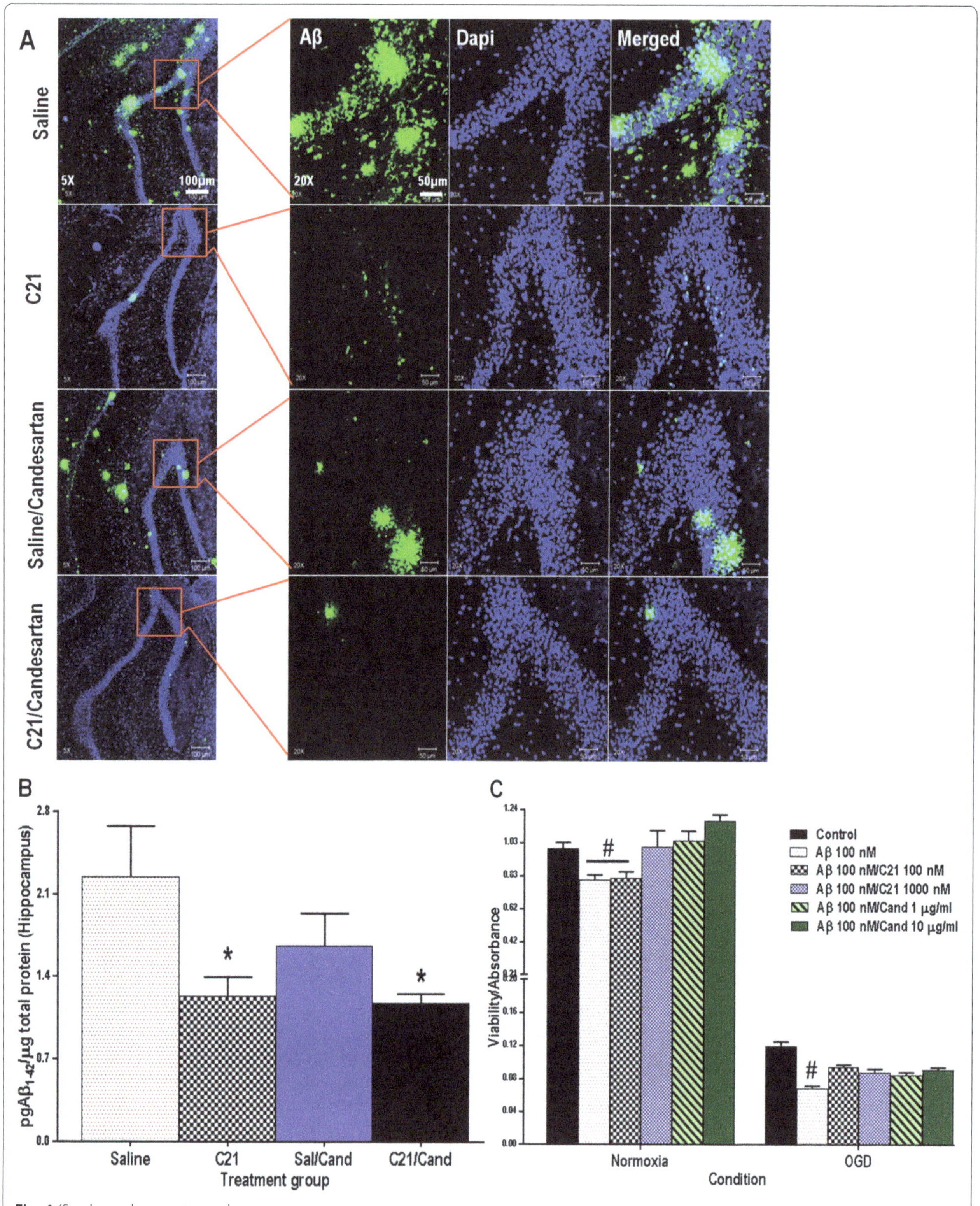

Fig. 4 (See legend on next page.)

(See figure on previous page.)

Fig. 4 RAS modulation prevented $A\beta_{42}$-mediated cytotoxicity in HBECs and C21 prevented hippocampal $A\beta_{42}$ accumulation in SHRs post-stroke. **a** Representative 5× and 20× immunofluorescent Aβ/green-stained images of SHR hippocampus with blue/dapi nuclear staining, scale bar represents 100 and 50 μm for 5× and 20× images, respectively. **b** An $A\beta_{1-42}$ ELISA analysis showed that animals treated with C21, for the first 7 days, had markedly lower hippocampal concentrations of $A\beta_{1-42}$ at 30 days post-stroke than those treated with saline. (C21 × candesartan interaction $F_{(1,18)} = 1.30$, $P = 0.2719$, $n = 5$–10 animals/group. **c** Cell viability (MTT conversion) was significantly reduced in cultured HBECs incubated with $A\beta_{1-42}$ compared with untreated controls, under similar conditions. This cytotoxicity was prevented when cells were co-treated with candesartan and higher dose C21 (condition by Aβ/C21/candesartan group interaction $F_{(5,89)} = 5.68$, $P = 0.0002$, $n = 6$–12 wells/group, error bars indicate SEM). Statistical significance for post hoc comparisons between groups using Tukey's multiple comparison procedure are denoted by $^*P < 0.05$ to indicate a difference from saline and **#**$P < 0.05$ to indicate a difference from all other treatment groups

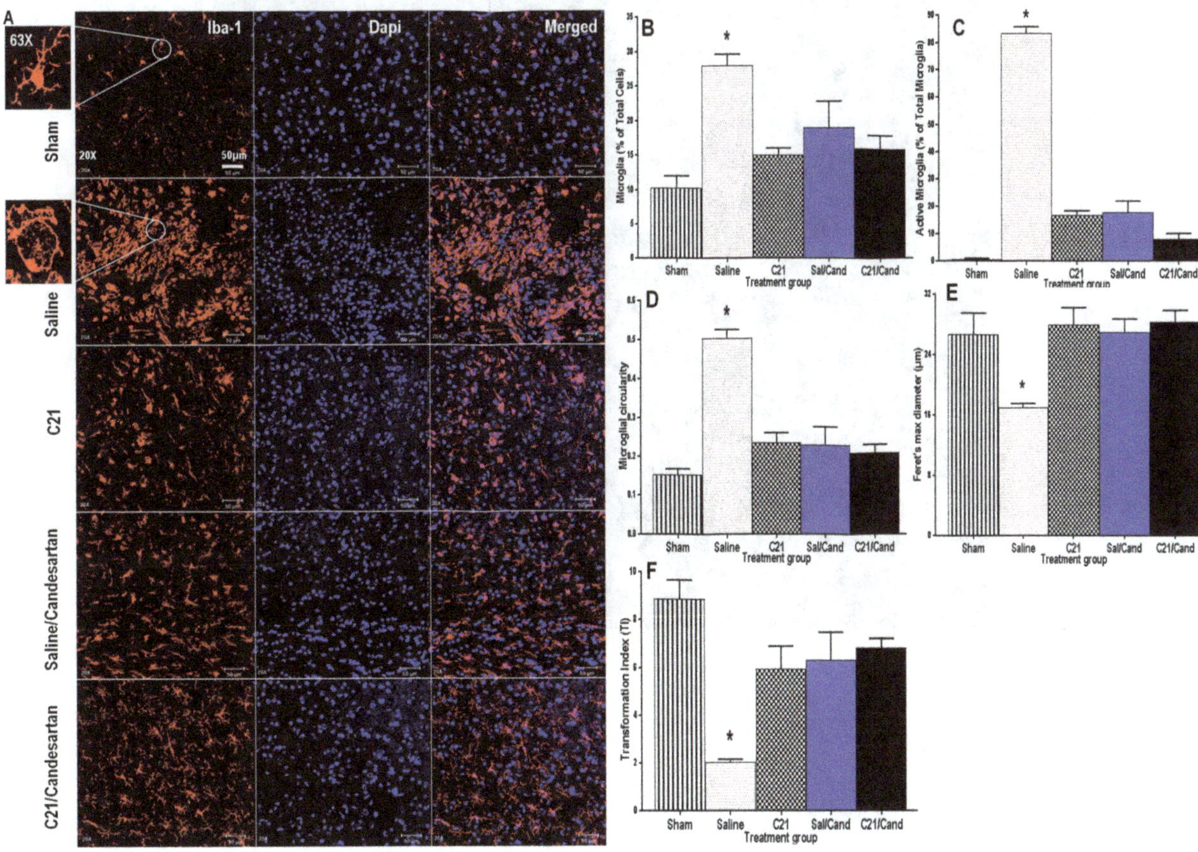

Fig. 5 RAS modulation reduced microglial accumulation, offset sustained activation and prevented chronic reactive microgliosis, in SHRs post-stroke. **a** Representative immunofluorescent images depicting microglial morphology/ramification status changes as illustrated Iba-1 positive (red stained) microglia with blue dapi nuclear staining, scale bar represents 50 and 20 μm for 20× and 63× images, respectively. Hypertensive controls (saline) subjected to tMCAO had, in the ischemic hemisphere, a significantly higher proportion of **b** total microglia ($F_{(4,14)} = 13.18$, $P < 0.05$) and **c** active, inflammatory microglia ($F_{(4,14)} = 249.1$, $P < 0.0001$) at 30 days post-stroke relative to shams and C21/candesartan-treated animals. These saline-treated controls also showed **d** increased circularity ($F_{(4,14)} = 33.52$, $P < 0.0001$), **e** reduced Feret's maximum diameter ($F_{(4,14)} = 7.314$, $P < 0.05$), and **f** reduced transformation index (TI) ($F_{(4,14)} = 14.02$, $P < 0.0001$), all consistent with a transformation of microglia from ramified to reactive amoeboid forms, at 30 days post-stroke relative to both sham and C21/candesartan-treated animals. However, C21 and candesartan-treated animals showed indices not much different from those of shams ($n = 3$–4 animals/group, error bars indicate SEM). Statistical significance for post hoc comparisons between groups using Tukey's multiple comparison procedure are denoted by $^*P < 0.05$ for differences in proportion of total microglia and Feret's maximum diameter and $^*P < 0.0001$ for differences in all other parameters. Feret's (maximum) diameter, a measure of cell length, is the greatest distance between any two points along the cell perimeter [51]. Circularity $= 4\pi \times$ [cell area (μm^2)]/[cell perimeter (μm)]^2 is unitless value that ranges from 0 (infinitely elongated)-1 (perfect circle) [51]. Transformation index (TI) = [perimeter of cell (μm)]^2/4π [cell area(μm^2)] [51]

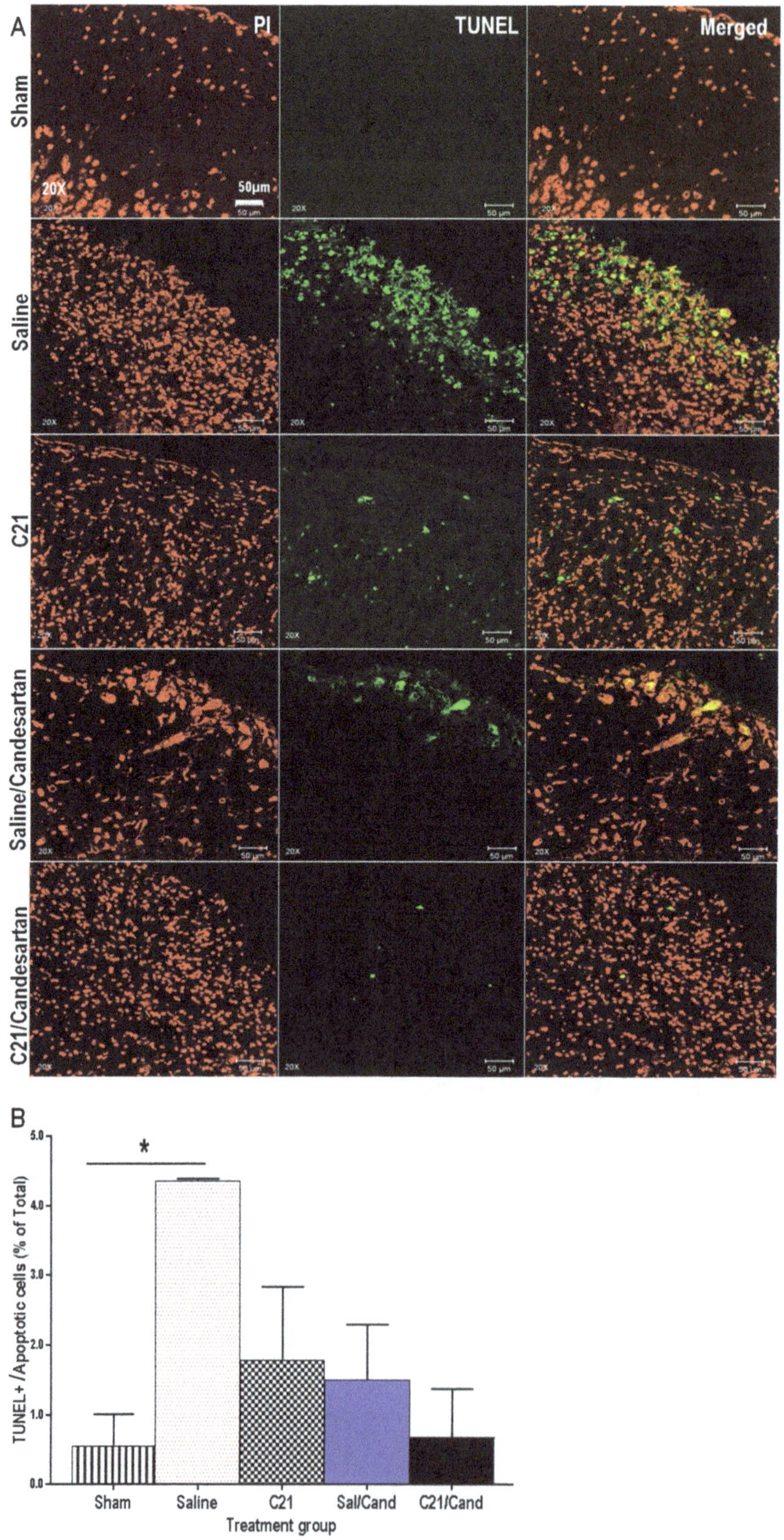

Fig. 6 (See legend on next page.)

(See figure on previous page.)
Fig. 6 RAS modulation reduced apoptotic cell death post-stroke. **a** Representative 20× immunofluorescent images depicting TUNEL positive (green stained) cortical cells with red propidium iodide nuclear staining, scale bar 50 μm. **b** Animals subjected to tMCAO had a significantly greater number of tunnel positive cells in the ischemic hemisphere than shams $F_{(4,7)} = 4.373$, $P = 0.0437$. Cell death was greatly reduced in animals treated long-term with C21 and candesartan ($n = 3$–4 animals/group, error bars indicate SEM). Statistical significance for post hoc comparisons between groups using Tukey's multiple comparison procedure are denoted by $^*P < 0.05$ to indicate a difference from unstroked/sham animals

post-stroke, compared to saline-treated animals, despite a lack of difference in sensorimotor recovery. We are the first to report this late therapeutic window for RAS modulation and the prevention of post-stroke cognitive impairment. Regarding the mechanism of this protection, our results showed that RAS modulators, both C21 and candesartan, maintained microglial salutary resting state and prevented the pathologically exaggerated microglial inflammatory response that otherwise persists in hypertensive animals post-stroke. This was also associated with reduced amyloid accumulation in the brains of C21-treated animals and less apoptotic cell death with both RAS modulators.

Both animal [6, 36, 37] and human [5] studies demonstrate an association between RAS modulation and preservation of cognitive function, with a wide range of potential mechanisms. These agents not only block brain AT1R but also indirectly stimulate AT2R signaling, a specific target of C21, hence promoting its protective effects. ARBs are also effective at preventing Aβ-induced cytotoxicity and vascular damage [8]. Although RAS modulation has been mechanistically linked to a reduction in $A\beta_{1-42}$ accumulation in studies of cognitive impairment [38, 39], our findings suggest other mechanisms of cognitive protection, so we investigated effects on cytotoxicity, apoptosis, and chronic inflammation.

C21, when administered for 7 days after ischemic stroke and either continued or replaced with low-dose candesartan, prevented accumulation of $A\beta_{1-42}$ in the hippocampus and ischemic borderzone of SHRs post-stroke, but animals whose treatment was delayed, were started on saline for the first 7 days post-stroke, displayed cognitive preservation despite elevations in hippocampal $A\beta_{1-42}$ at 30 days post-stroke. It has already been established that SHRs subjected to tMCAO tend to have Aβ accumulation of the ipsilateral cerebral cortex and hippocampus [40], but this is the first study to report the effect of C21 on brain $A\beta_{1-42}$ concentration post-stroke.

It is possible, however, that RAS modulators, candesartan and C21, prevent cognitive decline by reducing $A\beta_{1-42}$-mediated cytotoxicity. In hCMEC/D3, both doses of candesartan were equally effective at preventing $A\beta_{1-42}$-associated endothelial cell death under hypoxic conditions and only the higher dose of C21 was effective under normoxic conditions. Aβ damages both endothelial and neuronal cells by oxidative stress and free-radical generation and activates a variety of inflammatory and pro-apoptotic pathways, all of which may play an important role in the pathogenesis of AD (Additional file 6) [15, 41]. Accordingly, we conducted our dose-response studies with $A\beta_{1-42}$ concentrations in the nanomolar range (10–1000 nM) and chose the minimum toxic concentration (100 nM) for our cell culture studies. We also included OGD in order to simulate the ischemic conditions in the presence and absence of $A\beta_{1-42}$. The combination of Aβ and cerebrovascular disease, including either chronic cerebral hypoperfusion and/or acute ischemia, has been shown to negatively affect cognition [42].

RAS modulators have also been shown to prevent chronic reactive microgliosis, otherwise associated with ischemia-reperfusion in hypertensive animals. Conversion of microglia from the normal resting state (ramified phenotype) to an activated state (amoeboidal phenotype) is the initial step in the CNS inflammatory response [40]. This inflammatory response, which develops in the brain over a period of hours to days after the onset of cerebral ischemia, may impair neurogenesis and other reparative processes essential to functional recovery after stroke. Microglia can become chronically activated by a single stimulus (ischemic stroke) to result in cumulative neuronal loss with time [43], similar to the time frame we observed in the emergence of cognitive decline. Moreover, a sustained activation of microglia is one of the first pathological features of neurodegenerative disease and cognitive impairment, long before there is any evidence of actual neurodegeneration [38]. In fact, it was recently determined that microglia actively contribute to the neuronal loss observed in animal models of AD [44]. Moreover, elimination of microglia in these animals resulted in a significant recovery of contextual memory and overall cognitive function with a reversal of dendritic spine loss and prevention of neuronal loss, without any changes in amyloid-β levels or plaque loads [44]. Chronic microglial stimulation is associated with a perpetual pro-inflammatory, pro-oxidative state that causes neurotoxicity and eventually results in cognitive decline [44]. In fact, overactivation of microglia is solely capable of inducing neuronal death in the absence of other pathological stimulation [45]. With other studies, treatment is almost always initiated at very short time points after the onset of ischemia. This prevents any mechanistic distinction between agents that directly suppress microglial activation with those that simply reduce inflammation only as a result of reduced cell injury. This is a considerable strength of our study since although our findings are in line with others showing that RAS modulators suppress microglial activation, we were the first to show this to be true long-term and even when treatment is delayed.

Our findings are also consistent with recent reports of immune-mediated delayed cognitive impairment in a mouse model of experimental stroke [46]. Investigators demonstrated that the cognitive decline appearing at least 7 days after stroke could be prevented by depleting or deactivating B-lymphocytes [46]. It is possible that the increased reactive microglia that we report could be involved in the homing of B-lymphocytes to the brain, further worsening cognitive decline.

Clinical trial evidence strongly suggests that BP lowering with candesartan in the acute stroke period (first 7 days) is associated with worse stroke outcomes [47]. Therefore, this investigation was a randomized, double-blind, preclinical trial, designed to mimic how C21 and candesartan might be prescribed to stroke patients.

We found that C21 does not affect the BP of hypertensive animals, when administered systemically, in multiple doses, either before or immediately after tMCAO. These results are similar to what we and others have seen in normotensive and hypertensive animals in doses of up to 10 mg/kg/day [8, 43, 44, 48–50]. Another important finding of this study was that acute ischemic stroke increases the sensitivity of hypertensive animals to the blood pressure lowering effects of candesartan. In fact, a low dose of candesartan (0.3 mg/kg), even at 7 days after stroke onset, resulted in an average BP reduction of ≈ 20 mmHg, similar to that achieved with the higher dose (1 mg/kg/day) of candesartan in unstroked animals. This is consistent with what we had previously reported in our study showing that hypertensive animals were more sensitive to a single dose of candesartan, administered immediately after stroke, than normotensive rats [20]. This may indicate that restarting blood pressure medications in patients post-stroke may be dangerous if the same pre-stroke doses are used, even when therapy is delayed to 7 days post-stroke.

We included sham animals to demonstrate the natural history of cognitive changes over 28 days in these young adult, hypertensive animals. The fact that this group did not demonstrate impairment in the NOR and the PAT support the notion that the significant cognitive decline in the saline-treated stroked animals at 28 days was due to the stroke injury. It is likely that sham hypertensive animals treated with either C21 or candesartan would also exhibit preserved cognition upon chronic administration, as has been demonstrated by others [7, 44]. Since we were unable to detect significant decline in our untreated shams at 28 days, however, a longer period of follow-up may be required for future studies.

Conclusion

Our results clearly indicate that AT2R stimulation, either with the selective AT2R agonist C21, or the ARB, candesartan, may be beneficial in preventing the development of cognitive impairment after stroke, even when treatment is delayed to 7 days. This has important therapeutic implications and suggests therapy with C21 may be a valid approach for preserving cognition in various subsets of patients including certain elderly patients, those with severe carotid occlusive disease, and individuals with heart valve disorders, atrial fibrillation, and orthostatic hypotension. Although it is reasonable to withhold ARBs/BP lowering drugs during the acute period post-stroke, it may be appropriate and even advantageous to incorporate the novel, direct acting AT2 receptor agonist C21, as "bridge therapy," until antihypertensive therapy initiation/re-initiation. This would exploit the numerous protective benefits associated with AT2R stimulation, and hence sustain cognitive function, without lowering blood pressure. It may also be used in place of agents like candesartan in those with allergies or intolerance to other RAS modulators and are being treated with non-ACE/ARB blood pressure medications.

Additional files

Additional file 1: C21 ameliorates weight loss. C21 when administered daily, starting at 2 h after tMCAO and reperfusion, significantly ameliorated weight loss at day 7, compared to saline-treated controls, with animals showing most rapid recovery, between days 7 and 30, when treatment was followed with candesartan.

Additional file 2: Cognition declines over time after stroke. Despite complete recovery of sensorimotor function, the saline-treated animals demonstrated a continuous decline in cognition from baseline to day 14 to day 21. Statistical significance denoted by $*P < 0.0001$ for an effect of time, while $**P < 0.01$ indicates significance between the 2 treatment groups (C21 vs. saline), effect of treatment at 21 days post-stroke, and $\#P < 0.005$ indicates presence of a significant interaction between time and treatment effects.

Additional file 3: C21 reduces Aβ accumulation in the cortex after stroke. ELISA analysis showed that animals treated with C21, for the first 7 days, had markedly lower concentrations of $A\beta_{1-42}$ in their cortical ischemic borderzones, at 30 days post-stroke compared to those treated with saline. Statistical significance for post hoc comparisons between groups using Tukey's multiple comparison procedure are denoted by $*P < 0.01$ to indicate a difference from saline.

Additional file 4: RAS modulators reduced the total volume of injury after stroke. RAS modulation reduced infarct/cavitation size in SHRs post-stroke. The sections were stained with hematoxylin and eosin (H&E) stain and infarct/cavitation volumes quantified and expressed as a percentage of the contralateral side. Statistical significance for post hoc comparisons between groups using Tukey's multiple comparison procedure are denoted by $*P < 0.01$ to indicate a difference from all other treatment groups.

Additional file 5: RAS modulation reduces neuronal cytotoxicity. Cell viability was significantly reduced in primary neurons incubated with $A\beta_{1-42}$ compared with untreated controls, under similar conditions. This $A\beta_{1-42}$-mediated cytotoxicity was reduced when cells were co-treated with C21. This reached statistical significance only with the higher dose of C21. Statistical significance for post hoc comparisons between groups using Tukey's multiple comparison procedure are denoted by $*P < 0.05$ to indicate a viability substantially higher than that seen for $A\beta_{1-42}$-treated cells.

Additional file 6: Conceptual diagram. Acute cerebral hypoperfusion and hypoxia, due to stroke and/or chronic cerebral hypoperfusion, facilitates amyloid-β (Aβ) production by activating β-secretase enzyme, necessary for Aβ production. Aβ is a potent vasoconstrictor that worsens cerebral hypoperfusion by further reducing cerebral blood flow (CBF) and hence transvascular transport, thereby reducing its own clearance leading to additional accumulation and toxicity. Aβ also results in microglial activation, neuroinflammation, and endothelial dysfunction. It creates a vicious cycle whereby the endothelial dysfunction, which is associated with diminished vasodilation, leads to further reductions in cerebral blood flow (CBF) and hypoperfusion, BBB disruption, and alterations in permeability resulting in tissue edema which further reduces CBF, by compressing blood vessels. The resulting hypoperfusion leads to additional oxidative stress by inducing tissue hypoxia. The oxidative and pro-inflammatory environment induced by hypoperfusion and BBB breakdown results in demyelination, synaptic defects, and disruption of trophic coupling between neurovascular unit (NVU) components. Therefore, vascular dysfunction and stroke are tightly linked to Aβ accumulation and neuronal dysfunction. They are ultimately manifested as vascular cognitive impairment/dementia (VCID). Stimulation of the AT2R by C21 acts to reduce Aβ accumulation and possesses neurovascular benefits by virtue of its potent anti-inflammatory, antioxidant, and tissue-regenerating properties. ★ Pathways targeted by C21.

Abbreviations
AD: Alzheimer's disease; Ang II: Angiotensin II; ARBs: Angiotensin II type 1 receptor blockers; AT1R: Ang II type 1 receptor; AT2R: Ang II type 2 receptors; BDNF: Brain-derived neurotrophic factor; C21: Compound 21; CBF: Cerebral blood flow; ELISA: Enzyme linked immunosorbent assay; FDA: Food and Drug Administration; GAPDH: Glyceraldehyde 3-phosphate dehydrogenase; HBECs: Human brain endothelial cells; IACUC: Institutional Animal Care and Use Committee; IP: Intraperitoneal; NGF: Nerve growth factor; NIH: National Institute of Health; NOR: Novel object recognition; OGD: Oxygen glucose deprivation; PAT: Passive avoidance tests; RAS: Renin angiotensin system; SAP: Spontaneous alternation test; SHRs: Spontaneously hypertensive rats; tMCAO: Transient middle cerebral artery occlusion; VCID: Vascular cognitive impairment/dementia

Acknowledgements
We thank Ismail Kaddour, Almira Vazdarjanova, and Kristopher Bunting for their technical support and valuable advice.

Funding
This study was supported by R21-NS088016, VA Merit Review (BX000891), RO1-NS063965 to Susan C Fagan and by VA Merit Review (BX000347), VA Research Career Scientist Award, and R01NS083559 to Adviye Ergul.

Authors' contributions
HA designed and performed the research (administered coded treatments, monitored parameters, conducted behavior tests) and drafted the manuscript. TI performed the stroke surgeries and reviewed the manuscript. BP isolated the brain tissue and performed the molecular analyses. AF randomized the study and blinded study, prepared the coded treatments, and reviewed the manuscript. MS analyzed the behavior data from the recorded videos and reviewed the manuscript. WE reviewed the manuscript. JW performed the statistical analysis. AE interpreted the data and reviewed the manuscript. SCF designed the study, managed the experiments, interpreted the data, and reviewed the manuscript. All authors read and approved the final manuscript.

Consent for publication
Not applicable

Competing interests
Drugs were supplied from Astra-Zeneca and Vicore Pharma. The authors declared that they have no competing interests.

Author details
[1]Program in Clinical and Experimental Therapeutics, Charlie Norwood VA Medical Center and University of Georgia College of Pharmacy, HM Bldg., 1120 15th St, Augusta, GA 30912, USA. [2]Department of Anatomy and Neurobiology, College of Medicine, Neuroscience Institute, University of Tennessee Health Science Center, Memphis, TN, USA. [3]Department of Physiology, Augusta University, Augusta, GA, USA. [4]Department of Neurology, Augusta University, Augusta, GA, USA. [5]Department of Biostatistics and Epidemiology, Augusta University, Augusta, GA, USA.

References
1. Yang Y, Kimura-ohba S, Thompson J, Gary A. Rodent models of vascular cognitive impairment. Transl Stroke Res. 2016;7:407–14.
2. Iadecola C. The pathology of vascular dementia. Neuron. 2013;80:844–66.
3. Delavaran H, Jönsson A-C, Lövkvist H, Iwarsson S, Elmståhl S, Norrving B, et al. Cognitive function in stroke survivors: a 10-year follow-up study. Acta Neurol Scand. 2017;136:187–94.
4. Gorelick P, Scuteri A, Black S. Vascular contributions to cognitive impairment and dementia: a statement for healthcare professionals from the American Heart Association/American Stroke Association. Stroke. 2011;42:2672–713.
5. Rouch L, Cestac P, Hanon O, Cool C, Helmer C, Bouhanick B, et al. Antihypertensive drugs, prevention of cognitive decline and dementia: a systematic review of observational studies, randomized controlled trials and meta-analyses, with discussion of potential mechanisms. CNS Drugs. 2015;29:113–30.
6. Levine DA, Galecki AT, Langa KM, Unverzagt FW, Kabeto MU, Giordani B, et al. Trajectory of cognitive decline after incident stroke. JAMA. 2015;314:41–51.
7. Whitehead SN, Cheng G, Hachinski VC, Cechetto DF. Progressive increase in infarct size, neuroinflammation, and cognitive deficits in the presence of high levels of amyloid. Stroke. 2007;38:3245–50.
8. Wiesmann M, Kiliaan AJ, Claassen JA. Vascular aspects of cognitive impairment and dementia. J Cereb Blood Flow Metab. 2013;33:1696–706.
9. Füchtemeier M, Brinckmann MP, Foddis M, Kunz A, Po C, Curato C, et al. Vascular change and opposing effects of the angiotensin type 2 receptor in a mouse model of vascular cognitive impairment. J Cereb Blood Flow Metab. 2015;35:476–84.
10. Liu M, Guo H, Li C, Wang D, Wu J, Wang C, et al. Cognitive improvement of compound danshen in an Aβ25–35 peptide-induced rat model of Alzheimer's disease. BMC Complement Altern Med. 2015;15:382–90.
11. López-Gil X, Amat-Roldan I, Tudela R, Castañ A, Prats-Galino A, Planas AM, et al. DWI and complex brain network analysis predicts vascular cognitive impairment in spontaneous hypertensive rats undergoing executive function tests. Front Aging Neurosci. 2014;6:1–33.
12. Saavedra JM. Evidence to consider angiotensin II receptor blockers for the treatment of early Alzheimer's disease. Cell Mol Neurobiol. 2016;36:259–79.
13. Guimond M-O, Gallo-Payet N. The angiotensin II type 2 receptor in brain functions: an update. Int J Hypertens. 2012;2012:351758.
14. Alhusban A, Fouda AY, Pillai B, Ishrat T, Soliman S, Fagan SC. Compound 21 is pro-angiogenic in the brain and results in sustained recovery after ischemic stroke. J Hypertens. 2015;33:170–80.
15. Ahmed HA, Ishrat T, Pillai B, Bunting KM, Patel A, Vazdarjanova A, et al. Role of angiotensin system modulation on progression of cognitive impairment and brain MRI changes in aged hypertensive animals––a randomized double-blind pre-clinical study. Behav Brain Res. 2018;346:29–40.
16. Ishrat T, Fouda AY, Pillai B, Eldahshan W, Ahmed H, Waller JL, et al. Dose–response, therapeutic time-window and tPA-combinatorial efficacy of compound 21: a randomized, blinded preclinical trial in a rat model of thromboembolic stroke. J Cereb Blood Flow Metab. 2018:1–8 PMID: 29537907.
17. Wharton DP, Goldstein FC, Zhao L, Steenland K, Levey AI, Hajjar I. Rennin-angiotensin-system modulation may slow the convension from mild cognitive impairment to Alzheimer's disease. J Am Geriatr Soc. 2015;63: 1749–56.
18. Jusufovic M, Sandset EC, Bath PMW, Karlson BW, Berge E. Effects of blood pressure lowering in patients with acute ischemic stroke and carotid artery stenosis. Int J Stroke. 2015;10:1–6.
19. Freret T, Bouet V. Improvements of the stroke model guidelines––animal body weight and long-term functional concerns. J Exp Stroke Transl Med. 2009;2:28–31.
20. Kozak W, Kozak A, Johnson MH, Elewa HF, Fagan SC. Vascular protection

with candesartan after experimental acute stroke in hypertensive rats: a dose-response study. J pharmacol and exp ther. 2008;326:773–82.
21. Bederson JB, Pitts LH, Tsuji M, Nishimura MC, Davis RL, Bartkowski H. Rat middle cerebral artery occlusion: evaluation of the model and development of a neurologic examination. Stroke. 1986;17:472–6.
22. Ma J, Xiong JY, Hou WW, Yan HJ, Sun Y, Huang SW, et al. Protective effect of carnosine on subcortical ischemic vascular dementia in mice. CNS Neurosci Ther. 2012;18:745–53.
23. Wietrzych M, Meziane H, Sutter A, Ghyselinck N, Chapman PF, Chambon P, et al. Working memory deficits in retinoid X receptor gamma-deficient mice. Learn Mem. 2005;12:318–26.
24. Antunes M, Biala G. The novel object recognition memory: neurobiology, test procedure, and its modifications. Cogn Process. 2012;13:93–110.
25. Webster SJ, Bachstetter AD, Nelson PT, Schmitt FA, Van Eldik LJ. Using mice to model Alzheimer's dementia: an overview of the clinical disease and the preclinical behavioral changes in 10 mouse models. Front Genet. 2014;5:1–23.
26. Alonso M, Bekinschtein P, Cammarota M, Vianna MRM, Izquierdo I, Medina JH. Endogenous BDNF is required for long-term memory formation in the rat parietal cortex. Learn Mem. 2005;12:504–10.
27. Radahmadi M, Alaei H, Sharifi MR, Hosseini N. The effect of synchronized running activity with chronic stress on passive avoidance learning and body weight in rats. Int J Prev Med. 2013;4:430–7.
28. Albers GW, Goldstein LB, Hess DC, Wechsler LR, Furie KL, Gorelick PB, et al. Stroke treatment academic industry roundtable (STAIR) recommendations for maximizing the use of intravenous thrombolytics and expanding treatment options with intra-arterial and neuroprotective therapies. Stroke. 2011;42:2645–50.
29. Lapchak PA, Zhang JH, Noble-Haeusslein LJ. RIGOR guidelines: escalating STAIR and STEPS for effective translational research. Transl Stroke Res. 2013; 4:279–85.
30. Kilkenny C, Browne WJ, Cuthill IC, Emerson M, Altman DG. Improving bioscience research reporting: the ARRIVE guidelines for reporting animal research. PLoS Biol. 2010;8:1–5.
31. Soliman S, Ishrat T, Pillai A, Somanath PR, Ergul A, El-Remessy AB, et al. Candesartan induces a prolonged proangiogenic effect and augments endothelium-mediated neuroprotection after oxygen and glucose deprivation: role of vascular endothelial growth factors a and B. J Pharmacol Exp Ther. 2014;349:444–57.
32. Riss TL, Moravec RA, Niles AL, Benink HA, Worzella TJ, Minor L. Cell viability assays. Assay guidance manual; 2015. p. 1–23.
33. Palit P, Mukherjee D, Mandal SC. Reconstituted mother tinctures of *Gelsemium sempervirens* L. improve memory and cognitive impairment in mice scopolamine-induced dementia model. J Ethnopharmacol. 2015;159:274–84.
34. Ishrat T, Pillai B, Soliman S, Fouda AY, Kozak A, Johnson MH, Ergul A, Fagan SC. Low-dose candesartan enhances molecular mediators of neuroplasticity and subsequent functional recovery after ischemic stroke in rats. Mol Neurobiol. 2015;51:1542–53.
35. Van VanBruggen N, Thibodeaux H, Palmer JT, Lee WP, Fu L, Cairns B, et al. VEGF antagonism reduces edema formation and tissue damage after ischemia/reperfusion injury in the mouse brain. J Clin Invest. 1999;104:1613–20.
36. Kurata T, Lukic V, Kozuki M, Wada D, Miyazaki K, Morimoto N, et al. Long-term effect of telmisartan on Alzheimer's amyloid genesis in SHR-SR after tMCAO. Transl Stroke Res. 2014;6:107–15.
37. Kurata T, Lukic V, Kozuki M, Wada D, Miyazaki K, Morimoto N, et al. Telmisartan reduces progressive accumulation of cellular amyloid-β and phosphorylated Tau with inflammatory responses in aged spontaneously hypertensive stroke resistant rat. J Stroke Cerebrovasc Dis. 2014;23:2580–90.
38. Vincenti JE, Murphy L, Grabert K, Mccoll BW, Cancellotti E, Freeman TC, et al. Defining the microglia response during the time course of chronic neurodegeneration. J Virol. 2016;90:3003–17.
39. Szabo M, Gulya K. Development of the microglial phenotype in culture. Neuroscience. 2013;241:280–95.
40. Yenari MA, Kauppinen TM, Swanson RA. Microglial activation in stroke: therapeutic targets. Neurology. 2010;7:378–91.
41. Askarova S, Tsoy A, Shalakhmetova T, Lee JC-M. Effects of amyloid beta peptide on neurovascular cells. Cent Asian J Glob Health. 2013;1:1.
42. Lee MJ, Seo SW, Na DL, Kim C, Park JH, Kim GH, et al. Synergistic effects of ischemia and β-amyloid burden on cognitive decline in patients with subcortical vascular mild cognitive impairment. JAMA Psychiat. 2014;71:412–22.
43. Lull ME, Block ML. Microglial activation and chronic neurodegeneration. Neurotherapeutics. 2010;7:354–65.
44. Spangenberg EE, Lee RJ, Najafi AR, Rice RA, Elmore MRP, Blurton-Jones M, et al. Eliminating microglia in Alzheimer's mice prevents neuronal loss without modulating amyloid-β pathology. Brain. 2016;139:1265–81.
45. Luo X-G, Chen S-D, Farber K, Kettenmann H, Hanisch U, Kettenmann H, et al. The changing phenotype of microglia from homeostasis to disease. Transl Neurodegener. 2012;1:9.
46. Doyle KP, Quach LN, Montse S, Axtell RC, Nguyen TV, Soler-Llavina GJ, et al. B-lymphocyte-mediated delayed cognitive impairment following stroke. J Neurosc. 2015;35:2133–45.
47. Sandset EC, Murray GD, Bath PMW, Kjeldsen SE, Berge E. Relation between change in blood pressure in acute stroke and risk of early adverse events and poor outcome. Stroke. 2012;43:2108–14.
48. Gelosa P, Pignieri A, Fändriks L, de Gasparo M, Hallberg A, Banfi C, et al. Stimulation of AT2 receptor exerts beneficial effects in stroke-prone rats: focus on renal damage. J Hypertens. 2009;27:2444–51.
49. Sumners C, Horiuchi M, Widdop RE, Mccarthy C, Unger T, Steckelings UM. Protective arms of the renin-angiotensin-system in neurological disease. Clin Exp Pharmacol Physiol. 2013;40:580–8.
50. Jing F, Mogi M, Sakata A, Iwanami J, Tsukuda K, Ohshima K, et al. Direct stimulation of angiotensin II type 2 receptor enhances spatial memory. J Cereb Blood Flow Metab. 2012;32:248–55.
51. Caldeira C, Oliveira AF, Cunha C, Vaz AR, Falcão AS, Fernandes A, et al. Microglia change from a reactive to an age-like phenotype with the time in culture. Front Cell Neurosci. 2014;8:152.

The potassium channel KCa3.1 constitutes a pharmacological target for astrogliosis associated with ischemia stroke

Mengni Yi[1], Tianjiao Wei[1], Yanxia Wang[2], Qin Lu[1], Gaoxian Chen[1], Xiaoling Gao[1], Herbert M. Geller[3*], Hongzhuan Chen[1*] and Zhihua Yu[1*]

Abstract

Background: Reactive astrogliosis is one of the significantly pathological features in ischemic stroke accompanied with changes in gene expression, morphology, and proliferation. KCa3.1 was involved in TGF-β-induced astrogliosis in vitro and also contributed to astrogliosis-mediated neuroinflammation in neurodegeneration disease.

Methods: Wild type mice and KCa3.1$^{-/-}$ mice were subjected to permanent middle cerebral artery occlusion (pMCAO) to evaluate the infarct areas by 2,3,5-triphenyltetrazolium hydrochloride staining and neurological deficit. KCa3.1 channels expression and cell localization in the brain of pMCAO mice model were measured by immunoblotting and immunostaining. Glia activation and neuron loss was measured by immunostaining. DiBAC4 (3) and Fluo-4AM were used to measure membrane potential and cytosolic Ca^{2+} level in oxygen-glucose deprivation induced reactive astrocytes in vitro.

Results: Immunohistochemistry on pMCAO mice infarcts showed strong upregulation of KCa3.1 immunoreactivity in reactive astrogliosis. KCa3.1$^{-/-}$ mice exhibited significantly smaller infarct areas on pMCAO and improved neurological deficit. Both activated gliosis and neuronal loss were attenuated in KCa3.1$^{-/-}$ pMCAO mice. In the primary cultured astrocytes, the expressions of KCa3.1 and TRPV4 were increased associated with upregulation of astrogliosis marker GFAP induced by oxygen-glucose deprivation. The activation of KCa3.1 hyperpolarized membrane potential and, by promoting the driving force for calcium, induced calcium entry through TRPV4, a cation channel of the transient receptor potential family. Double-labeled staining showed that KCa3.1 and TRPV4 channels co-localized in astrocytes. Blockade of KCa3.1 or TRPV4 inhibited the phenotype switch of reactive astrogliosis.

Conclusions: Our data suggested that KCa3.1 inhibition might represent a promising therapeutic strategy for ischemia stroke.

Keywords: Astrocytes, Mouse, GFAP, Ischemia, Calcium

* Correspondence: geller@helix.nih.gov; hongzhuan_chen@hotmail.com; yuzhihua@shsmu.edu.cn
[3]Developmental Neurobiology Section, Division of Intramural Research, National Heart, Lung, and Blood Institute, National Institutes of Health, Bethesda, MD 20892, USA
[1]Department of Pharmacology, Institute of Medical Sciences, Shanghai Jiao Tong University School of Medicine, Shanghai 200025, China
Full list of author information is available at the end of the article

Background

During pathological brain insults such as cerebral ischemia, a rapid increase of intracellular calcium initiates apoptotic and necrotic cell death and reactive gliosis. Several lines of evidence suggest that $[Ca^{2+}]_i$ oscillations evoked by focal ischemia spread through the astrocytes and cause damage in distal regions of the central nervous system (CNS) [1]. KCa3.1, a Ca^{2+}-activated potassium channel, is involved in regulating membrane potential during activation of non-excitable inflammatory and structural cells, including astrocytes, in response to Ca^{2+} influx [2–4]. As such, KCa3.1 is a promising target to ameliorate the phenotype switch of astrocytes and microglia from resting to astrogliosis and microglia activation in ischemia, traumatic brain injury, Alzheimer's disease (AD) as well as spinal cord injury [5, 6].

Most recently, we reported that KCa3.1 was increased in reactive astrocytes as well as neurons in the brains of both mouse models of AD and AD patients. Furthermore, the blockade of KCa3.1 resulted in a decrease in astrogliosis and an attenuation of memory deficits in the AD mouse model [7]. After ischemic stroke in rats, blood-brain barrier endothelial cells exhibited KCa3.1 protein and activity, and pharmacological blockade of KCa3.1 significantly reduced Na^+ uptake and cytotoxic edema [8]. Moreover, in a mouse model of ischemia, genetic deletion and wild type mice treated with the KCa3.1 blocker TRAM-34 resulted in a decrease in infarct areas and improved neurological deficits [9]. These findings suggest that KCa3.1 channels are important in the process of stroke, and that their blockade might prove useful as therapy in stroke with upregulated KCa3.1 expression.

Over the past few years, a large number of studies suggested that astroglial calcium influx after ischemia could be mediated by the activation of Ca^{2+} permeable cation channels such as transient receptor potential (TRP) channels. The transient receptor potential vanilloid 4 (TRPV4) channel is widely expressed in the CNS, with demonstrated function not only in neurons and astrocytes but also in endothelial cells of cerebral arteries [10]. During cerebral ischemia, TRPV4 was overactivated by cytotoxic edema or the metabolites of arachidonic acid (AA), and TRPV4-mediated Ca^{2+} entry likely played a role in the intracellular Ca^{2+} overload [11]. Blockade of the TRPV4 channel reduced the damage to hippocampal pyramidal neurons and astrocytes upon oxidative stress [12] or oxygen-glucose deprivation [13] in vitro and reduced brain infarction in a mouse model of focal cerebral ischemia [14]. At present, the signal transduction pathways used by TRPV4 to induce astrogliosis are not well defined but seem mostly related to calcium overload of the cells, as TRPV4 channels are involved in ischemia-induced calcium entry in reactive astrocytes and thus, might participate in the pathogenic mechanisms of astroglial reactivity following ischemic insult [15].

The present study aims to investigate the mechanisms by which KCa3.1 regulates Ca^{2+} entry via TRPV4 channels, leading to reactive astrogliosis during ischemia stroke. We show, for the first time, a potential co-localization between KCa3.1 and TRPV4 channels in astrocytes. This co-localization allows KCa3.1 to maintain a negative membrane potential during astrogliosis, thus increasing the driving membrane potential for Ca^{2+} influx through TRPV4 channels. These strongly suggest that KCa3.1 is involved in reactive astrogliosis in the process of stroke, making it a promising target for the development of novel therapies.

Methods

Permanent focal cerebral ischemia

The study (ethics protocol number: A-2015-010) was approved by the Animal Care and Use Committee of the Shanghai Jiao Tong University School of Medicine, Shanghai, China. KCa3.1$^{-/-}$ mice were obtained from the Jackson Laboratory as described precisely [16–18]. 10–12 week old male C57BL/6 wild type mice and KCa3.1$^{-/-}$ mice were housed in a specific pathogen-free animal facility. A permanent focal cerebral ischemia model was prepared in accordance with the guidelines as described previously [19]. In brief, adult male mice weighing 23 to 27 g were anesthetized with 2% chloral hydrate and body temperature was maintained at 37 ± 0.5 °C throughout the surgery using a heating pad and lamp (ALC-HTP, Shanghai Alcott Biotech Co. Ltd). To induce permanent focal cerebral ischemia, a silicon rubbed-counted suture with a tip diameter of 0.22 mm (L2000, AAA, Guangzhou Jialing Biiotech Co, Ltd.) was inserted into the left external carotid artery to block the middle cerebral artery. Transcranial laser Doppler (moorVMS-LDF2) was used to monitor cerebral blood flow (CBF) to assure reduction of CBF through the surgery (Additional file 1: Figure S1). The sham-operated mice experienced the same surgical operations except for the silicon rubbed-counted suture inserted.

Stroke study population and quality control

The operators were not involved in data analysis and acquisition. The observers performed the surgeries, and parameters evaluation was unaware of the group to which each mouse belonged. The following conditions excluded mice from end-point analyses (exclusion criteria): (1) < 80% reduction in CBF; (2) subarachnoid hemorrhage or the brain parenchyma bleeding (as macroscopically assessed during brain sampling); (3) neurological score = 0 (6 h, 24 h after pMCAO); and (4) operation time > 10 min. In total, 158 mice (86 C57BL/6 WT, 72 KCa3.1$^{-/-}$) were used in this study. Of the 120 mice subjected to pMCAO, 12 mice (10%) met at least one exclusion criterion after randomization and, therefore, were withdrawn from the study.

Measurement of neurological deficits

Mice were studied for neurological deficits at 3, 6, and 24 h after pMCAO as described previously [20]. Briefly, neurological findings were scored on a 5-point scale: 0, no observable neurological deficits (normal); (1) failure to extend the right forepaw (mild); (2) circling to the contralateral side (moderate); (3) loss of walking or righting reflex (severe); (4) dead. The observers were unaware of the group to which each mouse belonged.

Determination of infarct volume

Groups of mice were euthanized at 3, 6, and 24 h after MCAO. Brains were quickly removed and chilled at – 20 ° C for 20 min to slightly harden the tissue. Then brains were sectioned into five 1 mm-thick coronal slices starting from the frontal pole. All sections were stained with 2% 2,3,5-triphenyltetrazolium hydrochloride in the dark for 20 min at 37°C and flipped every 5 min for staining of anterior and posterior faces [21]. Finally slices were fixed in 4% paraformaldehyde overnight at 4 °C. ImageJ was used to measure the infarct area of each brain.

Immunohistochemistry

For immunofluorescence staining of serial brain coronal sections (12 μm) and cultured cells, the tissues and cells were blocked with 1% bovine serum albumin and 1% goat normal serum 1 h at room temperature. Sections and cells were incubated at 4 °C overnight with primary antibodies: mouse anti-KCa3.1 (1:100; Alomone Labs), rabbit anti-GFAP (1:500; Dako); rabbit anti-Iba1 (1:500; Abcam); rabbit anti-NeuN antibody (1:500; Millipore), rabbit anti-TRPV4 (1:200; Alomone Labs). The sections and cells were incubated with following secondary antibodies: Alexa Fluor 555 goat anti-rabbit IgG (1:500; Invitrogen), Alexa Fluor 488 goat anti-mouse IgG (1:500; Invitrogen) for 1 h at room temperature. Then washed with PBS and stained with DAPI (4′, 6-diamidino-2-phenylindole).

Data collection and statistics of immunofluorescence

Twelve-micrometer-thick brain slices were collected from mice and four slices at 120 μm intervals from each brain were used to examine GFAP, Iba-1, and NeuN positive cells.

The average optical density of GFAP. At least three microscopic photographs of vision were selected in hippocampus or cortex of each immunofluorescence hemisphere slice. Leica·TCS·SP8 Laser scanning confocal microscope was used to capture photographs, which were obtained under the same confocal settings. The area of the AOI (area of interest, area) and the integral optical density (IOD) value was measured using the Image-Pro Plus 6.0 software as in previous study [22], and the IOD/ area was calculated to obtain the mean IOD in each image. At last, the final mean IOD of each slice was determined by the average of the mean IOD in each image.

Cell counting. At least three fields were captured in each slice with the same reference position for quantification. The numbers of Iba1$^+$ and NeuN$^+$ cells per 1 mm^2 in each slice were counted using the Image-Pro Plus 6.0 software. The data from at least three photographs of each hemisphere slice were averaged as one value and values from three slices were calculated.

Analysis of co-localization. For analysis of TRPV4 and KCa3.1 co-localization, images were processed and analyzed using Leica LAS AF Lite software (Leica, Germany). Pearson correlation was used to express the degree of co-localization as described early [23, 24]. The co-localization of KCa3.1 and TRPV4 in the overlap of the two channels was assessed using the co-localization tool in Leica LAS AF Lite software. The Pearson correlation values range from – 1 to + 1. A correlation of 1 indicates complete co-localization between the two proteins. A correlation of – 1 indicates a negative interaction, and a correlation of 0 indicates no co-localization between the two proteins [24].

Primary culture of astrocytes

Primary astrocyte cultures were prepared from neonatal (0–2 days old) C57BL/6 wild type or KCa3.1$^{-/-}$ mouse brains as described previously [17]. Briefly, the cerebral cortices were dissected out and dissociated into a single cell suspension. When cells grew to confluence (10-14 days later), flasks were shaken overnight (200 rpm, 37 °C) and the medium exchanged to remove adherent microglia and oligodendrocytes. The purified astrocytes were plated into plates in serum-containing DMEM. After once again reaching confluence, the medium was exchanged for serum-free DMEM for 24 h before treatments. In some cases, the cells were pretreated with the blockers 30 min before oxygen-glucose deprivation.

Oxygen-glucose deprivation and drug exposure

Confluent astrocytes were grown in serum-free DMEM for 24 h before OGD, at which time the culture medium was replaced with glucose/glutamine-free DMEM medium after a gentle cell washing with the same medium. The serum-free and glucose/glutamine-free DMEM medium was balanced for 30 min with 95% (*v/v*) N_2, 5% (*v/v*) CO_2 at 37°C before OGD. Then cells were exposed to hypoxia for different time points in a small anaerobic chamber filled with 95% (*v/v*) N_2 and 5% (*v/v*) CO_2 at 37 °C. Drugs and inhibitors were pretreated to the cells 30 min before OGD. A Cell

Counting Kit-8 (CCK-8, Dojindo Laboratories, Kumamoto, Japan) was used to measure cell viability [25].

Western blotting

Mouse brain tissues or astrocytes were homogenized in RIPA buffer (25 mM Tris pH 7.4, 150 mM NaCl, 1% NP-40) containing 0.1% sodium dodecyl sulfate (SDS) and 4% protease inhibitor (complete protease inhibitor cocktail, Roche). Tissue lysates were centrifuged at 13500 rpm for 30 min at 4 °C, and supernatants were collected. Total lysates were diluted in 2 × SDS sample buffer (120 mM Tris/HCl, 10% SDS, 20% glycerine, 20% 2-mercaptoethanol, pH 6.8) to a final concentration of 2 μg/μl and were used for western blotting. The following primary antibodies were used: anti-KCa3.1 (1:500; Abcam), anti-TRPV4 (1:500; Alomone Labs), anti-GFAP (1:2000; Z0334, Dako), and anti-β-actin (1:1000; Santa Cruz). HRP-conjugated anti-rabbit or anti-mouse IgG secondary antibodies (1:3000; Amersham Biosciences) were used for 1 h at room temperature. ImageJ software was used to quantify the protein bands and normalized to the actin band, which served as loading control [26].

Cell viability

Cell viability was assessed using a Cell Counting Kit-8 (CCK-8, Dojindo Molecular Technologies) as previously described [4]. Briefly, the confluent astrocytes were cultured in serum-free media for 24 h and were then treated with OGD for different time points (1, 3, 4 6, 12 h). Ten microliter CCK-8 was added to each well of the 96-well plate and then was placed in a CO_2 incubator for 2 h. Measure the absorbance at 450 nm with a microplate reader.

Membrane potential measurement

Bis-(1,3-dibutylbarbituric acid) trimethine oxonol [DiBAC4(3)], the potentiometric fluorescent dye, was used to measure membrane potential as described previously [27]. Briefly, primary cultured astrocytes were loaded with 100 nmol/l DiBAC4 (3) for 20 min to ensure dye distribution across the cell membrane at 37 °C in an incubator. 1-EBIO (200 μM) or RN1747 (10 μM) was added to the cells at 60 s. A TCS SP8 confocal laser-scanning microscope (Leica, Germany) was used to evaluate relative changes in membrane potential by monitoring DiBAC4(3) fluorescence. TRAM-34 (1 and 10 μM) or HC 067047 (10 μM) was added 1 h before the experiment. DiBAC4(3) fluorescence was measured at 530 nm with excitation at 488 nm. Confocal images were taken and stored every 1 s for 1800 s.

$[Ca^{2+}]_i$ measurement

Cytosolic Ca^{2+} ($[Ca^{2+}]_i$) was measured as described previously [27]. Briefly, astrocytes were loaded with 5 μM Fluo-4 AM (MAIBIO, Shanghai, China) for 30 min at 37 °C in an incubator, rinsed, and incubated in DMEM with the appropriate test reagents. Baseline fluorescence was measured for the first 60 s, and then 1-EBIO (200 μM) or RN1747 (10 μM) was added to the cell plate. A TCS SP8 confocal laser-scanning microscope (Leica, Germany) was used to evaluate relative changes in intracellular calcium concentration ($[Ca^{2+}]_i$) by monitoring Fluo-4 fluorescence. TRAM-34 (1 and 10 μM) or HC 067047 (10 μM) was added 1 h before the experiment. Fluo-4 fluorescence was measured at 510 nm, with excitation at 488 nm. Confocal images were taken and stored every 1 s for 360 s.

Statistical analysis

All data are presented as means ± SEM. Statistical analyses were performed using Prism software (GraphPad Software, Inc., La Jolla, CA, USA). Data were tested for Gaussian distribution with the Kolmogorov–Smirnov normality test and then analyzed by one-way ANOVA and Dunnett's post hoc tests. Data were analyzed with unpaired, two-tailed Student's t test when comparing between two groups, or the non-parametric Mann–Whitney test was applied. Statistical significance was set at $p < 0.05$.

Results

Upregulation of KCa3.1 expression in the brains of pMCAO mice

Most recently, we reported KCa3.1 was increased in reactive astrocytes in the brains of both mouse models of AD and AD patients, and pharmacological inhibition or genetic deletion of KCa3.1 reduced astrogliosis-induced neuronal loss in the AD mouse model [7]. Based on this, we hypothesized that KCa3.1 is also mechanistically involved in astrogliosis-mediated neuronal damage following ischemic stroke. Here, we chose a mouse model of pMCAO as described previously [19]. Following MCAO blockage, the expression of both KCa3.1 and GFAP was significantly increased in the infarcted hemisphere of pMCAO mice as detected by western blotting (Fig. 1a, b) for up to 12 h (Additional file 2: Figure S2).

Co-immunostaining of KCa3.1 with specific for neurons, astrocytes, and microglia was performed on brain sections of control and 6 h pMCAO mice. KCa3.1 expression was found in NeuN$^+$ neurons in the brains of both control and 6 h pMCAO mice (Fig. 1c). Less KCa3.1 expression was detected in the neurons of pMCAO mice because of the cells loss during the pathology process of ischemia compared to the control group, but there was no obviously difference in the percentage of the co-localization between pMCAO and control group. In control mice, a low level of expression of KCa3.1 was detected in GFAP$^+$ astrocytes (Fig. 1d). However, at 6 h pMCAO, we detected a clear co-localization between KCa3.1 and GFAP$^+$ reactive

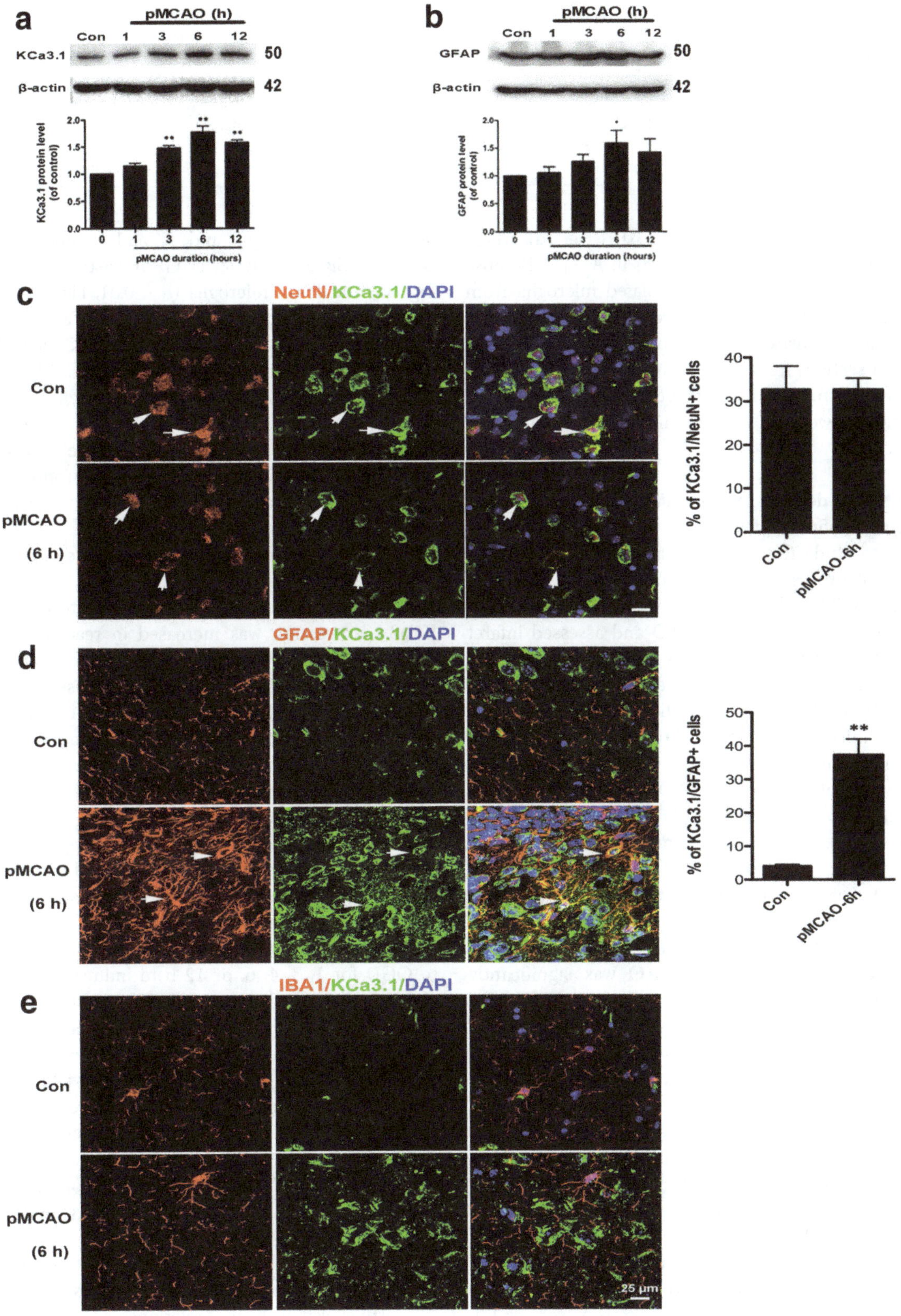

Fig. 1 (See legend on next page.)

(See figure on previous page.)

Fig. 1 Upregulation of KCa3.1 channels and GFAP in mouse brains following pMCAO. **a**, **b** Western blot analysis of lysates from 10-week-old male WT mice following 1, 3, 6, or 12 h of pMCAO analyzed by antibodies to KCa3.1 (**a**) and GFAP (**b**). Data represent the means ± SEM of KCa3.1 and GFAP density normalized to β-actin values for $n = 3$. $^{*}p < 0.05$, $^{**}p < 0.01$, one-way ANOVA followed by the Dunnett's multiple comparison test compared with control. Con control. **c–e** Cellular localization of KCa3.1 channels in mouse brains following pMCAO. Double immunofluorescence analysis of KCa3.1 (green) levels in (**c**) neurons (NeuN, red), (**d**) astrocytes (GFAP, red), and (**e**) microglia (Iba1, red) of control and 6 h pMCAO mouse brain. DAPI (blue) was used to label nuclei. Quantification of the percentage of $NeuN^{+}$ (**c**) or $GFAP^{+}$ (**d**) cells colabeled for KCa3.1 at 6 h pMCAO compared with the control group. $^{**}p < 0.01$, unpaired, two-tailed Student's t test compared with control mice ($n = 4$). Scale bar: 25 μm. Con control

astrocytes in the infarct regions ($p < 0.01$, Fig. 1d), which is consistent with our previous reports in AD [7]. Because Chen et al. [9] reported acutely isolated microglia from the brains of transient MCAO mice with 8 days of reperfusion exhibit increased function of KCa3.1 channels, so we labeled sections from the 6 h pMCAO for KCa3.1 and the microglial marker Iba1. There was no obvious co-localization between KCa3.1 and microglia at 6 h pMCAO (Fig. 1e).

Genetic KCa3.1 deletion reduces infarct area and improve neurological deficit in pMCAO

In order to study the role of KCa3.1 deficiency on the pathological processes of ischemic stroke, we subjected wild type (WT) and KCa3.1 gene deletion ($KCa3.1^{-/-}$) mice to 3, 6, and 24 h of pMCAO and assessed infarct volumes and neurological deficits (Fig. 2). As shown in Fig. 2a–f, the infarct area measurements by TTC staining in pMCAO brains indicated that infarct volumes in $KCa3.1^{-/-}$ mice was smaller than those in WT mice, and infarct areas in $KCa3.1^{-/-}$ mice were significantly reduced by 19% at 6 h after pMCAO compared with those in WT mice ($p < 0.05$, Fig. 2c, d) but there was no significant difference in infarct measurement at 3 h ($p = 0.3085$, Fig. 2a, b) and 24 h after stroke ($p = 0.0951$, Fig. 2e, f). Furthermore, the neurological deficit scores of $KCa3.1^{-/-}$ mice were significantly lower than those of WT mice at 24 h after pMCAO ($p < 0.05$, Fig. 2g). The survival rate of 24 h after pMCAO was significantly higher in $KCa3.1^{-/-}$ mice than that in WT mice ($p < 0.05$, 66.7% (12/18) vs 37.5% (6/16), Fig. 2g).

Genetic KCa3.1 deficiency reduces neuron loss and gliosis induced by pMCAO

It is well documented that reactive gliosis of both astrocytes and microglia are two hallmark features of ischemia and its penumbral region [28]. We previously showed in primary astrocyte cultures and an AD mouse model that inhibition of KCa3.1 attenuated the reactive glial response [7]. Furthermore, we also demonstrated that deletion or inhibition of KCa3.1 reduced astrogliosis-induced neurotoxicity in a co-culture system of neurons-astrocytes [7]. To assess the role of KCa3.1 in the process of ischemic stroke, neuron survival and glial activation were measured by immunostaining with markers of neurons, astrocyte, and microglia in WT and $KCa3.1^{-/-}$ mice 6 h after pMCAO. Significantly fewer $GFAP^{+}$ astrocytes ($p < 0.05$, Fig. 3a) and $Iba1^{+}$ microglia ($p < 0.01$, Fig. 3b) were detected in the 6 h pMCAO brains of $KCa3.1^{-/-}$ mice as compared to WT mice, while more $NeuN^{+}$ neurons were detected in the 6 h pMCAO brains of $KCa3.1^{-/-}$ mice as compared to WT mice ($p < 0.01$, Fig. 3c). As shown in Fig. 3d, the images of Fig. 3a–c were taken from CA1 (Additional file 3: Figure S3). Overall, these results suggest that targeted deletion of KCa3.1 has neuroprotective effects against cerebral ischemic injury induced by pMCAO.

KCa3.1 and TRPV4 mediate oxygen-glucose deprivation induced astrogliosis

We previously found in primary astrocyte cultures that KCa3.1 expression was increased in reactive astrocytes induced by TGF-β, while pharmacological blockade or genetic deletion of KCa3.1 attenuated astrogliosis [17]. Butenko et al. [15] reported that TRPV4 was markedly enhanced in astrocytes of the CA1 region after hypoxia/ischemia and that increased TRPV4 expression coincided with the development of astrogliosis. We therefore investigated the hypothesis that KCa3.1 regulates Ca^{2+} entry via the TRPV4 channel leading to reactive astrogliosis-induced neuronal damage during ischemia stroke. We firstly evaluated the expression of KCa3.1 and TRPV4 during the process of OGD-induced astrogliosis in vitro. Primary cultured astrocytes were subject to OGD for 1, 3, 4, 6, or 12 h to induce reactive astrogliosis as described previously [29]. As shown in Fig. 4, OGD induced a time-dependent upregulation of KCa3.1 and TRPV4 channels, which was consistent with the upregulation of GFAP (Fig. 4a–c). The cell viability analysis showed a significant decrease in astrocytes viability during 1–12 h after OGD treatment (Fig. 4d). These data suggested that the increase in KCa3.1 and TRPV4 occurred concomitantly with upregulation of GFAP during the process of OGD-induced reactive astrogliosis.

KCa3.1 channels hyperpolarize reactive astrocytes membrane potential during oxygen-glucose deprivation

To further establish the relationship between KCa3.1 and TRPV4 in regulating reactive astrocytes during ischemia stroke, we investigated the role of TRPV4 in the process of KCa3.1 regulated membrane potential. As

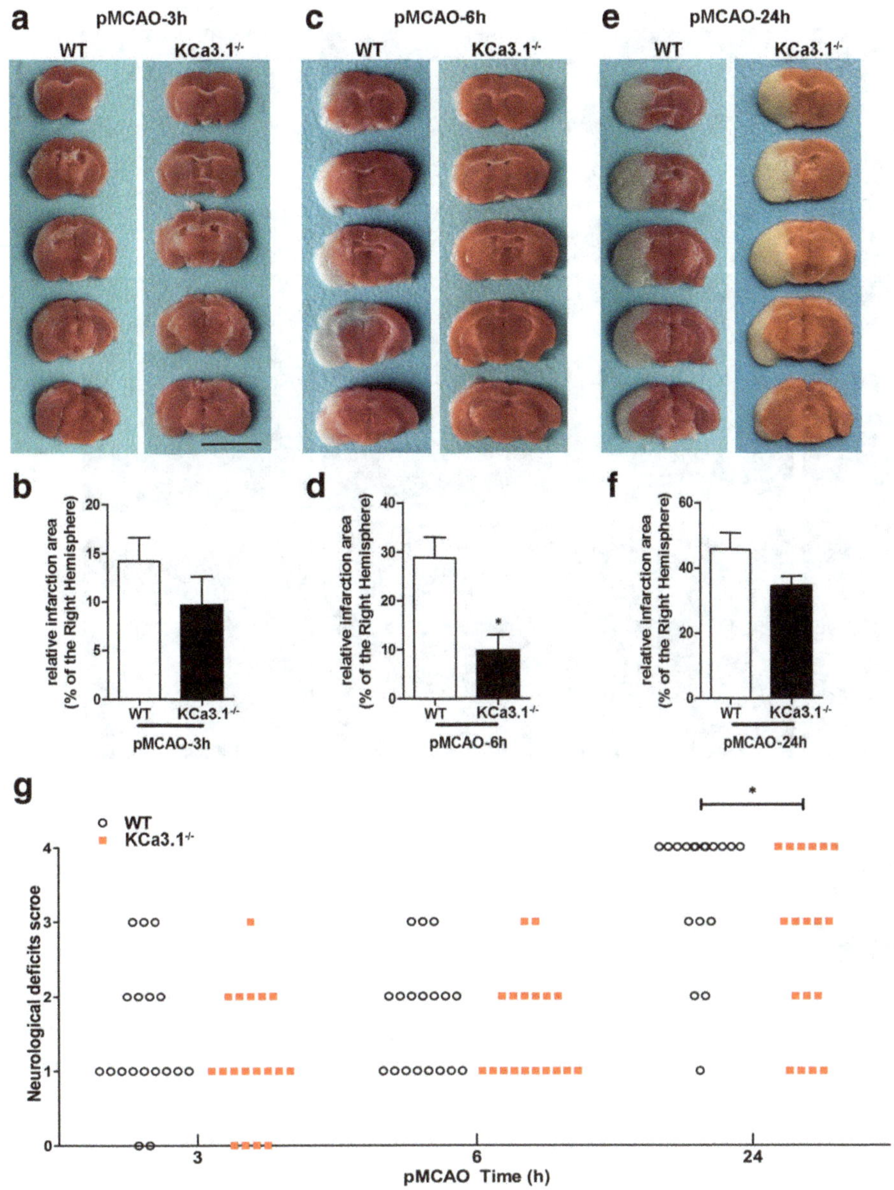

Fig. 2 KCa3.1 deficiency reduces infarction volume and improves of neurological conditions. Focal cerebral ischemia was induced by pMCAO. **a**, **c**, and **e** Representative TTC staining of five corresponding coronal brain sections of a 10-week-old male WT mouse and a 10 week-old male KCa3.1$^{-/-}$ mouse after 3 h (**a**), 6 h (**c**), and 24 h (**e**) of pMCAO. **b**, **d**, and **f**. Quantitative analysis of infarction volume in a, c, and e, respectively. Data are presented as means ± SEM. $n = 6$. $^{*}p < 0.05$, unpaired, two-tailed Student's t test compared with ischemic WT group. **g** Neurological deficits were assessed at 3, 6, and 24 h after pMCAO. Significance: $^{*}p < 0.05$ vs WT group ($n = 18$). Mann–Whitney test compared with WT mice. The survival rate of 24 h after pMCAO was obviously higher in the KCa3.1$^{-/-}$ group than that in the WT group (66.7 vs 37.5%, respectively), and significant differences was observed ($p = 0.0486$, chi-square test)

reported before, activation of KCa3.1 hyperpolarizes non-excitable cells such as airway smooth muscle cells [25] and pancreatic cancer cells [30]; this hyperpolarization enhances the driving force for Ca^{2+} influx. To evaluate the role of KCa3.1 in OGD activation of astrocytes, the KCa3.1 pharmacological activator 1-ethylbenzimidazolinone (EBIO) was used to activate KCa3.1 [31] with and without OGD. As shown in Fig. 5a, 200 μM 1-EBIO induced a larger hyperpolarization (as measured by DiBAC4(3) fluorescence intensity) in the 1 h OGD-treated astrocytes as compared to control cells, likely due to enhanced K^{+} efflux upon increased KCa3.1 activation. We then used the TRPV4 channel antagonist HC 067047 to test the role of TRPV4 channels in regulating membrane potential during 1-EBIO-induced KCa3.1 activation. Blockade of TRPV4 attenuated the level of 1-EBIO-mediated membrane hyperpolarization in OGD-induced astrocytes ($p < 0.001$, Fig. 5a, b). In addition, 10 μM, but not 1 μM, KCa3.1 selective blocker

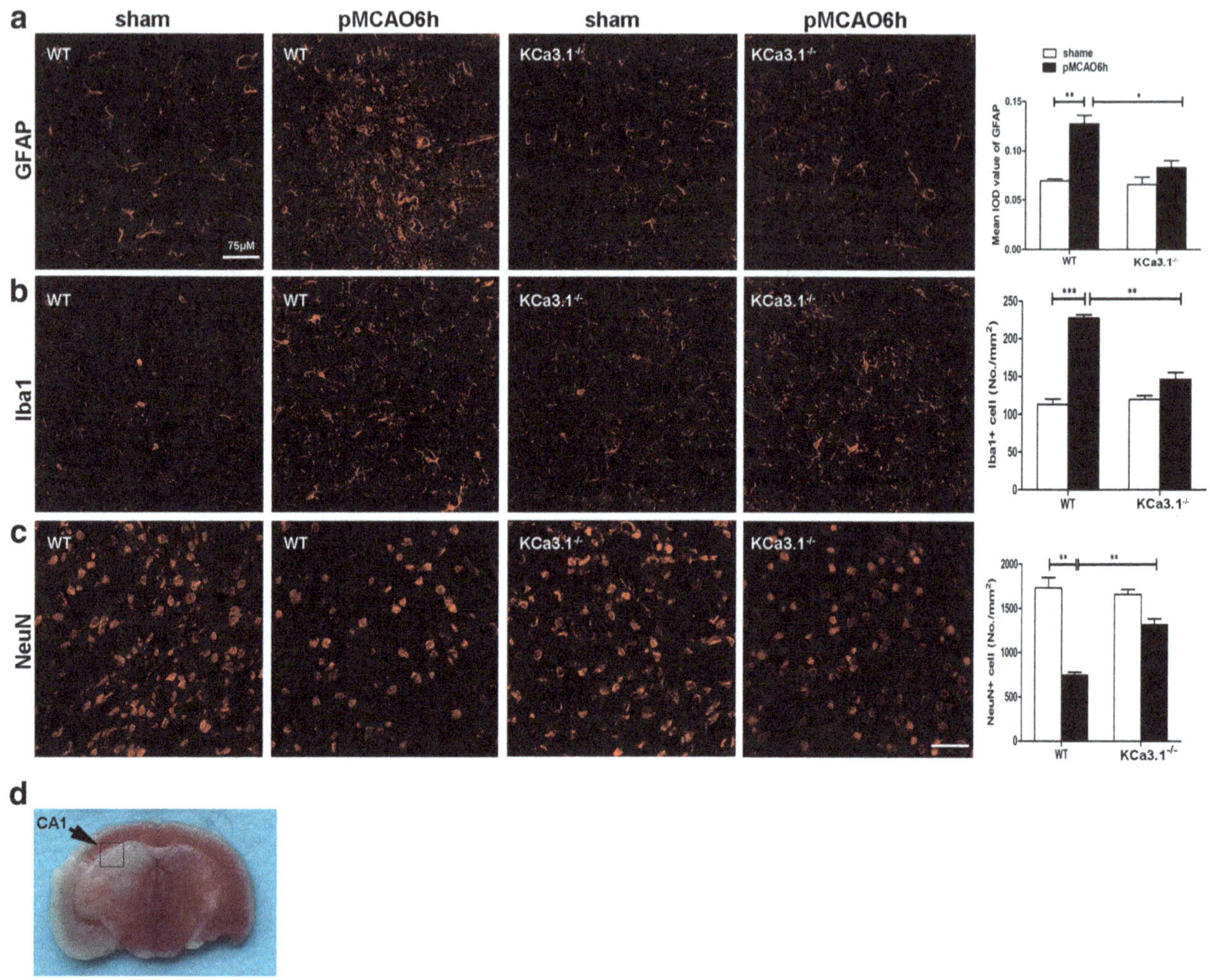

Fig. 3 Decreased glial activation and neuronal loss in brains of KCa3.1 deletion mice following pMCAO. Reactive astrocytes (**a**), activated microglia (**b**), and neurons (**c**) from the hippocampal CA1 regions of WT or KCa3.1$^{-/-}$ mice at 6 h after pMCAO were visualized by GFAP, Iba1, and NeuN immunostaining, respectively. At least four coronal slices from each mouse brain and at least three brains of each genotype were used for immunostaining and counting. $n = 4$ per group. Scale bar: 75 μm. Data represent means ± SEM. $^{*}p < 0.05$, $^{**}p < 0.01$, $^{***}p < 0.001$, unpaired, two-tailed Student's *t* test. **d** Images of Fig. 3a–c were taken from CA1 regions (black box). WT, wild type

TRAM-34 attenuated 200 μM 1-EBIO-induced membrane hyperpolarization in 1 h OGD-treated astrocytes ($p < 0.001$, Fig. 5c, d).

It was reported that as the downstream component of the TRPV4 transduction pathway, a genetic deficit of KCa3.1 reduced lung damage and pulmonary circulatory collapse induced by TRPV4 channel activation [32]. We therefore measured the change in membrane potential in both WT and KCa3.1 KCa3.1$^{-/-}$ astrocytes following the addition of the TRPV4 channel agonist 10 μM RN1747 along with OGD. We found that hyperpolarization in response to RN1747 was reduced in the KCa3.1$^{-/-}$ astrocytes, compared with the WT cells ($p < 0.001$, Fig. 5e, f), both in normoxia and in response to OGD.

KCa3.1 activation induces calcium entry in astrocytes through TRPV4 calcium channel during oxygen-glucose deprivation

It has been suggested that the Ca^{2+} influx resulting from activation of TRPV4 channels is leveraged by the high Ca^{2+} sensitivity of KCa3.1 and KCa2 to cause vascular endothelium vasodilation [33]. To evaluate the potential activation of KCa3.1 channels by OGD, we measured $[Ca^{2+}]_i$ in response to activation of KCa3.1 channels by 1-EBIO in control astrocytes and in astrocytes subjected to 1 h of OGD. We found that 200 μM 1-EBIO induced a larger increase in $[Ca^{2+}]_i$ in the 1 h OGD-treated astrocytes as compared to the control cells ($p < 0.001$, Fig. 5g, h). We then used HC 067047 to test the role of TRPV4 channels in the Ca^{2+} influx during OGD and 1-EBIO-induced KCa3.1

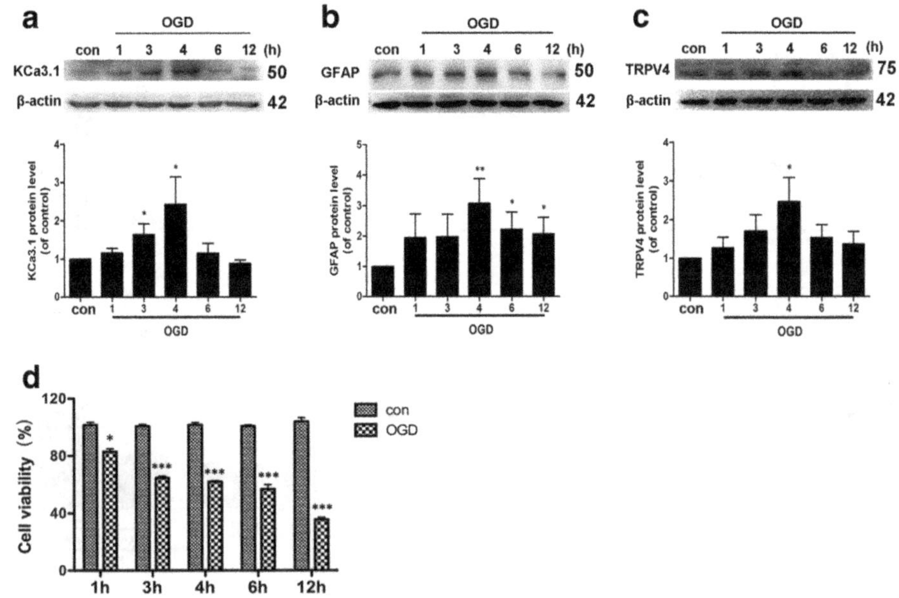

Fig. 4 Upregulation of KCa3.1, GFAP, and TRPV4 channels following OGD in cultured astrocytes. Western blot analysis of (**a**) KCa3.1, (**b**) GFAP, and (**c**) TRPV4 expression after OGD-treatment for 0, 1, 3, 4, 6, 12 h. Data represent the means ± SEM of KCa3.1, GFAP, and TRPV4 density normalized to β-actin values for $n = 3$ cultures. $^{*}p < 0.05$, $^{**}p < 0.01$, one-way ANOVA followed by the Dunnett's multiple comparison test compared with control. (**d**) Cell viability was determined by the CCK-8 assay. The values represent the percentage of cells viability induced by 1, 3, 4, 6, or 12 h of OGD ($n = 4$). Data represent means ± SEM. $^{*}p < 0.05$, $^{***}p < 0.001$, unpaired, two-tailed Student's t test compared with control. Con control, OGD oxygen-glucose deprivation

activation; we found that blockade of TRPV4 channels attenuated the level of 1-EBIO-mediated Ca^{2+} increase in OGD-induced astrocytes ($p < 0.001$, Fig. 5g, h). To further confirm that KCa3.1 activation induced the $[Ca^{2+}]_i$ increase, TRAM-34 (1 and 10 μM) was used in the same experiments. In the presence of 1 and 10 μM TRAM-34, the $[Ca^{2+}]_i$ increase induced by 200 μM 1-EBIO was attenuated in both the 1 μM ($p < 0.01$, Fig. 5i, j) and 10 μM ($p < 0.001$, Fig. 5i, j) TRAM-34 treatment of 1 h OGD-astrocytes.

To evaluate the effect of OGD on TRPV4 channels, we used 10 μM RN1747 in WT and KCa3.1$^{-/-}$ astrocytes with and without OGD. $[Ca^{2+}]_i$ was measured before and after the application of OGD 1 h. In the KCa3.1$^{-/-}$ astrocytes, the Ca^{2+} influx induced by RN1747 was drastically reduced as compared with the WT cells ($p < 0.001$, Fig. 5k, l). Taken together, our data showed that TRPV4 channels mediated the plasma membrane hyperpolarization-evoked $[Ca^{2+}]_i$ increase due to activation of KCa3.1.

KCa3.1 and TRPV4 channels regulated astrogliosis

The above results indicate that KCa3.1 and TRPV4 are functionally linked. The question then arises as to whether they are physically associated with each other. The physical interaction between KCa3.1 and TRPV4 channels was further tested. Confocal analysis of double-labeled staining showed that KCa3.1 and TRPV4 channels co-localized in normal mouse brain (Fig. 6a, b) and primary cultured astrocytes (Fig. 6c, d). Histograms represent the ratio of the mean Pearson correlation coefficient using Leica LAS AF Lite software. The Pearson correlation values range from − 1 to + 1. A correlation of 1 indicates complete co-localization between the two proteins. A correlation of − 1 indicates a negative interaction, and a correlation of 0 indicates no co-localization between the two proteins. When double-labeled staining of KCa3.1 and TRPV4 channels, co-localization was observed in normal mouse brain (Fig. 6a, b) and primary cultured astrocytes (Fig. 6c, d). As shown in Fig. 6e, Pearson correlation coefficients are 0.57 (mouse brain) and 0.49 (astrocytes), confirming co-localization between KCa3.1 and TRPV4.

The involvement of the KCa3.1 and TRPV4 in regulating the emergence of astrogliosis induced by 4 h OGD was studied by using antagonists of these two channels. In the presence of either TRAM-34 (1 μM) or HC 067047 (10 μM), upregulation of GFAP was attenuated ($p < 0.05$, Fig. 7a, b). Moreover, astrocytes from KCa3.1 KCa3.1$^{-/-}$ mice exhibited a decrease in GFAP expression induced by 4 h OGD treatment ($p < 0.001$, Fig. 7c, d) as compared to WT astrocytes. These results suggested that KCa3.1 and TRPV4 are both involved in the process of astrogliosis induced by OGD.

Discussion

The major findings of this study are that the KCa3.1 channel contributes to reactive astrogliosis following

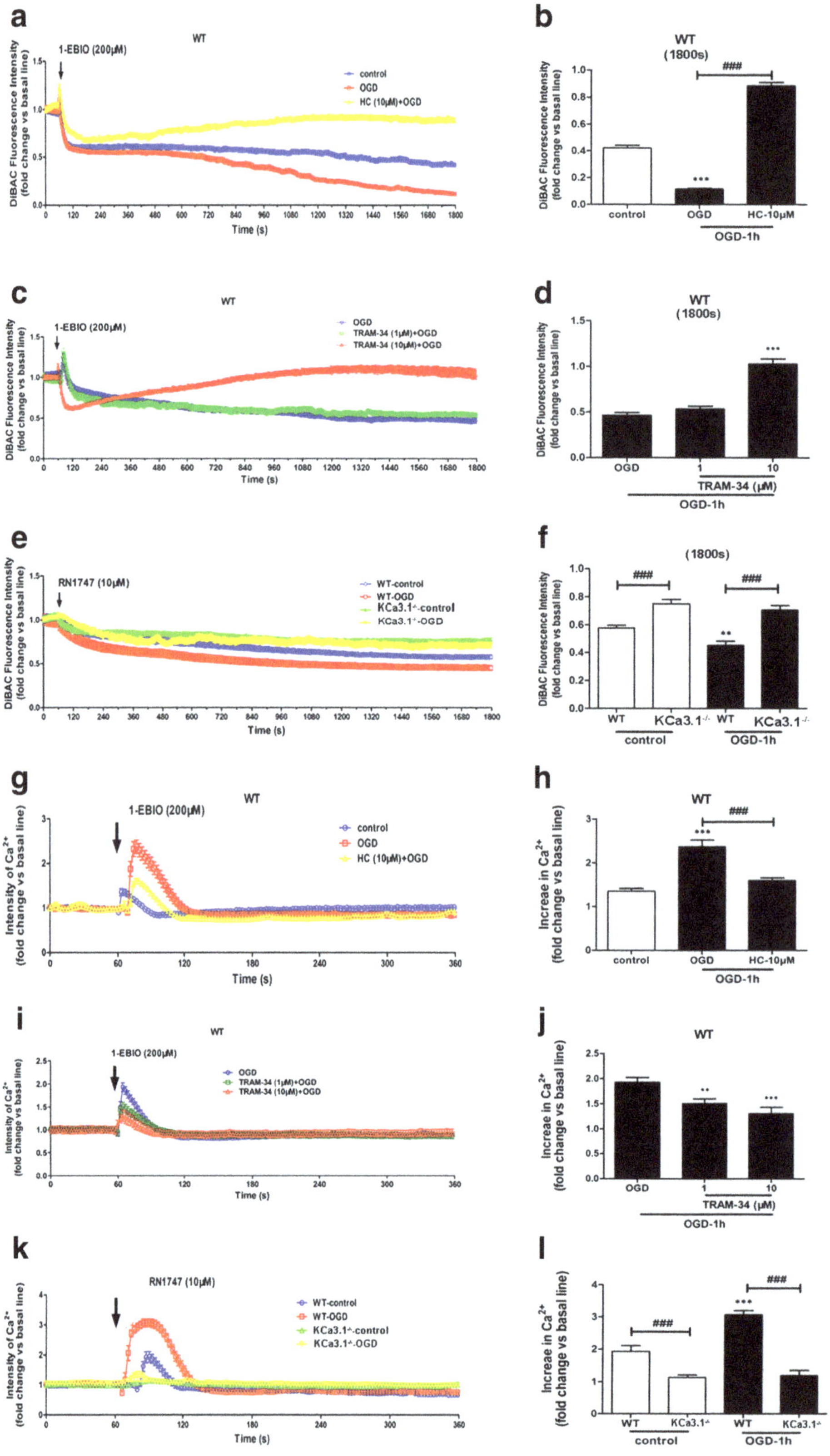

Fig. 5 (See legend on next page.)

(See figure on previous page.)
Fig. 5 Role of TRPV4 and KCa3.1 in alteration of membrane potential and Ca^{2+} entry in astrocytes following OGD. **a–f** Changes in membrane potential in response to activation of KCa3.1 channels and TRPV4 channels in astrocytes exposed to OGD 1 h. **a**, **b** 1-EBIO was added to WT astrocytes and membrane potential measured with or without OGD or HC 067047. Data are presented as means ± SEM. $n = 10–20$. $^{***}p < 0.001$ vs control. $^{###}p < 0.001$ vs OGD. **c**, **d** 1-EBIO was added to WT astrocytes and membrane potential measured with or without OGD or TRAM-34 (1 and 10 μM). Data are presented as means ± SEM. $n = 10–20$. $^{***}p < 0.001$ vs OGD. **e**, **f** RN1747 was added to WT or KCa3.1 KCa3.1$^{-/-}$ astrocytes and membrane potential measured with or without OGD. **b**, **d**, **f** Summary of data showing the membrane potential in **a**, **c**, and e at 1800s. Data are presented as means ± SEM. $n = 10–20$. $^{**}p < 0.01$ vs WT control, $^{###}p < 0.001$ vs WT control or WT OGD. **g–l** Changes in $[Ca^{2+}]_i$ in response to activation of KCa3.1 channels and TRPV4 channels in astrocytes exposed to OGD 1 h. **g**, **h** 1-EBIO was added to WT astrocytes and $[Ca^{2+}]_i$ measured with or without OGD or HC 067047. Data are presented as means ± SEM. $n = 10–20$. $^{***}p < 0.001$ vs control. $^{###}p < 0.001$ vs OGD. **i**, **j** 1-EBIO was added to WT astrocytes and $[Ca^{2+}]_i$ measured with or without OGD or TRAM-34 (1 and 10 μM). Data are presented as means ± SEM. $n = 10–20$. $^{**}p < 0.01$, $^{***}p < 0.001$ vs OGD. **k**, **l** RN1747 was added to WT or KCa3.1 KCa3.1$^{-/-}$ astrocytes and $[Ca^{2+}]_i$ measured with or without OGD. **h**, **j**, **l** Summary of data showing the $[Ca^{2+}]_i$ in **h**, **j**, and **l** at 70–80 s. Data are presented as means ± SEM. $n = 10–20$. $^{***}p < 0.001$ vs WT control, $^{###}p < 0.001$ vs WT control or WT OGD. Statistical analysis was performed using unpaired, two-tailed Student's *t* test. 1-EBIO, 1-ethyl-2-benzimidazolinone, OGD oxygen-glucose deprivation, WT wild type, HC HC 067047

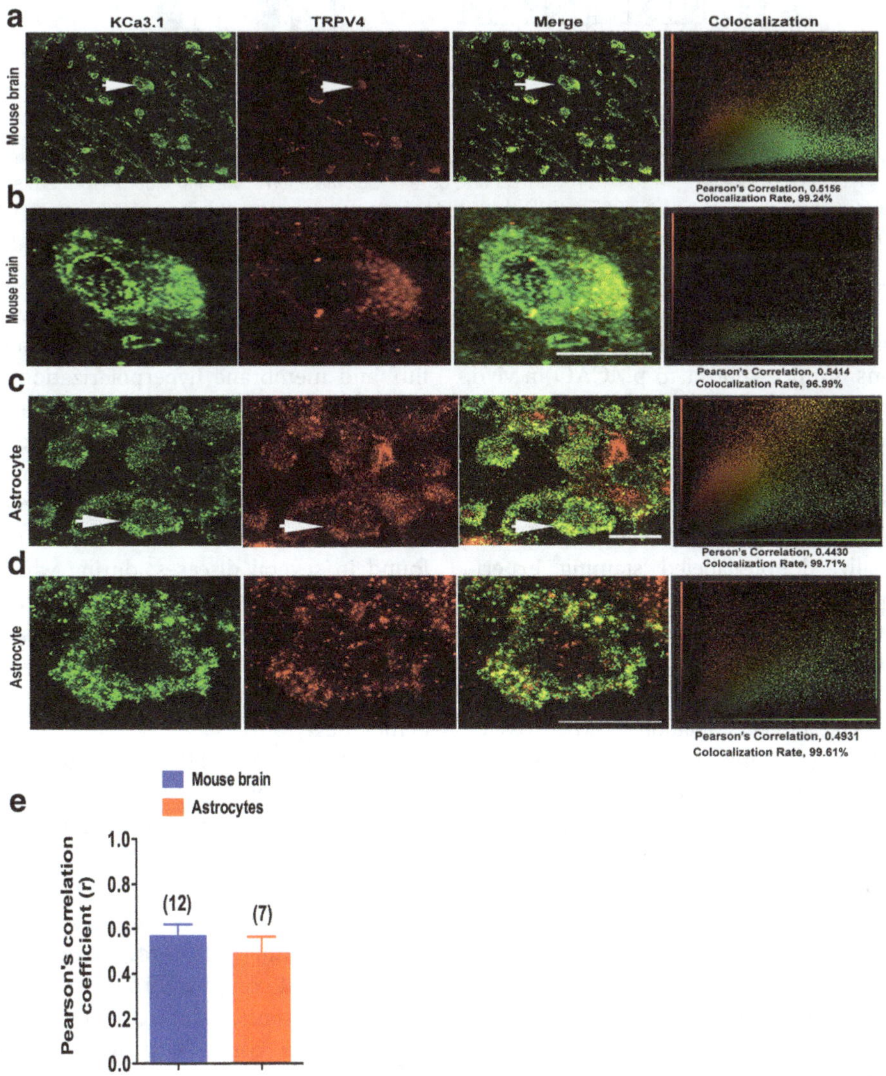

Fig. 6 KCa3.1 and TRPV4 co-localized in primary cultured astrocytes and mouse brain cortex. Double immunofluorescence images of KCa3.1 (green) and TRPV4 (red) in normal mouse brains (**a**, **b**), and primary cultured astrocytes (**c**, **d**). Note the strong co-localization indicated by merge yellow fluorescence, quantification of the co-localization observed in experiments as shown in g. (**e**) The histograms represent the ratio of the mean Pearson correlation coefficient calculated from the co-labeling in a number of samples, as indicated above the bar. Scale bar: 25 μm

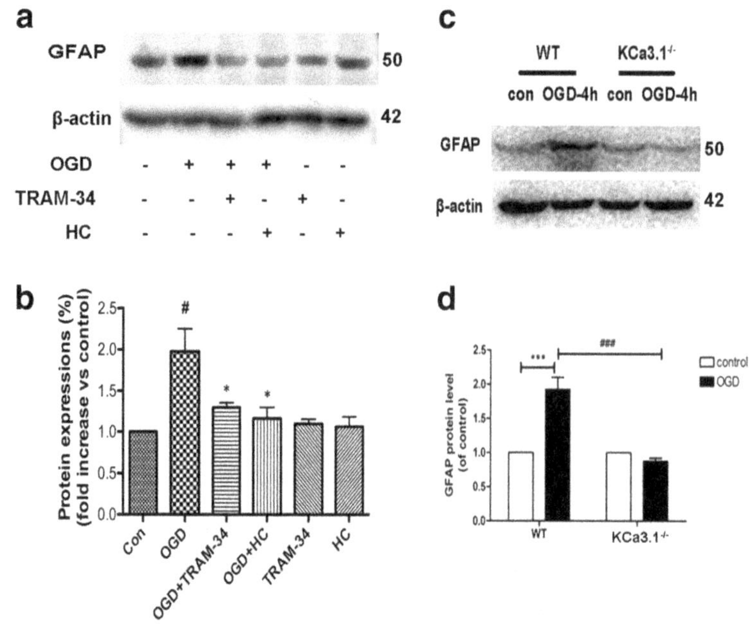

Fig. 7 Involvement of KCa3.1 in OGD-induced reactive astrogliosis. **a**, **b** Representative western blot showing GFAP expression in cultured astrocytes treated with OGD for 4 h in the presence of 1 μM TRAM-34 and 10 μM HC 067047. Quantification of western blot for GFAP expression ($n = 3$). Data are presented as means ± SEM. $^{\#}p < 0.05$ vs control, $^{*}p < 0.05$ vs OGD alone. **c**, **d** Representative western blot and quantification of GFAP expression after 4 h OGD treatment in WT and KCa3.1 KCa3.1$^{-/-}$ astrocytes ($n = 3$–4). $^{***}p < 0.001$, $^{\#\#\#}p < 0.001$. One-way ANOVA followed by the Dunnett's multiple comparison test. Con control, WT wild type

ischemia, as shown in both OGD-treated astrocytes in vitro and the brains of mice subject to pMCAO in vivo, that KCa3.1 regulated Ca^{2+} influx and membrane potential by functional cooperation with the TRPV4 channel in OGD-treated astrocytes. The expression of both channels was increased during astrogliosis and blockade either KCa3.1 or TRPV4 attenuated the astrogliosis process. Additionally, double-labeled staining experiments showed the co-localization between TRPV4 and KCa3.1 in mouse brain and primary astrocytes, where they might cooperate to regulate the reactive astrogliosis.

We provided genetic target validation of the role of KCa3.1 by demonstrating that mice with a gene deletion of KCa3.1 exhibited significantly reduced pathology after pMCAO. This was manifested as both reduced infarct area after the insult as well as reduced astrogliosis, microglial activation and neuron loss. This is consistent with recent studies that demonstrated that pharmacological blockade of KCa3.1 or gene silence reduces infarct size and other neurological deficits in rats or mice [34]. Moreover, in the present study, we extended this hypothesis to show that KCa3.1 acted as an endogenous sensor of Ca^{2+} influx caused by activation of TRPV4. We found that blockade of either channel could reduce astrogliosis. In addition, we found that these channels could be co-localization.

The lack of voltage-gated Ca^{2+} channels in non-excitable cells allows KCa3.1 to act as Ca^{2+} detectors and Ca^{2+} amplifiers. Activation of KCa3.1 induced K^{+} efflux and membrane hyperpolarization, which ultimately upregulated the driving force for Ca^{2+} influx [35, 36], and further KCa3.1 channels will be activated in a positive feedback loop. KCa3.1-Ca^{2+} channels were involved in non-excitable cells activation process [35]. An interaction between KCa3.1 and TRPV4 channels has been found in several diseases, during which Ca^{2+} dynamics induced by KCa3.1 were dependent on Ca^{2+} influx via TRPV4 channels [37, 38]. There was a functional co7-upling between KCa3.1 and TRPV4 to regulate Ca^{2+} levels leading to pulmonary circulatory collapse and hemorrhage [39].

An interaction of TRPV4 and KCa channels has been found in several other brain functions. In retinal ganglion cells, activation of TRPV4 induced apoptosis due to Ca^{2+} overload [40]. Shi et al. [41] reported that Ca^{2+} influx via TRPV4 channels involved in infrasound-induced activation of astrocytes and microglia, and then neuronal death. Astrocytes volume was regulated by TRPV4/AQP4 complex through water transport and calcium homeostasis. Over activation of the interaction of TRPV4/AQP4 complex would trigger the pathological swelling and reactive gliosis [42]. Ca^{2+} influx through TRPV4 channels activated the large Ca^{2+}-activated K^{+} channel (BK), and TRPV4/BK functional coupling regulated bladder contractility in the storage phase [43]. Gene deletion of KCa3.1 channels attenuated lung damage and pulmonary circulatory collapse caused by TRPV4 activation. In addition, these data are consistent with recent studies that suggested that the KCa channels might serve as amplifiers of the Ca^{2+} signaling through TRP channels [44] and data demonstrating a coupling of the two types of channels in osmosensors in the paraventricular nucleus [45]. Recently, it was reported that calcium-gated K^+ channels of the KCa1.1- and KCa3.1-type couple intracellular Ca^{2+} signals to membrane hyperpolarization in mesenchymal stromal cells from the human adipose tissue (Tarasov et al. 2017). It might explain the reason that stimulation of TRPV4 agonist RN1747 still caused membrane hyperpolarization in the KCa3.1$^{-/-}$ astrocytes as shown in Fig. 6e.

Reactive astrocytes are involved in many pathological processes of CNS diseases, such as stroke, traumatic brain injury, and AD [46]. During the process of neuroinflammation, activated microglia induce the phenotypic switch of astrocytes from a quiescent to a reactive phenotype. Neurotoxic reactive astrocytes, termed A1 astrocytes, are induced by activated microglia, which lose the ability to support neurons and oligodendrocyte survival and synaptogenesis [47]. In our previous studies, we showed that a similar phenotype can be induced in culture using TGF-β [17], and that blockade or deletion of the KCa3.1 channel prevented the emergence of the reactive phenotype. Whether this mechanism of astrocyte activation depends upon the astrocytic TRPV4 channels is a subject for future investigation.

KCa3.1 is thought to regulate microglial activation such as migration and neurotoxicity induced by activated microglia in vitro [48, 49]. Higher densities of Kv1.3, KCa3.1, and Kir2.1 currents were detected in microglia from the infarcted area of reversible MCAO than that from non-infarcted control brains. Similarly, strong KCa3.1 immunoreactivity was also found on activated microglia/macrophages of human infarcts [34]. However, we did not find any obvious co-localization between KCa3.1 and microglia in the brains of pMCAO mice by immunofluorescence staining. It may be that the different model of ischemic stroke (reversible MCAO vs pMCAO) as well as the different detection method (patch clamp vs immunofluorescence staining) might be the reason.

Conclusions

In conclusion, these data suggested that KCa3.1 and TRPV4 channels forms a signaling complex involved in maintaining abnormally high $[Ca^{2+}]_i$ levels to drive phenotype switch of astrogliosis during ischemia stroke. Gene deletion of KCa3.1 attenuated infarct area and reduced neuron loss and gliosis in pMCAO, which may have therapeutic utility in ischemia stroke associated with abnormally high $[Ca^{2+}]_i$ in astrogliosis.

Additional files

Additional file 1: Figure S1. Cerebral blood flow (CBF) of ischemic brain hemisphere before and during permanent middle cerebral artery occlusion (pMCAO) was monitored by transcranial laser Doppler. The arrow depicted the start of pMCAO.

Additional file 2: Figure S2. Western blot analysis of lysates from 10-week-old male WT mice following 1, 3, 6, or 12 h of pMCAO analyzed by antibodies to KCa3.1 (A) and GFAP (B).

Additional file 3: Figure S3. $GFAP^+$ reactive astrocytes and $Iba1^+$ activated microglia from the cortex and hippocampal regions of WT or KCa3.1$^{-/-}$ mice brain at 6 h after pMCAO were visualized by immunostaining. Scale bar: 200 μm. WT, wild type.

Abbreviations

1-EBIO: 1-Ethylbenzimidazolinone; GFAP: Glial fibrillary acidic protein; KCa3.1: Intermediate-conductance calcium-activated potassium channel; pMCAO: Permanent middle cerebral artery occlusion; TRAM-34: 1-((2-chlorophenyl) (diphenyl) methyl)-1H–pyrazole; TRPV4: Transient receptor potential vanilloid 4

Acknowledgements

We thank Dr. Tianle Xu and Dr. Jingjing Wang (Department of Anatomy, Histology and Embryology, Collaborative Innovation Center for Brain Science, Shanghai Key Laboratory for Tumor Microenvironment and Inflammation, Shanghai Jiao Tong University School of Medicine, Shanghai, China.) for kindly providing the Transcranial laser Doppler.

Funding

This work was supported by Science and Technology Commission of Shanghai Municipality grant 16ZR1418700, National Natural Science Foundation of China grant 81773699. The authors declare that the research was conducted in the absence of any commercial or financial relationships that could be construed as a potential conflict of interest.

Authors' contributions

ZY supervised the entire project, designed the research, and wrote the paper. HC and HG conceived and designed the experiments, interpreted and analyzed the data, and supervised all the experimental procedure. MY and TW conceived and designed the experiments, performed the research interpreted, and analyzed the data. QL and XG performed the research and analyzed the data. GC and YW analyzed the data and critically revised the manuscript. All authors read and approved the final manuscript.

Consent for publication

Not applicable.

Competing interests

The authors declare that they have no competing interests.

Author details

[1]Department of Pharmacology, Institute of Medical Sciences, Shanghai Jiao Tong University School of Medicine, Shanghai 200025, China. [2]Experimental Teaching Center of Basic Medicine, School of Medicine, Shanghai Jiao Tong University, Shanghai 200025, China. [3]Developmental Neurobiology Section,

Division of Intramural Research, National Heart, Lung, and Blood Institute, National Institutes of Health, Bethesda, MD 20892, USA.

References

1. Nedergaard M, Rodriguez JJ, Verkhratsky A. Glial calcium and diseases of the nervous system. Cell Calcium. 2010;47:140–9.
2. Di L, Srivastava S, Zhdanova O, Ding Y, Li Z, Wulff H, Lafaille M, Skolnik EY. Inhibition of the k+ channel kca3.1 ameliorates t cell-mediated colitis. Proc Natl Acad Sci U S A. 2010;107:1541–6.
3. Toyama K, Wulff H, Chandy KG, Azam P, Raman G, Saito T, Fujiwara Y, Mattson DL, Das S, Melvin JE, Pratt PF, Hatoum OA, Gutterman DD, Harder DR, Miura H. The intermediate-conductance calcium-activated potassium channel kca3.1 contributes to atherogenesis in mice and humans. J Clin Invest. 2008;118:3025–37.
4. ZH Y, Wang YX, Song Y, HZ L, Hou LN, Cui YY, Chen HZ. Up-regulation of kca3.1 promotes human airway smooth muscle cell phenotypic modulation. Pharmacol Res. 2013;77:30–8.
5. Bouhy D, Ghasemlou N, Lively S, Redensek A, Rathore KI, Schlichter LC, David S. Inhibition of the ca(2)(+)-dependent k(+) channel, kcnn4/kca3.1, improves tissue protection and locomotor recovery after spinal cord injury. J Neurosci. 2011;31:16298–308.
6. Mauler F, Hinz V, Horvath E, Schuhmacher J, Hofmann HA, Wirtz S, Hahn MG, Urbahns K. Selective intermediate–/small-conductance calcium-activated potassium channel (kcnn4) blockers are potent and effective therapeutics in experimental brain oedema and traumatic brain injury caused by acute subdural haematoma. Eur J Neurosci. 2004;20:1761–8.
7. Wei T, Yi M, Gu W, Hou L, Lu Q, Yu Z, Chen H. The potassium channel kca3. 1 represents a valid pharmacological target for astrogliosis-induced neuronal impairment in a mouse model of alzheimer's disease. Front Pharmacol. 2016;7:528.
8. Chen YJ, Wallace BK, Yuen N, Jenkins DP, Wulff H, O'Donnell ME. Blood-brain barrier kca3.1 channels: Evidence for a role in brain na uptake and edema in ischemic stroke. Stroke. 2015;46:237–44.
9. Chen YJ, Nguyen HM, Maezawa I, Grossinger EM, Garing AL, Kohler R, Jin LW, Wulff H. The potassium channel kca3.1 constitutes a pharmacological target for neuroinflammation associated with ischemia/reperfusion stroke. J Cerebral Blood Flow Metab. 2016;36:2146–61.
10. Shibasaki K, Hosoi N, Kaneko R, Tominaga M, Yamada K. Glycine release from astrocytes via functional reversal of glyt1. J Neurochem. 2017;140:395–403.
11. Jie P, Lu Z, Hong Z, Li L, Zhou L, Li Y, Zhou R, Zhou Y, Du Y, Chen L, Chen L. Activation of transient receptor potential vanilloid 4 is involved in neuronal injury in middle cerebral artery occlusion in mice. Mol Neurobiol. 2016;53:8–17.
12. Bai JZ, Lipski J. Differential expression of trpm2 and trpv4 channels and their potential role in oxidative stress-induced cell death in organotypic hippocampal culture. Neurotoxicology. 2010;31:204–14.
13. Lipski J, Park TI, Li D, Lee SC, Trevarton AJ, Chung KK, Freestone PS, Bai JZ. Involvement of trp-like channels in the acute ischemic response of hippocampal ca1 neurons in brain slices. Brain Res. 2006;1077:187–99.
14. Li L, Qu W, Zhou L, Lu Z, Jie P, Chen L, Chen L. Activation of transient receptor potential vanilloid 4 increases nmda-activated current in hippocampal pyramidal neurons. Front Cell Neurosci. 2013;7:17.
15. Butenko O, Dzamba D, Benesova J, Honsa P, Benfenati V, Rusnakova V, Ferroni S, Anderova M. The increased activity of trpv4 channel in the astrocytes of the adult rat hippocampus after cerebral hypoxia/ischemia. PLoS One. 2012;7:e39959.
16. Yi M, Dou F, Lu Q, Yu Z, Chen H. Activation of the kca3.1 channel contributes to traumatic scratch injury-induced reactive astrogliosis through the jnk/c-jun signaling pathway. Neurosci Lett. 2016;624:62–71.
17. Yu Z, Yu P, Chen H, Geller HM. Targeted inhibition of kca3.1 attenuates tgf-beta-induced reactive astrogliosis through the smad2/3 signaling pathway. J Neurochem. 2014;130:41–9.
18. Begenisich T, Nakamoto T, Ovitt CE, Nehrke K, Brugnara C, Alper SL, Melvin JE. Physiological roles of the intermediate conductance, ca2+–activated potassium channel kcnn4. J Biol Chem. 2004;279:47681–7.
19. Chu HX, Kim HA, Lee S, Broughton BR, Drummond GR, Sobey CG. Evidence of ccr2-independent transmigration of ly6c(hi) monocytes into the brain after permanent cerebral ischemia in mice. Brain Res. 2016;1637:118–27.
20. Tanaka Y, Fukumitsu H, Soumiya H, Yoshimura S, Iwama T, Furukawa S. 2-decenoic acid ethyl ester, a compound that elicits neurotrophin-like intracellular signals, facilitating functional recovery from cerebral infarction in mice. Int J Mol Sci. 2012;13:4968–81.
21. Konig S, Browne S, Doleschal B, Schernthaner M, Poteser M, Machler H, Wittchow E, Braune M, Muik M, Romanin C, Groschner K. Inhibition of orai1-mediated ca(2+) entry is a key mechanism of the antiproliferative action of sirolimus in human arterial smooth muscle. Am J Phys Heart Circ Phys. 2013;305:H1646–57.
22. Sun S, Chen G, Xu M, Qiao Y, Zheng S. Differentiation and migration of bone marrow mesenchymal stem cells transplanted through the spleen in rats with portal hypertension. PLoS One. 2013;8:e83523.
23. Bradley H, Shaw CS, Bendtsen C, Worthington PL, Wilson OJ, Strauss JA, Wallis GA, Turner AM, Wagenmakers AJ. Visualization and quantitation of glut4 translocation in human skeletal muscle following glucose ingestion and exercise. Physiol Rep. 2015;3(5):e12375.
24. YY W, Singer CA, Buxton IL. Variants of stretch-activated two-pore potassium channel trek-1 associated with preterm labor in humans. Biol Reprod. 2012;87:96.
25. ZH Y, JR X, Wang YX, GN X, ZP X, Yang K, DZ W, Cui YY, Chen HZ. Targeted inhibition of kca3.1 channel attenuates airway inflammation and remodeling in allergic asthma. Am J Respir Cell Mol Biol. 2013;48:685–93.
26. Schneider CA, Rasband WS, Eliceiri KW. Nih image to imagej: 25 years of image analysis. Nat Methods. 2012;9:671–5.
27. Gopalakrishnan SM, Moreland RB, Kofron JL, Helfrich RJ, Gubbins E, McGowen J, Masters JN, Donnelly-Roberts D, Brioni JD, Burns DJ, Warrior UA. cell-based microarrayed compound screening format for identifying agonists of g-protein-coupled receptors. Anal Biochem. 2003;321:192–201.
28. Iglesias J, Morales L, Barreto GE. Metabolic and inflammatory adaptation of reactive astrocytes: Role of ppars. Mol Neurobiol. 2017;54:2518–38.
29. Wang LP, Cheung G, Kronenberg G, Gertz K, Ji S, Kempermann G, Endres M, Kettenmann H. Mild brain ischemia induces unique physiological properties in striatal astrocytes. Glia. 2008;56:925–34.
30. Lallet-Daher H, Roudbaraki M, Bavencoffe A, Mariot P, Gackiere F, Bidaux G, Urbain R, Gosset P, Delcourt P, Fleurisse L, Slomianny C, Dewailly E, Mauroy B, Bonnal JL, Skryma R, Prevarskaya N. Intermediate-conductance ca2+–activated k+ channels (ikca1) regulate human prostate cancer cell proliferation through a close control of calcium entry. Oncogene. 2009;28: 1792–806.
31. Devor DC, Singh AK, Frizzell RA, Bridges RJ. Modulation of cl- secretion by benzimidazolones. I. Direct activation of a ca(2+)-dependent k+ channel. Am J Phys. 1996;271:L775–84.
32. Wandall-Frostholm C, Dalsgaard T, Bajoriunas V, Olivan-Viguera A, Sadda V, Beck L, Mogensen S, Stankevicius E, Simonsen U, Kohler R. Genetic deficit of kca 3.1 channels protects against pulmonary circulatory collapse induced by trpv4 channel activation. Br J Pharmacol. 2015;172:4493–505.
33. Sonkusare SK, Bonev AD, Ledoux J, Liedtke W, Kotlikoff MI, Heppner TJ, Hill-Eubanks DC, Nelson MT. Elementary ca2+ signals through endothelial trpv4 channels regulate vascular function. Science. 2012;336:597–601.
34. Chen YJ, Nguyen HM, Maezawa I, Grossinger EM, Garing AL, Kohler R, Jin LW, Wulff H. The potassium channel kca3.1 constitutes a pharmacological target for neuroinflammation associated with ischemia/reperfusion stroke. J Cerebral Blood Flow Metab. 2016;36:2146–61.
35. Gueguinou M, Chantome A, Fromont G, Bougnoux P, Vandier C, Potier-Cartereau M. Kca and ca(2+) channels: The complex thought. Biochim Biophys Acta. 2014;1843:2322–33.
36. Gueguinou M, Gambade A, Felix R, Chantome A, Fourbon Y, Bougnoux P, Weber G, Potier-Cartereau M, Vandier C. Lipid rafts, kca/clca/ca2+ channel complexes and egfr signaling: Novel targets to reduce tumor development by lipids? Biochim Biophys Acta. 2015;1848:2603–20.
37. Li Y, Hu H, Tian JB, Zhu MX, O'Neil RG. Dynamic coupling between trpv4 and ca2+–activated sk1/3 and ik1 k+ channels plays a critical role in regulating the k+–secretory bk channel in kidney collecting duct cells. Am J Physiol Renal Physiol. 2017;312:F1081–9.
38. Qian X, Francis M, Kohler R, Solodushko V, Lin M, Taylor MS. Positive feedback regulation of agonist-stimulated endothelial ca2+ dynamics by kca3.1 channels in mouse mesenteric arteries. Arterioscler Thromb Vasc Biol. 2014;34:127–35.
39. Simonsen U, Wandall-Frostholm C, Olivan-Viguera A, Kohler R. Emerging roles of calcium-activated k channels and trpv4 channels in lung oedema and pulmonary circulatory collapse. Acta Physiol. 2017;219:176–87.
40. Ryskamp DA, Witkovsky P, Barabas P, Huang W, Koehler C, Akimov NP, Lee SH, Chauhan S, Xing W, Renteria RC, Liedtke W, Krizaj D. The polymodal ion

channel transient receptor potential vanilloid 4 modulates calcium flux, spiking rate, and apoptosis of mouse retinal ganglion cells. J Neurosci. 2011; 31:7089–101.
41. Shi M, Du F, Liu Y, Li L, Cai J, Zhang GF, XF X, Lin T, Cheng HR, Liu XD, Xiong LZ, Zhao G. Glial cell-expressed mechanosensitive channel trpv4 mediates infrasound-induced neuronal impairment. Acta Neuropathol. 2013; 126:725–39.
42. Benfenati V, Caprini M, Dovizio M, Mylonakou MN, Ferroni S, Ottersen OP, Amiry-Moghaddam M. An aquaporin-4/transient receptor potential vanilloid 4 (aqp4/trpv4) complex is essential for cell-volume control in astrocytes. Proc Natl Acad Sci U S A. 2011;108:2563–8.
43. Isogai A, Lee K, Mitsui R, Hashitani H. Functional coupling of trpv4 channels and bk channels in regulating spontaneous contractions of the guinea pig urinary bladder. Pflugers Archiv. 2016;468:1573–85.
44. Parikh J, Kapela A, Tsoukias NM. Stochastic model of endothelial trpv4 calcium sparklets: Effect of bursting and cooperativity on edh. Biophys J. 2015;108:1566–76.
45. Feetham CH, Nunn N, Lewis R, Dart C, Barrett-Jolley R. Trpv4 and k(ca) ion channels functionally couple as osmosensors in the paraventricular nucleus. Br J Pharmacol. 2015;172:1753–68.
46. Sofroniew MV. Multiple roles for astrocytes as effectors of cytokines and inflammatory mediators. Neuroscientist. 2014;20:160–72.
47. Liddelow SA, Guttenplan KA, Clarke LE, Bennett FC, Bohlen CJ, Schirmer L, Bennett ML, Munch AE, Chung WS, Peterson TC, Wilton DK, Frouin A, Napier BA, Panicker N, Kumar M, Buckwalter MS, Rowitch DH, Dawson VL, Dawson TM, Stevens B, Barres BA. Neurotoxic reactive astrocytes are induced by activated microglia. Nature. 2017;541:481–7.
48. Ferreira R, Lively S, Schlichter LC. Il-4 type 1 receptor signaling up-regulates kcnn4 expression, and increases the kca3.1 current and its contribution to migration of alternative-activated microglia. Front Cell Neurosci. 2014;8:183.
49. Kaushal V, Koeberle PD, Wang Y, Schlichter LC. The ca2+–activated k+ channel kcnn4/kca3.1 contributes to microglia activation and nitric oxide-dependent neurodegeneration. J Neurosci. 2007;27:234–44.

11

Choroid plexus-cerebrospinal fluid route for monocyte-derived macrophages after stroke

Ruimin Ge, Daniel Tornero, Masao Hirota, Emanuela Monni, Cecilia Laterza, Olle Lindvall and Zaal Kokaia*

Abstract

Background: Choroid plexus (CP) supports the entry of monocyte-derived macrophages (MDMs) to the central nervous system in animal models of traumatic brain injury, spinal cord injury, and Alzheimer's disease. Whether the CP is involved in the recruitment of MDMs to the injured brain after ischemic stroke is unknown.

Methods: Adult male C57BL/6 mice were subjected to focal cortical ischemia by permanent occlusion of the distal branch of the right middle cerebral artery. Choroid plexus tissues were collected and analyzed for Vcam1, Madcam1, Cx_3cl1, Ccl2, Nt5e, and Ifnγ expression at different timepoints after stroke using qPCR. Changes of MDMs in CP and cerebrospinal fluid (CSF) at 1 day and 3 days after stroke were analyzed using flow cytometry. Infiltration of MDMs into CP and CSF were validated using β-actin-GFP chimeric mice and Fgd5-CreERT2 x Lox-stop-lox-Tomato mice. CD115+ monocytes were isolated using a magnetic cell separation system from bone marrow of Cx_3cr1-GFP or wild-type C57BL/6 donor mice. The freshly isolated monocytes or M2-like MDMs primed in vitro with IL4 and IL13 were stereotaxically injected into the lateral ventricle of stroke-affected mice to trace for their migration into ischemic hemisphere or to assess their effect on post-stroke recovery using open field, corridor, and active avoidance behavioral tests.

Results: We found that CP responded to cortical stroke by upregulation of gene expression for several possible mediators of MDM trafficking and, concomitantly, MDMs increased in CP and cerebrospinal fluid (CSF). We then confirmed that MDMs infiltrated from blood into CP and CSF after the insult using β-actin-GFP chimeric mice and Fgd5-CreERT2 x Lox-stop-lox-Tomato mice. When MDMs were directly administered into CSF following stroke, they homed to the ischemic hemisphere. If they had been primed in vitro prior to their administration to become M2-like macrophages, they promoted post-stroke recovery of motor and cognitive function without influencing infarct volume.

Conclusions: Our findings suggest the possibility that autologous transplantation of M2-like MDMs into CSF might be developed into a new strategy for promoting recovery also in patients with stroke.

Keywords: Stroke, Inflammation, Choroid plexus, Transplantation, Functional recovery

* Correspondence: zaal.kokaia@med.lu.se
Laboratory of Stem Cells and Restorative Neurology, Lund Stem Cell Center, University Hospital, SE-221 84 Lund, Sweden

Background

Ischemic stroke is caused by occlusion of a cerebral artery, leading to focal ischemia and cell death. Although most survivors improve to some degree, stroke is a leading cause of long-term disability in humans and effective therapies to promote recovery in the chronic phase are lacking [11]. Recent studies in animal models have indicated that monocyte-derived macrophages (MDMs) play an important role for the spontaneous functional restoration. Following a stroke, resident microglia are activated and MDMs and other blood-borne leukocytes are recruited to the ischemic hemisphere [8, 22]. Infiltration of MDMs occurs mainly over the first week and peaks at 3 days after the insult both in a transient [35] and a permanent ischemia model [21] in mice. We have shown that ablation of monocytes during the first week after stroke abolishes long-term behavioral recovery [35].

Macrophages are known to express a wide spectrum of activity, ranging from pro-inflammatory (M1-like) to anti-inflammatory (M2-like) state, depending on their microenvironment [20]. After myocardial infarction, pro-inflammatory M1-like macrophages are the dominant phenotype in the early phase digesting damaged tissue, followed by dominance of anti-inflammatory M2-like macrophages that promote healing in the second phase [23]. Recently, it was reported that myeloid-derived growth factor, produced by monocytes and macrophages, promotes repair after myocardial infarction [15]. Similar to the heart, infiltrating anti-inflammatory M2-like MDMs were shown to improve recovery following injury to the mouse spinal cord [29]. Over the first week following an ischemic stroke in mice, MDMs exhibit a similar switch from pro-inflammatory to anti-inflammatory activity [35]. Interestingly, Hu and colleagues found that expression of M2 markers peaked earlier than that of M1 markers [14]. However, these authors did not distinguish microglia from blood-borne macrophages. Anti-inflammatory M2-like MDM-derived factors, such as Ym1 and TGFβ, were proposed to contribute to the observed spontaneous post-stroke recovery. In line with these animal experimental data, the level of a subtype of monocytes, which expresses surface markers similar to those of mouse anti-inflammatory macrophages [12], was inversely related to poor outcome in stroke patients [34].

Blood-borne leukocytes can enter the diseased central nervous system (CNS) not only via a leaking blood-brain barrier but also through other routes. For example, effector T cells were found to infiltrate the CNS parenchyma via the leptomeninges in a rat multiple sclerosis model [28]. Apart from its canonical function of secreting cerebrospinal fluid (CSF), the choroid plexus (CP) has recently been reported to mediate both immunosurveillance of the healthy CNS and trafficking of leukocytes in several CNS diseases [16, 17, 26, 29]. After traumatic brain injury, CP mediates infiltration of blood-borne monocytes and neutrophils into the lesion site [31, 32]. CP plays a similar role in Alzheimer's disease, and manipulating this selective gateway for immune cells results in increased infiltration of MDMs and clearance of amyloid plaques [1, 2]. Importantly, it has been shown that CP specifically orchestrates recruitment of monocytes that give rise to beneficial M2-like MDMs in the injured area of the spinal cord, whereas monocytes that enter through the leptomeninges display M1-like activity at the lesion site [29]. Whether CP is involved in the recruitment of MDMs to the injured brain after ischemic stroke is unknown.

Here, we show that CP responds to an ischemic stroke located in the cerebral cortex by upregulation of gene expression for some adhesion molecules and chemokines concomitantly with an increase of monocytes in CSF. We demonstrate that MDMs can infiltrate from blood into CP and CSF after stroke. We then provide evidence that both freshly isolated monocytes and in vitro-polarized M2-like macrophages delivered in CSF can migrate into the ischemic hemisphere and that the polarized M2-like macrophages improve motor and cognitive function without influencing infarct volume. Our findings highlight the importance of M2-like MDMs, which reach CSF and infiltrate the injured parenchyma, for functional restoration after stroke.

Methods

Animals

All procedures were carried out in accordance with the guidelines set by the Malmö-Lund Ethical Committee for the use of laboratory animals and were conducted in accordance with the European Union directive on the subject of animal rights. Procedures were carried out on C57BL/6 mice (25–30 g, Charles River, Germany), β-actin-GFP mice (25–30 g, The Jackson Laboratory stock No. 006567), Fgd5-CreERT2 mice (25–30 g, The Jackson Laboratory stock No. 027789), Lox-stop-lox-Tomato mice (25–30 g, The Jackson Laboratory stock No. 007909), and male Cx3cr1-GFP mice (The Jackson Laboratory stock No. 005582), housed under 12 h light/12 h dark cycle with ad libitum access to food and water. For generation of chimeric mice, wild type C57BL/6 recipient mice received 900 cGy irradiation (Cesium source). Bone marrow cells isolated from femur, tibia, and hips of β-actin-GFP mice were then intravenously injected into the tail vein of recipient mice. Transplanted mice were kept under antibiotic treatment in drinking water. Successful generation of chimeric mice was confirmed 2 weeks later by FACS analysis of peripheral blood. Fgd5-CreERT2 x Lox-stop-lox-Tomato mice were generated by crossing Fgd5-CreERT2 mice with Lox-stop-lox-Tomato mice and treated with tamoxifen for over 1 year in order to label all hematopoietic stem cell-derived cells.

Choroid plexus tissue was collected at 6 h, 1 day, 3 days, 7 days, and 14 days after stroke from male C57BL/6 mice and analyzed using qPCR. For delivery of Cx_3cr1-GFP non-primed freshly isolated monocytes or primed M2-like MDMs into lateral ventricle, injection was carried out 1 day after stroke on male C57BL/6 mice and analysis was performed 3 days after transplantation (4 days after stroke).

Surgical procedures

Animals were anesthetized with isoflurane (3.0% induction; 1.5% maintenance) mixed with air. All animals received locally injected marcaine for pain relief. While under anesthesia and in the early recovery period (2 h), animals were placed on a heating pad maintained at 37 °C.

Permanent occlusion of the distal branch of the right middle cerebral artery (dMCAO) was performed on adult 25–30 g C57BL/6 mice under anesthesia as described elsewhere [25]. In brief, after shaving the skin, a scission was made between the right eye and the right ear. Muscles covering the cranium were cut and opened, and a small hole was then drilled in the cranium at the level of the distal portion of the right middle cerebral artery. The dura mater was removed, and the artery was visualized and occluded by cauterization. The artery was then cut off to make sure there was no remaining blood flow to the corresponding cortical region. After the skin had been sutured, mice were injected with 1.5 ml Ringer's solution, returned to their cages, and put on a heating pad. For sham-operated mice, the distal portion of the middle cerebral artery was exposed in the same way as in dMCAO surgery, but without occlusion of the artery using cauterization.

For macrophages administration, phosphate-buffered saline (PBS) solutions with or without cells (vehicle) were stereotaxically injected using a glass microneedle into the lateral ventricle (coordinates: −0.1 mm rostral, −1.0/+1.0 mm lateral to bregma, 2.2 mm ventral from brain surface). Injection was carried out 1 day after MCAO. Mice were randomly allocated to Cell or PBS groups using a random sequence generated (https://www.random.org/sequences/). In total, 5 μl PBS with or without 3 million cells were injected using a speed of 1 μl/min. Microneedle was left in place for 5 min after all solution had been injected, and was then slowly removed in 1 min. Finally, wound was cleaned and sutured, and mice were returned to cages with heating pad.

Choroid plexus tissue and cerebrospinal fluid collection

For choroid plexus (CP) tissue collection, mice were deeply anesthetized with an overdose of pentobarbital and transcardially perfused with at least 150 ml 4 °C saline to thoroughly remove blood from CP. Brain was removed, and CP tissues were collected under surgical microscope. CP in the 4th ventricle was first collected, followed by the ones in 3rd ventricle and in lateral ventricles. CP tissues were then transferred into pre-cooled Eppendorf tube on dry ice for RNA collection or in 4 °C L-15 medium for FACS analysis. For immunohistochemical analysis of CP, freshly isolated tissue was fixed in 4% paraformaldehyde (PFA) overnight and washed in PBS for further analysis.

Cerebrospinal fluid (CSF) was collected from cisterna magna [18]. In brief, mice were anesthetized using isoflurane (3.0% induction; 1.5% maintenance) mixed with air, and were then fixed on a stereotaxic frame. A scission over the back of the neck was made, and muscles covering cisterna magna were separated using a pair of cotton anti-bleeding bars. Body of the mouse was bent at 135° to the head. Cisterna magna was visualized under microscope. A glass pipette was carefully inserted into cisterna magna with avoidance of arteria spinalis dorsalis. On average, 2 μl CSF were collected from each mouse. Any CSF contaminated with blood was discarded. The collected CSF was blown out from the glass pipette using a syringe and was kept at 4 °C for further analysis.

Immunohistochemistry and microscopical analysis

Mice were deeply anesthetized with an overdose of pentobarbital and transcardially perfused with saline followed by 4% PFA. Brains were post-fixed overnight in 4% PFA and then placed in 20% sucrose for 24 h before coronal sectioning (30 μm) on dry ice. Brain sections were kept in anti-freezing solution before staining. For the staining, free-floating sections were washed in KPBS lasting 10 min for three times and then pre-incubated with the appropriate serum for 1 h. Sections were then incubated with primary antibodies overnight at 4 °C. After incubation, sections were washed in KPBS with 0.25% Triton X-100 lasting 10 min for three times, then incubated for 2 h in the dark with secondary antibodies conjugated with Cy3, Alexa Fluor 647 or Alexa Fluor 488 (1:200, Molecular Probes, Life Technologies). The following antibodies were used: goat anti-CD206 (1:100, R&D), rat anti-VCAM1 (1:50, Santa Cruz), rat anti-CD11b (1:200, AbD Serotec), chicken anti-GFP (1:400, Merck Millipore), rat anti-CD16/32 (1:200, BD Biosciences), rabbit anti-YM1 (1:100, Abcam), rabbit anti-NeuN (1:2000, Abcam), rabbit anti-IGF1 (1:50, Abcam), rabbit anti ZO-1 (1:200, Life Technologies), rabbit anti-IBA1 (1:1000, Wako), Cy3, Alexa Fluor 647 or Alexa Fluor 488-conjugated donkey anti-chicken, goat, rat or rabbit (all 1:200, Jackson ImmunoResearch), and biotinylated horse anti-rabbit (1:200, Vector Laboratories).

Nuclei were then stained with Hoechst 33342 (1:4000, Molecular Probes or Jackson Laboratories) for 10 min followed by three rinses and sections were mounted with Dabco (Sigma) on gelatin-coated slides.

Single labeling for NeuN was performed with biotinylated horse anti-rabbit antibody and visualized with avidin-biotin-peroxidase complex (Elite ABC kit, Vector Laboratories), followed by peroxidase-catalyzed diaminobenzidine reaction.

Visualization of IBA1+/CD206+, IBA1+/CD16/32+, GFP+/CD206+, GFP+/CD16/32+, GFP+/YM1+ double positive cells was done using a confocal microscope (ZEISS LSM 780, Zees, Germany). Pictures were taken using ZEN software (Zeiss, GERMANY).

For infarct volume estimation, area of uninjured tissue in ipsilateral and contralateral hemisphere was measured using Visiopharm software (Visopharm, Denmark). The area of uninjured tissue in the ipsilateral hemisphere was subtracted from that of the contralateral hemisphere to get infarct area, and this infarct area was subsequently multiplied with section thickness (30 μm) and series numbers (8 series) to get infarct volume. The assessment was performed in a blinded manner.

Flow cytometry

Choroid plexus tissue was diced and re-suspended in a +37 °C papain, neutral protease (dispase II), DNAse (PPD) solution and incubated for 30 min at +37 °C. The PPD solution was prepared as follows: 2.5 U/ml papain (Worthington Biochemical Corporation), 250 U/ml DNAse I (Worthington Biochemical Corporation), and 1 U/ml dispase II (Roche) were dissolved in DMEM containing 4.5 g/l glucose at +37 °C, filter sterilized and stored at −20 °C prior to use. Tissue was then triturated, and excess DMEM/F12 with glutamine (500 μl/50 ml) and 10% fetal bovine serum (FBS) medium was added. Cells were washed by centrifugation, re-suspended in FACS block buffer (2% FBS in PBS), and strained through a 40-μm strainer. Cells were re-centrifuged and re-suspended in FACS block buffer with CD16/32 antibody (1:100, BD Biosciences) for 10 min at +4 °C. Cells were then incubated with antibodies for 30 min at +4 °C. Brilliant Violet 421-conjugated rat anti-mouse/human CD11b (1:100, BioLegend) and Brilliant Violet 510-conjugated rat anti-mouse CD45 (1:100, BioLegend) were used. Cells were washed by centrifugation at +4 °C and re-suspended in 200 μl FACS buffer (1% BSA in PBS) to be ready for FACS analysis (BD FACS LSRII, Becton Dickinson, Franklin lakes, NJ). Because of the small volume of CSF samples, 20 μl FACS block buffer were first added to CSF. Then, the samples were incubated with antibodies as mentioned above. After incubation, 100 μl FACS buffer were added. DRAQ5 (1:200, Thermo Scientific) and 2 μl propidium iodide (PI) were added to the CP and CSF samples before analysis for the identification of live cells.

RNA extraction and quantitative PCR

Total RNA was extracted from cells or tissue using a RNeasy Plus micro kit (Qiagen) and then reversed to cDNA using a qScript cDNA Synthesis Kit (QuantaBio). For quantitative PCR, TaqMan Gene expression master mix (Life Technologies) and TaqMan probes (Life Technologies) were used (Table 1). Cycle threshold values of target genes were normalized to geometric mean of housekeeping HPRT and GAPDH to get ΔCt. Two to the power of −ΔCt were calculated for final analysis. Because choroid plexus samples collected from different time-points after MCAO (6 h, 1d, 3d, 7d, and 14d) were run at different plates, MCAO sample values were normalized to the corresponding uninjured mouse sample values in each plate and presented as fold change relative to uninjured (Fig. 1).

Monocyte isolation and culture

Bone marrow cells were collected from male Cx_3cr1-GFP or wildtype C57BL/6 donor mice by crushing the femurs, tibiae, and hips. Cells were passed through a 40-μm strainer and rinsed with PBS supplemented with 2% FBS. CD115+ cells were isolated using a magnetic cell separation system and biotinylated anti-CD115 antibody combined with streptavidin-magnetic beads (Miltenyi Biotec, Germany). The freshly isolated monocytes were used for direct transplantation or further culture.

For M2-like macrophage generation, monocytes were isolated as mentioned above and then cultured at 0.5 × 10^6 cells/ml in RPMI-1640 medium supplemented with 10% FBS, 1 mM L-glutamine, 1 mM sodium pyruvate,

Table 1 Taqman probes used for qPCR analysis

Gene name	Gene function	Taqman probe number
Hprt	Housekeeping gene	Mm03024075_m1
Gapdh	Housekeeping gene	Mm99999915_g1
Nt5e	Leukocyte transmigration mediator	Mm00501910_m1
Ifnγ	Choroid plexus activator	Mm01168134_m1
Ccl2	Chemokine	Mm00441242_m1
Cx_3cl1	Chemokine	Mm00436454_m1
Madcam1	Adhesion molecule	Mm00522088_m1
Vcam1	Adhesion molecule	Mm01320970_m1
Tnfα	M1-like macrophage marker	Mm00443258_m1
Igf1	M2-like macrophage marker	Mm00439560_m1
Ym1	M2-like macrophage marker	Mm00657889_mH
Tgfβ1	M2-like macrophage marker	Mm01178820_m1
Arg1	M2-like macrophage marker	Mm00475988_m1

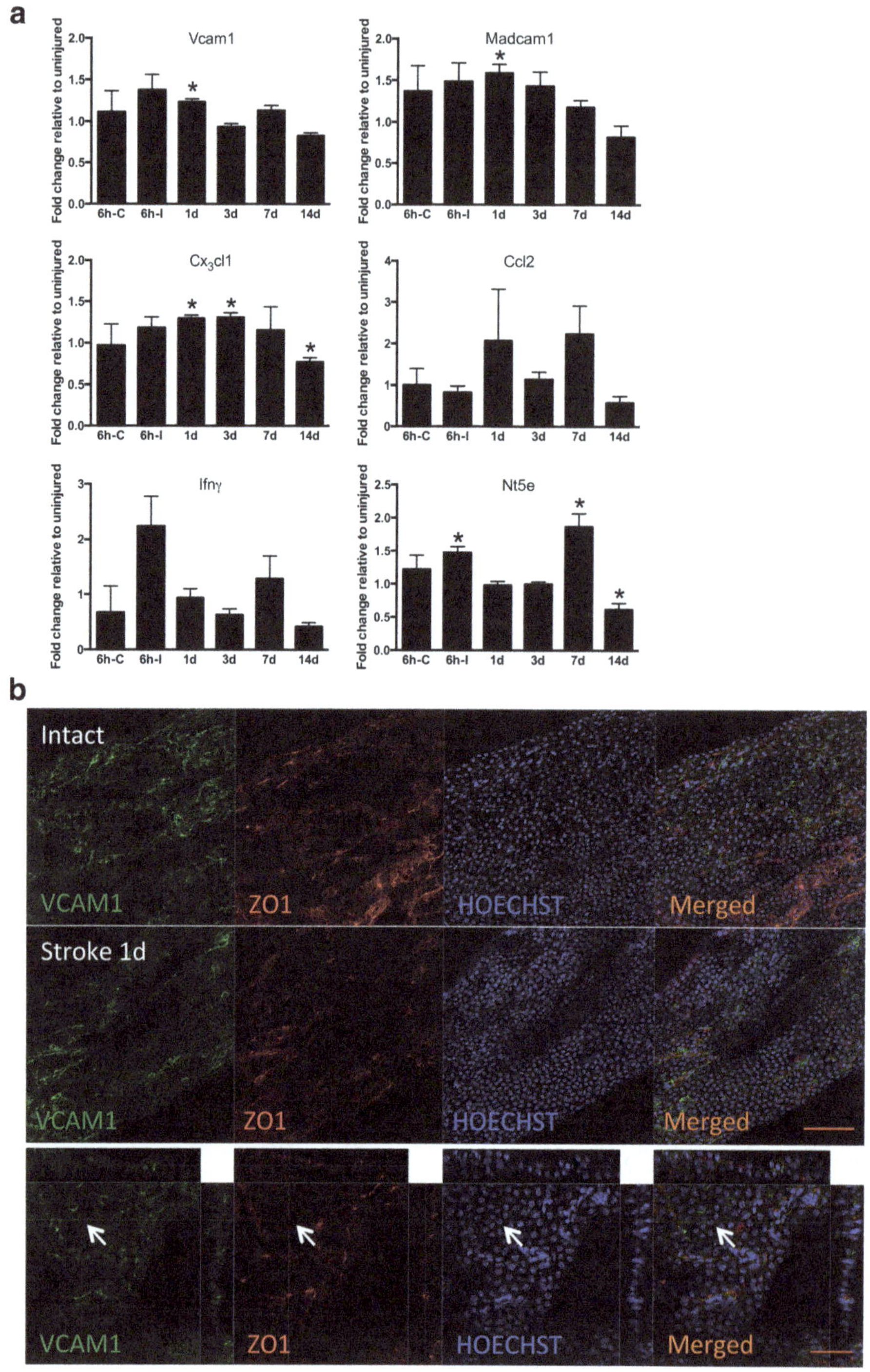

Fig. 1 Cortical stroke upregulates adhesion molecule and chemokine gene expression in choroid plexus (CP). **a** qPCR analysis of adhesion molecule and chemokine gene expression in choroid plexus (CP). The sample values from MCAO-subjected mice were normalized to and presented as fold-change relative to the corresponding uninjured mouse sample values in each plate. Measurements at different time-points after the insult using qPCR were performed on pooled CP tissue from both lateral ventricles and third and fourth ventricle except at 6 h when CP ipsi- and contralateral to the ischemic lesion were analyzed separately. Means ± SEM. *Asterisk*: significant difference compared to corresponding samples from uninjured animals, unpaired *t* test, $n = 4–5$. 6 h-C = 6 h contralateral and 6 h-I = 6 h ipsilateral to injury. **b** Expression of VCAM1 protein on ZO-1 positive CP epithelium in intact mice and at 1 day after stroke. Scale bar 100 μm (*upper images*), 50 μm (*lower images*). *Arrows* depict colocalization of VCAM1 with ZO-1

100 U/ml penicillin, 100 mg/ml streptomycin, 50 ng/ml M-CSF (Peprotech), 50 ng/ml IL4 (Peprotech), and 25 ng/ml IL13 (Peprotech). Five days later, macrophages were collected, washed, and resuspended in PBS for transplantation.

Behavioral test

All behavioral tests were done in a blinded manner.

For open field test, mice were brought into the test room 30 min before the test to acclimate the mice to the environment. During the whole 1-h test, the test room was kept in darkness. For the test, mice were kept in a black box equipped with a camera. Movements of the mice were automatically recorded using ANY-MAZE software (Stoelting Co., UK). Various parameters of mice movement, such as total movement distance, time spent on movement (Time immobile), mobile episode number, clockwise rotation number, anti-clockwise rotation number, time freezing, rearing number, and central zone entries number, were obtained automatically by the software. Twelve sessions of individual 5-min test were acquired and averaged for further analysis.

The corridor test adapted to mice was used to assess sensorimotor impairment [6, 13]. Briefly, animals were food deprived 12 h before the first testing day and kept on a restricted food intake (2.5–3.5 g/day) so that the body weight did not fall below 85% of initial value. Food was provided only after the daily test session. At the first time point, mice were habituated to the corridor by scattering sugar pellets along the floor and allowing them to freely explore for 10 min on 2 consecutive days before testing. When testing began, the mice were transferred to one end of the testing corridor. The numbers of ipsilateral and contralateral retrievals were counted until a maximum time of 5 min had elapsed. A "retrieval" was defined as an exploration into a pot, whether or not a pellet was eaten, and a new retrieval could only be made by investigating a new pot. Two sessions of the test were done for each mouse in one test day. Retrieval average was calculated for the total five testing days. Contralateral side touches (% of total) were expressed as percentage of pellets eaten or smelled on the contralateral side out of those on contralateral and ipsilateral sides combined.

The cognitive function of mouse was assessed based on their escape behavior [27] in an automated step-through type system (GEMINI, San Diego Instruments Inc., San Diego, CA, USA). The equipment software controls the opening of the gate between the two boxes and the electrical shocks on grid floor. On the first day (pre-training day), the tested mouse was allowed to habituate to the environment with both boxes in darkness and gate opened for 10 min. For active avoidance test training, the light turned on in the box opposite to where the mouse was. When the mouse stayed in the dark box over 30 s, it received an electrical shock of 1 mA for 5 s. This was repeated 30 times during the first training day, and the number of moving to the illuminated box was counted as the number of avoidances. This training was performed in all mice for a total of 3 days in the same way. Five days after last day of training, mice were tested in the same way as in the training but without any electric shock and the number of avoidances was counted. This trial test was repeated for 4 days.

Statistical analysis

Comparisons were performed using Prism 6 software (GraphPad Software, Inc.) by Student's unpaired t test or two-way ANOVA followed by Bonferroni's post hoc test. Data are presented as means ± SEM, and differences are considered significant at $p < 0.05$.

Results

Cortical stroke upregulates expression of leukocyte trafficking molecules by the brain choroid plexus

In the first experiment, we determined whether brain CP responds to stroke by changing gene expression for factors that might be involved in homing and trafficking of monocytes. We used a model of cortical stroke in mice in which a distal branch of the middle cerebral artery is occluded, resulting in permanent cortical ischemia without reperfusion. This model was chosen because in our standard middle cerebral artery occlusion model [35], we also interrupt blood flow in the anterior choroidal artery, which provides blood supply to the CP in the lateral ventricle. This would result in ischemia in the CP and be a confounding factor in the interpretation of the CP response to a stroke-induced lesion in the brain parenchyma [10].

We used qPCR to measure changes in gene expression at different time-points following cortical stroke. We focused on six genes that were found to be upregulated in CP after spinal cord injury: the adhesion molecules Vcam1 and Madcam1, the chemokines Cx_3cl1 and Ccl2, Nt5e that mediates macrophage transmigration [29], and Ifnγ that can activate CP for immune surveillance and repair [17, 26]. For the qPCR analysis, we pooled CP from the two lateral ventricles and the third and fourth ventricle. At 6 h after stroke, none of the examined factors showed significant change of gene expression compared to uninjured mice (data not shown). However, when we analyzed CP ipsi- and contralateral to the ischemic lesion separately, we found that Nt5e was upregulated at 6 h on the ipsilateral side (Fig. 1a, Nt5e). At 1 day after stroke, Vcam1, Madcam1, and Cx_3cl1 showed upregulation (Fig. 1a, Vcam1, Madcam1, and Cx_3cl1), and this change of Cx_3cl1 expression remained 2 days later (Fig. 1a, Cx3cl1). At 7 days, Nt5e was upregulated compared to uninjured condition (Fig. 1a, Nt5e), but, similar to Cx3cl1, showed downregulation at 2 weeks (Fig. 1a, Cx3cl1, Nt5e). We detected no changes of gene expression of Ccl2 or Ifnγ at any of the examined timepoints (Fig. 1a, Ccl2, Ifnγ). Using immunohistochemistry, we observed VCAM1 protein expression in CP of intact mice and 1 day after stroke (Fig. 1b). Taken together, our findings show that although CP is located distant to the ischemic lesion, it responds to cortical stroke by upregulation of adhesion molecule and chemokine genes, mainly during the first 3 days after the insult.

Monocyte-derived macrophages infiltrate into choroid plexus and cerebrospinal fluid after cortical stroke

It has been described that monocyte-derived macrophages (MDMs) are recruited through the CP into the cerebrospinal fluid (CSF) following spinal cord injury [29]. To provide evidence whether such a mechanism can operate also after stroke, we first identified CD45+CD11b+ MDMs in CP and CSF using FACS. We found that the percentage of CD45+CD11b+ MDMs out of the total number of live cells in the CP was increased at 3 days after stroke, whereas at 1 day, it was similar to that in uninjured condition (Fig. 2a). In CSF, the density of CD45+CD11b+ MDMs was increased already at 1 day after stroke, while at 3 days, it had returned to control level (Fig. 2a). These data suggested that MDMs might infiltrate CP and CSF after stroke. To provide further evidence for this hypothesis, we used β-actin-GFP chimeric mice in which blood cells were labeled with GFP. We subjected these chimeric mice to MCAO and, at 1 day after stroke, detected a substantial number of GFP+CD11b+ MDMs in CP and CSF (Fig. 2b). To rule out the possibility that the irradiation procedure per se had induced MDM infiltration into CP and CSF, we utilized Fgd5-CreERT2 mice [7] crossed to Lox-stop-lox-Tomato mice. In this model, Tamoxifen administration leads to Tomato labeling of endothelial and blood cells, which can be distinguished from one another by ZsGreen fluorescence. At 1 day after stroke, we detected, besides FGD5+(ZsGreen+)Tomato+ endothelial cells, also CD11b+Tomato+ZsGreen- MDMs (Fig. 2c). Infiltrating Tomato+CD11b+ MDMs were in close vicinity of Tomato+ vascular endothelium. Taken together, these data provide strong evidence that CP-CSF acts as a possible route for MDM entry into the ischemic brain.

We also analyzed the expression of pro-inflammatory M1-like and anti-inflammatory M2-like markers in macrophages in CP and CSF at 3 days after stroke. Immunohistochemistry showed that almost all Iba1+ macrophages in CP expressed the M1-like marker CD16/32 and 31.9 ± 5.2% the M2-like marker CD206 (Fig. 2b, $n = 3$). Using FACS, we found that 13.3 ± 6.7% ($n = 3$) of all CD45+CD11b+ MDMs were Cx3cr1^{hi}Ly6-C^{lo} M2-like MDMs in CSF. Taken together, these data indicate that MDM could infiltrate into CP and CSF, where some of them express an M2-like marker, following a cortical stroke.

Monocyte-derived macrophages from CSF home to ischemic hemisphere after cortical stroke

We then asked whether once the monocytes had reached the CSF could they home into the ischemic hemisphere after stroke. To address this, we utilized Cx3cr1-GFP mice in which monocytes are labeled with GFP. We isolated with MACS GFP+ monocytes from the bone marrow using CD115 antibody conjugated with magnetic beads. We directly injected the freshly isolated monocytes into the lateral ventricle ipsilateral to ischemia 1 day after the insult and perfused the mice 3 days thereafter. Using immunohistochemistry, a large number of GFP+ MDMs were found in the area around the ischemic core (Fig. 3a, arrow). Many GFP+ cells, possibly migrating MDMs, were located between the lateral ventricle and the ischemic core (Fig. 3a, arrow head). Some of the GFP+ MDMs in the area around the ischemic core had downregulated GFP and adopted a more round morphology, indicating an activated phenotype (Fig. 3b, arrow), whereas others expressed high GFP protein level and maintained a ramified phenotype (Fig. 3b, arrow head).

We did not find any GFP+ cells in the contralateral hemisphere of stroke-injured animals or, with the exception of a few GFP+ cells around the needle track, in the brains of mice subjected to sham procedure and injected with GFP+ monocytes (data not shown). To further confirm the homing of MDMs, administered into CSF, to the ischemic hemisphere, we injected freshly isolated GFP+ monocytes also into the contralateral lateral ventricle 1 day after stroke. Again we found many GFP+ MDMs in the ischemic hemisphere 3 days later (Fig. 3c). We also injected GFP+ monocytes deficient in Cx3cr1 into CSF of ipsilateral lateral ventricle 1 day after stroke and could still detect GFP+ MDMs in the ischemic hemisphere 3 days thereafter. This finding suggests that the Cx3cr1 pathway plays at most a minor role in mediating the migration of MDMs from CSF into the ischemic hemisphere.

We examined the GFP+ MDMs in the area around the ischemic core with respect to their phenotype. Neither the GFP^{high} ramified nor the GFP^{low} round MDMs expressed marker characteristics of M1-like or M2-like phenotype such as CD16/32 or CD206 (Fig. 3d). Taken together, our data using delivery of monocytes into CSF provide evidence that also MDMs which have increased

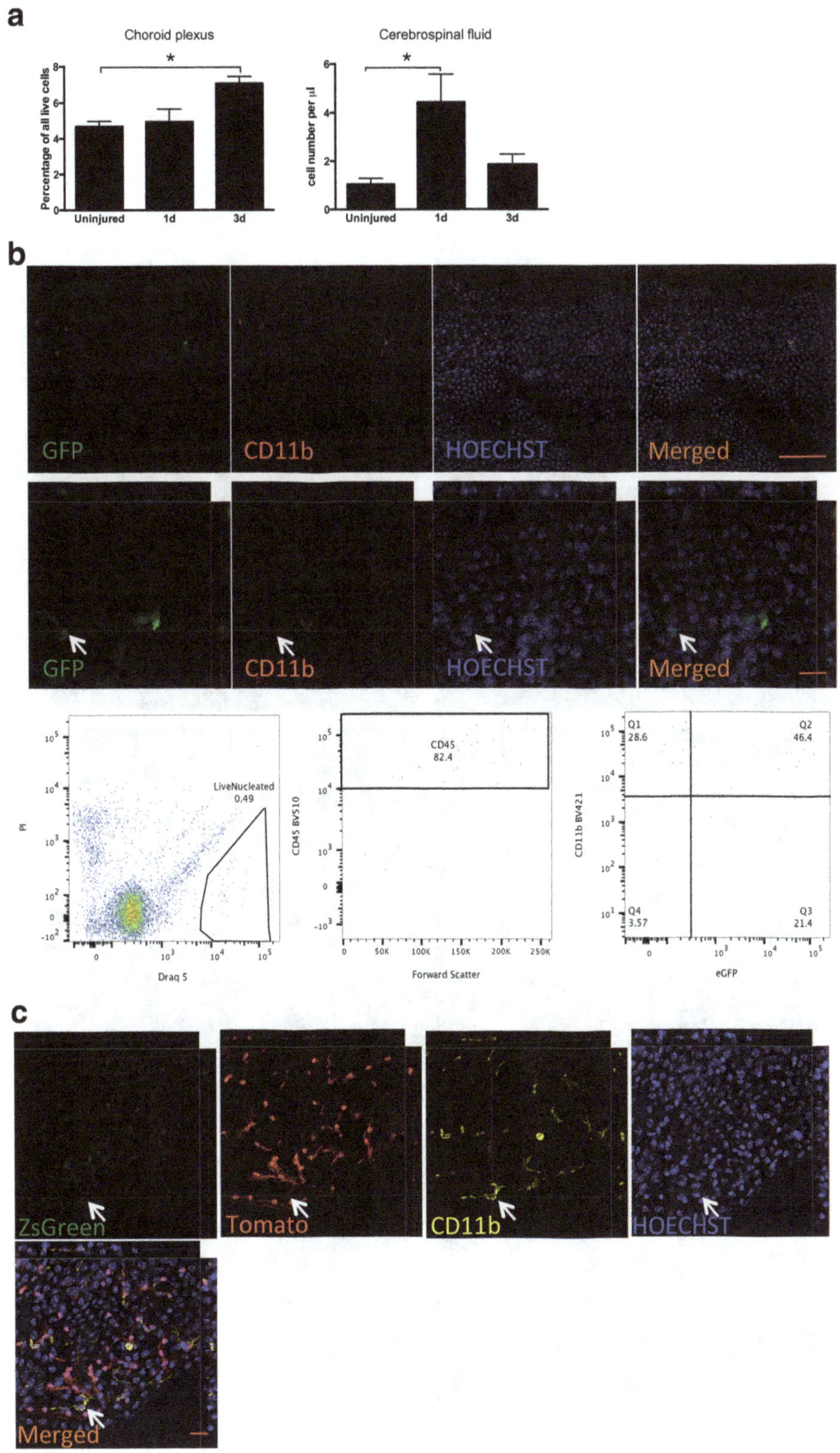

Fig. 2 (See legend on next page.)

(See figure on previous page.)

Fig. 2 Infiltration of MDMs into choroid plexus (CP) and cerebrospinal fluid (CSF) after cortical stroke. **a** Quantification using FACS of CD45+CD11b+ monocyte-derived macrophages in CP and CSF in uninjured mice, and at 1 day and 3 days after cortical stroke. Means ± SEM. *Asterisk*: significant difference compared to corresponding samples from uninjured animals, unpaired *t* test, $n = 4–5$. **b** Photomicrographs and FACS plots showing infiltration of GFP+CD11b+ MDMs into CP and CSF at 1 day after stroke in β-actin-GFP chimeric mice. Scale bar 100 μm (*upper images*), 20 μm (*lower images*). **c** Photomicrographs showing infiltration of TOMATO+CD11b+ MDMs into CP at 1 day after stroke in Fgd5-CreERT2 x Lox-stop-lox-Tomato mice. Scale bar 20 μm

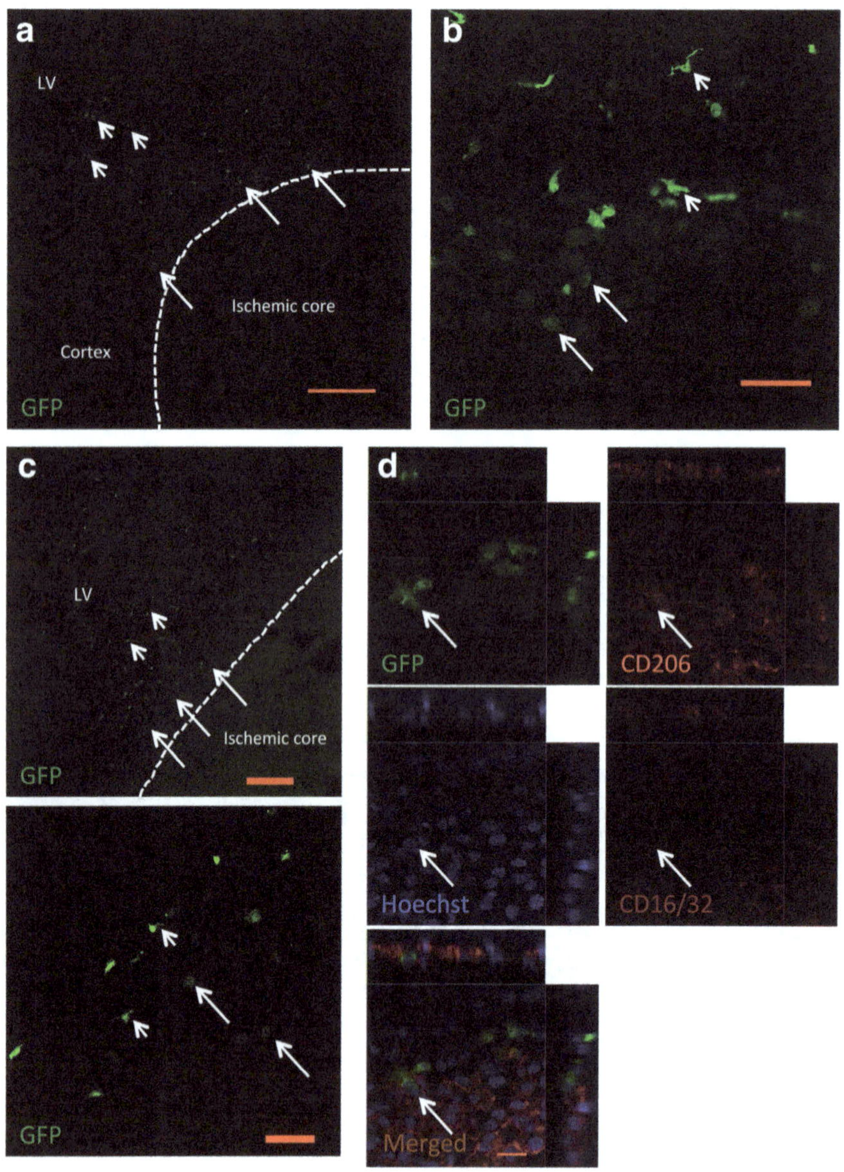

Fig. 3 Monocyte-derived macrophages in cerebrospinal fluid (CSF) infiltrate ischemic hemisphere after cortical stroke. **a**–**c** Photomicrographs showing representative images of GFP+ monocyte-derived macrophages (MDMs) in ischemic hemisphere. Monocytes were injected into CSF of ipsilateral (**a**, **b**) or contralateral (**c**) lateral ventricle 1 day after stroke, and the animals were analyzed 3 days later. *Arrows* depict GFP+ MDMs (**a**, **c** *upper image*) and, at high magnification, round MDMs (**b**, **c** *lower image*), in area around ischemic core. *Arrow heads* indicate GFP+ MDMs located between lateral ventricle and ischemic core (**a**, **c** *upper image*) and, at high magnification, ramified MDMs in area around ischemic core (**b**, **c** *lower image*). **d** Photomicrographs showing confocal images illustrating colocalization of GFP with M2-like marker CD206 and M1-like marker CD16/32. *Arrows* indicate GFP+ MDMs (**d**). Scale bar 200 μm (**a**, **c** *upper image*), 50 μm (**b**, **c** *lower image*), 15 μm (**d**). *LV* lateral ventricle

in CSF after cortical stroke can migrate into the ischemic hemisphere after stroke.

Anti-inflammatory M2-like monocyte-derived macrophages derived in vitro can infiltrate ischemic hemisphere from CSF

Next, we investigated if we could take advantage of the CSF route to enhance the infiltration of MDMs that are biased towards anti-inflammatory phenotype prior to their administration to the CSF. Freshly isolated Cx_3cr1-GFP monocytes from the bone marrow were cultured in the presence of IL4 and IL13 to prime them towards an anti-inflammatory fate. After 5 days in culture, many M2-like markers, such as YM1, ARG1, IGF1, and TGFβ1, were upregulated, whereas the M1-like marker TNFα was downregulated (Fig. 4a). Thus, the freshly isolated monocytes had been activated and adopted an M2-like phenotype. These M2-like MDMs were then injected into the lateral ventricle on the ischemic side at 1 day after cortical stroke, i.e., concomitantly with the observed increase of endogenous MDMs in the CSF at the same time-point (Fig. 2a). Three days later, numerous GFP+ MDMs were found around the ischemic core (Fig. 4b), $47.9 \pm 8.5\%$ ($n = 2$) of all ED+ cells are GFP+ M2-like MDMs. Almost all GFP+ MDMs expressed the M2-like markers YM1, IGF1, and CD206, while the M1-like marker CD16/32 was only very weakly expressed, providing evidence that the injected primed MDMs homed to lesion site and maintained their M2-like phenotype at this time-point (Fig. 4b). Taken together, our findings show that M2-like MDMs migrate into the ischemic hemisphere and retain their M2-like phenotype 3 days after delivery into CSF.

Administration of M2-like monocyte-derived macrophages promotes behavioral recovery after cortical stroke

Finally, we explored if enhancement of the infiltration of M2-like MDMs into the ischemic hemisphere, caused by delivery of the cells into the CSF through the ipsilateral lateral ventricle, could influence the magnitude of behavioral recovery following stroke. Mice were subjected to distal MCAO and randomly allocated to injection of either in vitro-derived M2-like MDMs or vehicle 1 day later. In some animals, we assessed the infarct volume at 7 days after cell or vehicle injection. As expected from our previous work of monocyte depletion after stroke [35], the infarct volume was not affected by the injected MDMs (vehicle: 12.4 ± 2.1 mm^3, $n = 5$; MDMs: 13.7 ± 1.8 mm^3, $n = 6$; unpaired t test), indicating that the infiltrating M2-like MDMs had not influenced the extent of ischemic damage.

We then investigated the effect of M2-like MDM delivery into CSF on post-stroke recovery using various behavioral tests: open-field and corridor tests and active avoidance test to assess restoration of motor and cognitive function, respectively. At 3 weeks, mice transplanted with M2-like MDMs showed more pronounced anticlockwise rotation in the open-field test compared to vehicle-injected ones (Fig. 5a), indicating improvement of the deficit in rotational movements previously reported after stroke [5]. Also, cell-injected mice showed increased preference of smelling or eating pellet on the contralateral side in corridor test (Fig. 5b). Notably, at 3 months after transplantation, the difference between the two groups had disappeared (Fig. 5a, b). At both 3 weeks and 3 months, mice that had received M2-like MDMs showed enhanced locomotor activity in the open field test, as evidenced by the increased distance moved (Fig. 5a). In the active avoidance test, there was no difference between cell- and vehicle-injected mice in learning curve at 2 weeks after injection (Fig. 5c). However, at 3 months after injection, mice with M2-like MDMs showed significantly better learning curve than mice with vehicle injection, indicating better memory skills (Fig. 5c). After we finished the behavioral tests at 3 months, we examined the infarct volume between the cell transplantation and vehicle injection groups. Consistent with the result at 7 days after transplantation, the two groups showed no difference in infarct volume (vehicle: 4.84 ± 1.34 mm^3, $n = 5$; MDMs: 5.14 ± 1.02 mm^3, $n = 6$; unpaired t test).

Next, we then asked whether the in vitro priming of the monocytes to M2-like MDMs before delivery was important for the effect on post-stroke behavioral performance. To this end, we injected either freshly isolated non-primed monocytes or vehicle into the ipsilateral ventricle at 1 day after distal MCAO as in the previous experiment. In contrast to the findings with primed M2-like MDMs, injection of non-primed monocytes did not give rise to any improvement as compared to vehicle in performance of open-field test or corridor test at 3 weeks or of active avoidance test at 3 months after stroke (Fig. 5d). Taken together, these data indicate that intraventricular injection of M2-like MDMs increases post-stroke recovery of both motor and cognitive impairments.

Discussion

In this study, we have shown that CP responds to a cortical ischemic lesion by transiently elevated gene expression for adhesion molecules and chemokines. Vcam1, Madcam1, Cx_3cl1, and Nt5e were transiently upregulated up to 1 week after the insult. During the same time period, MDMs increased in CP and CSF, and MDMs could infiltrate from blood into CP and CSF. We then demonstrate that MDMs when delivered into CSF infiltrate the ischemic hemisphere and, if they have been primed in vitro to beneficial M2-like phenotype,

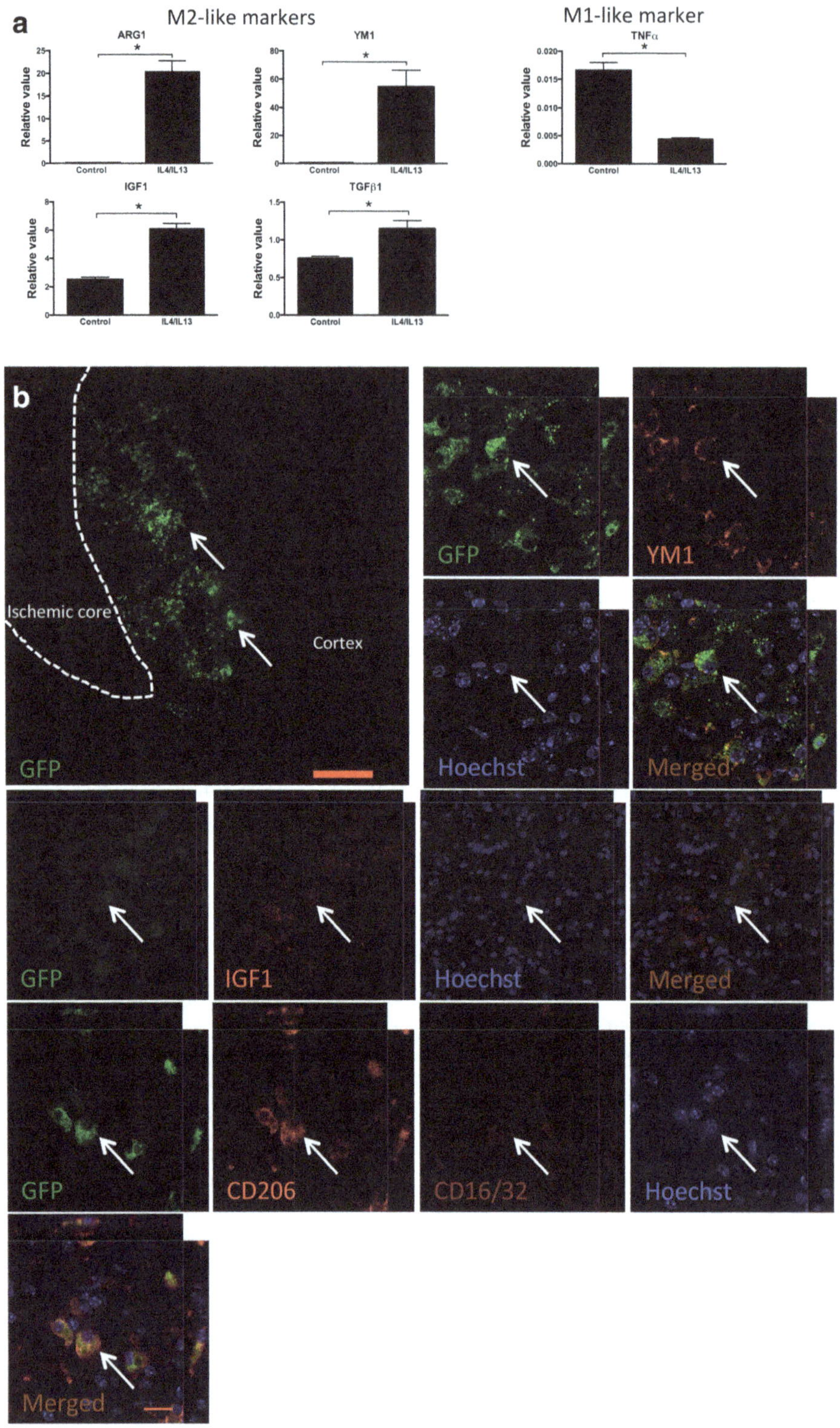

Fig. 4 Anti-inflammatory M2-like monocyte-derived macrophages primed in vitro infiltrate ischemic hemisphere from cerebrospinal fluid (CSF). **a** Upregulation of M2-like markers and downregulation of M1-like marker in macrophages cultured with IL4 and IL13 for 5 days as measured using qPCR. Means ± SEM. *Asterisk*: significant difference compared to control macrophages cultured without IL4 and IL13, unpaired *t* test, $n = 4$. **b** Photomicrographs showing infiltration of GFP+ monocyte-derived macrophages co-expressing M2-like markers YM1, IGF1, and CD206 in the ischemic hemisphere at 3 days after injection into ipsilateral lateral ventricle. *Arrows* indicate GFP+ MDMs (**b**). Scale bar 200 μm (**b** *upper left image*), 15 μm (**b** Other)

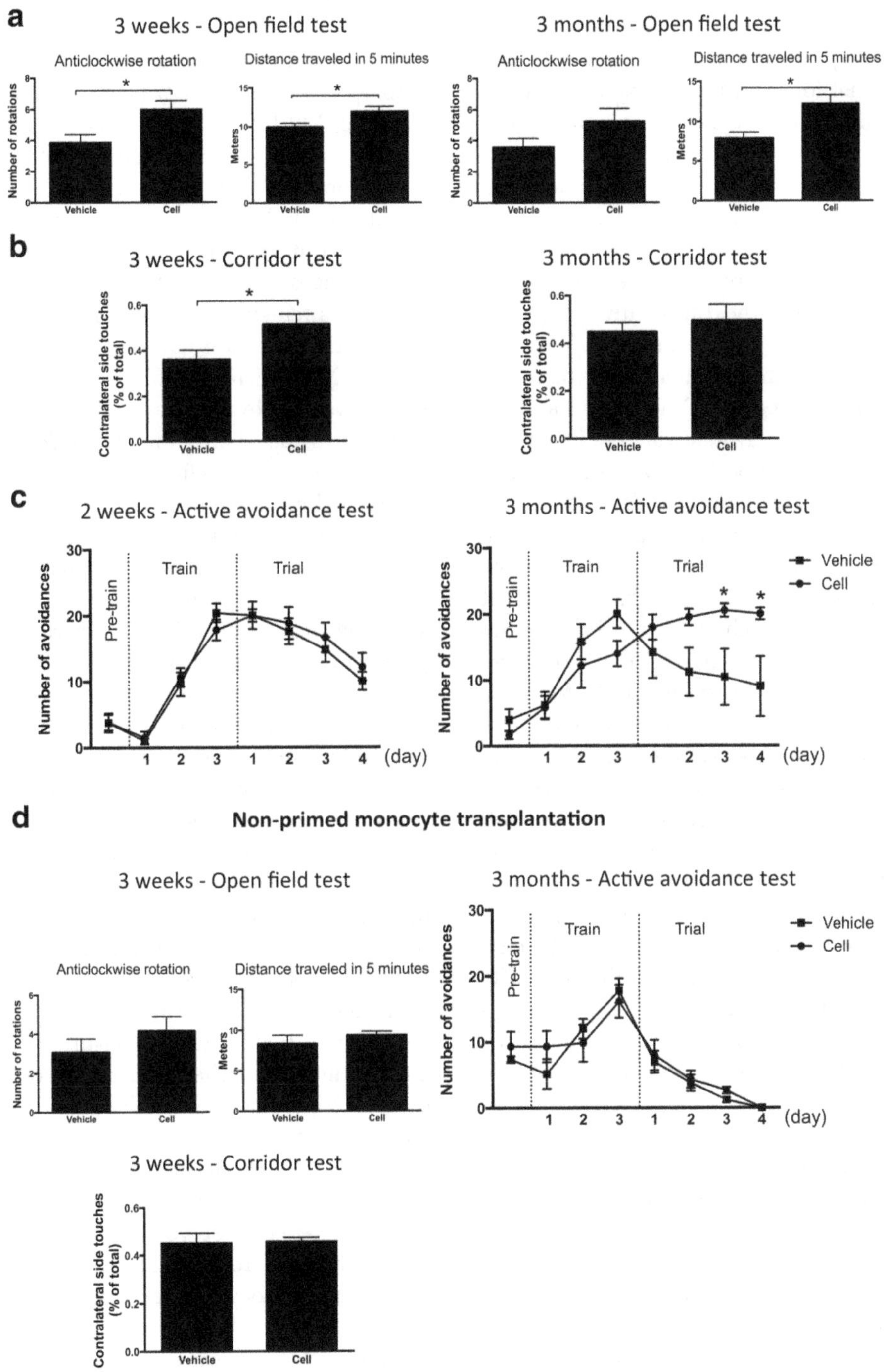

Fig. 5 Effects of intraventricular administration of M2-like monocyte-derived macrophages or non-primed monocytes on post-stroke behavioral recovery. Performance in open-field test, corridor test, and active avoidance test at 2 or 3 weeks and 3 months after injection of M2-like monocyte-derived macrophages ($n = 6$, **a**–**c**), or non-primed monocytes ($n = 6$, **d**) or vehicle ($n = 5$, **a**–**d**) into the ipsilateral lateral ventricle 1 day after cortical stroke. Means ± SEM. *Asterisk*: significant difference compared to vehicle-injected animals, unpaired *t* test (**a**, **b** open-field test and corridor test in **d**) and two-way ANOVA with Bonferroni's post hoc test (**c** active avoidance test in **d**). Contralateral side touches (% of total) indicate percentage of pellets eaten or smelled on the contralateral side out of those on contralateral and ipsilateral sides combined (**b**, corridor test in **d**). Pre-train, Train, and Trial indicate pre-training stage (for 1 day), training stage (for 3 days), and trial test (for 4 days) of active avoidance test, respectively (**c** active avoidance test in **d**)

promote post-stroke recovery of motor and cognitive function.

Several of the upregulated factors have previously been shown to be essential for MDM infiltration via the CP-CSF route after spinal cord injury [29]. In line with a similar role after cortical stroke, we detected Vcam1, Madcam1, and Cx_3cl1 upregulation in CP concomitant with increased MDMs in CSF at 1 day following the insult and Cx_3cl1 was upregulated in CP also at 3 days. The MDMs in the CSF could reflect those that had trafficked through the CP via the transiently upregulated Vcam1, Madcam1, and Cx_3cl1. The increased density of MDMs in CSF returned to baseline at 3 days after stroke, indicating that the peak of MDM infiltration via CSF route occurs around 1 day following the insult. This time-point is earlier than the peak of overall MDM infiltration into ischemic hemisphere at 4 days after stroke [21]. The upregulation of Vcam1, Madcam1, Cx_3cl1, and Nt5e in CP following spinal cord injury was maintained at 14 days [29]. In contrast, the response of the CP to cortical ischemia, which was characterized by upregulation of the same factors, was transient and occurred mainly during the first 3 days after the insult. Moreover, we found that only 30% of the total number of Iba1+ macrophages in the CP expressed the M2-like marker CD206 at 3 days after stroke, whereas almost all of them expressed the M1-like marker CD16/32. And 13.3 ± 6.7% ($n = 3$) of all CD45+CD11b+ MDMs were $Cx_3cr1^{hi}Ly6C^{lo}$ M2-like MDMs in CSF at 3 days after stroke. After spinal cord injury, the majority of macrophages in CP were found to be in M2-like state [29]. Taken together, these findings indicate that compared to the role of CP as the main port of entry for M2-like macrophages after spinal cord injury, the CP probably plays only a minor role as a route for M2-like macrophage infiltration after stroke.

We further found that both non-primed monocytes and M2-like macrophages derived in vitro homed into the injured hemisphere after injection into CSF. This finding raises the possibility that once monocytes had reached the CSF, they could home to the lesion site. We did not observe any migration of MDMs into the hemispheres when monocytes were injected into animals which had not been subjected to stroke but to sham procedure, apart from some MDMs left in the needle track. One potential candidate molecule for recruiting MDMs from CSF towards the ischemic lesion is the chemokine CCL2 [33], which was found to be increased in the ischemic cortex of mice and in the CSF of stroke patients [19, 21]. Another potential mechanism is signaling through the Cx_3cl1 receptor Cx_3cr1, which is a known chemotactic factor to monocytes/macrophages [9]. Arguing against this possibility, we found that GFP+ monocytes with deficiency in Cx_3cr1 which were injected into CSF could still migrate into the ischemic hemisphere.

Several lines of evidence have suggested that M2-like macrophages may have a beneficial effect in stroke. For example, M2-like microglia/macrophages were found to protect neurons from ischemic death in vitro [14], and IL-4 promoted long-term recovery after stroke in mice, possibly by inducing an M2-like macrophage phenotype [18]. In contrast, intravenous administration of M2-like macrophages had no effect on motor recovery up to 2 weeks after stroke in rats [4]. However, whether the intravenous injection had resulted in significant infiltration of M2-like macrophages into the ischemic hemisphere was not examined.

We provide here direct evidence supporting a recovery-promoting effect of M2-like MDMs following focal cerebral ischemia. Thus, we show that M2-like MDMs delivered into CSF infiltrate the ischemic hemisphere and promote recovery of both motor and cognitive function after a cortical ischemic lesion. At 3 weeks after the insult, the MDM-injected mice showed more pronounced anticlockwise rotation in the open-field test and higher preference for smelling and eating pellets on the contralateral side in the corridor test as compared to vehicle-injected animals. This difference was transient which may indicate that the MDMs had induced a more rapid recovery of these functional deficits. Locomotor activity was better in cell-injected mice at both time-points, providing evidence of both a rapid and stable improvement. In line with these findings, intrathecal injection of macrophages with M2-like phenotype derived in vitro has been reported to improve neurological performance in stroke patients [3].

We found that although non-primed monocytes could migrate into the ischemic hemisphere, they did not express M2-like markers and had no effect on recovery of motor function at 3 weeks or cognitive function at 3 months post-insult. These data indicate that the M2-like state of MDMs is essential for the recovery-promoting effect observed in our study. This is in agreement with our recent findings following depletion of infiltrating monocytes after stroke [35]. We obtained no evidence that the behavioral improvement after delivery of M2-like MDMs was due to an effect on the extent of the ischemic damage. Therefore, the recovery-promoting effect is most likely due to secreted factors from M2-like MDMs that can promote cellular and synaptic plasticity of remaining neurons. Supporting this hypothesis, we found that at 3 days after transplantation, the M2-like MDMs expressed IGF1, a factor shown to enhance axonal growth of corticospinal motor neurons [24]. Interestingly, we found that at 18 days after delivery of M2-like MDMs into ipsilateral lateral ventricle, hardly any GFP+ M2-like MDMs were detected in the ischemic hemisphere (data not shown). This observation indicates that persistent presence of M2-like MDMs is not necessary for long-term recovery, which is in line with our previous findings showing that depletion of circulating monocytes during the first week after stroke causes impaired functional recovery at 2 months following the insult [35]. Although our data indicate that M2-like MDMs can use the CSF route to infiltrate the ischemic hemisphere and promote recovery, it cannot be excluded that M1-like MDMs, possibly taking other routes such as a leaking blood-brain barrier, convert in situ to M2-like MDMs and contribute to functional restoration. Also, it would be interesting to determine in the future whether CP mediates infiltration also of other leukocytes such as neutrophils and T cells [30, 32] into the stroke-injured brain.

Conclusions

Our findings suggest the possibility that delivery of M2-like MDMs into CSF could be developed into a new therapeutic strategy for promoting post-stroke recovery. A potential advantage is that M2-like MDMs can easily be obtained from the stroke patient's own peripheral blood in large numbers, and autologous transplantation into CSF will not require immunosuppressive treatment. Here, we administered 3 million MDMs at 1 day after the insult. However, it will be important in future studies to determine if these cells can give rise to improvement also when delivered at later stages of recovery and to identify the optimum dose of cells for inducing maximum functional restoration. In the clinical translation, autologous human MDMs should be labeled and it should be clarified whether they can efficiently infiltrate the ischemically injured tissue in the stroke patient's brain and give rise to a measurable therapeutic effect.

Abbreviations

CP: Choroid plexus; CSF: Cerebrospinal fluid; dMCAO: Distal middle cerebral artery occlusion; GFP: Green fluorescent protein; IL13: Interleukin 13; IL4: Interleukin 4; MDMs: Monocyte-derived macrophages; PBS: Phosphate-buffered saline; PFA: Paraformaldehyde

Acknowledgements

We are grateful to Prof. Michal Schwartz (Weizman Institute, Rehovot, Israel) for valuable discussions and to Alexander Kertser and Kuti Baruch (Weizman Institute, Rehovot, Israel) for advice and support with methodology. We acknowledge Talía Velasco and Isabel Hidalgo for advice and assistance with the generation of the chimeric mice and Petter Säwén and David Bryder for providing recombined Fgd5-CreERT2 x Lox-stop-lox-Tomato mice. We thank Zhi Ma and Teona Roschupkina for help with cell sorting and Linda Jansson for technical assistance.

Funding

This work was supported by the Swedish Research Council, European Union project TargetBraIn (279017), AFA Foundation, Swedish Brain Foundation, Torsten Söderberg Foundation, Region Skåne, Sparbanksstiftelsen Färs & Frosta, and Swedish Government Initiative for Strategic Research Areas (StemTherapy).

Authors' contributions

RG, DT, MH, CL, and EM conducted experiments and data analysis. RG, OL, and ZK designed the study, made the figures, and wrote the manuscript. All authors critically read and approved the final manuscript.

Consent for publication

Not applicable.

Competing interests

The authors declare that they have no competing interests.

References

1. Baruch K, Deczkowska A, Rosenzweig N, Tsitsou-Kampeli A, Sharif AM, Matcovitch-Natan O, Kertser A, David E, Amit I, Schwartz M. PD-1 immune checkpoint blockade reduces pathology and improves memory in mouse models of Alzheimer's disease. Nat Med. 2016;22:135–7.
2. Baruch K, Rosenzweig N, Kertser A, Deczkowska A, Sharif AM, Spinrad A, Tsitsou-Kampeli A, Sarel A, Cahalon L, Schwartz M. Breaking immune tolerance by targeting Foxp3(+) regulatory T cells mitigates Alzheimer's disease pathology. Nat Commun. 2015;6:7967.
3. Chernykh ER, Shevela EY, Starostina NM, Morozov SA, Davydova MN, Menyaeva EV, Ostanin AA. Safety and therapeutic potential of M2 macrophages in stroke treatment. Cell Transplant. 2016;25:1461–71.
4. Desestret V, Riou A, Chauveau F, Cho TH, Devillard E, Marinescu M, Ferrera R, Rey C, Chanal M, Angoulvant D, Honnorat J, Nighoghossian N, Berthezene Y, Nataf S, Wiart M. In vitro and in vivo models of cerebral ischemia show discrepancy in therapeutic effects of M2 macrophages. PLoS One. 2013;8:e67063.
5. Desland FA, Afzal A, Warraich Z, Mocco J. Manual versus automated rodent behavioral assessment: comparing efficacy and ease of Bederson and Garcia neurological deficit scores to an open field video-tracking system. J Cent Nerv Syst Dis. 2014;6:7–14.
6. Dowd E, Monville C, Torres EM, Dunnett SB. The Corridor Task: a simple test of lateralised response selection sensitive to unilateral dopamine deafferentation and graft-derived dopamine replacement in the striatum. Brain Res Bull. 2005;68:24–30.
7. Gazit R, Mandal PK, Ebina W, Ben-Zvi A, Nombela-Arrieta C, Silberstein LE, Rossi DJ. Fgd5 identifies hematopoietic stem cells in the murine bone marrow. J Exp Med. 2014;211:1315–31.
8. Gelderblom M, Leypoldt F, Steinbach K, Behrens D, Choe CU, Siler DA, Arumugam TV, Orthey E, Gerloff C, Tolosa E, Magnus T. Temporal and spatial dynamics of cerebral immune cell accumulation in stroke. Stroke. 2009;40:1849–57.
9. Gevrey JC, Isaac BM, Cox D. Syk is required for monocyte/macrophage chemotaxis to CX3CL1 (Fractalkine). J Immunol. 2005;175:3737–45.
10. Gillardon F, Lenz C, Kuschinsky W, Zimmermann M. Evidence for apoptotic cell death in the choroid plexus following focal cerebral ischemia. Neurosci Lett. 1996;207:113–6.
11. Go AS, Mozaffarian D, Roger VL, Benjamin EJ, Berry JD, Blaha MJ, Dai S, Ford ES, Fox CS, Franco S, Fullerton HJ, Gillespie C, Hailpern SM, Heit JA, Howard VJ, Huffman MD, Judd SE, Kissela BM, Kittner SJ, Lackland DT, Lichtman JH, Lisabeth LD, Mackey RH, Magid DJ, Marcus GM, Marelli A, Matchar DB, McGuire DK, Mohler 3rd ER, Moy CS, Mussolino ME, Neumar RW, Nichol G, Pandey DK, Paynter NP, Reeves MJ, Sorlie PD, Stein J, Towfighi A, Turan TN, Virani SS, Wong ND, Woo D, Turner MB, C. American Heart Association Statistics, S. Stroke Statistics. Heart disease and stroke statistics—2014 update: a report from the American Heart Association. Circulation. 2014;129: e28–292.
12. Gordon S, Taylor PR. Monocyte and macrophage heterogeneity. Nat Rev Immunol. 2005;5:953–64.
13. Grealish S, Mattsson B, Draxler P, Bjorklund A. Characterisation of behavioural and neurodegenerative changes induced by intranigral 6-hydroxydopamine lesions in a mouse model of Parkinson's disease. Eur J Neurosci. 2010;31:2266–78.
14. Hu X, Li P, Guo Y, Wang H, Leak RK, Chen S, Gao Y, Chen J. Microglia/macrophage polarization dynamics reveal novel mechanism of injury expansion after focal cerebral ischemia. Stroke. 2012;43:3063–70.

15. Korf-Klingebiel M, Reboll MR, Klede S, Brod T, Pich A, Polten F, Napp LC, Bauersachs J, Ganser A, Brinkmann E, Reimann I, Kempf T, Niessen HW, Mizrahi J, Schonfeld HJ, Iglesias A, Bobadilla M, Wang Y, Wollert KC. Myeloid-derived growth factor (C19orf10) mediates cardiac repair following myocardial infarction. Nat Med. 2015;21:140–9.
16. Kunis G, Baruch K, Miller O, Schwartz M. Immunization with a myelin-derived antigen activates the brain's choroid plexus for recruitment of immunoregulatory cells to the CNS and attenuates disease progression in a mouse model of ALS. J Neurosci. 2015;35:6381–93.
17. Kunis G, Baruch K, Rosenzweig N, Kertser A, Miller O, Berkutzki T, Schwartz M. IFN-gamma-dependent activation of the brain's choroid plexus for CNS immune surveillance and repair. Brain. 2013;136:3427–40.
18. Liu L, Duff K. A technique for serial collection of cerebrospinal fluid from the cisterna magna in mouse. J Vis Exp. 2008;10(21):960.
19. Losy J, Zaremba J. Monocyte chemoattractant protein-1 is increased in the cerebrospinal fluid of patients with ischemic stroke. Stroke. 2001;32:2695–6.
20. Mantovani A, Biswas SK, Galdiero MR, Sica A, Locati M. Macrophage plasticity and polarization in tissue repair and remodelling. J Pathol. 2013; 229:176–85.
21. Miro-Mur F, Perez-de-Puig I, Ferrer-Ferrer M, Urra X, Justicia C, Chamorro A, Planas AM. Immature monocytes recruited to the ischemic mouse brain differentiate into macrophages with features of alternative activation. Brain Behav Immun. 2016;53:18–33.
22. Moskowitz MA, Lo EH, Iadecola C. The science of stroke: mechanisms in search of treatments. Neuron. 2010;67:181–98.
23. Nahrendorf M, Swirski FK, Aikawa E, Stangenberg L, Wurdinger T, Figueiredo JL, Libby P, Weissleder R, Pittet MJ. The healing myocardium sequentially mobilizes two monocyte subsets with divergent and complementary functions. J Exp Med. 2007;204:3037–47.
24. Ozdinler PH, Macklis JD. IGF-I specifically enhances axon outgrowth of corticospinal motor neurons. Nat Neurosci. 2006;9:1371–81.
25. Perez-de Puig I, Miro F, Salas-Perdomo A, Bonfill-Teixidor E, Ferrer-Ferrer M, Marquez-Kisinousky L, Planas AM. IL-10 deficiency exacerbates the brain inflammatory response to permanent ischemia without preventing resolution of the lesion. J Cereb Blood Flow Metab. 2013;33:1955–66.
26. Raposo C, Graubardt N, Cohen M, Eitan C, London A, Berkutzki T, Schwartz M. CNS repair requires both effector and regulatory T cells with distinct temporal and spatial profiles. J Neurosci. 2014;34:10141–55.
27. Sansone M, Castellano C, Palazzesi S, Battaglia M, Ammassari-Teule M. Effects of oxiracetam, physostigmine, and their combination on active and passive avoidance learning in mice. Pharmacol Biochem Behav. 1993;44: 451–5.
28. Schlager C, Korner H, Krueger M, Vidoli S, Haberl M, Mielke D, Brylla E, Issekutz T, Cabanas C, Nelson PJ, Ziemssen T, Rohde V, Bechmann I, Lodygin D, Odoardi F, Flugel A. Effector T-cell trafficking between the leptomeninges and the cerebrospinal fluid. Nature. 2016;530:349–53.
29. Shechter R, Miller O, Yovel G, Rosenzweig N, London A, Ruckh J, Kim KW, Klein E, Kalchenko V, Bendel P, Lira SA, Jung S, Schwartz M. Recruitment of beneficial M2 macrophages to injured spinal cord is orchestrated by remote brain choroid plexus. Immunity. 2013;38:555–69.
30. Strazielle N, Creidy R, Malcus C, Boucraut J, Ghersi-Egea JF. T-Lymphocytes traffic into the brain across the blood-CSF barrier: evidence using a reconstituted choroid plexus epithelium. PLoS One. 2016;11:e0150945.
31. Szmydynger-Chodobska J, Strazielle N, Gandy JR, Keefe TH, Zink BJ, Ghersi-Egea JF, Chodobski A. Posttraumatic invasion of monocytes across the blood-cerebrospinal fluid barrier. J Cereb Blood Flow Metab. 2012;32: 93–104.
32. Szmydynger-Chodobska J, Strazielle N, Zink BJ, Ghersi-Egea JF, Chodobski A. The role of the choroid plexus in neutrophil invasion after traumatic brain injury. J Cereb Blood Flow Metab. 2009;29:1503–16.
33. Takeya M, Yoshimura T, Leonard EJ, Kato T, Okabe H, Takahashi K. Production of monocyte chemoattractant protein-1 by malignant fibrous histiocytoma: relation to the origin of histiocyte-like cells. Exp Mol Pathol. 1991;54:61–71.
34. Urra X, Villamor N, Amaro S, Gomez-Choco M, Obach V, Oleaga L, Planas AM, Chamorro A. Monocyte subtypes predict clinical course and prognosis in human stroke. J Cereb Blood Flow Metab. 2009;29:994–1002.
35. Wattananit S, Tornero D, Graubardt N, Memanishvili T, Monni E, Tatarishvili J, Miskinyte G, Ge R, Ahlenius H, Lindvall O, Schwartz M, Kokaia Z. Monocyte-derived macrophages contribute to spontaneous long-term functional recovery after stroke in mice. J Neurosci. 2016;36:4182–95.

12

Cell permeable HMGB1-binding heptamer peptide ameliorates neurovascular complications associated with thrombolytic therapy in rats with transient ischemic stroke

Miaodan Li[1], Shumin Chen[1], Xue Shi[1], Chenfei Lyu[1], Yongfang Zhang[1], Miaoqin Tan[1], Chen Wang[1], Nailiang Zang[1], Xiaoxi Liu[1], Yafang Hu[1], Jiangang Shen[2*], Liang Zhou[1*] and Yong Gu[1*]

Abstract

Background: Blood–brain barrier (BBB) breakdown and inflammatory responses are the major causes of tissue-type plasminogen activator (tPA)-induced hemorrhagic transformation (HT), while high-mobility group box 1 (HMGB1) exacerbates inflammatory damage to BBB during the process of brain ischemia/reperfusion. This study aimed to investigate the change of HMGB1 after thrombolytic therapy and whether blocking HMGB1 could ameliorate the neurovasculature complications secondary to tPA treatment in stroke rats.

Methods: Sera from acute stroke patients and rats with thrombolytic therapy were collected to investigate HMGB1 secretion. Male Sprague-Dawley rats with 2 h or 4.5 h middle cerebral artery occlusion were continuously infused with tPA followed by administration of membrane permeable HMGB1-binding heptamer peptide (HBHP). The mortality rate, neurological score, HT, brain swelling, BBB permeability, and inflammatory factors were determined.

Results: The results revealed that HMGB1 levels were elevated in both stroke patients and rats after tPA treatment. Blocking HMGB1 signaling by HBHP in the rat model of 4.5 h brain ischemia significantly attenuated tPA-related complications, including mortality rate, the degree of hemorrhage, brain swelling, neurological deficits, BBB impairment, microglia activation, and the expressions of inflammatory cytokines.

Conclusions: tPA treatment might induce HMGB1 secretion while blocking HMGB1 with HBHP could markedly reduce the risk of thrombolysis-associated brain hemorrhage and mortality through attenuating BBB damage and inflammatory reactions. These results indicate that HMGB1 may potentiate the risk of HT in tPA administration and that blocking HMGB1 signaling would be helpful in preventing complications brought by thrombolysis in ischemic stroke.

Keywords: Ischemic stroke, Tissue-type plasminogen activator, Blood–brain barrier, Hemorrhagic transformation, HMGB1, HMGB1-binding heptamer peptide, Inflammation

* Correspondence: shenjg@hku.hk; zhouliang_1963@126.com; yonggu@smu.edu.cn
[2]School of Chinese Medicine, The University of Hong Kong, Hong Kong, People's Republic of China
[1]Department of Neurology, Nanfang Hospital, Southern Medical University, Guangzhou, Guangdong 510515, People's Republic of China

Background

Ischemic stroke is the second leading cause of death worldwide while the therapeutic approaches are limited [1]. Tissue-type plasminogen activator (tPA) is the only FDA-approved drug for ischemic stroke, but its use is finite due to the narrow therapeutic time window (within 3 h or 4.5 h) and the increased risk of severe neurovascular complications, such as hemorrhagic transformation (HT) and edema [2], resulting in the fact that more than 95% of stroke patients cannot benefit from thrombolytic therapy [3]. The leakage of blood–brain barrier (BBB) is a critical factor causing tPA-associated HT and edema [4]. Therefore, exploring a combination therapy that can preserve BBB integrity is a promising therapeutic strategy to reduce the risk of neurovasculature complications.

Although the mechanisms underlying BBB breakdown and tPA-induced neurovascular complications are not fully understood, it has been suggested that they occur as a result of exaggeration of neuroinflammation [5]. Danger signals, such as high-mobility group box 1 (HMGB1) and ATP, were released into the environment from dying cells, leading to the activation of microglia and the expression of inflammatory factors in ischemic brain [6]. HMGB1, a non-histone DNA-binding protein localized in the nucleus, can be either actively secreted by immune cells or passively released from necrotic cells in response to infections and tissue injuries [7, 8]. Studies conducted by us and others revealed that the binding of extracellular HMGB1 to pattern recognition receptors of microglia could induce a significant elevation of cytokines expression, thereby eliciting inflammatory responses during brain ischemia/reperfusion [9, 10]. Moreover, HMGB1 serves as an extracellular inflammatory cytokine and contributes to neuronal injury and BBB disruption. HMGB1 level was elevated in patients with ischemic stroke [11, 12]. Anti-HMGB1 monoclonal antibody reduces infarct volume by 90% and potently reduces BBB permeability in stroke animal models [13, 14]. Administration of low-dose HMGB1-binding heptamer peptide (HBHP) significantly suppressed HMGB1-mediated neuronal damage [15]. But the relationship between HMGB1 and tPA-induced complications is unclear. Given that neuroinflammation contributes to the BBB disruption and tPA's neurovascular complications, we logically hypothesize that HMGB1 may potentiate the risk of tPA-associated complications, while blocking HMGB1-induced inflammation could protect BBB integrity, subsequently reducing tPA-induced hemorrhage during thrombolytic therapy for ischemic stroke.

Methods

Patients

Participants were selected from acute stroke patients admitted to the Department of Neurology, Nanfang Hospital, Southern Medical University. Enrollment criteria included subjects who were diagnosed with acute cerebral ischemia caused by occlusion of middle cerebral artery and met the criteria for thrombolysis. Excluded patients were those suffering from acute inflammatory illness, autoimmune diseases, or cancer. Patients who recently took anti-inflammatory drugs, glucocorticoid, or embolectomy were also ruled out. The study was approved by the ethics committee of the Nanfang Hospital, Southern Medical University (NO. NFEC-2016-171). Written informed consent was provided by patients or legally authorized representatives, and we obtained the consent from every participants or representatives to publish and report the data.

Animals and ethics statement

Male Sprague-Dawley rats weighing 250~300 g were obtained from the Experimental Animal Center, Southern Medical University. All animals were housed in a standard light-dark cycle with an average temperature of 23 °C. Food and water were provided ad libitum. All procedures were approved by the committee on Animal Care and Use of Nanfang Hospital, Southern Medical University, and followed the guide and care for the use of laboratory animals published by US NIH. A total of 166 rats were employed in the study. All efforts were made to minimize the number of animals used and their pain suffered.

Transient focal brain ischemia/reperfusion model

Middle cerebral artery occlusion (MCAO) model was employed as we previously described [16] to induce transient focal brain ischemia/reperfusion. Briefly, rats were anesthetized by inhalation of 5% isoflurane and maintained by 2% isoflurane in a mixture of 70% N2O and 30% O2. A piece of 3/0 monofilament nylon suture with its tip lapped round by silicone was introduced via lumen of right external carotid artery stump to embed into right anterior cerebral artery so that right MCA was occluded at its origin. Rats in sham-operated group underwent the same procedures except occluding the MCA. The temperature was maintained at 37 ± 0.1 °C until animals woke up completely. Animal operations and preclinical stroke study were followed ARRIVE guidelines [17]. Cerebral blood flow velocity of the right MCA territory (core cortex, 2 mm posterior and 6 mm lateral to the bregma) was assessed by the laser Doppler blood flow assessment (Moor Instruments, Wilmington, DE). After 2 h or 4.5 h occlusion, suture was removed to induce blood reperfusion whose flow velocity was monitored again (Fig. 1b). To confirm the success of MCAO, a 2-mm-thick brain coronal section 6 mm away from the tip of the frontal lobe was stained with 2,3,5-triphenyltetrazolium chloride (TTC) [18].

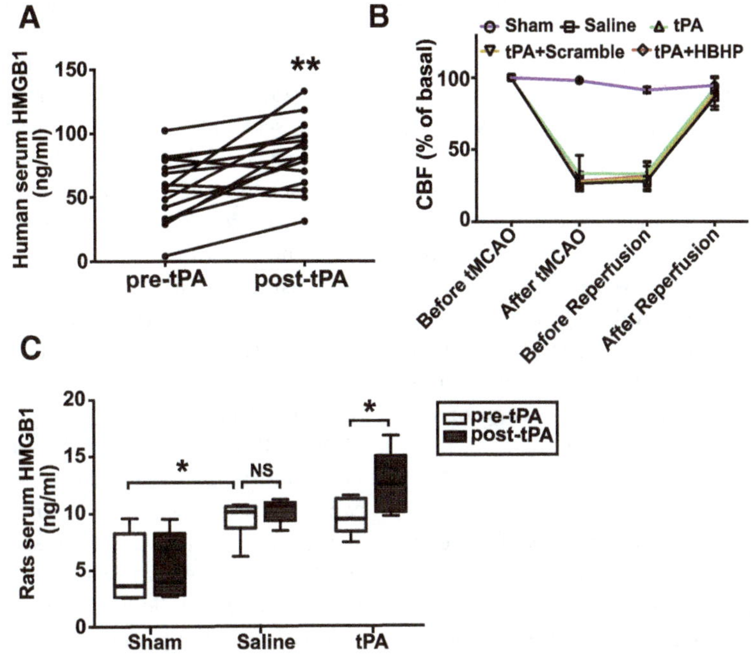

Fig. 1 Serum HMGB1 levels were elevated after thrombolysis in stroke patients and rats. **a** ELISA data of HMGB1 concentrations in patients' sera collected pre- and 2 h post-thrombolysis ($n = 15$). **b** Cerebral blood flow (CBF) of each rat subjected to ischemia/reperfusion was detected by laser-Doppler and expressed as percentage of basal level. ***c.*** *ELISA* result of serum HMGB1 levels at 30 min pre- and 4 h post-treatment of vehicle saline or tPA in 4.5 h MCAO rats ($n = 6$). NS: not significant; $^*P < 0.05$, $^{**}P < 0.01$. Data were shown as mean ± SD

Detection of HMGB1 and interleukin (IL)-1β in sera from patients and rats

Blood samples from patients were collected pre- and 2 h post-tPA treatment for self-comparison. Rat blood samples were collected pre- and 4 h post-tPA administration. Sera from patients and rats were obtained and the levels of HMGB1 were detected by enzyme-linked immunosorbent assay (ELISA) kits (Chondrex, Redmond, WA). Meanwhile, sera were incubated with Protein A/G MagBeads (GenScript, Piscataway, NJ) to remove immunoglobins followed by Western blot to observe HMGB1 levels. IL-1β in the sera from rats at 8 h after ischemia were also detected by ELISA kits (eBioscience, Austria). Tests were performed by investigators blinded to the origin of samples.

Experimental groups and drug treatment

MCAO rats were randomly divided into four groups with randomized number table and, respectively, administered saline, tPA only, tPA plus scramble peptide or tPA plus HBHP. tPA (Actilyse, 5 mg/kg, Boehringer Ingelheim, German) was injected (10% bonus, 90% continuous infusion for 30 min) via right femoral vein of MCAO rats. The suture was withdrawn to induce reperfusion at 15 min after tPA injection. Different doses of TAT-HBHP (YGRKKRRQRRR-HMSKPVQ, 1, 5, 10 mg/kg) were intravenously administered after tPA treatment within 30 min (Fig. 3a) [15, 19]. TAT-scramble peptide (YGRKKRRQRRR-PMQSKHV, 5 mg/kg) was employed as vehicle control. Peptides were synthesized by China-Peptides, Shanghai, China.

Measurement of survival rate and neurological deficit

Rats were monitored by video camera after surgery, and the time of death was recorded. Neurological deficits at 24 h after MCAO were assessed using modified Neurological Severity Score (mNSS) [20]. Neurological function was graded on a series of scales from 0 to 18 with higher scores indicating more severe neurologic deficits. Tests were independently performed by two investigators blinded to animal grouping.

Measurement of brain swelling and brain hemorrhage

At 24 h after ischemia, rats were transcardially perfused with cold PBS. The hemispheric area of each 2-mm-thick brain slice was measured to calculate the brain swelling by using ImageJ software (NIH, Bethesda, MD). The swelling index was calculated using the following equation: extent of brain swelling = (volume of ischemia ipsilateral hemisphere/volume of contralateral hemisphere − 1) × 100%. After taking photographs, the brain tissues were homogenized and centrifuged. QuantiChrom Hemoglobin Assay Kit (BioAssay Systems, Hayward, CA) was used to calculate the levels of hemoglobin in supernatants at 400 nm optical density. Hemoglobin contents of hemispheres were calculated based on optical density and expressed as microgram per gram brain.

Extravasation of Evans blue

Blood–brain barrier (BBB) integrity was assessed by measuring the extravasation of Evans blue dye. Briefly, Evans blue (2% in saline, 4 ml/kg; Sigma-Aldrich) was administered 90 min before sacrifice followed by transcardially perfused with saline to remove the residual dye from the vessels. The hemispheres were weighed and incubated in methanamide (Sigma-Aldrich) in 60 °C water bath overnight. After that, Evans blue content was determined in supernatants at 632 nm and expressed as microgram per gram brain. Gradient concentrations of Evans blue were used to build standard curve.

Western blot analysis

Proteins were prepared from the same regions of ischemic cerebral hemisphere (bregma 0 to + 2 mm) from different treatment groups, or serum proteins after magnetic separation. Fifty micrograms of total proteins were separated on 8 to 12% SDS-PAGE gel. After blocking, the membranes were incubated overnight at 4 °C with the primary antibodies including anti-occludin (1:1000; Invitrogen, Camarillo, CA), anti-COX-2 (1:1000; CST, Beverly, MA), anti-IL-1β, anti-iNOS (1:200; Santa Cruz Biotech, CA), anti-β-actin (1:500; ZSGB-Bio, Beijing, China) or anti-HMGB1 (1:1000; Proteintech, UK), followed by incubation with horseradish peroxidase-conjugated secondary antibodies (1:5000; Santa Cruz Biotech). Bands were detected by ECL advance Western blotting detection reagents (Millipore, Billercia, MA). The band intensities were normalized to β-actin using the ImageJ.

RNA preparation and reverse transcription-PCR

Total RNA was isolated from brains of 4.5 h MCAO rats at 8 h after ischemia onset (bregma – 1 to + 1 mm), and reverse-transcribed to complementary DNA (cDNA) using PrimeScript™ RT Master Mix Kit (Takara, Japan). cDNA samples were then amplified by quantitative real-time PCR on ABI-Prism 7500 Real-Time PCR System (Applied Biosystems, Carlsbad, CA) using SYBR® Premix Ex Taq™ II (Takara). The expression of mRNA was normalized with the internal standard β-actin.

Histological examination

Cryosections cut from rat brains (0~2.0 mm posterior to the bregma) were immunolabeled by primary antibody against IgG (Alexa647; 1:500; Abcam, Cambridge, UK) to evaluate the permeability of BBB at 24 h. Meanwhile, sections collected at 8 h after ischemia were postfixed with 4% formaldehyde, permeabilized with Triton X-100, and blocked with donkey serum, followed by incubation with anti-Iba-1 or CD68 (a marker of activated microglia cells; 1:200; Abcam) overnight at 4 °C, then with the donkey anti-goat (1:500; Abcam) or goat anti-mouse (ZSGB-BIO) secondary antibody. Three serial sections of each brain sample were observed, nine fields were randomly selected in the brain section region surrounded by black solid line (Fig. 6d) under Olympus Fluoview laser scanning confocal microscope (Olympus, Japan). The mean counts of Iba-1- and CD68-positive cells per field under × 40 magnification were automatically calculated using Image-Pro Plus version 6.0 (Media Cybernetics, Warrendale, PA). All counts were performed blind to the investigator on coded sections.

Statistical analysis

Online Power and Sample Size Calculators (http://powerandsamplesize.com/) was used to confirm the sample size needed for comparisons to yield statistical significance. Data were expressed as mean ± SD. Statistical significance was evaluated using one-way analysis of variance and followed by Dunnett test for two group comparisons. Nonparametric paired test was adopted for self-comparison. All statistical analyses were performed using SPSS 20.0 (IBM, Armonk, NY) or GraphPad Prism 6.05 (GraphPad, La Jolla, CA). P values less than 0.05 were considered to be significant.

Results

Treatment of tPA significantly elevates the serum HMGB1 levels in stroke patients and rats

We firstly determined whether HMGB1 secretion was changed after tPA treatment. Fifteen patients diagnosed with MCAO-induced acute ischemic stroke were enrolled in the study. The characteristics of enrolled patients were summarized in Table 1. Blood samples from patients were collected pre- and 2 h post-tPA treatment for self-comparison. ELISA data revealed that the serum HMGB1 level was significantly elevated after tPA treatment (56.31 ± 25.54 ng/mL before, vs 82.71 ± 26.72 ng/mL after, tPA treatment; $P < 0.01$; Fig. 1a).

Then, animal studies were conducted to further clarify the change of HMGB1 release in response to thrombolysis. Although the embolic stroke model can closely mimic the clinical situation, it produces big variations of infarct size and locations among individuals [18, 21]. Transient filament occlusion model would be more stable for us to

Table 1 Patient characteristics

Traits		Risk factors	
Men/women	10/5	Diabetes	10
Age (mean ± SD, years)	61.93 ± 7.79	Hypertension	10
NIHSS	7.67 ± 4.05	Smoking	7
Anti-inflammatory drugs	0	Dyslipidemia	9
Glucocorticoid	0	High homocysteine	1

specifically investigate tPA-induced complications. A total of 166 rats were employed in the study. Only the rats that displayed more than 70% reduction of cerebral blood flow during ischemia and paralysis of the contralateral limb after reperfusion were selected (Fig. 1b). In line with the data of human study, the rat serum HMGB1 level was also found to be increased after tPA treatment (from 9.84 ± 1.62 to 12.62 ± 2.78 ng/mL; $P < 0.05$; Fig. 1c). Considering ischemic injury itself can also induce HMGB1 release, to eliminate the possibility that timely accumulated HMGB1 release after ischemia leads to HMGB1 elevation, we compared its dynamic change in stroke rats with saline injection. Results in Fig. 1c showed that HMGB1 was not significantly altered at 4 h after saline injection. Based on these evidences, it seems that tPA treatment induces HMGB1 release. To eliminate the potential interference brought by non-specificity of HMGB1 antibody in purchased ELISA kits, sera proteins were magnetic separated and immunoblotted by HMGB1 antibody. Results revealed that HMGB1 could be detected by Western blot and it was also increased after tPA treatment, although a relatively deep background was observed (Additional file 1: Figure S1).

HBHP alleviates HT in MCAO rats with tPA treatment

To explore the correlation between elevated HMGB1 and tPA-induced complications, we next investigated whether blocking HMGB1 signaling with HBHP could improve the complication after tPA treatment. HT is the most severe side effect of thrombolytic therapy. We quantified hemorrhage volume in rats 24 h after experimental ischemia. Early tPA infusion at 2 h did not induce obvious HT (Fig. 2a, b) which is consistent with the previous finding [22]. Meanwhile, delayed tPA treatment at 4.5 h resulted in evident HT in the ischemic brain (Fig. 2c, d). Notably, co-treatment of HBHP (5 mg/kg) significantly reduced delayed tPA-induced

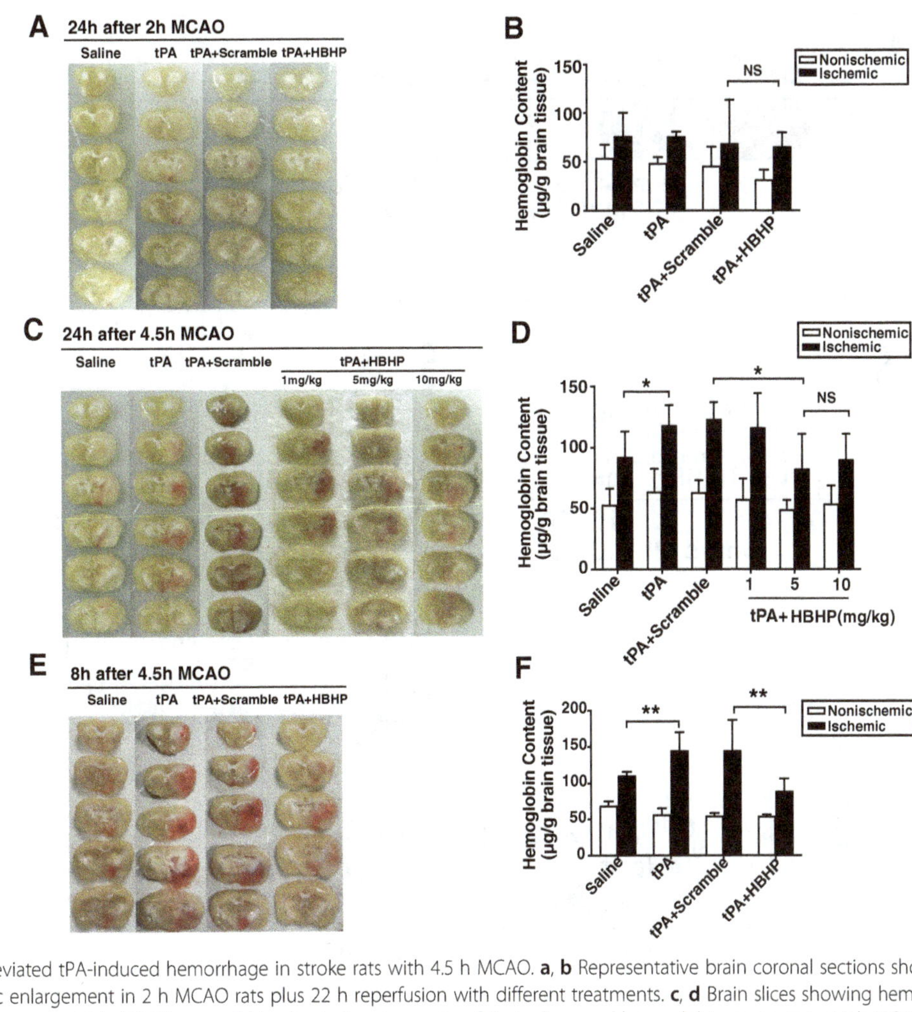

Fig. 2 HBHP alleviated tPA-induced hemorrhage in stroke rats with 4.5 h MCAO. **a**, **b** Representative brain coronal sections showing hemorrhage and hemispheric enlargement in 2 h MCAO rats plus 22 h reperfusion with different treatments. **c**, **d** Brain slices showing hemorrhage and brain hemoglobin contents in 4.5 h MCAO rats at 24 h after ischemia onset. **e**, **f** Brain slices and hemoglobin contents in 4.5 h MCAO rats at 8 h after ischemia onset. Hemoglobin content was quantified and presented as bar graph. NS: not significant; $^*P < 0.05$, $^{**}P < 0.01$; $n = 5$–8. Data were shown as mean ± SD

hemorrhage, while scramble peptide and HBHP (1 mg/kg) did not. Hemoglobin quantification assay further confirmed this finding. There was no statistical difference between 5 and 10 mg/kg. Therefore, we selected 5 mg/kg as the minimum dose of maximum efficacy in the following experiments.

Since most 4.5 h-tPA rats who had more volume of brain hemorrhage might not survive to 24 h, the determination of survived rats at 24 h was inaccurate. Therefore, we quantified the contents of hemoglobin in 4.5 h-MCAO rats at 8 h after ischemia onset and found tPA administration caused severe hemorrhage, which could also be mitigated by HBHP (Fig. 2e, f). These results indicate that HBHP can alleviate tPA-induced HT in ischemic rats.

HBHP decreases mortality of rats treated with tPA after brain ischemia

Higher volume of hemorrhage in the brain brings poor prognosis. As shown in Fig. 3b, c, rats receiving 4.5 h ischemia followed by tPA administration (4.5 h-tPA) had a much higher mortality (73.91%, 17 out of 23) than the vehicle saline-treated group rats (40.91%, 9 out of 22). In contrast, HBHP markedly lowered the mortality to 44.44% at 24 h after ischemia (8 of 18; Fig. 3c) and improved 24 h survival outcome after 4.5 h ischemia followed by tPA administration (Fig. 3b). In 2 h ischemia model, the mortality was not statistically different in different treatment groups (Fig. 3c).

HBHP improves neurological outcome and attenuates brain swelling in MCAO rats with tPA treatment

Similar effects were observed for mNSS score estimation. Rats in 4.5 h-tPA group displayed more severe neurological impairment than in saline group, and the neural deficits were ameliorated by HBHP (Fig. 4a). No statistical differences in neurological outcome were noted in 2 h-MCAO groups. Expectedly, HBHP treatment significantly reduce ischemia hemispheric enlargement caused

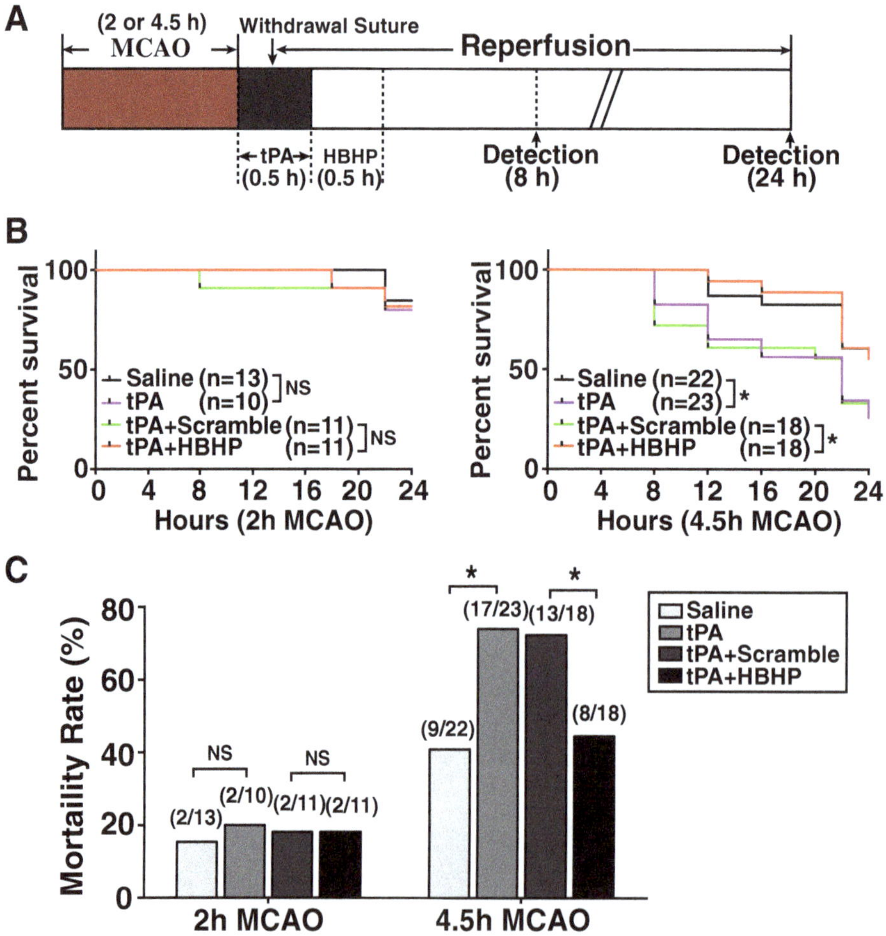

Fig. 3 HBHP decreased the mortality of 4.5 h MCAO rats with tPA administration. **a** Schematic diagram of the overall experimental design. **b** The 24 h survival curves of rats with 2 h or 4.5 h MCAO treated with vehicle or tPA in combination of HBHP or scramble peptide. The rat number in each group was labeled. **c** The mortality of each group rats at 24 h post ischemia. Numbers in parentheses mean "the dead rats/the total number of rats" in each group. NS: not significant; $*P < 0.05$

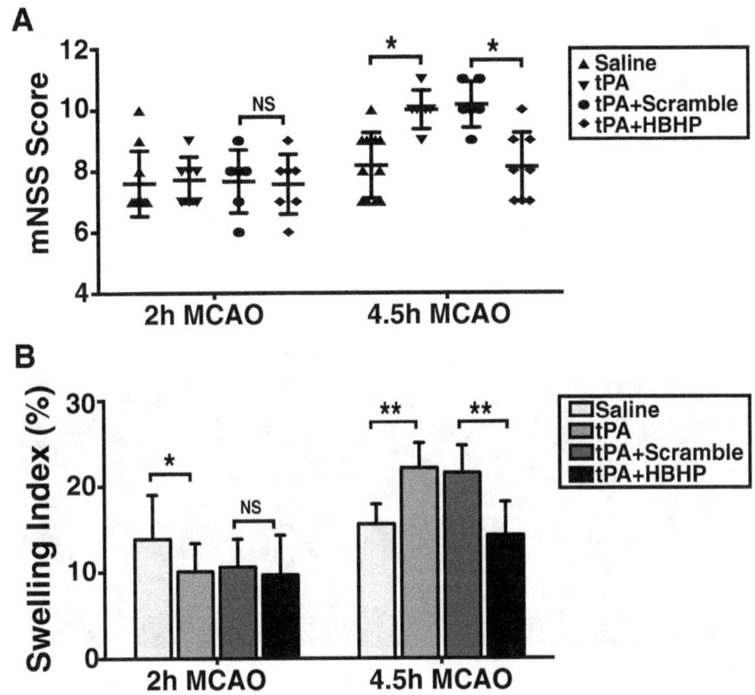

Fig. 4 HBHP improved neurological outcome and brain swelling of 4.5 h MCAO rats with tPA treatment. **a** Modified Neurological Severity Scores (mNSS) at 24 h post ischemia. **b** The ratio of brain swelling at 24 h after ischemia of stroke rats. NS: not significant; $*P < 0.05$, $**P < 0.01$; $n = 5–8$. Data were shown as mean ± SD

by 4.5 h-tPA (Fig. 4b). Together, these results suggest that HBHP treatment improves prognosis in rats after experimental 4.5 h ischemia followed by tPA administration.

HBHP alleviates BBB disruption in MCAO rats with tPA treatment

Thrombolytic therapy has been reported to exaggerate BBB breakdown, leading to the HT in animal stroke models [4, 5]. BBB permeability in 4.5 h-MCAO rats was evaluated via the observation of the Evans blue dye and IgG leakage to brain parenchyma, as well as the loss of tight junction protein occludin. Because 2 h-MCAO did not cause high mortality and severe HT, the following experiments were conducted on 4.5 h-MCAO model. Results showed that Evans blue content in ipsilateral ischemic hemispheres was remarkably decreased in the HBHP treatment group compared with scramble group (6.409 ± 4.514 vs 21.298 ± 8.233 μg/g) (Fig. 5a). Immunofluorescence staining assay showed that a large number of IgG permeated in cortex and striatum regions of the ischemic ipsilateral hemispheres after tPA treatment, which was significantly decreased by HBHP treatment (Fig. 5b). Consistently, the tPA-induced reduction of occludin was rescued by HBHP (Fig. 5c), suggesting that HBHP protects BBB integrity in tPA-treated rats.

HBHP downregulates inflammatory cytokine expressions and inhibits microglia activation in ischemic brains with tPA treatment

Considering residential inflammation has been reported to be involved in the disruption of BBB, we finally investigated whether the protective effect of HBHP is related to inflammatory reactions. Activation of microglia and the expression of cytokines were observed at 8 h after ischemia onset. Data revealed that inflammatory cells were further activated by tPA, as evident by more CD68- and Iba-1-positive cells [23] in peri-infarct area in tPA-treated rats, which was ameliorated by HBHP treatment (Fig. 6a–c). Quantitative real-time PCR, Western blot, and ELISA assay were performed to detect cytokine expression or release. Results showed that HBHP decreased mRNA expressions of IL-1β, IL-6, and IL-12b, while TNF-α did not change after treatment (Fig. 7b). HBHP treatment significantly downregulated the protein expressions of iNOS, COX-2, and IL-1β in the ischemic hemisphere from tPA-treated rats compared with scramble control (Fig. 7c). The secretion of IL-1β, determined by ELISA, was also inhibited after HBHP treatment (Fig. 7a). Taken together, HBHP can reduce inflammatory response secondary to tPA administration, contributing to the attenuation of neurovascular complications.

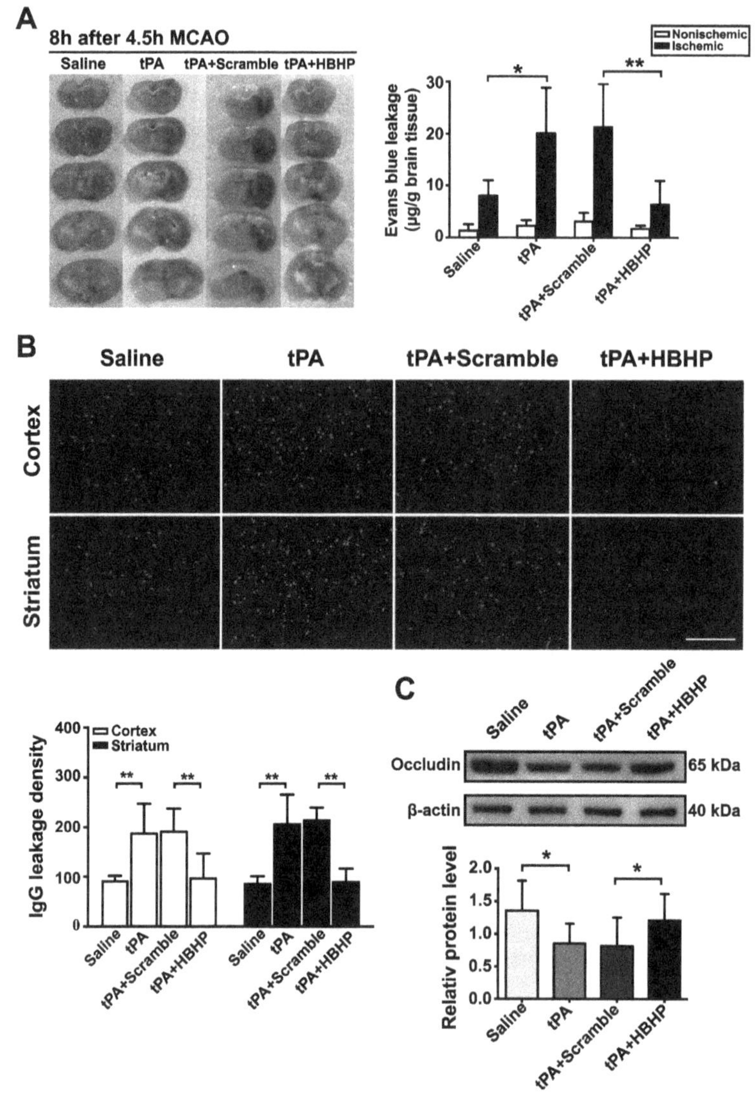

Fig. 5 HBHP decreased the BBB permeability in tPA-treated MCAO rats. **a** Representative images of Evans blue leakage from 4.5 h MCAO rats. The contents of Evans blue leakage were measured and expressed as microgram per gram brain. $*P < 0.05$, $**P < 0.01$; $n = 4–6$. **b** Immunofluoresence staining with IgG antibody (red) in the cerebral cortex and striatum from 4.5 h MCAO rats. The leaked IgG was quantified. Scale bar = 200 μm. $**P < 0.01$, $n = 3–4$. **c** Western blot and quantified data of occludin in ischemic ipsilateral hemispheres from 4.5 h MCAO rats. $*P < 0.05$, $**P < 0.01$; $n = 4$. Data were shown as mean ± SD

Discussion

Presently, tPA is still a highly effective therapy to salvage potentially reversible ischemic tissue and early improve neurological deficits. However, tPA application is limited by narrow therapeutic time window and severe neurovascular complications. Stroke patients with tPA treatment have about 10-fold higher risk of suffering HT than untreated patients. A recent study indicates 28% had hemorrhages in the ischemic area and 44.6% developed cerebral microbleeds using susceptibility-weighted imaging (SWI), a magnetic resonance imaging (MRI) sequence [24]. HT is a severe complication after thrombolysis which dramatically worsens patient outcome. Exploring strategies that can prevent HT occurrence and reduce hemorrhage volume is especially urgent for thrombolytic therapy. Given that HMGB1 has been reported to deteriorate neurovascular complications in stroke and might be elevated after tPA treatment evidenced in our present study, preventing HMGB1 signaling might provide a good strategy to attenuate the side effects caused by tPA. Here, we firstly demonstrate that HMGB1 blocking peptide reduced the tPA-associated mortality, brain hemorrhage, swelling, and BBB disruption in an animal model of ischemic stroke.

Extracellular HMGB1 in its reduced form with a disulfide bond connecting C23 and C45 exhibits a cytokine-inducing activity [25, 26] and participates in the pathological processes of numerous inflammatory and autoimmune diseases [25, 27]. Recently, it was paid particular attention on

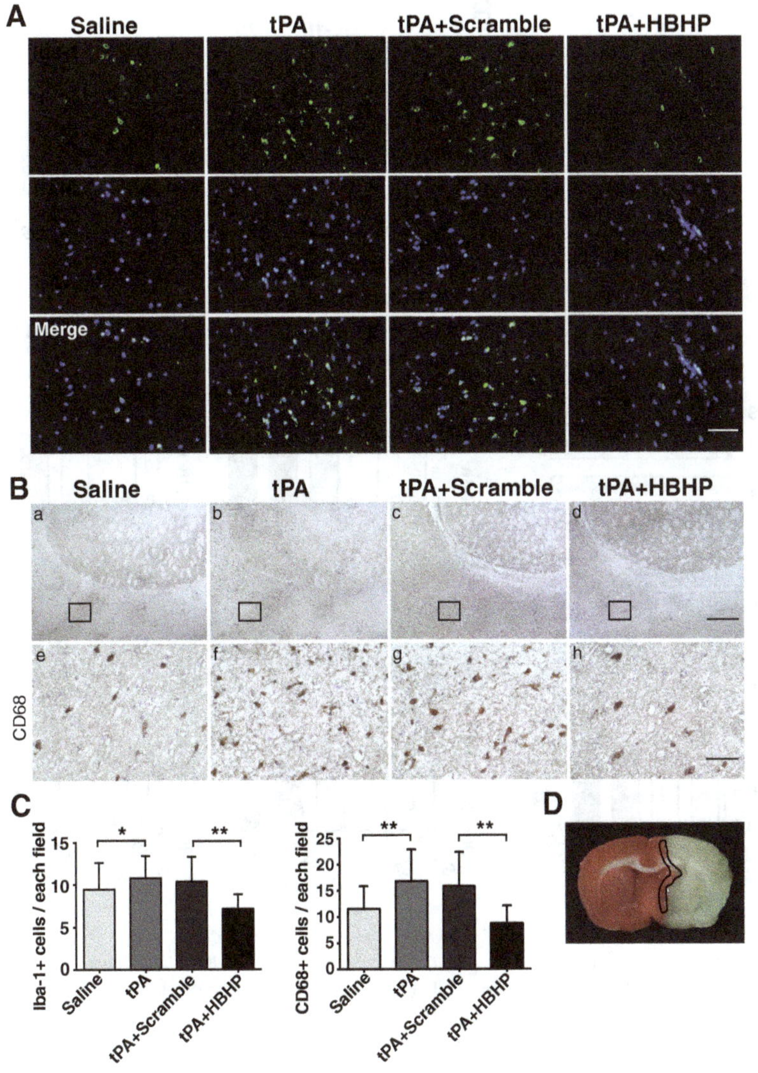

Fig. 6 HBHP inhibited microglia activation in tPA-treated MCAO rats. **A** Representative graphs of immunofluorescence staining with anti-Iba-1 antibodies (green) and DAPI (blue) in the peri-infarct cortex from 4.5 h MCAO rats. Scale bar = 50 μm. **B** Representative graphs of immunohistochemistry staining with CD68 antibodies. The volumes of **e**–**h** were the amplification of **a**–**d**. Scale bar = 500 μm in **a**–**d** (4×); Scale bar = 50 μm in **e**–**h** (40×). **C** The number of Iba-1- and CD68-positive cells was quantified. **D** 2-3-5-Triphenyl tetrazolium chloride staining of ischemic brain indicated the position where the corresponding images were obtained. The brain region surrounded by black solid line indicates the areas where the typical Iba-1-positive cells were observed. $^{*}P < 0.05$, $^{**}P < 0.01$; $n = 3$–4. Data were shown as mean ± SD

its significant role in brain ischemia/reperfusion. As one of the damage-associated molecular pattern molecules, extracellular HMGB1 binds to pattern recognition receptors of microglia and subsequently leads to synthesis and release of pro-inflammatory mediators, aggravating neuronal injury and BBB disruption [9]. In addition, extracellular HMGB1 also acts on its target receptors on endothelial progenitor cells (EPCs) to promote peri-infarct angiogenesis [28] which is related to ischemia/reperfusion-induced HT [29]. Here, we step forward to show that serum HMGB1 was increased in both patients and rats after tPA treatment and that blocking HMGB1 signaling significantly reduced neurovascular complications, emphasizing the critical role of HMGB1 in tPA-induced HT and the pathological importance during cerebral ischemia/reperfusion.

Brain ischemia/reperfusion can induce HMGB1 translocation and release. According to a previous report, HMGB1 level in cerebrospinal fluid was approximately twofold at 2 h, and increased to sixfold higher at 12 h after reperfusion in MCAO rats than sham-operated animals [14], indicating the time-dependent elevation of serum HMGB1 after reperfusion. To investigate tPA, rather than reperfusion time, induced serum HMGB1 increase, we collected patients' sera at 2 h post-tPA

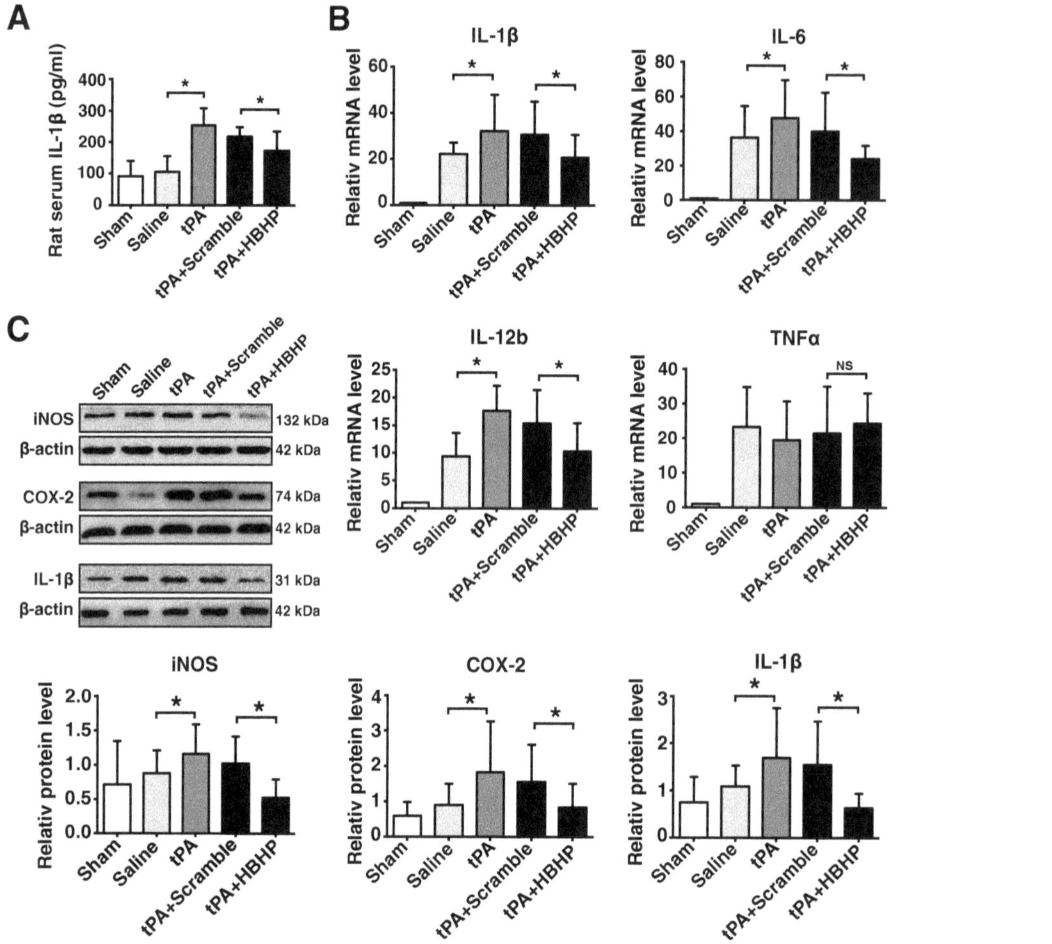

Fig. 7 HBHP alleviated inflammatory reactions in tPA-treated stroke rats. **a** ELISA data of serum IL-1β levels in stroke rats at 8 h after ischemia, $n = 5–7$. **b** Quantitative real-time PCR analysis of mRNA expressions of IL-1β, IL-6, IL-12b, and TNF-α in the peri-infarct cortex from 4.5 h MCAO rats or in the same regions of sham-operated rats, $n = 3–4$. **c** Western blot and quantified data of iNOS, COX-2, and IL-1β in ischemic ipsilateral hemispheres at 8 h after ischemia, $n = 3–4$. NS: not significant; $*P < 0.05$. Data were shown as mean ± SD

treatment in order to reduce the effect caused by reperfusion time. Meanwhile, we compared the changes of HMGB1 in tPA and saline-treated MCAO rats within the same time durations. Our data revealed that serum HMGB1 levels seemed to be elevated after tPA treatment within a short time. In the MCAO rat model, serum HMGB1 level was also increased after tPA treatment, but did not obviously alter in vehicle-treated rats. It would be better to detect HMGB1 in cerebrospinal fluid where HMGB1 play the role in central nervous system diseases. Due to the technical limitation in our lab, serum HMGB1, rather than CSF HMGB1, was determined. How tPA treatment induces HMGB1 release is unknown. Some indirect evidences may imply this finding. For example, tPA could upregulate the expression of inflammatory mediators in cultured human cerebral microvascular endothelial cells [30], which might then mediate inflammatory cell death and the subsequent passive HMGB1 release.

Currently, there are several approaches to block HMGB1-mediated inflammation and thereby protecting neurovascular unit, including neutralizing monoclonal antibody (mAb) [13, 14], N-terminal domain of HMGB1 (competitively binds to receptors) [31], non-specific inhibitors like glycyrrhizin [32], and blocking peptide (HBHP) [15, 19, 33]. Among them, mAb requires intracerebroventricular injection, whereas HMGB1 N -terminal domain and glycyrrhizin lack target specificity. Fortunately, Kim et al. reported that HBHP binds directly to HMGB1 A box, confers anti-inflammation effect, and suppresses the synergistic effect of LPS and HMGB1 [33]. More importantly, intranasal delivery of low-dose HBHP effectively reduces infarct volume and improves neurological outcome after cerebral ischemia [15]. These elegant works suggest that HBHP would be a good drug candidate for stroke therapy. In the present study, intravenous injection of TAT-fused HBHP could pass BBB to get to brain parenchyma [34], maybe directly block

HMGB1-mediated glial cell activation and inflammatory response, and subsequently dramatically reduce BBB disruption, HT and mortality after thrombolysis, although the drug bioactivity and pharmacological mechanisms are not fully observed and require in-depth investigation.

Since most 4.5 h-tPA rats who might have more amount of brain bleeding could not survive to 24 h, the results of hemoglobin quantification and BBB permeability detected in the survived rats at 24 h were inaccurate, and the results of surviving animals (24 h after MCAO) would have bias. Therefore, we calculated the hemoglobin contents of hemispheres again before the death time of most rats (8 h after ischemia), and found that tPA administration caused more severe hemorrhage, and further indicated the protective effect of HBHP on hemorrhagic transformation.

The loss of BBB leakage is a critical factor inducing HT after the ischemia/reperfusion [35]. Pretreatment determination of BBB permeability can predict post-treatment intracranial hemorrhage in patients receiving intravenous tPA or endovascular therapy [36, 37]. Meanwhile, HMGB1 was reported to exaggerate BBB insult [13, 14]. In line with these findings, we showed here, tPA exacerbated the extravasation of Evans blue and the impairment of tight junction proteins, the markers of BBB leakage. HBHP significantly attenuated tPA-mediated exaggeration of BBB impairment. However, an opposite finding was observed in an in vitro study, in which, HMGB-1 reduced tPA-driven BBB leakage [38]. The inconsistency might be explained by a much lower metabolic rate and the lack of micro-environment producing inflammatory factors in cell culture system compared with in vivo conditions.

Moreover, neuroinflammation is one of the main causes of BBB breakdown and HT [39]. Consistently, HBHP significantly alleviated the activated microglia and reduced the mRNA or protein levels of IL-1β, IL-6, IL-12b, iNOS, and COX-2 in the ischemic brains with tPA treatment. Considering the induction of iNOS, COX-2 has been reported to be involved in the disruption of BBB [40], our findings suggest that the activation of microglia and cytokine expression contribute to HMGB1-induced BBB disruption and HT development after thrombolysis in ischemic stroke. Therefore, it is reasonable that HBHP, which has the ability to reduce the expression of proinflammatory factors, exerted profound therapeutic effects on tPA-associated complications. In addition, the present study indicated that HBHP and purified HMGB1 could not directly interact with tPA (Additional file 2: Figure S2), possibly represents that they did not alter the protease activity. However, we could not exclude other potential underlying mechanisms that mediate this therapeutic effect of HBHP, such as the disturbance of other protein-tPA interaction. Clear mechanisms are expected to be uncovered in our following studies.

Conclusions

In conclusion, the levels of serum HMGB1 seemed increased after thrombolysis in stroke patients and animals. Furthermore, HBHP treatment could reduce cerebral hemorrhage, brain swelling and mortality in tPA treatment after stroke. Our findings indicate that HMGB1-mediated inflammation and BBB breakdown may contribute to tPA-induced occurrence of HT and death in ischemic stroke, and that blocking HMGB1 signaling would be helpful to prevent the complications brought by thrombolysis. However, rationally designed clinical studies with well-defined patient population are needed to validate whether HBHP can be developed as an efficacious adjuvant therapy for ischemic stroke.

Additional files

Additional file 1: Figure S1. Western blot analysis indicated serum HMGB1 levels were elevated after thrombolysis in stroke patients and rats. Sera from human and rats received thrombolysis were incubated with Protein A/G MagBeads (GenScript, Piscataway, NJ) to remove immunoglobins and then the proteins were separated in SDS-PAGE gels and immunolabeled with HMGB1 antibody.

Additional file 2: Figure S2. HBHP and HMGBP could not directly interact with tPA. Biolayer interferometry binding measurements using BLItz system from ForteBio were used to detect the binding affinity of HBHP and HMGBP with tPA. (A) Proteins were biotinylated and immobilized on streptavidin-coated biosensor tips. After equilibration, the tips were probed with the interacting analytes. The complexes were dissociated by immersing the sensor into sample dilution buffer. Data were generated automatically by the Octet User Software. (B) tPA binding measurements with HMGB1 were analyzed. The results showed that the combined signals were the same as those of uncured sensor, indicating HMGB1 has no specific binding with tPA. (C) HBHP binding measurements with tPA were analyzed. The combined signals were the same as those of the uncured sensor, indicating HBHP also has no specific binding with tPA.

Abbreviations

BBB: Blood–brain barrier; ELISA: Enzyme-linked immunosorbent assay; EPCs: Endothelial progenitor cells; HBHP: HMGB1-binding heptamer peptide; HMGB1: High-mobility group box 1; HT: Hemorrhagic transformation; mAb: Neutralizing monoclonal antibody; MCAO: Middle cerebral artery occlusion; mNSS: Modified Neurological Severity Score; SLE: Systemic lupus erythematosus; tPA: Tissue-type plasminogen activator; TTC: 2,3,5-Triphenyltetrazolium chloride

Acknowledgements

The work was supported by grants from the National Natural Science Foundation of China (No.81400990), the Natural Science Foundation of Guangdong Province of China (No. 2014A030310197), the Science and Technology Plan of Guangdong Province of China (No. 2016A020215113), the President Funding of Nanfang Hospital, Southern Medical University (No. 2016B017), and Hong Kong RGC GRF Grant (Ref No.17102915).

Funding

The study received the following grants: No.81400990 (the National Natural Science Foundation of China), No. 2014A030310197 (the Natural Science Foundation of Guangdong Province of China), No. 2016A020215113 (the Science and Technology Plan of Guangdong Province of China), No. 2016B017 (the President Funding of Nanfang Hospital, Southern Medical University), and Ref No.17102915 (Hong Kong RGC GRF Grant).

Authors' contributions
LZ, YG, JS, and ML planned and designed the research. ML, SC, XS, CL, YZ, MT, CW, XL, NZ, and YH performed the experiments. YG and ML analyzed the data, prepared the figures, and wrote the manuscript. All authors read and approved the final manuscript.

Consent for publication
Not applicable.

Competing interests
The authors declare that they have no competing interests.

References

1. Mathers CD, Boerma T, Ma FD. Global and regional causes of death. Br Med Bull. 2009;92:7–32.
2. Group TNI of ND and S rt-PSS. Tissue plasminogen activator for acute ischemic stroke. N Engl J Med. 1995;333:1581–7.
3. Fonarow GC, Smith EE, Saver JL, Reeves MJ, Bhatt DL, Grau-Sepulveda MV, et al. Timeliness of tissue-type plasminogen activator therapy in acute ischemic stroke: patient characteristics, hospital factors, and outcomes associated with door-to-needle times within 60 minutes. Circulation. 2011; 123:750–8.
4. Wang X, Tsuji K, Lee SR, Ning M, Furie KL, Buchan AM, et al. Mechanisms of hemorrhagic transformation after tissue plasminogen activator reperfusion therapy for ischemic stroke. Stroke. 2004;35:2726–30.
5. Eltzschig HK, Eckle T. Ischemia and reperfusion--from mechanism to translation. Nat Med. 2011;17:1391–401.
6. Iadecola C, Anrather J. The immunology of stroke: from mechanisms to translation. Nat Med. 2011;17:796–808.
7. Lotze MT, Tracey KJ. High-mobility group box 1 protein (HMGB1): nuclear weapon in the immune arsenal. Nat Rev Immunol. 2005;5: 331–42.
8. Lu B, Wang C, Wang M, Li W, Chen F, Tracey KJ, et al. Molecular mechanism and therapeutic modulation of high mobility group box 1 release and action: an updated review. Expert Rev Clin Immunol. 2014; 10:713–27.
9. Liesz A, Dalpke A, Mracsko E, Antoine DJ, Roth S, Zhou W, et al. DAMP signaling is a key pathway inducing immune modulation after brain injury. J Neurosci. 2015;35:583–98.
10. Liu XX, Wang C, Huang SF, Chen Q, Hu YF, Zhou L, et al. Regnase-1 in microglia negatively regulates high mobility group box 1-mediated inflammation and neuronal injury. Sci Rep. 2016;6:24073.
11. Goldstein RS, Gallowitsch-Puerta M, Yang L, Rosas-Ballina M, Huston JM, Czura CJ, et al. Elevated high-mobility group box 1 levels in patients with cerebral and myocardial ischemia. Shock. 2006;25:571–4.
12. Sims GP, Rowe DC, Rietdijk ST, Herbst R, Coyle AJ. HMGB1 and RAGE in inflammation and cancer. Annu Rev Immunol. 2010;28:367–88.
13. Liu K, Mori S, Takahashi HK, Tomono Y, Wake H, Kanke T, et al. Anti-high mobility group box 1 monoclonal antibody ameliorates brain infarction induced by transient ischemia in rats. FASEB J. 2007;21:3904–16.
14. Zhang J, Takahashi HK, Liu K, Wake H, Liu R, Maruo T, et al. Anti-high mobility group box-1 monoclonal antibody protects the blood-brain barrier from ischemia-induced disruption in rats. Stroke. 2011;42:1420–8.
15. Kim ID, Shin JH, Lee HK, Jin YC, Lee JK. Intranasal delivery of HMGB1-binding heptamer peptide confers a robust neuroprotection in the postischemic brain. Neurosci Lett. 2012;525:179–83.
16. Gu Y, Zheng G, Xu M, Li Y, Chen X, Zhu W, et al. Caveolin-1 regulates nitric oxide-mediated matrix metalloproteinases activity and blood-brain barrier permeability in focal cerebral ischemia and reperfusion injury. J Neurochem. 2012;120:147–56.
17. Kilkenny C, Browne W, Cuthill IC, Emerson M, Altman DG, Group NCRGW. Animal research: reporting in vivo experiments: the ARRIVE guidelines. Br J Pharmacol. 2010;160:1577–9.
18. Liu W, Hendren J, Qin XJ, Liu KJ. Normobaric hyperoxia reduces the neurovascular complications associated with delayed tissue plasminogen activator treatment in a rat model of focal cerebral ischemia. Stroke. 2009; 40:2526–31.
19. Kim ID, Lee JK. HMGB1-binding heptamer confers anti-inflammatory effects in primary microglia culture. Exp Neurobiol. 2013;22:301–7.
20. Chen J, Sanberg PR, Li Y, Wang L, Lu M, Willing AE, et al. Intravenous administration of human umbilical cord blood reduces behavioral deficits after stroke in rats. Stroke. 2001;32:2682–8.
21. Carmichael ST. Rodent models of focal stroke: size, mechanism, and purpose. NeuroRx. 2005;2:396–409.
22. Fagan SC, Garcia JH. Hemorrhagic transformation in focal cerebral ischemia: influence of time to artery reopening and tissue plasminogen activator. Pharmacotherapy. 1999;19:139–42.
23. Jeong H, Ji K, Kim J, Jou I, Joe E. Repair of astrocytes , blood vessels , and myelin in the injured brain: possible roles of blood monocytes. Mol. Brain. 2013;6:1.
24. Ozbek D, Ozturk O, Ekinci G, Midi I. Risk of hemorrhage in ischemic stroke and its relationship with cerebral microbleeds. Clin Neurol Neurosurg Elsevier. 2018;168:112–7.
25. Antoine D, Harris H. A systematic nomenclature for the redox states of high mobility group box (HMGB) proteins. Mol Med. 2014;20:1.
26. Kang R, Chen R, Zhang Q, Hou W, Wu S, Cao L, et al. HMGB1 in health and disease. Mol Aspects Med Elsevier Ltd. 2014;40:1–116.
27. Musumeci D, Roviello GN, Montesarchio D. An overview on HMGB1 inhibitors as potential therapeutic agents in HMGB1-related pathologies. Pharmacol Ther. 2014;141:347–57.
28. Hayakawa K, Pham LDD, Katusic ZS, Arai K, Lo EH. Astrocytic high-mobility group box 1 promotes endothelial progenitor cell-mediated neurovascular remodeling during stroke recovery. Proc Natl Acad Sci U S A. 2012;109: 7505–10.
29. Jickling GC, Liu D, Stamova B, Ander BP, Zhan X, Lu A, et al. Hemorrhagic transformation after ischemic stroke in animals and humans. J Cereb Blood Flow Metab. 2014;34:185–99.
30. Wang X, Lee SR, Arai K, Lee SR, Tsuji K, Rebeck GW, et al. Lipoprotein receptor-mediated induction of matrix metalloproteinase by tissue plasminogen activator. Nat Med. 2003;9:1313–7.
31. Arumugam T, Ramachandran V, Gomez SB, Schmidt AM, Logsdon CD. S100P-derived RAGE antagonistic peptide reduces tumor growth and metastasis. Clin Cancer Res. 2012;18:4356–64.
32. Mollica L, De Marchis F, Spitaleri A, Dallacosta C, Pennacchini D, Zamai M, et al. Glycyrrhizin binds to high-mobility group box 1 protein and inhibits its cytokine activities. Chem Biol. 2007;14:431–41.
33. Kim ID, Luo L, Lee HB, Lee HK, Lee JK. HMGB1-binding heptamer suppresses the synergistic effect of HMGB1 and LPS by interacting directly with HMGB1. Neurosci Lett. 2015;593:40–4.
34. Shi X, Li M, Huang K, Zhou S, Hu Y, Pan S, et al. HMGB1 binding heptamer peptide improves survival and ameliorates brain injury in rats after cardiac arrest and cardiopulmonary resuscitation. Neurosci IBRO. 2017;360:128–38.
35. Latour LL, Kang DW, Ezzeddine MA, Chalela JA, Warach S. Early blood-brain barrier disruption in human focal brain ischemia. Ann Neurol. 2004;56:468–77.
36. Leigh R, Jen SS, Hillis AE, Krakauer JW, Barker PB, Stir, et al. Pretreatment blood-brain barrier damage and post-treatment intracranial hemorrhage in patients receiving intravenous tissue-type plasminogen activator. Stroke. 2014;45:2030–5.
37. Leigh R, Christensen S, Campbell BC, Marks MP, Albers GW, Lansberg MG, et al. Pretreatment blood-brain barrier disruption and post-endovascular intracranial hemorrhage. Neurology. 2016;87:263–9.
38. Roussel BD, Mysiorek C, Rouhiainen A, Jullienne A, Parcq J, Hommet Y, et al. HMGB-1 promotes fibrinolysis and reduces neurotoxicity mediated by tissue plasminogen activator. J Cell Sci. 2011;124:2070–6.
39. Obermeier B, Daneman R, Ransohoff RM. Development, maintenance and disruption of the blood-brain barrier. Nat Med. 2013;19:1584–96.
40. Iadecola C, Niwa K, Nogawa S, Zhao X, Nagayama M, Araki E, et al. Reduced susceptibility to ischemic brain injury and N-methyl-D-aspartate-mediated neurotoxicity in cyclooxygenase-2-deficient mice. Proc Natl Acad Sci U S A. 2001;98:1294–9.

Chronic cerebral hypoperfusion induces post-stroke dementia following acute ischemic stroke in rats

Dong Bin Back[1], Kyoung Ja Kwon[1,2], Dong-Hee Choi[2], Chan Young Shin[3], Jongmin Lee[4], Seol-Heui Han[1] and Hahn Young Kim[1,5*]

Abstract

Background: Post-stroke dementia (PSD) is one of the major consequences after stroke. Chronic cerebral hypoperfusion (CCH) can induce vascular cognitive impairment and potentiate amyloid pathology. We investigated how CCH contributes to the development of PSD after stroke in the context of neuroinflammation and amyloid pathology.

Methods: We designed a unique animal model for PSD. We performed middle cerebral artery occlusion (MCAO) surgery in rats mimicking acute territorial infarct, which was followed by bilateral common carotid artery occlusion (BCCAo) surgery mimicking CCH. We performed behavioral tests including neurologic function test and water maze task and histological investigations including neuroinflammation, neuronal cell death, amyloid pathology, and aquaporin 4 (AQP4) distribution.

Results: Spatial memory was synergistically impaired when BCCAo was superimposed on MCAO. Neuroinflammation with astroglial or microglial activation and amyloid pathology were enhanced in the ipsilateral cortex, thalamus, and hippocampus when BCCAo was superimposed on MCAO. Glymphatic pathway-related AQP4 distribution changed from perivascular to parenchymal pattern.

Conclusions: Our experimental results suggest that CCH may contribute to the development of PSD by interfering with amyloid clearance through the glymphatic pathway and concomitant neuroinflammation. Therapeutic strategy to clear brain metabolic waste through the glymphatic pathway may be a promising approach to prevent PSD after stroke.

Keywords: Post-stroke dementia, Chronic cerebral hypoperfusion, Neuroinflammation, Glymphatic pathway, Amyloid pathology, Animal model

Background

Stroke is the third leading cause of death following cancer and cardiovascular disease in most of the developed countries [1]. More than half of stroke survivors experience residual physical disability or cognitive decline [2]. Even in physically independent survivors, cognitive decline can be a major hurdle in returning to the premorbid social life. A quarter of stroke patients develop dementia within 3 months post stroke [3]. Any dementia developed or aggravated after stroke can be considered as post-stroke dementia (PSD) by the definition "post-stroke". Although this concept is simple and useful to define PSD, its clinical manifestations are diverse from unmasking of a pre-stroke cognitive impairment to the newly developed dementia resulting from recurrent multiple infarcts or a single strategic infarct [4].

The pathophysiology of dementia is complicated and heterogeneous including vascular dementia (VD), Alzheimer's disease (AD), or mixed dementia [5]. Considering the nature of PSD developing after stroke, PSD may be more related to VD including strategic infarct dementia, multi-infarct dementia, subcortical ischemic vascular dementia, hypoperfusion dementia, or mixed dementia rather than pure neurodegenerative dementia such as AD [4]. Single or recurrent cortical infarcts can

* Correspondence: hykimmd@gmail.com
[1]Department of Neurology, Konkuk University School of Medicine, Research Institute of Medical Science, Seoul, Republic of Korea
[5]Konkuk University Medical Center, 120-1 Neungdong-ro, Gwangjin-gu, Seoul 05030, Republic of Korea
Full list of author information is available at the end of the article

lead to strategic infarct dementia or multi-infarct dementia [6], whereas subcortical infarcts such as lacunes or white matter lesions can be associated with subcortical ischemic vascular dementia or hypoperfusion dementia [6]. Pathology related to AD such as amyloid deposits can be observed in ischemic lesions or surrounding penumbra in animal experiments [7–10] or patients with stroke [11]. More complex interaction among white matter lesions, hypertensive angiopathy, and amyloid deposit in the brain parenchyma and vessels may contribute to the development of PSD rather than direct effect of stroke lesions [12]. Considering the complex interaction of AD and vascular pathology [13], pathophysiology of PSD may be complicated by the interaction between ischemic lesions and amyloid deposit.

Mechanism-mediating amyloid clearance have been reported, including enzymatic degradation, receptor-mediated blood-brain barrier clearance, cerebrospinal fluid (CSF) absorption clearance, and interstitial fluid (ISF) bulk flow clearance [14]. Recently, glymphatic pathway has drawn attention as an ISF bulk flow clearance for brain metabolic wastes such as amyloid, tau, and synuclein [14–17]. In addition, impaired clearance is associated with the development of neurodegenerative disease such as AD [14–17]. Considering that AD-related pathology was reported in the brain of patients with PSD [11], glymphatic pathway may provide a possible link among VD, AD, and mixed dementia comprising a diverse nature of PSD.

Previously, we showed that cognitive impairments in rats with permanent occlusion of bilateral common carotid arteries (BCCAo) suggest its usefulness as an animal model for VD induced by chronic cerebral hypoperfusion (CCH) [18–20]. Cognitive impairments in this animal model were associated with white matter disintegration [18, 20]. Considering that white matter lesions induced by CCH are one of the predisposing factors for PSD, we hypothesized that CCH may play a key role in the development of PSD after stroke.

To simulate interaction between stroke and underlying CCH in the development of PSD, we designed a unique animal model for PSD. We performed transient occlusion of the middle cerebral artery (MCAO) for 90 min in rats mimicking a territorial infarct, which was followed by BCCAo mimicking a CCH. Using this model, we investigated how CCH contributes to the development of PSD after stroke in the context of neuroinflammation and amyloid pathology.

Methods

Experimental design

Male Wistar rats were used in these experiments (aged 3 months; 300–350 g; Orient Bio, Seoul, Republic of Korea). All rats resided in the vivarium at Konkuk University for 2 weeks before the beginning of the experiment. The rats were housed at a controlled temperature (22 ± 1 °C) and humidity (50 ± 10%) on a 12-h alternate light-dark cycle. Food and water were provided ad libitum throughout the experiment. All animal experimental procedures were performed in accordance with the approved guidelines of the Institutional Animal Care and Use Committee of Konkuk University (Approval number KU16070) and ARRIVE guidelines (https://www.nc3rs.org.uk/arrive-guidelines). Sequential surgeries, i.e., initial MCAO surgery followed by BCCAo surgery after 2 weeks, were performed (Fig. 1a). The rats were divided into four groups as follows: MCAO followed by BCCAo (M + B) or sham operation of BCCAo (M + S) and sham operation of MCAO followed by BCCAo (S + B) or sham operation of BCCAo (S + S). Based on the calculation using previous data of mortality and blindness after surgery [18, 20], the rats were allocated randomly to sham operation or MCAO at a ratio of 1:2 (Fig. 1b). Transient MCAO was achieved with a standard intraluminal suture approach for 90 min as described elsewhere [21]. The BCCAo was performed as described elsewhere [18–20]. Briefly, the bilateral common carotid arteries were carefully exposed through a midline incision and were permanently double-ligated with silk sutures. As time went on after the BCCAo, cerebral blood flow decreased chronically down to 70% of the baseline in our previous study [20]. Rats were anesthetized using a 5% isoflurane/oxygen mix and maintained on 3% isoflurane/oxygen during the surgery. The rectal temperature was maintained between 37 ± 0.5 °C with a heating pad during the surgery. The timeline of the experiment is shown in Fig. 1a. Motor function recovery was serially measured by modified neurologic severity scores (mNSS). After excluding rats with impaired vision by blind test, Morris water maze task was performed for 2 weeks, starting from 10 weeks after the initial surgery. For histological evaluation, rats were sacrificed after all behavioral experiments were performed. Rats were coded with numbers, and all investigators were blinded to the treatment groups until the end of the data analysis.

Neurologic function test

The mNSS, ranging from 0 to 14, is a composite scoring system for the neurologic function composed of motor status, abnormal movements, sensory tests, and reflexes [22]. For each individual task, one point is awarded for the inability to correctly perform. The higher the score is, the more severe neurological injury it suggests.

Blind test

Prior to the water maze task, blind test was performed as previously described [20]. Rats were placed in a

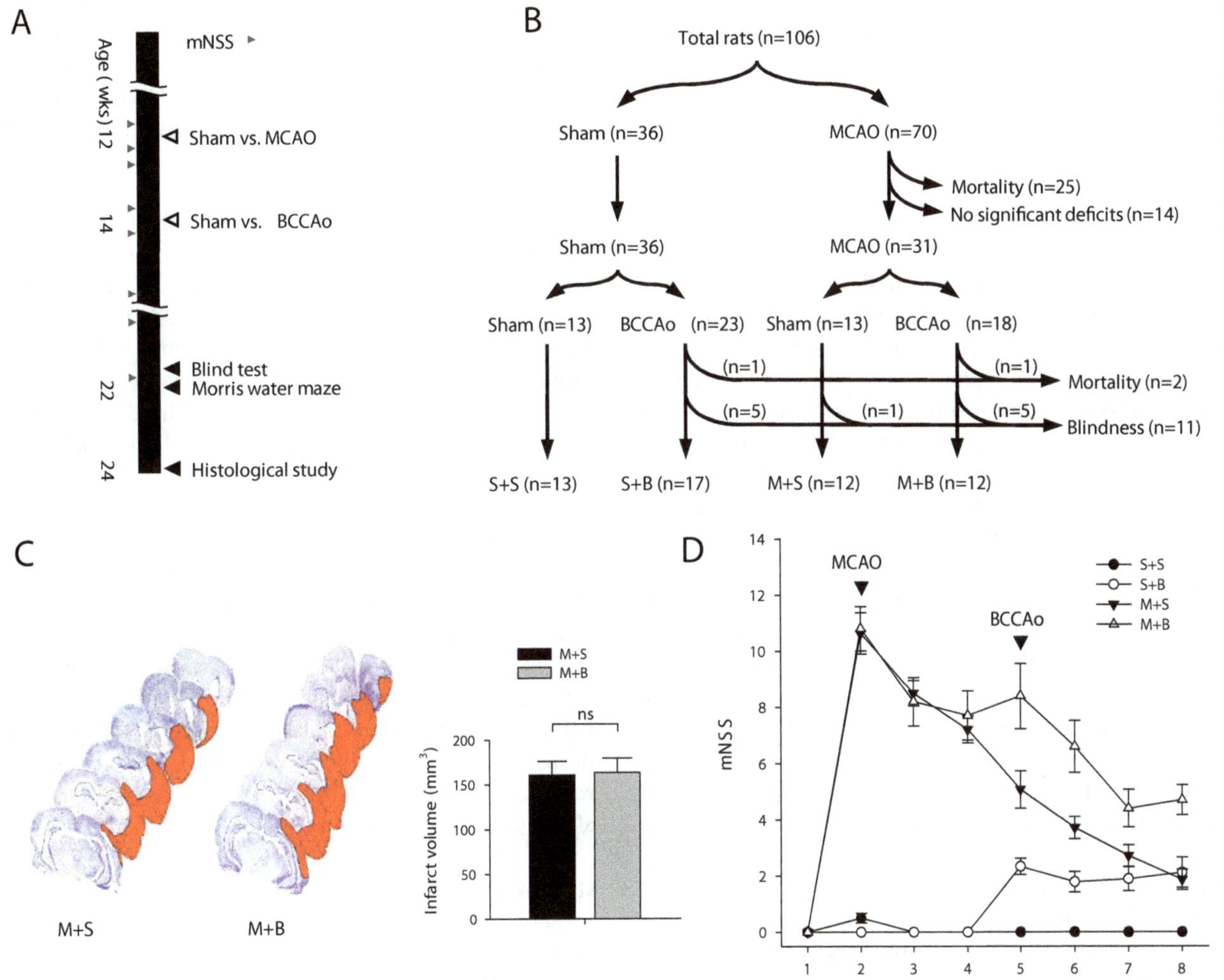

Fig. 1 **a** The timeline of the experiment. **b** Allocation of rats into groups. **c** Representative images of cresyl violet staining and quantification of infarct volume in M + S and M + B groups. $n = 10$ in both groups. **d** Serial neurologic function test. $n = 12$ to 17 in each group. MCAO middle cerebral artery occlusion, BCCAo bilateral common carotid artery occlusion, S + S sham + sham, S + B sham + BCCAo, M + S MCAO + sham, M + B MCAO + BCCAo, mNSS modified neurologic severity scores, ns not significant

90 cm × 45 cm × 32 cm (height) sized box separated by a wall with an open path in the middle (18 cm × 32 cm). The floor of one space was gridded with electrodes and that of another space was flat. After free exploration of the space for 5 min, rats were put into the grid space and given a foot shock with 3 mA for 1 s. Under daylight, rats with normal vision could escape to a safe space through the open path immediately after the shock, while blinded rats were unable to find the path and turned around repeatedly in the grid space. Escape latency longer than the mean plus three standard deviations of sham-operated rats was used as an arbitrary cut-off to determine blindness.

Water maze task

Rats were evaluated in a Morris water maze as previously described [18–20]. The maze was a round tank with 1.83 m of diameter and 0.58 m deep, filled to a depth of 35.5 cm with tepid (26 ± 1 °C) water made opaque by the addition of white paint. A moveable circular platform with 12 cm of diameter was located 2 cm below the surface of water. The maze was surrounded by white curtains on which black visual stimuli of various shapes and sizes were placed. A camera which relayed images to a videocassette recorder and an HVS Image Analysis Computer System (Hampton, UK) was located above the center of the maze. Four consecutive sessions, each consisting of five trials for 2 days (alternating two or three trials per day), were conducted on eight consecutive days. The hidden platform was constantly located in the southeast quadrant of the pool. Rats were gently submerged in water, facing the inside wall of the tank. Every trial started at different points, alternating among four quadrants. Rats were gently handled for 10 min daily for 7 days before the test. In the maze, the rats were allowed to swim for a maximum of 90 s. Further, they were allowed to remain on the platform for 30 s at the end of each trial. Performance accuracy was evaluated by the analysis of search error, time latency, and path length data of all trials. Measurement of the search error was based on a computation of the average distance from the platform during the trial. The distance between the rat and the platform was sampled 10 times/s during each trial, and these distances were averaged in 1-s bins. Cumulative search error is the sum of these 1-s averages of the proximity measure corrected for the specific platform location and start location by subtracting the proximity score that would be produced by a perfect performance in the trial. A probe trial was conducted 1 min after every 10th training trial. Therefore, rats took the second probe trial after finishing 10 more training trials over 4 days after the first probe trial. The entire training procedure included two probe trials for each rat, during which the rats swam with the platform retracted to the bottom of the pool for 30 s. After recording the swimming path, the platform was raised to its normal position for completion of the trial. The swimming time spent in the target quadrant and the number of crossings above the retracted platform were used as parameters for the retention of spatial memory.

Tissue preparation

After all behavioral experiments, the rats were intracardially perfused with 0.01 M phosphate-buffered saline (PBS) and subsequently with 4% paraformaldehyde (PFA) under deep anesthesia. The brain was removed quickly and post-fixed in 4% PFA for 2 days, cryoprotected in PBS containing 30% sucrose for 48 h, frozen in powdered dry ice, and sectioned using a microtome at a thickness of 30 μm.

Cresyl violet staining

Sections were mounted onto resin-coated slide glass, dried for 10 days, hydrated through descending concentrations of ethanol, and subsequently dipped twice in distilled water. Sections were immersed in cresyl violet acetate (Sigma Aldrich) dissolved at 0.5% (*w*/*v*) in distilled water for 5 min and then dehydrated through ascending concentrations of ethanol. Finally, they were defatted in xylene and coverslipped with permount reagent.

Immunohistochemistry

The sections were washed in PBS with 0.3% Triton X-100 and then incubated in blocking serum, 5% normal donkey serum in 0.15% triton with PBS. Subsequently, they were incubated in primary antibody solution for 1 h at room temperature and overnight at 4 °C as follows: mouse anti-glial fibrillary acidic protein (GFAP) (1:1000, BD Bioscience), rabbit anti-ionized calcium-binding adapter molecule-1 (Iba-1) (1:1000, Wako), rabbit anti-NeuN (1:1000, EMD Millipore), and mouse anti-amyloid beta$_{17\text{-}24}$ (4G8) (1:100, Covance), rabbit anti-collagen IV (1:1000, Abcam), and mouse anti-aquaporin 4 (AQP4) (1:100, Abcam). Then, the sections were washed in PBS with 0.15% Triton X-100 and incubated in a secondary antibody solution for 3 h at room temperature as follows: anti-mouse Alexa Fluor 488 and 568; anti-rabbit Alexa Fluor 488 and 568; all from donkey (1:200, Invitrogen). Stained sections were mounted on resin-coated slides and dried for 30 min. Slides were then coverslipped with ProLong® Gold antifade reagent (Invitrogen).

The histological staining of amyloid beta was confirmed by the approach of 3, 3′-diaminobenzidine (DAB) staining. The sections were incubated with 3% hydroxide and 3% methyl alcohol for quenching endogenous peroxidase activity. They were then blocked and incubated with 4G8 (1:100, Covance) overnight at 4 °C. The sections were subsequently washed and incubated in a secondary antibody solution (biotinylated horse anti-mouse antibody, Vector, 1:200) for 1 h at room temperature. Finally, peroxidase activity was visualized using DAB solution (Vector SG kit, Vector).

Quantitative analysis

Signal intensity of GFAP and Iba-1 immunoreactivity was evaluated from the section at bregma 0.20 mm for the cortex and striatum and at bregma − 3.30 mm for the thalamus and hippocampus. Images encompassing a region of interest (ROI) were captured using a confocal microscope (Olympus FV1000). Ipsilateral ROIs in the cortex and striatum of M + S and M + B rats were selected in the peri-infarct area. Contralateral ROIs were selected as symmetrical regions in the contralateral hemisphere. The ROIs were pictured with a 20X/0.75 NA objective in 1024 × 1024 pixels (field size 653.283 × 653.283 μm^2 for the cortex, striatum, and thalamus) and a 4X/0.16 NA in 1024 × 1024 pixels (field size 3178.461 × 3178.461 μm^2 for the hippocampus). Fluorescence signal intensity in the ROIs was evaluated using the FluoView v.3.1 software (Olympus) and expressed as the relative percentage change compared to those of S + S rats.

Amyloid deposit

Number and area of amyloid plaques in the cortex were summed from sections at bregma 0.20 and − 3.30 mm. An amyloid plaque was defined as a conglomeration comprised of degenerated neurons surrounded by amyloid fibrils stained by 4G8. Single degenerated neuron occupying less than 10 μm^2 was not considered as an amyloid plaque. The number of amyloid plaques was manually counted, and the area of each amyloid plaque was manually drawn and calculated using NIH Image J (Bethesda, MD, USA).

Distribution of AQP4

Distribution patterns of AQP4 immunoreactivity were analyzed. The AQP4 signals colocalized with collagen IV were considered as vascular AQP4 and those not-colocalized with collagen IV were considered as parenchymal AQP4. An arbitrary low stringency threshold was set to define the total area of AQP4 immunoreactivity, whereas a high stringency threshold was set to define an area of vascular AQP4 which was colocalized with collagen IV. The ratio between the areas of vascular and parenchymal AQP4 was compared among groups. Moreover, the area ratio of vascular AQP4 to collagen IV was defined as AQP4/Col IV colocalization index, reflecting perivascular astrocytic end feet coverage of microvessels. Area calculations were performed using images converted into black and white by an equal threshold to all individual images using NIH Image J (Bethesda, MD, USA).

Infarct volume

The infarct volume was calculated using an indirect method based on six representative cresyl violet-stained slices selected with 2-mm interval.

Hippocampus

The number of viable or degenerative neurons in the hippocampus was evaluated by cresyl violet or 4G8, respectively. Rectangular ROIs occupying 100 × 100 μm^2 were selected in the CA1 and CA3 regions selected from section at bregma −3.30 mm. The neurons were counted using a cell counter available in NIH Image J (Bethesda, MD, USA) and expressed as the number of cells per mm^2.

Statistical analysis

Parameters for spatial memory including search error, time latency, path length, and swimming speed were analyzed by one-way repeated-measure ANOVA followed by a post hoc Tukey's honest significant difference test. One-way ANOVA was conducted to compare results of the probe trials and the quantitative data of the immunohistochemistry (mean ± SE). A value of $p < 0.05$ was considered to be statistically significant. Data analyses were performed with the SPSS Statistics 24.0.

Results

Experimental groups

One-hundred and six rats were distributed into four groups with sizes ranging from 12 to 17 per group (Fig. 1b). Mortality rate for MCAO and BCCAo surgeries was 35.7% (25 of 70) and 4.9% (2 of 41), respectively. Rats without significant neurological deficits (mNSS 0 to 2) after MCAO surgery (n = 14) were excluded due to the possibility of no infarct. Rats that failed to pass blind test were excluded from the water maze task, which depends on intact visual function (n = 11).

Infarct volume and neurologic function

Although infarct volume was slightly larger in M + B rats than in M + S rats, it was not statistically significant (p = 0.895, Fig. 1c). Additional BCCAo surgery did not increase the infarct volume of MCAO surgery. The neurologic functions of the rats deteriorated immediately after MCAO or BCCAo surgery. However, functions recovered enough to perform the water maze task (Fig. 1d).

Spatial memory

Four experimental groups showed statistically significant difference in the performance of the water maze task ($p < 0.001$ in search error, time latency, and path length, Fig. 2a). Post hoc analysis revealed that M + B rats showed poorer performance in the search error than did S + S and M + S rats ($p < 0.001$) or S + B rats (p = 0.007). However, the search error was not different between S + S and M + S rats (p = 0.216). Other parameters including time latency and path length showed similar pattern. Swimming speed was not different among groups (p = 0.377, Fig. 2b). In the first probe trial, the time in the target quadrant and the number of crossings were not different among groups (p = 0.253 and p = 0.876, respectively; Fig. 2c, d). However, in the second probe trial, the time in the target quadrant and the number of crossings were significantly different among groups (p = 0.004 and p = 0.006, respectively; Fig. 2c, d) suggesting most effective learning in S + S rats.

Neuroinflammation

Astroglial activation localized with GFAP increased in the ipsilateral cortex of M + B rats followed by the ipsilateral cortex of M + S rats and the contralateral cortex of M + B rats ($p < 0.001$, Fig. 3a). Post hoc analysis revealed that the astroglial activation significantly increased in the ipsilateral cortex of M + B rats compared to that in S + S rats ($p < 0.001$). Microglial activation localized with Iba-1 increased in the ipsilateral cortex of M + B rats followed by the ipsilateral cortex of M + S rats and the contralateral cortex of M + B rats (p = 0.001, Fig. 3b). Compared with S + S rats, M + B rats showed a significant increase in microglial activation in the ipsilateral cortex (p = 0.001). Both neuroinflammatory markers showed similar patterns in the striatum and in the thalamus as those in the cortex.

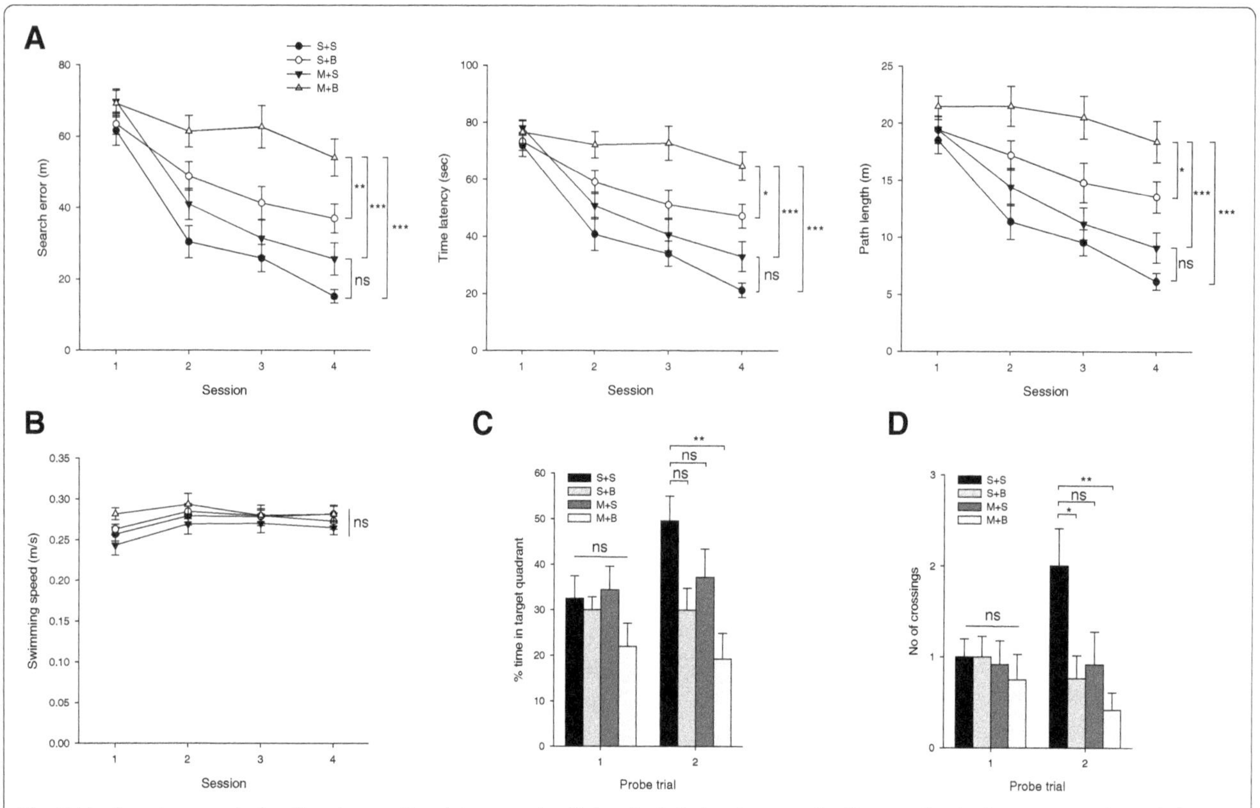

Fig. 2 Morris water maze task. **a** Search error, time latency, and path length. **b** Swimming speed. **c** Time staying in the target quadrant during probe trials. **d** Number of crossings over the removed platform during probe trials. $n = 12$ to 17 in each group; *$p < 0.05$, **$p < 0.01$, and ***$p < 0.001$ on post hoc analysis; MCAO middle cerebral artery occlusion, BCCAo bilateral common carotid artery occlusion, S + S sham + sham, S + B sham + BCCAo, M + S MCAO + sham, M + B MCAO + BCCAo, ns not significant

Amyloid deposit

Amyloid deposit was investigated in the cortex (Fig. 4a). The number and area of amyloid plaques were the highest in the ipsilateral cortex of M + B rats ($p < 0.001$). Compared with that in S + S rats, the number of amyloid plaques significantly increased in the cortex of both hemispheres in M + B rats ($p < 0.001$ in the ipsilateral cortex and $p = 0.035$ in the contralateral cortex). Moreover, this number was higher in the ipsilateral cortex of M + B rats than in the ipsilateral cortex of M + S rats ($p = 0.023$, Fig. 4b). Compared with that in S + S rats, the area of amyloid plaques significantly increased in the ipsilateral cortex of M + S rats ($p = 0.045$) and M + B rats ($p < 0.001$). In M + B rats, the area increased in the ipsilateral cortex compared to the contralateral cortex ($p = 0.008$, Fig. 4c). Densely conglomerated amyloid plaques in the ipsilateral thalamus, which were reported as secondary neurodegeneration after MCAO, were more frequently observed in M + B rats (5/12, 41.7%) than in M + S rats (2/12, 16.7%), although this result did not reach statistical significance ($p = 0.178$, Fig. 5).

Distribution of AQP4

Along with increased neuroinflammation, AQP4 distribution changed from normal perivascular pattern to scattered parenchymal pattern (Fig. 6a). Vascular AQP4 comprising more than 90% in S + S rats decreased to 20% in the ipsilateral cortex of M + B rats, whereas the opposite effect was observed for the parenchymal AQP4 ($p < 0.001$, Fig. 6b). Compared with that in S + S rats, this pattern shift was significant in the ipsilateral cortex of M + S and both cortex of M + B rats. Colocalization of AQP4 with collagen IV decreased in the ipsilateral cortex of M + B rats followed by the ipsilateral cortex of M + S and contralateral cortex of M + B ($p = 0.009$, Fig. 6c). Compared with that in S + S rats, the AQP4 colocalization index significantly decreased in the ipsilateral cortex of M + B rats ($p = 0.025$).

Hippocampus

Neuroinflammation, neuronal cell death, and amyloid-positive degenerative neurons in the hippocampus were investigated (Fig. 7a). Neuroinflammation increased in the ipsilateral cortex of M + B rats, which was significantly higher than that of S + S rats ($p = 0.042$ in GFAP and $p = 0.002$ in Iba1, Fig. 7b). Both neuronal cell death and number of amyloid-positive degenerative neurons were significantly different among groups ($p < 0.001$ in CA1 and CA3, Fig. 7c and d, respectively). Compared to

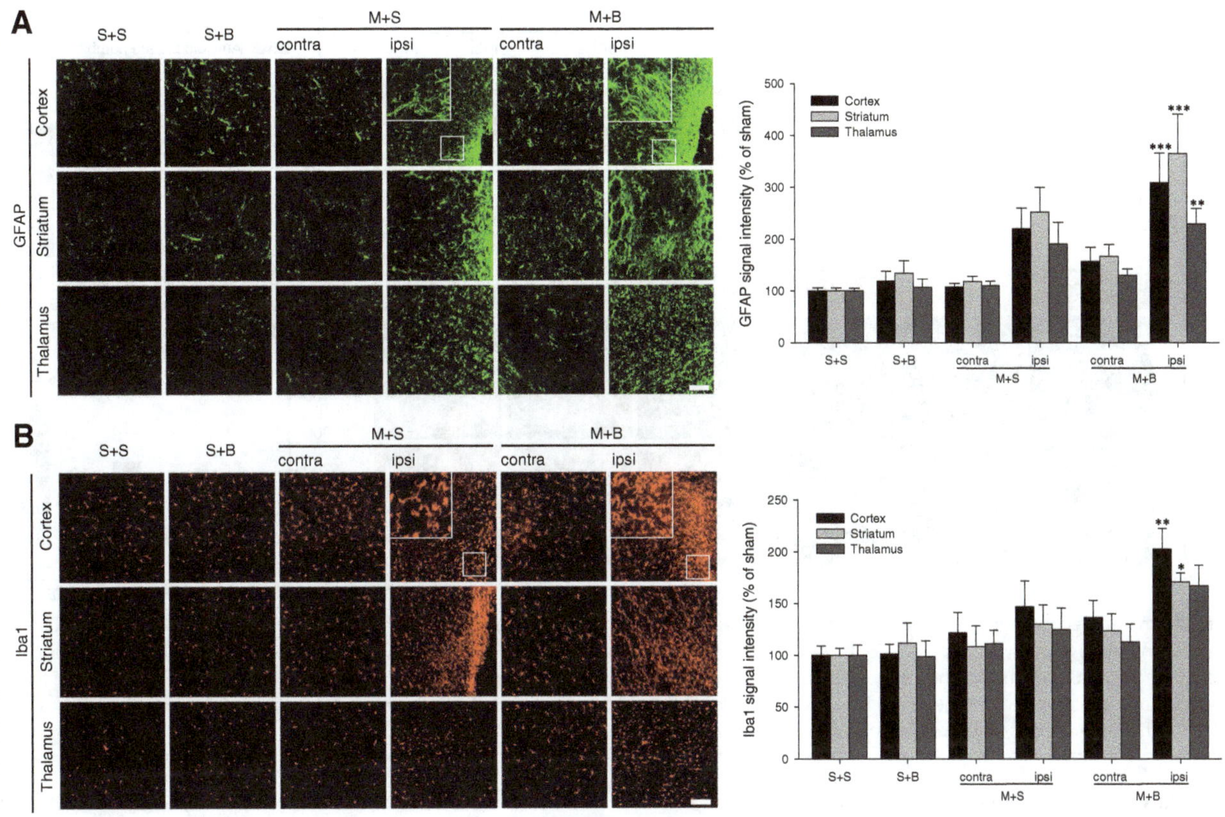

Fig. 3 Neuroinflammation measured by astroglial and microglial activation. **a** Glial fibrillary acidic protein (GFAP) immunoreactivity and its quantification. **b** Iba1 immunoreactivity and its quantification. $n = 6$ to 8 in each group; scale bar = 100 µm; $^{*}p < 0.05$, $^{**}p < 0.01$, and $^{***}p < 0.001$ on the post hoc analysis compared to S + S; MCAO middle cerebral artery occlusion, BCCAo bilateral common carotid artery occlusion, S + S sham + sham, S + B sham + BCCAo, M + S MCAO + sham, M + B MCAO + BCCAo

that in S + S rats, neuronal cell death was prominent in S + B ($p < 0.05$) and M + B rats ($p < 0.01$) and the number of amyloid-positive degenerative neurons was higher in all groups ($p < 0.001$).

Discussion

Our experimental results suggest that CCH may contribute to the development of PSD by interfering with amyloid clearance through the glymphatic pathway and concomitant neuroinflammation. Therapeutic strategy alleviating these pathologies may be a promising approach to prevent PSD in patients who experienced stroke.

Although the prevalence of PSD is relatively high, reaching up to 30% of the stroke survivors as they age [2, 6], not all the patients who experienced a stroke develop PSD. Clinical factors including aging, low education level, pre-stroke cognitive decline, hypertension, diabetes, and atrial fibrillation or neuroimaging findings including silent infarcts, global cerebral atrophy, medial temporal lobe atrophy, and white matter changes are suggested as risk factors or predictors of the development of PSD [6]. Long-standing exposure to vascular risk factors such as hypertension, diabetes, or atrial fibrillation can deteriorate cerebral microperfusion [23]. Neuroimaging findings associated with cognitive impairments such as silent infarcts, global cerebral atrophy, and white matter changes can be consequences of CCH [24, 25]. We hypothesized that underlying CCH may be one of the main predisposing factors for the development of PSD among stroke survivors.

To test this hypothesis, we used a unique experimental design that can show how CCH contributes to the development of PSD after stroke. Most of the previous experimental studies on post-stroke cognitive impairment were performed using animal stroke models such as MCAO [26, 27]. However, these animal models may be insufficient to reflect complex clinical settings for the development of PSD that occurs more frequently when underlying CCH was combined. In our study, M + B rats mimicking a clinical setting where CCH is superimposed after stroke may be more appropriate to study complex interactions between CCH and territorial infarction for the development of PSD than a simple stroke model. M + B rats showed the worst performance in water maze task compared to other groups, whereas the performance of M

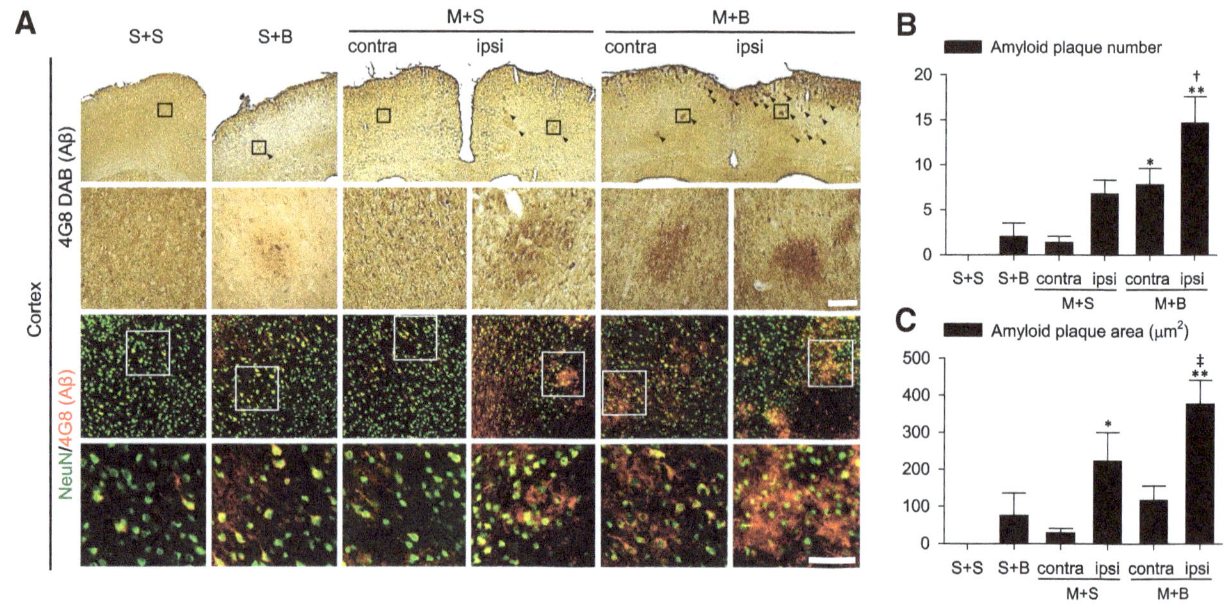

Fig. 4 Amyloid deposit in the cortex. **a** Amyloid plaques are indicated in 4G8 DAB staining (arrow heads) and double immunofluorescent labeled by neuron (NeuN) and amyloid deposit (4G8). **b** Quantification of amyloid plaque number and **c** area. $n = 6$ to 8 in each group; scale bar = 100 μm; *$p < 0.05$, **$p < 0.001$ on the post hoc analysis compared to S + S; †$p < 0.05$ on the post hoc analysis compared to ipsilateral M + S; ‡$p < 0.05$ on the post hoc analysis compared to contralateral M + B; MCAO middle cerebral artery occlusion, BCCAo bilateral common carotid artery occlusion, S + S sham + sham, S + B sham + BCCAo, M + S MCAO + sham, M + B MCAO + BCCAo

+ S rats was not impaired compared to that of S + S rats. In other words, performance based on spatial memory was synergistically impaired when BCCAo was superimposed on MCAO. These experimental findings suggest that cognitive impairment can be significantly aggravated when CCH is combined with territorial infarcts. Predisposing conditions such as CCH can be more important in PSD development than stroke itself.

The infarct volume was not different between M + S and M + B rats. Although the recovery of the motor function measured by mNSS was delayed in M + B rats, the swimming speed during the water maze task was not different among groups. The worst performance of M + B rats in water maze task may be the consequence of a post-stroke neurodegenerative process rather than larger infarct volume or impaired motor function. These findings appear to be consistent with clinical findings reporting that some stroke patients develop PSD and some do not, although they had similar infarct volume. In addition, PSD can develop even in stroke survivors with

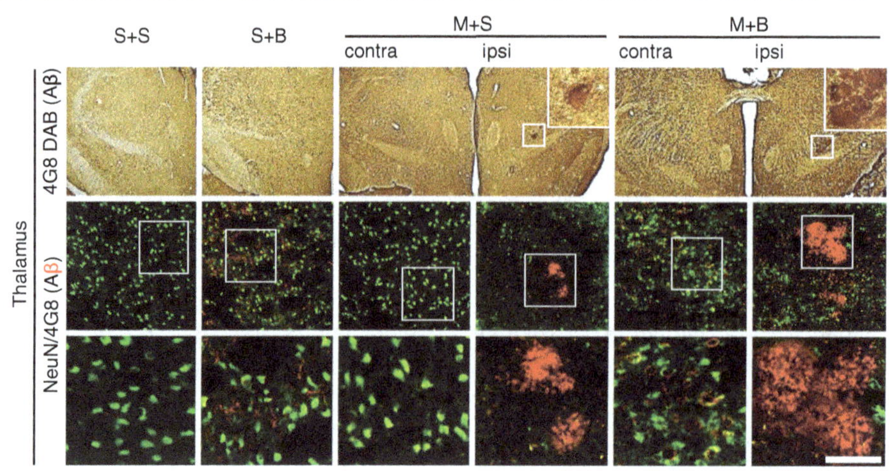

Fig. 5 Amyloid deposit in the thalamus. Amyloid plaques are indicated in 4G8 DAB staining (insets in the first column) and double immunofluorescent labeled by neuron (NeuN) and amyloid deposit (4G8). $n = 12$ in each group; scale bar = 100 μm; MCAO middle cerebral artery occlusion, BCCAo bilateral common carotid artery occlusion, S + S sham + sham, S + B sham + BCCAo, M + S MCAO + sham, M + B MCAO + BCCAo

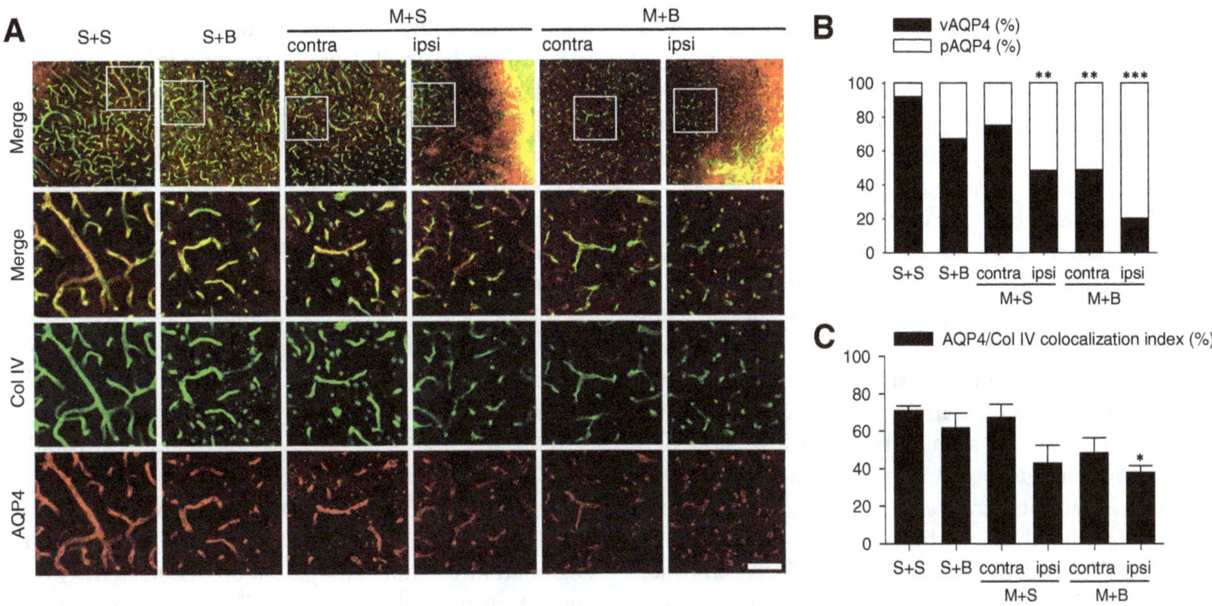

Fig. 6 a Distribution patterns of AQP4 immunoreactivity. **b** Ratio of vascular and parenchymal AQP4. **c** AQP4/Col IV colocalization index. $n = 5$ to 7 in each group; scale bar = 50 μm; *$p < 0.05$, **$p < 0.01$, and ***$p < 0.001$ on post hoc analysis compared to S + S; vAQP4 vascular AQP4, pAQP4 parenchymal AQP4, Col IV collagen IV, MCAO middle cerebral artery occlusion, BCCAo bilateral common carotid artery occlusion, S + S sham + sham, S + B sham + BCCAo, M + S MCAO + sham, M + B MCAO + BCCAo

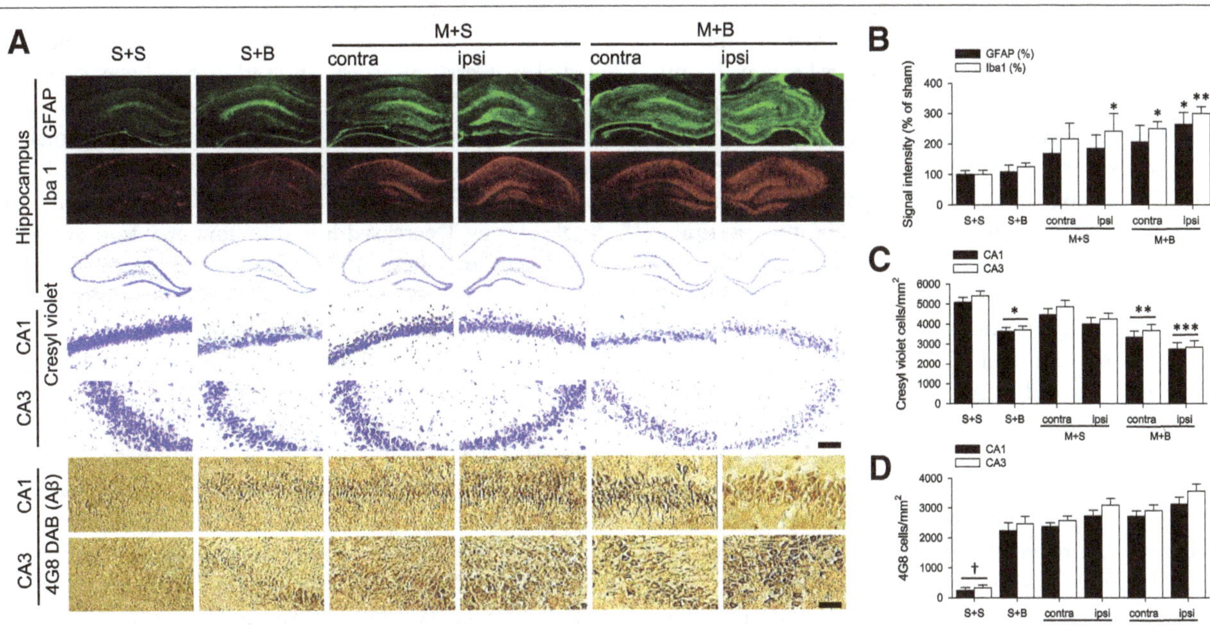

Fig. 7 a Hippocampus and its magnification in CA1 and CA3 regions. Scale bar = 100 μm. **b** Neuroinflammation measured by astroglial (GFAP) and microglial (Iba1) activation ant its quantification. $n = 7$ to 8 in each group; *$p < 0.05$ and **$p < 0.01$ on post hoc analysis compared to S + S. **c** Neuronal cell death measured by cresyl violet and its quantification. $n = 8$ to 10 in each group; *$p < 0.05$, **$p < 0.01$, and ***$p < 0.001$ on post hoc analysis compared to S + S. **d** Amyloid-positive degenerative neurons measured by 4G8 and its quantification. $n = 6$ to 8 in each group, †$p < 0.001$ on post hoc analysis compared to other groups; MCAO middle cerebral artery occlusion, BCCAo bilateral common carotid artery occlusion, S + S sham + sham, S + B sham + BCCAo, M + S MCAO + sham, M + B MCAO + BCCAo

complete motor recovery. Hence, we asked which pathology could be a culprit to trigger or aggravate a post-stroke neurodegenerative process in the development of PSD other than infarct volume itself.

Here, we showed that amyloid deposit along with neuroinflammation was significantly enhanced in the ipsilateral cortex of M + B rats compared to that in M + S rats. CCH induced by BCCAo may have enhanced neuroinflammation and amyloid pathology leading to the neurodegenerative process in the ipsilateral cortex of stroke, especially in the peri-infarct area. Interestingly, amyloid deposit in M + B rats was enhanced not only in the ipsilateral cortex but also in the contralateral cortex and ipsilateral thalamus. In a rat model of transient MCAO, stress proteins such as heat shock protein were reported to be inducible not only in the peri-infarct area but also in remote contralateral cortex areas beyond the vascular territory through the mechanism of spreading depression [28]. Amyloid deposit in the ipsilateral thalamus after MCAO in rats was reported as a secondary neurodegeneration with amyloid pathology [7, 29–31]. In our study, this phenomenon was strongly enhanced in M + B rats compared to that in M + S rats, suggesting that CCH may also work as an aggravating factor for the secondary neurodegeneration in the ipsilateral thalamus after stroke. In our study, neuronal cell death and amyloid-positive degenerative neurons along with neuroinflammation in the hippocampus increased when CCH was superimposed on the stroke. Although the underlying mechanism needs further investigation, the effect of CCH on amyloid deposit after stroke may be more diffuse than expected, involving whole brain hemispheres beyond the peri-infarct area.

Post-stroke neurodegenerative processes including amyloid pathology may be more dynamic than expected. Rapid increase of amyloid plaques in the peri-infarct area within a week after the experimental stroke and subsequent clearance over the next few weeks were reported in transgenic mouse models of amyloid deposit [32, 33]. In the transient MCAO rat model, amyloid precursor protein and amyloid staining increased in the peri-infarct area for 1 week after stroke and faded over the following months [7–10]. Amyloid deposit in the peri-infarct area increased more in older than in younger rats, suggesting that the aged brain is more susceptible to the amyloid deposit after stroke [10]. A human study using amyloid positron-emission tomographic (PET) scan showed that amyloid deposit was higher in the ipsilateral peri-infarct area in patients with recent infarcts [34]. However, a further study performed by same authors showed no significant increase of amyloid deposit in the peri-infarct area [35]. Although further studies are needed to explain these conflicting results, the dynamic nature of amyloid deposit and clearance suggested by experimental animal studies may explain this discrepancy. Even though amyloid deposit occurred after stroke in a human brain, if it was cleared rapidly, amyloid PET scan could not have detected any increase of amyloid deposit. If amyloid PET scan could be performed in selected patients who have underlying pathologies such as AD, VD, or white matter lesions that are well-known risk factors for PSD, results of amyloid PET scan could be positive in these patients who are more susceptible to amyloid deposit after stroke. This hypothesis appears consistent with the clinical finding that stroke patients with underlying amyloid deposit showed a more severe and rapid cognitive decline over 3 years compared to those without underlying amyloid deposit [36].

Next, we questioned how CCH accelerates amyloid deposit in the peri-infarct area. Among various mechanisms mediating amyloid clearance, we hypothesized that ISF bulk flow clearance rather than other enzymatic degradation clearance may be more associated with vascular factors such as CCH. Glymphatic pathway has been reported as a brain interstitial metabolic solute clearance system comprised of a para-arterial CSF influx, a para-venous ISF clearance, and a trans-parenchymal pathway that is dependent on astroglial water transport via AQP4 water channel [14–17]. Metabolic waste proteins such as amyloid, tau, and synuclein can be targets for the clearance of glymphatic pathway and its impairments can lead to pathologic accumulation in the brain leading to neurodegenerative diseases such as AD, Parkinson's disease, and traumatic brain encephalopathy [14–17]. Cerebral arterial pulsation has been suggested as a possible driving force for glymphatic pathway maintaining ISF bulk flow [14, 37]. In our study, a permanent ligation of both common carotid arteries (i.e. BCCAo surgery) may have attenuated arterial pulsation in cerebral arteries. Decreased ISF bulk flow may have hindered interstitial metabolic solute clearance through the glymphatic pathway. Consequently, perturbed amyloid clearance through the glymphatic pathway may have been attributed to the amyloid deposit in the peri-infarct area in M + B rats. Hence, we investigated the distribution of AQP4 water channels, which play a key role for the astroglial water transport in the glymphatic pathway. Perivascular distribution of AQP4 in S + S rats, implicating normal functioning water channel in the glymphatic pathway, changed to scattered parenchymal pattern in M + B rats. Moreover, colocalization of AQP4 over vascular collagen IV signal decreased. Dislocation of AQP4 water channels from perivascular expression on the end-feet of astrocytes to scattered parenchymal patterns may reflect dysfunction of glymphatic pathway. Taken together, perturbed glymphatic pathway suggested by the aberrant dislocation of AQP4 water channel along with neuroinflammation may have contributed to the post-stroke amyloid deposit in M + B rats. However, detailed mechanisms of PSD in our study need further investigation. First, the dynamics of amyloid deposit after stroke over time remain to be addressed. Second, the mechanism of how CCH affects the functional and structural changes of glymphatic pathway related to the amyloid clearance warrants further study. Third, further experiments using aged animals with comorbidities such as atherosclerosis, hypertension, diabetes, obesity, or metabolic syndrome are needed to investigate neurodegeneration which occurs mostly in elderly patients with these chronic disease conditions [38–40]. Mechanism focused on the interaction between neuroinflammation and cerebral perfusion deficits in patients with PSD also warrants further study [41].

Conclusions

Our proof-of-concept study provides experimental evidence for the mechanism of PSD, suggesting that CCH may contribute to the development of PSD by interfering with amyloid clearance after stroke through the glymphatic pathway and concomitant neuroinflammation. Therapeutic strategies to improve brain metabolic waste clearance through glymphatic pathway may be promising approaches to prevent PSD after stroke.

Abbreviations

4G8: Amyloid beta$_{17\text{-}24}$; AD: Alzheimer's disease; AQP4: Aquaporin 4; BCCAo: Occlusion of bilateral common carotid arteries; CCH: Chronic cerebral hypoperfusion; CSF: Cerebrospinal fluid; DAB: Diaminobenzidine; GFAP: Glial fibrillary acidic protein; Iba-1: Ionized calcium-binding adapter molecule-1; ISF: Interstitial fluid; MCAO: Occlusion of the middle cerebral artery; mNSS: Modified neurologic severity scores; PBS: Phosphate-buffered saline; PET: Positron-emission tomographic; PFA: Paraformaldehyde; PSD: Post-stroke dementia; ROI: Region of interest; VD: Vascular dementia

Acknowledgements

Not applicable.

Funding

This work was supported by the Basic Science Research Program through the National Research Foundation of Korea (NRF) funded by the Ministry of Education (2014R1A1A2057042 and 2017R1D1A1B03030906) and the Korea Health Technology R&D Project through the Korea Health Industry Development Institute (KHIDI) funded by the Ministry of Health & Welfare, Republic of Korea (HI17C0368).

Authors' contributions

DBB, KJK, and HYK participated in the conception and design of the study. DBB and HYK drafted the manuscript and participated in the general management. DBB, KJK, and DC helped in the acquisition and analysis of the data. CYS, JL, and SH helped to draft the manuscript. All authors reviewed and approved the final manuscript.

Consent for publication

Not applicable.

Competing interests

The authors declare that they have no competing interests.

Author details

[1]Department of Neurology, Konkuk University School of Medicine, Research Institute of Medical Science, Seoul, Republic of Korea. [2]Department of Medicine, Konkuk University School of Medicine, Seoul, Republic of Korea. [3]Department of Pharmacology, Konkuk University School of Medicine, Seoul, Republic of Korea. [4]Department of Rehabilitation Medicine, Konkuk University School of Medicine, Seoul, Republic of Korea. [5]Konkuk University Medical Center, 120-1 Neungdong-ro, Gwangjin-gu, Seoul 05030, Republic of Korea.

References

1. Murray CJ, Lopez AD. Global mortality, disability, and the contribution of risk factors: Global Burden of Disease Study. Lancet. 1997;349:1436–42.
2. Ivan CS, Seshadri S, Beiser A, Au R, Kase CS, Kelly-Hayes M, et al. Dementia after stroke: the Framingham study. Stroke. 2004;35:1264–8.
3. Censori B, Manara O, Agostinis C, Camerlingo M, Casto L, Galavotti B, et al. Dementia after first stroke. Stroke. 1996;27:1205–10.
4. O'Brien JT, Thomas A. Vascular dementia. Lancet. 2015;386:1698–706.
5. Langa KM, Foster NL, Larson EB. Mixed dementia: emerging concepts and therapeutic implications. JAMA. 2004;292:2901–8.
6. Leys D, Henon H, Mackowiak-Cordoliani MA, Pasquier F. Poststroke dementia. Lancet Neurol. 2005;4:752–9.
7. van Groen T, Puurunen K, Maki HM, Sivenius J, Jolkkonen J. Transformation of diffuse beta-amyloid precursor protein and beta-amyloid deposits to plaques in the thalamus after transient occlusion of the middle cerebral artery in rats. Stroke. 2005;36:1551–6.
8. Hiltunen M, Makinen P, Peraniemi S, Sivenius J, van Groen T, Soininen H, et al. Focal cerebral ischemia in rats alters APP processing and expression of Abeta peptide degrading enzymes in the thalamus. Neurobiol Dis. 2009;35:103–13.
9. Nihashi T, Inao S, Kajita Y, Kawai T, Sugimoto T, Niwa M, et al. Expression and distribution of beta amyloid precursor protein and beta amyloid peptide in reactive astrocytes after transient middle cerebral artery occlusion. Acta Neurochir. 2001;143:287–95.
10. Popa-Wagner A, Schroder E, Walker LC, Kessler C. Beta-amyloid precursor protein and ss-amyloid peptide immunoreactivity in the rat brain after middle cerebral artery occlusion: effect of age. Stroke. 1998;29:2196–202.
11. Pasquier F, Leys D. Why are stroke patients prone to develop dementia? J Neurol. 1997;244:135–42.
12. Hennerici MG. What are the mechanisms for post-stroke dementia? Lancet Neurol. 2009;8:973–5.
13. Zlokovic BV. Neurovascular pathways to neurodegeneration in Alzheimer's disease and other disorders. Nat Rev Neurosci. 2011;12:723–38.
14. Tarasoff-Conway JM, Carare RO, Osorio RS, Glodzik L, Butler T, Fieremans E, et al. Clearance systems in the brain-implications for Alzheimer disease. Nat Rev Neurol. 2015;11:457–70.
15. Kress BT, Iliff JJ, Xia M, Wang M, Wei HS, Zeppenfeld D, et al. Impairment of paravascular clearance pathways in the aging brain. Ann Neurol. 2014;76:845–61.
16. Iliff JJ, Nedergaard M. Is there a cerebral lymphatic system? Stroke. 2013;44:S93–5.
17. Bakker EN, Bacskai BJ, Arbel-Ornath M, Aldea R, Bedussi B, Morris AW, et al. Lymphatic clearance of the brain: perivascular, paravascular and significance for neurodegenerative diseases. Cell Mol Neurobiol. 2016;36:181–94.
18. Choi BR, Kim DH, Back DB, Kang CH, Moon WJ, Han JS, et al. Characterization of white matter injury in a rat model of chronic cerebral hypoperfusion. Stroke. 2016;47:542–7.
19. Choi BR, Kwon KJ, Park SH, Jeon WK, Han SH, Kim HY, et al. Alternations of septal-hippocampal system in the adult Wistar rat with spatial memory impairments induced by chronic cerebral hypoperfusion. Exp Neurobiol. 2011;20:92–9.
20. Choi BR, Lee SR, Han JS, Woo SK, Kim KM, Choi DH, et al. Synergistic memory impairment through the interaction of chronic cerebral hypoperfusion and amlyloid toxicity in a rat model. Stroke. 2011;42:2595–604.
21. Kim HY, Singhal AB, Lo EH. Normobaric hyperoxia extends the reperfusion window in focal cerebral ischemia. Ann Neurol. 2005;57:571–5.
22. Li Y, Chen J, Wang L, Lu M, Chopp M. Treatment of stroke in rat with intracarotid administration of marrow stromal cells. Neurology. 2001;56:1666–72.
23. Skoog I. Vascular aspects in Alzheimer's disease. J Neural Transm Suppl. 2000;59:37–43.

24. Norrving B. Evolving concept of small vessel disease through advanced brain imaging. J Stroke. 2015;17:94–100.
25. Kim BJ, Lee SH. Prognostic impact of cerebral small vessel disease on stroke outcome. J Stroke. 2015;17:101–10.
26. Yonemori F, Yamada H, Yamaguchi T, Uemura A, Tamura A. Spatial memory disturbance after focal cerebral ischemia in rats. J Cereb Blood Flow Metab. 1996;16:973–80.
27. Andersen MB, Zimmer J, Sams-Dodd F. Specific behavioral effects related to age and cerebral ischemia in rats. Pharmacol Biochem Behav. 1999;62:673–82.
28. Popp A, Jaenisch N, Witte OW, Frahm C. Identification of ischemic regions in a rat model of stroke. PLoS One. 2009;4:e4764.
29. Zhang J, Zhang Y, Xing S, Liang Z, Zeng J. Secondary neurodegeneration in remote regions after focal cerebral infarction: a new target for stroke management? Stroke. 2012;43:1700–5.
30. Zhang Y, Xing S, Zhang J, Li J, Li C, Pei Z, et al. Reduction of beta-amyloid deposits by gamma-secretase inhibitor is associated with the attenuation of secondary damage in the ipsilateral thalamus and sensory functional improvement after focal cortical infarction in hypertensive rats. J Cereb Blood Flow Metab. 2011;31:572–9.
31. Loos M, Dihne M, Block F. Tumor necrosis factor-alpha expression in areas of remote degeneration following middle cerebral artery occlusion of the rat. Neuroscience. 2003;122:373–80.
32. Garcia-Alloza M, Gregory J, Kuchibhotla KV, Fine S, Wei Y, Ayata C, et al. Cerebrovascular lesions induce transient beta-amyloid deposition. Brain. 2011;134:3697–707.
33. Van Nostrand WE, Davis J, Previti ML, Xu F. Clearance of amyloid-beta protein deposits in transgenic mice following focal cerebral ischemia. Neurodegener Dis. 2012;10:108–11.
34. Ly JV, Rowe CC, Villemagne VL, Zavala JA, Ma H, Sahathevan R, et al. Subacute ischemic stroke is associated with focal 11C PiB positron emission tomography retention but not with global neocortical Aβ deposition. Stroke. 2012;43:1341–6.
35. Sahathevan R, Linden T, Villemagne VL, Churilov L, Ly JV, Rowe C, et al. Positron emission tomographic imaging in stroke: cross-sectional and follow-up assessment of amyloid in ischemic stroke. Stroke. 2016;47:113–9.
36. Liu W, Wong A, Au L, Yang J, Wang Z, Leung EY, et al. Influence of amyloid-beta on cognitive decline after stroke/transient ischemic attack: three-year longitudinal study. Stroke. 2015;46:3074–80.
37. Iliff JJ, Wang M, Zeppenfeld DM, Venkataraman A, Plog BA, Liao Y, et al. Cerebral arterial pulsation drives paravascular CSF-interstitial fluid exchange in the murine brain. J Neurosci. 2013;33:18190–9.
38. Buga AM, Ciobanu O, Badescu GM, Bogdan C, Weston R, Slevin M, et al. Up-regulation of serotonin receptor 2B mRNA and protein in the peri-infarcted area of aged rats and stroke patients. Oncotarget. 2016;7:17415–30.
39. Buga AM, Di Napoli M, Popa-Wagner A. Preclinical models of stroke in aged animals with or without comorbidities: role of neuroinflammation. Biogerontology. 2013;14:651–62.
40. Sandu RE, Buga AM, Uzoni A, Petcu EB, Popa-Wagner A. Neuroinflammation and comorbidities are frequently ignored factors in CNS pathology. Neural Regen Res. 2015;10:1349–55.
41. Popa-Wagner A, Buga AM, Tica AA, Albu CV. Perfusion deficits, inflammation and aging precipitate depressive behaviour. Biogerontology. 2014;15:439–48.

14

Ischaemic stroke and the recanalization drug tissue plasminogen activator interfere with antibacterial phagocyte function

Antje Vogelgesang[1*], Claudia Lange[1], Lara Blümke[1], Georg Laage[1], Sarah Rümpel[1], Sönke Langner[3], Barbara M. Bröker[2], Alexander Dressel[1,4] and Johanna Ruhnau[1]

Abstract

Background: Stroke induces immune alterations such as impaired oxidative burst and reduced release of neutrophil extracellular traps (NETs). We hypothesised that key enzymes of these defence mechanisms may be altered in ischaemic stroke. Therefore, we analysed the intra- and extracellular amounts of myeloperoxidase (MPO) and neutrophil elastase (NE) in patient sera and granulocytes and monocytes. Because the autonomous nervous system is thought to mediate stroke-induced immune alterations, we also studied the influence of stress hormones and acetylcholine on MPO and NE. Rapid recanalization by recombinant tissue plasminogen activator (r-tPA) is the only available treatment for ischaemic stroke besides thrombectomy, and its influence on antibacterial defence mechanisms of granulocytes and monocytes were addressed here.

Methods: *Ex vivo:* Intracellular and serum MPO and NE were measured on days 0, 1, 3 and 5 post-stroke by either flow cytometry or enzyme-linked immunosorbent assay (ELISA) and compared to controls. *In vitro:* Blood from healthy donors was incubated with catecholamines, dexamethasone and acetylcholine, and the percentage of NET-producing cells and the area covered by NETs were quantified immunohistochemically. Intra- and extracellular MPO and NE were quantified by flow cytometry or ELISA. Blood samples from healthy donors were incubated with r-tPA, and oxidative burst, phagocytosis, NETosis, cytokine release, MPO and NE were quantified by flow cytometry, ELISA and microscopy.

Results: MPO was reduced in granulocytes but increased in sera obtained from stroke patients compared to controls. NE was not altered intracellularly but was elevated in patient sera. The percentage of NET-producing neutrophils was decreased by stress hormones and increased by acetylcholine. Neither intracellular MPO nor NE was altered by hormone treatment; however, adrenaline and acetylcholine induced NE release.
r-tPA led to reduced phagocytosis and oxidative burst in granulocytes and monocytes in vitro. NETosis, MPO release and cytokines were not altered, whereas NE release was enhanced by r-tPA.

Conclusions: Intracellular reduction of MPO might be responsible for reduced NETosis in stroke patients. The impact of enhanced MPO and NE serum levels in stroke patients should be addressed in future studies.
r-tPA impaired antibacterial defence function in vitro. Therefore, patients who undergo unsuccessful recanalization therapy might be at higher risk for infection, which should be analysed in future investigations. Immune alterations due to r-tPA effects in stroke patients should also be investigated.

Keywords: Stroke, r-tPA, NETosis, Oxidative burst, Phagocytosis, Innate immune response, Hormones

* Correspondence: antje.vogelgesang@uni-greifswald.de
[1]Department of Neurology, University Medicine Greifswald, Fleischmannstraße 41, FC3, 17475 Greifswald, Germany
Full list of author information is available at the end of the article

Background

Stroke induces profound immune alterations, which include the suppression of innate antibacterial defence mechanisms predisposing patients to post-stroke infections [1–3]. Such infections are reported in approximately 30% of stroke patients and are associated with worse outcomes and increased post-stroke mortality [4]. These immune alterations are thought to be initialized by high concentrations of catecholamines and glucocorticoids, which are regularly observed post-stroke in mice and in humans [5–9]. In animal models, inhibition of the sympathetic nervous system by propranolol or interruption of the parasympathetic nervous system by vagotomy reversed lymphocytic dysfunction and lowered the incidence of bacteraemia and pneumonia, whereas blocking the hypothalamus-pituitary gland axis by Ru486 normalised lymphocyte numbers and HLA-DR expression in monocytes [10, 11]. We previously reported that the oxidative burst, a mechanism that produces free oxygen radicals to kill phagocytosed bacteria, is impaired in ischaemic stroke patients in both granulocytes and monocytes. In addition, the amount of neutrophil extracellular traps (NETs) released by neutrophils in post-stroke patients is lower than in healthy subjects [1]. These traps, formed of DNA, prevent bacteria from further spreading and kill bacteria via high local concentrations of enzymes and bactericidal molecules that are attached to the DNA [12].

The enzymes myeloperoxidase (MPO) and neutrophil elastase (NE) are involved in the key steps of oxidative burst and NETosis. MPO produces antibacterial hypochlorous acid. Upon reactive oxygen species (ROS) production, NE escapes the azurophilic granules and translocates to the nucleus. MPO binds to chromatin in later stages, and both enzymes cooperatively enhance chromatin decondensation, leading to cell rupture and NETosis [13].

Recombinant tissue plasminogen activator (r-tPA) is the only available treatment for stroke patients besides mechanical thrombectomy, which both target rapid recanalization of the blocked vessels. The beneficial effect of recanalization by r-tPA is undisputed; however, experimental stroke studies have also reported neurotoxic effects of r-tPA [14, 15]. It was previously reported that r-tPA leads to degranulation of neutrophils, thus increasing NE and MPO in serum [16], and that r-tPA reduces stroke lesion size or outcomes independent of successful recanalization [17, 18]. Potential off-target effects of r-tPA on innate bacterial defence mechanisms of granulocytes and monocytes have not yet been studied; they could, however, be relevant for patient outcomes.

We therefore investigated the influence of (i) ischaemic stroke, (ii) stress hormones and the neurotransmitter acetylcholine and (iii) r-tPA on intra- and extracellular NE and MPO levels in patient blood samples and in cell cultures.

Methods

Study aim, design and setting

Ex vivo analyses of patient-derived samples

This prospective explorative study recruited patients from the dedicated stroke unit of the University Medicine Greifswald. We investigated the effects of ischaemic stroke on the key enzymes of NETosis and oxidative burst ex vivo. MPO and NE were quantified intracellularly and in sera in peripheral blood samples obtained within 12 h of stroke onset and thereafter on days 1, 3 and 5.

Patients aged ≥18 years suffering from middle cerebral artery (MCA) infarct were eligible for this study within 12 h after the onset of symptoms if their National Institute of Health Stroke Scale Score (NIHSS) was ≥6 and if no signs of systemic infection were detected on admission (C-reactive protein ≤50 mg/L and procalcitonin ≤0.5 ng/mL). Patients receiving immunosuppressive drugs or diagnosed with a malignancy were not recruited. Patients were treated with the best medical care. Recanalization with r-tPA and/or thrombectomy was carried out as clinically indicated. Age-matched control individuals were either healthy volunteers or were recruited from the ophthalmology clinics among patients scheduled to receive cataract surgery. Controls were neurologically and immunologically healthy. See the participants' characteristics in Tables 1 and 2.

Determination of stroke lesion size

Routine cerebral computed tomographic (cCT) images (sequential cCT native, 4.5 mm layer thickness supra- and infratentorial; mAs = 50; kV = 120) were acquired on a 16-row multislice CT scanner (Somatom 16, Siemens Medical Systems, Erlangen, Germany). Images were analysed using OSIRIX 5.6. To calculate the infarct size, the regions of interest were defined manually and the lesion volume was calculated semi automatically.

In vitro studies

To analyse whether catecholamines, dexamethasone or acetylcholine account for the observed alterations in NETosis post-stroke, blood samples from healthy donors were incubated with the specified hormones and transmitters for 4 h. NETosis was induced, and the NET area and percentage of NET-releasing cells were immunohistochemically quantified. Additionally, intracellular MPO and NE were determined by flow cytometry and ELISA after 24 h of co-culture.

To analyse the influence of r-tPA on antibacterial defence, peripheral blood mononuclear cells (PBMCs) from healthy subjects were incubated with 0, 0.5 or

Table 1 Subjects characteristics: myeloperoxidase (MPO) extra- and intracellular

		Total no.	Age (years)[a]	NIHSS[b]	Lesion volume (mm^3)[c]	Male	Female	Thrombolysis	Thrombectomy
Extracellular[f] (Fig. 1a)	Control subjects	11	79 (69–86)	NA	NA	6	5	NA	NA
	Stroke patients	23	73 (52–92)	9 (6–22)	55.97 (3.69–411.49)[e]	15	8	10	1
Intracellular (Fig. 1b)	Control subjects	14	75 (67-83)	NA	NA	8	6	NA	NA
	Stroke patients	20	75 (52–89)	9 (6–20)	21.61 (2.82–104.15)[d]	10	10	16	0

NA not applicable
[a]Mean (range)
[b]Median (range)
[c]Median (range)
[d]11 without demarkated infarct area
[e]8 without demarkated infarct area
[f]Experiments were conducted using the same study population

1 µg/ml r-tPA for 4 h, and oxidative burst, phagocytosis, NETosis, MPO and NE were quantified by flow cytometry, ELISA and microscopy. The release of cytokines was analysed after 72 h of incubation with r-tPA. r-tPA dosage was chosen to mimic the levels that are found in patients.

Phagocytosis

During phagocytosis, bacteria are engulfed by specialised phagocytes such as monocytes and neutrophils. After labelling cells with anti-CD14 antibody to distinguish monocytes (hCD14 APC; clone M5E2; BD Biosciences), a Phagotest Kit® (Biotechnology GmbH, Heidelberg, Germany) was used according to the manufacturer's instructions to quantify phagocytosis. Cells were incubated with FITC-labelled opsonized *Escherichia coli.* Engulfment of *E. coli* was stopped by placing the samples on ice after 10 min, and the FITC-signal of non-engulfed *E. coli* was quenched. The percentage of phagocytosing cells and the amount of engulfed *E. coli* per single cell were determined by flow cytometry. The results were evaluated using FlowJo Software 7.6.5 (Tree Star Inc., Ashland, OR, USA).

Oxidative burst

The intracellular production of free oxygen radicals during oxidative burst is a key bacterial defence mechanism. After labelling cells with anti-CD14 antibody (hCD14 APC; clone M5E2; BD Biosciences) to identify monocytes, the respiratory burst was measured using a Phagoburst Kit® (Glycotope Biotechnology GmbH) according to the manufacturer's instructions. Cells were left unstimulated or were incubated with *E. coli*, phorbol 12-myristate 13-acetate (PMA), or *N*-formylmethionine-leucyl-phenylalanine (fMLP) as stimulants for 10 min at 37 °C. Conversion of dihydrorhodamine 123 to rhodamine 123 enabled quantification of reactive oxygen species by flow cytometry. The percentage of phagocytes that underwent oxidative burst and the enzymatic activity per cell, given by the mean fluorescence intensity (MFI), were quantified and evaluated using FlowJo Software 7.6.5 (Tree Star Inc., Ashland, OR, USA).

Quantification of NETosis

To determine the capacity of neutrophils to release NETs, cells were isolated and cultured as described previously [1]. NETosis was induced by incubating either fMLP (455 nmol/l) or PMA (736 nmol/l) for 2 h at 37 °C in 5% CO_2. Unstimulated neutrophils served as a negative control. DNA was stained with *SYTOX*®-Green Nucleic Acid Stain (Invitrogen, Eugene), and both the total cells and NET-forming cells were quantified by microscopy (LEICA DBMI-4000b). NET-releasing cells were defined by a fluorescent area of ≥300 μm^2. The percentage of cells

Table 2 Subjects characteristics: neutrophil elastase (NE) extra- and intracellular

		Total No.	Age (years)[a]	NIHSS[b]	Lesion Volume (mm^3)[c]	Male	Female	Thrombolysis	Thrombectomy
Extracellular[f] (Fig. 1c)	Control subjects	11	79 (69–86)	NA	NA	6	5	NA	NA
	Stroke patients	23	73 (52–92)	9 (6–22)	55.97 (3.69–411.49)[e]	15	8	10	1
Intracellular (Fig. 1d)	Control subjects	10	73 (63–86)	NA	NA	4	6	NA	NA
	Stroke patients	12	71 (30–85)	18 (8–22)	52.12 (1.67–312.43)[d]	5	7	7	5

NA not applicable
[a]Mean (range)
[b]Median (range)
[c]Median (range)
[d]11 without demarkated infarct area
[e]8 without demarkated infarct area
[f]Experiments were conducted using the same study population

releasing NETs and the total area covered by NETs/cell were calculated Additional file 1.

Intracellular NE and MPO staining

NE and MPO are essential enzymes involved in oxidative burst and NET formation. To measure the intracellular NE and MPO amount, these enzymes where stained for flow cytometric analysis. Whole venous blood anticoagulated with ethylenediaminetetraacetic acid (EDTA) was lysed in accordance with the instructions of Human FoxP3 Buffer Set (BD Biosciences, Heidelberg, Germany). Non-specific binding was blocked by Fc Receptor Blocking Reagent for human samples (Miltenyi Biotec GmbH, Bergisch Gladbach, Germany). MPO was stained by fluorescein isothiocyanate (FITC)-labelled antibody according to the manufacturer's instructions for the FITC anti-human flow kit (Biolegend, San Diego, CA, USA). For NE staining, cells were incubated with anti-human-NE as a primary antibody (DAKO, Glostrup, Denmark). Phycoerythrin (PE)-labelled goat anti-mouse immunoglobulin G (minimal-x-reactivity, Biolegend, San Diego, CA, USA) served as a secondary antibody. CD14 surface expression was detected by allophycocyanin (APC)-coupled anti-human CD14 antibody (Biolegend, San Diego, CA, USA). Intracellular amounts of NE and MPO were measured using a BD LSR II flow cytometer (BD Biosciences, San Jose, CA, USA) by determining the MFI. Isotype controls and FMO controls were used as appropriate.

In vitro hormone and neurotransmitter assays

Transmitters of the sympathetic and parasympathetic nervous systems and cortisol as an effector of the hypothalamic–pituitary–adrenal axis have been shown to induce immune alterations post-stroke. To determine their in vitro effects on NETosis and oxidative burst, whole blood from healthy donors was pre-incubated for 4 h (for NETosis at room temperature; for oxidative burst at 37 °C) in 5% CO_2 (for NETosis, 0.04% CO_2) in the presence of either adrenaline (1×10^{-7} mol/l; 1×10^{-5} mol/l), noradrenaline (1×10^{-7} mol/l; 1×10^{-5} mol/l), acetylcholine (5.5×10^{-6} mol/l; 5.5×10^{-4} mol/l) (adrenaline, noradrenaline, acetylcholine from Sigma, Deisenhofen, Germany) or dexamethasone (2.5×10^{-7} mol/l; 2.5×10^{-6} mol/l) (MerckPharmaGmbH, Darmstadt) followed by neutrophil isolation and induction of NETosis or oxidative burst. In addition, we quantified intracellular and extracellular MPO and NE by flow cytometry and ELISA after 24 h of hormone or acetylcholine exposure. RPMI (supplemented with 2% glutamine, 2% penicillin/streptomycin, 10% AB-Sera, 1% HEPES (4-(2-hydroxyethyl)-1-piperazineethanesulfonic acid) without hormones or acetylcholine served as controls. Hormone concentration was chosen to span the range that is found in patients' post-stroke.

In vitro r-tPA assays

r-tPA is the most commonly used treatment for rapid recanalization in the acute phase of cerebral ischaemia. To study its impact on antibacterial immune defence mechanisms, whole blood samples from healthy donors were incubated for 4 h with 0.5 or 1 μg/ml r-tPA or control buffer alone in vitro. The phagocytes were tested for phagocytosis, oxidative burst and NETosis as described above. Intracellular amounts of MPO and NE were examined by flow cytometry.

To determine the effect of r-tPA on cytokine patterns, cells were incubated for 72 h before supernatants were obtained.

MPO-ELISA and NE-ELISA

Commercially available kits were used to measure MPO and NE in the supernatants of samples incubated with or without r-tPA as described above according to the manufacturer's instructions (MPO: Biolegend, San Diego, CA, USA; NE: Assaypro, St. Charles, MO, USA).

Cytokine assay

Venous blood was sampled into (i) EDTA or (ii) heparin vacutainers, and PBMCs were isolated by standard density centrifugation (Biocoll Separating Solution, Biochrom AG, Berlin, Germany). Then, 200,000 cells per well were (i) stimulated with PHA (1 μg/ml) in 96-well round-bottom plates or (ii) placed in anti-CD3/anti-CD28 (purified NA/LE mouse anti-human CD3 and purified NA/LE mouse anti-human CD28, both BD Pharmingen, San Jose, USA) pre-coated 96-well flat-bottom plates and incubated with r-tPA for 72 h. The production of INF-γ, IL-2, IL-4, IL-5, IL-6, IL-9, IL-10, IL-13, IL-17A, IL-17F, IL-21, IL-22 and TNF-α was measured using a LegendplexTM Multi-Analyte Flow Assay Kit (Biolegend, San Diego, CA, USA) in the supernatants of PBMCs according to the manufacturer's instructions.

Statistical analyses

All datasets were tested for adherence to a Gaussian distribution via the Kolmogorov–Smirnov test. Multiple comparisons of Gaussian-distributed data were performed using analysis of variance, and the Bonferroni correction for multiple comparisons was used as a post-test. When some of the experimental data failed the normality test, non-parametric testing was used throughout. ANOVA or repeated measures ANOVA, the Kruskal–Wallis test with Dunn's multiple comparison test as a post-test or the Friedman test were used as appropriate. Post-tests were only performed when initial testing revealed significant differences between groups. Correlations were determined by Spearman analysis. GraphPad-PRISM 5.0 (GraphPad Software Inc., San Diego, CA, USA) was used for all analyses. A p value <0.05 was regarded as significant. Gaussian-distributed data are shown as the mean ± SD. Other data are shown as the median [min–max].

Results

Intracellular MPO reduction and increased NE and MPO release in stroke patients

To explain the reduced respiratory burst and impaired NETosis after stroke, we analysed the intracellular amounts of MPO and NE in patients' granulocytes and monocytes and compared the results to those obtained with cells from age- and sex-matched healthy subjects.

On day 1 post-stroke intracellular MPO was significantly reduced in stroke patients' granulocytes compared to controls ($MPO{-}MFI_{d1(mean\ \pm\ SD)}$: 4598 ± 1642 vs. $MPO{-}MFI_{Control}$: 6580 ± 1955; $p = 0.0136$) (Fig. 1a). The reduction was transient. The same trend was observed in monocytes (see Additional file 2A). By contrast, MPO serum levels steadily increased during the observation period, and differences with controls became significant from day 3 post-stroke ($MPO_{d3(median\ [min\text{-}max])}$ 422 ng/ml [118–1952 ng/ml], $MPO_{d5(median\ [min\text{-}max])}$ 441 ng/ml [101–1656 ng/ml] vs. $MPO_{Control(median\ [min\text{-}max])}$ 115 ng/ml [13–1453 ng/ml]; $p = 0.0176$ (Fig. 1b).

Intracellular NE amounts were not altered in stroke patients' granulocytes (Fig. 1c) ($NE{-}MFI_{d1(mean\ \pm\ SD)}$ 4136 ± 1343; $NE{-}MFI_{d3}$ 4639 ± 1259; $NE{-}MFI_{d5}$ 4610 ± 1368 vs. $NE{-}MFI_{Control}$ 4055 ± 1473) nor monocytes ($NE{-}MFI_{d1(mean\ \pm\ SD)}$ 2457 ± 1002; $NE{-}MFI_{d3}$ 3027 ± 725; $NE{-}MFI_{d5}$ 2839 ± 737 vs. $NE{-}MFI_{Control}$ 3211 ± 1056) (see Additional file 2B). NE in the sera of stroke patients was significantly increased after stroke on all days investigated ($NE_{Control(median\ [min-max]}$ 98 ng/ml [26–430 ng/ml], $NE_{d0(median\ [min-max]}$: 565 ng/ml [64–1542 ng/ml], $NE_{d1(median\ [min-max]}$ 584 ng/ml [188–3678 ng/ml], $NE_{d3(median\ [min-max]}$ 619 ng/ml [27–3874 ng/ml], $NE_{d5(median\ [min-max]}$ 697 ng/ml [49–1772 ng/ml]; $p = 0.0007$) (Fig. 1d). None of the intra- und extracellular MPO and NE parameters correlated with stroke severity or neutrophil numbers.

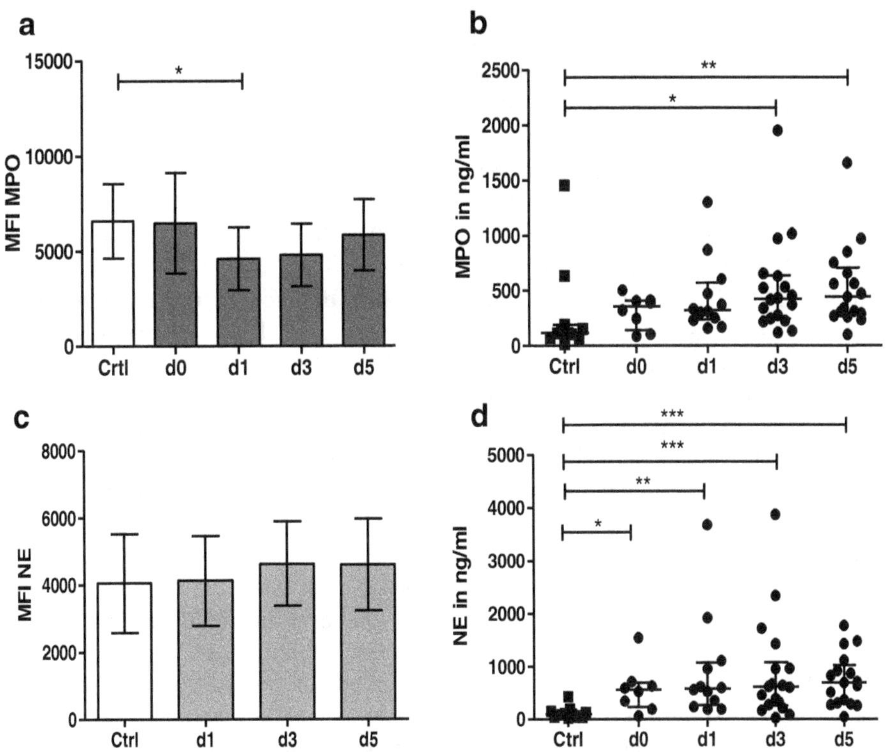

Fig. 1 NE and MPO in stroke patients versus controls. Stroke patients were analysed and compared to healthy controls. MPO and NE levels were measured intracellularly in granulocytes by flow cytometry (**a, c**) and are reported as MFI and in the sera of patients using ELISA (**b, d**) and reported in ng/ml. MPO was estimated on the day of stroke admission (d0), day 1 (d1), day 3 (d3) and day 5 (d5) by flow cytometry (**a**; $n_{crtl} = 14$, $n_{d0} = 14$, $n_{d1} = 18$, $n_{d3} = 14$, $n_{d5} = 15$). The extracellular amount of MPO was measured by ELISA (d0, d1, d3, d5) (**b**; $n_{crtl} = 11$, $n_{d0} = 8$, $n_{d1} = 12$, $n_{d3} = 18$, $n_{d5} = 17$). The intracellular amount of NE was measured on the day after stroke (d1) and on days 3 and 5 (d3, d5) (**c**, $n_{crtl} = 10$, $n_{d1} = 10$, $n_{d3} = 10$, $n_{d5} = 10$). NE in the sera was analysed on the day of stroke admission (d0) and on days 1, 3 and 5 after stroke (d1, d3, d5) (**d**; $n_{crtl} = 11$, $n_{d0} = 8$, $n_{d1} = 12$, $n_{d3} = 18$, $n_{d5} = 17$). *$p < 0.05$; **$p < 0.01$; ***$p < 0.005$. Mean and SD ranges for **a** and **c** and medians and interquartile ranges for **b** and **d** are given. ANOVA and Bonferroni comparisons as post hoc tests were used for data in **a** and **c**; data in **b** and **d** were assessed by Kruskal-Wallis test and Dunn's multiple comparison test

Hormones and acetylcholine do not influence intracellular MPO or NE but increase NE release in vitro

To determine whether the stroke-induced loss of intracellular MPO and the enhanced levels of MPO and NE in sera could be mediated by catecholamines, acetylcholine or dexamethasone, we determined the effect of each of the compounds in vitro. Healthy donors' whole venous blood samples were incubated with each of the compounds for 24 h. These treatments did not alter intracellular MPO (see Additional file 3A) or NE content (see Additional file 3B) in granulocytes or monocytes.

In supernatants, there was a small but statistically significant increase in NE concentration following treatment with 1×10^{-7} mol/l adrenaline ($p < 0.0001$), which was not confirmed at the higher concentrations of 1×10^{-5} mol/l adrenaline. Acetylcholine induced NE release at the highest concentration tested at 5.5×10^{-4} mol/l ($p = 0.0259$). MPO release was not induced under any of the conditions investigated (see Additional file 4).

Catecholamines and dexamethasone decreased NET release in vitro, acetylcholine had an opposite effect

We reported earlier that NET area is significantly reduced post-stroke [1]. Here, we investigate the in vitro effect of hormones and neurotransmitters, which are highly increased after stroke, on NETosis; (i) adrenaline, (ii) noradrenaline, (iii) dexamethasone, a glucocorticoid substitute, and (iv) acetylcholine were tested. Neutrophil of healthy donor's samples were isolated, and NETosis was induced in vitro by PMA and fMLP and compared to unstimulated conditions (Unstim). PMA is a strong inducer of NET, whereas fMLP has a moderate potency [19]. The percentage of NET-releasing cells in response to PMA was significantly downregulated by adrenaline (PMA_{Epi}: $p = 0.0003$), noradrenaline (PMA_{Norepi}: $p = 0.0033$), and dexamethasone (PMA_{Dexa}: $p = 0.0087$) in a dose-dependent manner. The same tendency was observed in unstimulated and fMLP-treated samples ($Unstim_{Epi}$: $p = 0.0106$; $Unstim_{Norepi}$: $p = 0.0448$; $Unstim_{Dexa}$: $p = 0.5880$; $fMLP_{Epi}$: $p = 0.0149$; $fMLP_{Norepi}$: $p = 0.0317$; $fMLP_{Dexa}$: $p = 0.0376$) (Fig. 2a–c). In line with these findings, the area covered by PMA-induced NETs was significantly reduced by 1×10^{-5} M adrenaline ($Unstim_{Epi}$: $p = 0.9669$; PMA_{Epi}: $p = 0.0161$; $fMLP_{Epi}$: $p = 0.0545$) (see Additional file 5). Stimulation with acetylcholine induced the opposite effect. The percentage of cells that released NETs was significantly and dose-dependently increased in unstimulated and stimulated samples ($Unstim_{ACh}$: $p = 0.012$; PMA_{ACh}: $p = 0.029$; $fMLP_{ACh}$: $p = 0.0081$) (Fig. 2d). The area covered by NETs was significantly increased under unstimulated conditions and with fMLP treatment ($Unstim_{Ach}$: $p = 0.0167$; PMA_{ACh}: $p = 0.1741$; $fMLP_{ACh}$: $p = 0.0431$) (see Additional file 5).

r-tPA reduces the efficiency of phagocytosis and the oxidative burst and increases NE release

Exposure to r-tPA is common in ischaemic stroke patients. Potential immunological effects of r-tPA may influence patients' clinical courses and skew the results of immunological studies performed in stroke patients. Here, we analysed the effects of r-tPA on MPO, NE, phagocytosis, oxidative burst, NETosis and cytokine production in healthy donor's samples in vitro.

r-tPA treatment significantly increased the in vitro release of NE into the supernatant in a dose-dependent manner but did not influence intracellular MPO or NE amounts. ($NE_{0\ \mu g/ml(mean\ \pm\ SD)}$ 21.26 ± 2.28 ng/ml; $NE_{0.5\ \mu g/ml}$ 24.55 ± 3.42 ng/ml, $NE_{1\ \mu g/ml}$ 27.75 ± 3.75 ng/ml; $p < 0.0001$). In addition, MPO release was not altered (see Additional file 6).

Whereas the percentage of reacting phagocytes was only minimally affected, (granulocytes: $phagocytosis_{0\ \mu g/ml(mean\ \pm\ SD)}$ $79.52 \pm 8.99\%$; $phagocytosis_{0.5\ \mu g/ml(mean\ \pm\ SD)}$ $81.09 \pm 8.87\%$; $phagocytosis_{1\ \mu g/ml(mean\ \pm\ SD)}$ $81.90 \pm 9.31\%$; $p = 0.0422$; monocytes: $phagocytosis_{0\ \mu g/ml\ (mean\ \pm\ SD)}$ $64.88 \pm 9.37\%$; $phagocytosis_{0.5\ \mu g/ml(mean\ \pm\ SD)}$ $66.93 \pm 6.21\%$; $phagocytosis_{1\ \mu g/ml(mean\ \pm\ SD)}$ $68.47 \pm 6.48\%$; $p = 0.0185$) (Fig. 3a, b), high- and low-r-tPA concentrations significantly decreased the numbers of phagocytosed *E. coli* per monocyte or granulocyte (granulocytes: $MFI_{0\ \mu g/ml(mean\ \pm\ SD)}$ 10123 ± 2874; $MFI_{0.5\ \mu g/ml(mean\ \pm\ SD)}$ 8990 ± 2734; $MFI_{1\ \mu g/ml(mean\ \pm\ SD)}$ 8751 ± 2671; $p < 0.0001$; monocytes: $MFI_{0\ \mu g/ml\ (mean\ \pm\ SD)}$ 5863 ± 927.8; $MFI_{0.5\ \mu g/ml(mean\ \pm\ SD)}$ 4766 ± 742.0; $MFI_{1\ \mu g/ml(mean\ \pm\ SD)}$ 4577 ± 454.3; $p < 0.0001$) (Fig. 3c, d).

r-tPA did not alter the percentages of unstimulated, fMLP-treated, PMA-treated or *E. coli*-treated cells that underwent oxidative burst, although general increases in the percentages of cells that underwent bursts due to fMLP, PMA and *E. coli* stimuli were observed (data not shown). However, there were less radicals per granulocyte in fMLP-stimulated cells treated with 0.5 μg/ml r-tPA (fMLP $MFI_{0\ \mu g/ml:\ (mean\ \pm\ SD)}$ 1376 ± 471.9; fMLP $MFI_{0.5\ \mu g/ml}$ 1067 ± 360.0; fMLP $MFI_{1\ \mu g/ml}$ 1244 ± 373.9; $p = 0.0004$) even though fMLP did not increase the amount of radicals per cell over unstimulated levels (Fig. 4a). Using more powerful stimuli, PMA and *E. coli*, a similar tendency was observed but did not reach statistical significance for granulocytes. In monocytes, all three stimulants reached statistical significance (Fig. 4b) (fMLP $MFI_{0\ \mu g/ml:\ (mean\ \pm\ SD)}$ 773.5 ± 126.1; fMLP $MFI_{0.5\ \mu g/ml}$ 740 ± 113; fMLP $MFI_{1\ \mu g/ml}$ 699 ± 90.23; $p = 0.0086$; PMA $MFI_{0\ \mu g/ml:\ (mean\ \pm\ SD)}$ 4236 ± 1659; PMA $MFI_{0.5\ \mu g/ml}$ 3291 ± 979; PMA $MFI_{1\ \mu g/ml}$ 3625 ± 1250; $p = 0.0033$; *E. coli* $MFI_{0\ \mu g/ml:\ (mean\ \pm\ SD)}$ 4000 ± 1725; *E. coli* $MFI_{0.5\ \mu g/ml}$ 3283 ± 1261; *E. coli* $MFI_{1\ \mu g/ml}$ 2952 ± 998.3; $p = 0.0427$).

The percentages of NET-releasing cells and the area covered by NETs remained unchanged by preincubating

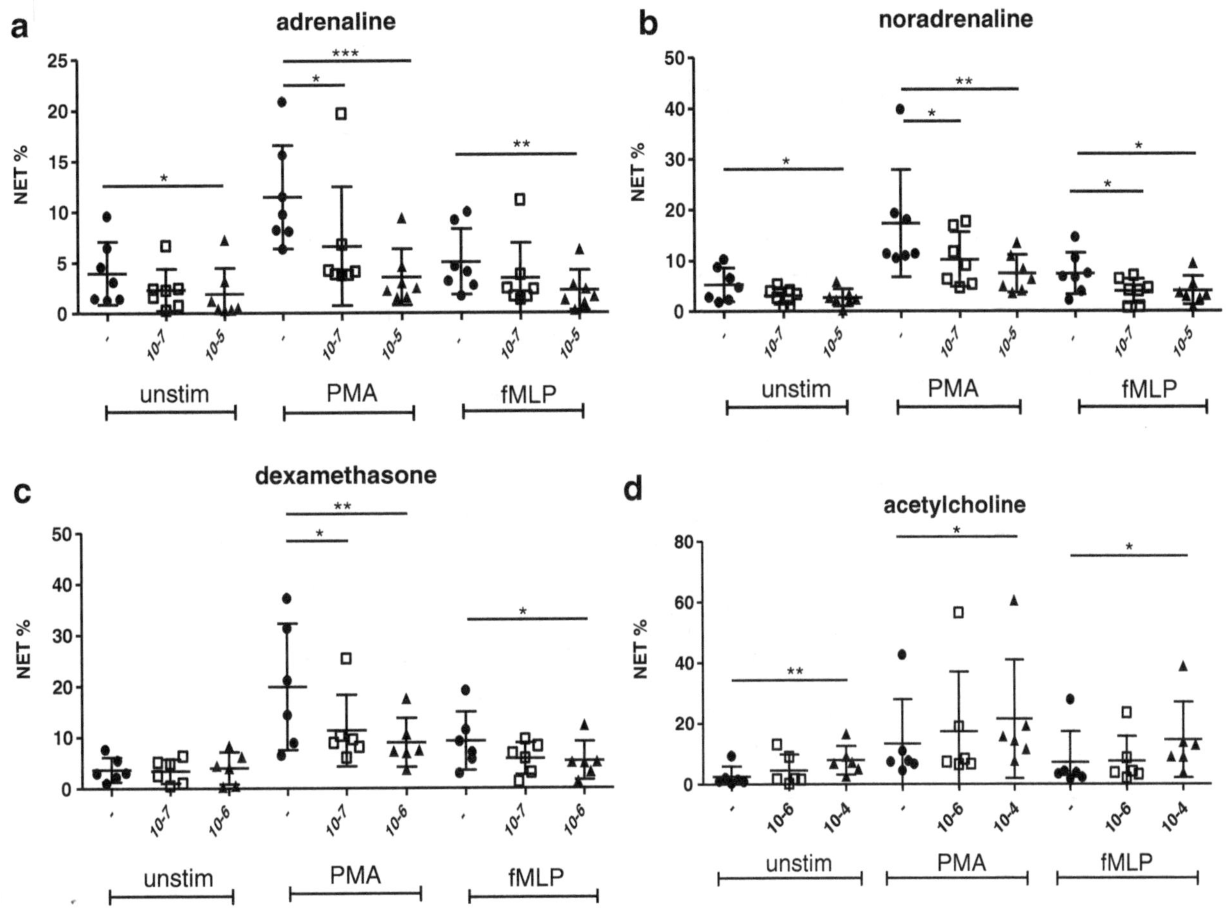

Fig. 2 NET percentage after incubation with adrenaline, noradrenaline, dexamethasone and acetylcholine. Effect of in vitro administration of 1×10^{-7} M and 1×10^{-5} M adrenaline (**a**) and noradrenaline (**b**); 2.5×10^{-7} M and 2.5×10^{-6} M dexamethasone (**c**); and 5.5×10^{-6} M and 5.5×10^{-4} M acetylcholine (**d**) on the percentage of NET-producing cells. After incubating blood of healthy donors with hormones and acetylcholine for 4 h at room temperature, neutrophils were isolated, and NETs were induced using PMA or fMLP or left unstimulated ($n_{a,b} = 7$; $n_{c,d} = 6$). $^{*}p < 0.05$; $^{**}p < 0.01$; $^{***}p < 0.005$. The mean and SD ranges are given. For **a–c**, ANOVA and Bonferroni comparisons as post hoc tests were used. Data in **d** were assessed by Friedman test and Dunn's multiple comparison test. Repeated measures tests were used within each of the three stimulation conditions

with r-tPA (data not shown). In addition, no significant changes in cytokine secretion were measured in PHA- or anti-CD3/anti-CD28-stimulated PBMCs incubated with r-tPA for 72 h (see Additional file 7A + B).

Discussion

Stroke induces immune alterations such as suppression of antibacterial defences by the innate immune system. As previously published, two key antibacterial defence steps, the oxidative burst and NETosis, are impaired in stroke patients [1]. Furthermore, the molecular mechanisms linking this functional loss to cerebral ischaemia remain unknown. Here, we investigated the intra- and extracellular levels of two key enzymes, MPO and NE, that are involved in NETosis and the oxidative burst post-stroke.

In stroke patients, intracellular MPO was reduced in granulocytes, and a similar finding was also observed in monocytes. MPO is the key enzyme involved in free radical generation during oxidative burst, and the enzyme is also involved in chromatin decondensation, a key step in NETosis. Thus, the reduction of intracellular MPO could contribute to the impaired oxidative burst as well as the reduced NET area in stroke patients.

Although the intracellular amount of MPO was reduced, which may result in impaired intracellular killing of engulfed bacteria, the extracellular levels of MPO and NE were elevated in stroke patients. This result is in line with an earlier report [20]. The increased amounts of MPO and NE post-stroke might be caused by increased release due to phagocyte cell death including NETosis by degradation of NET and post-stroke granulocytosis [21]. It is known that secreted NE plays a role in the

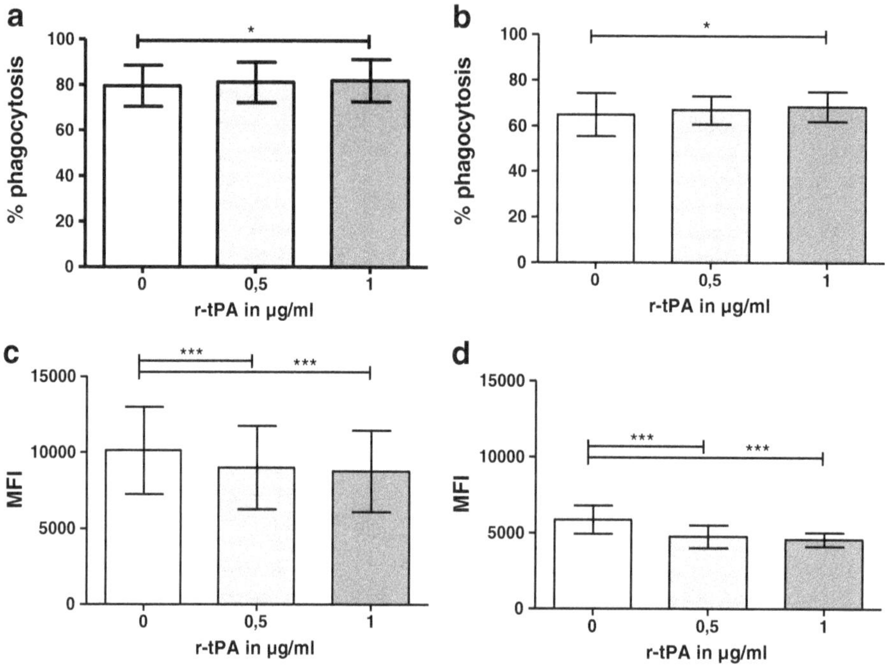

Fig. 3 Influence of r-tPA on phagocytosis. PBMCs of healthy donors were incubated with 0.5 or 1 µg/ml r-tPA for 4 h at 37 °C in 5% CO_2. Phagocytosis was then induced using FITC-labelled opsonized *E. coli*. The percentage of phagocytosing cells (**a, b**) and the efficacy of phagocytosis defined as the MFI (**c, d**) were investigated for granulocytes (**a, c**) and monocytes (**b, d**) ($n = 10$). $^{*}p < 0.01$; $^{***}p < 0.005$. The mean and SD ranges are given. Repeated measures ANOVA and Bonferroni comparisons as post hoc tests were used

regulation of local inflammatory immune responses via the proinflammatory cytokine degradation, MMP-9 activation, TGF-β generation and tissue remodelling [22, 23]. Substrates of NE include fibrin, fibronectin and coagulation factors [24]. NE also promotes microvascular injury of the lungs [25]. However, the impact of extracellular MPO and NE on post-stroke immune responses and patient outcomes still needs to be determined. In addition, sample size within our study has to be regarded as limitation.

To identify the factors that trigger MPO and NE modulation in stroke, we investigated the role of catecholamines, dexamethasone and acetylcholine. None of these factors altered the amounts of intracellular MPO or NE, although adrenaline and acetylcholine increased NE release into the supernatant. This mechanism could contribute to the elevated levels of NE in patient sera. Moreover, catecholamines and dexamethasone decreased NETosis while acetylcholine was a stimulator. Catecholamines mediate their effects through adrenergic receptors which include α_1, α_2 and β subtypes [26]. Glucocorticoids bind to the cytoplasmatic glucocorticoid receptor [27] and acetylcholine to nicotinic acetylcholine receptors [28] and muscarinic acetylcholine receptors [29]. It is known that hormone concentrations also span a wide range in patients within the first 24 h post-stroke [5] and that hormone effects can vary depending on receptor subtype, hormone concentration and receptor expression. Future experiments should be investigating combined hormone or selective receptor effects.

Many stroke patients are exposed to r-tPA, which is a common recanalization therapy for cerebral ischaemia. We observed significant r-tPA-induced inhibition of phagocytosed bacteria and radical production per cell in vitro, whereas we detected no r-tPA effect on the pattern of cytokines released by lymphocytes.

It is difficult to assess r-tPA effects in vivo, as patients who receive thrombolysis are by definition distinct from patients who do not receive this treatment. Although the clinical relevance of this finding remains to be determined, r-tPA treatment may be an unrecognised confounder in studies designed to determine stroke-induced immune alterations. In addition to neurotoxicity rt-PA exerts within the brain it might have beneficial effects in regard to neutrophil function by reducing the ability of the cells to produce free radicals within this compartment.

Conclusions

Reduced intracellular MPO could explain the impaired oxidative burst and reduced NET area in stroke patients.

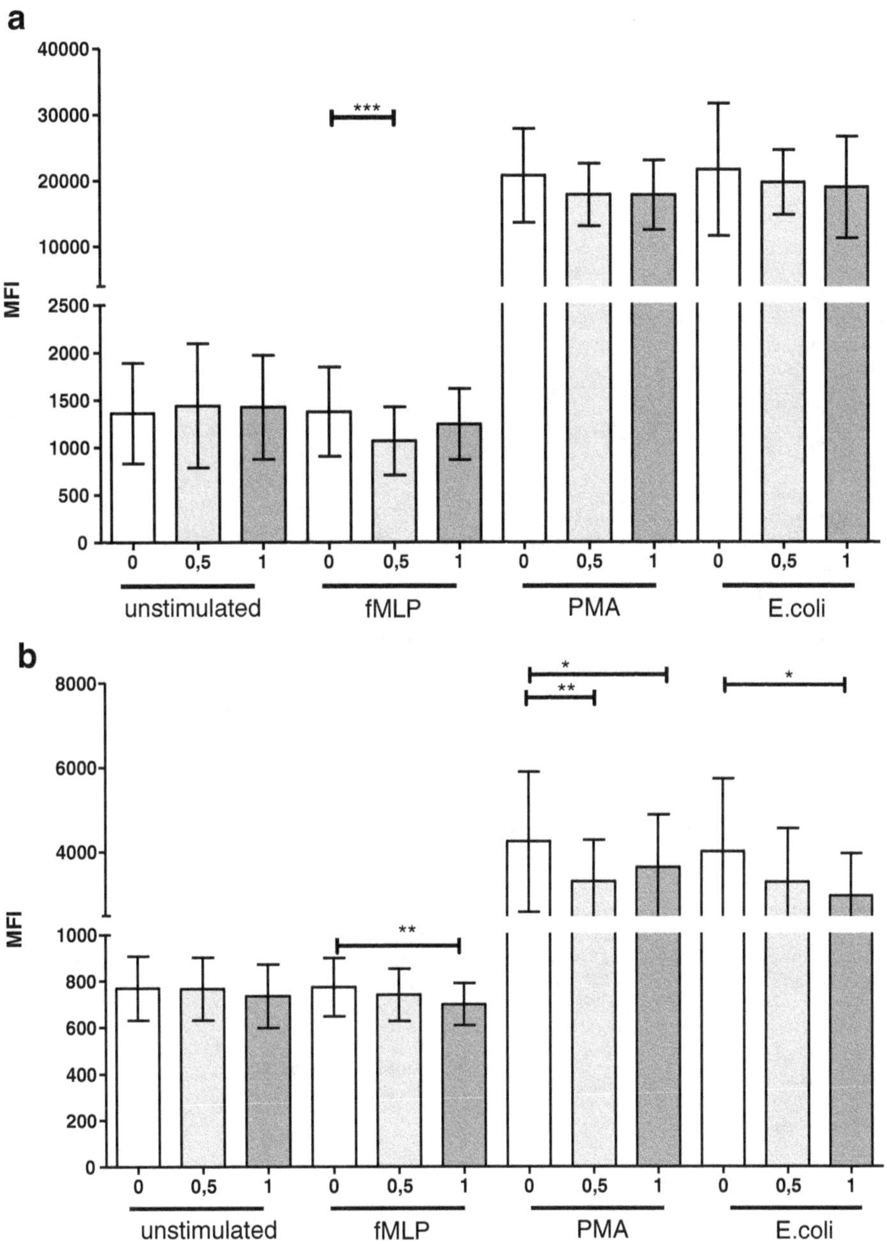

Fig. 4 Influence of r-tPA on oxidative burst. Oxidative burst analysis was performed using blood from healthy donors for granulocytes (**a**) and monocytes (**b**). Blood samples of healthy donors were incubated with 0.5 or 1 μg/ml r-tPA for 4 h at 37 °C in 5% CO_2. The oxidative burst was then induced using fMLP or PMA, and the efficacy (defined as the mean fluorescence intensity, MFI) of ROS was measured by flow cytometry ($n = 10$). $^*p < 0.05$; $^{**}p < 0.01$; $^{***}p < 0.005$. The mean and SD ranges are given. Repeated measures ANOVA and Bonferroni comparisons as post hoc tests were used within each of the four stimulation conditions

This mechanism should be targeted in future studies. The novel finding that r-tPA impairs bactericidal defences in vitro raises the question as to whether this treatment may increase the risk of developing a post-stroke infection. Patients treated successfully with r-tPA were not reported to be at a higher risk for infection. The beneficial effects of timely recanalization clearly outweigh potential off-target effects of r-tPA in this patient group. However, this outcome may be different among patients who undergo failed recanalization, who should therefore be closely monitored for infection or even receive preventive treatment. A clinical study should be carried out to test this hypothesis, and existing data from studies of stroke patients should be retrospectively subanalysed to determine the effects of r-tPA.

Additional files

Additional file 1: Netosis in an adult control. In vitro imaging of NETs forming neutrophils with representative images for one control subject. A brightfield image allowed quantification of total cells, SYTOX® Green allowed quantification of NETosis based on size of events and comparison of different stimuli. One representative example of the unstimulated and one PMA stimulated sample is shown. Fiji Software was used to measure NET area. Images of SYTOX® Green stained cells were taken with a Leica DMI 4000 B microscope; exposure time = 170 ms.

Additional file 2: Monocytic intracellular expression (MFI) of NE and MPO per cell in stroke patients versus controls. Stroke patients were analysed and compared to healthy controls. MPO (A) and NE (B) were measured intracellularly in monocytes using flow cytometry and are expressed in MFI. MPO was measured on the day of stroke admission (d0) and on days 1, 3 and 5 after stroke (d1, d3, d5) (A; $n_{crtl} = 14$, $n_{d0} = 14$, $n_{d1} = 18$, $n_{d3} = 14$, $n_{d5} = 16$). NE was measured on day 1 (d1) after stroke onset, day 3 (d3) and day 5 (d5) by flow cytometry (B, $n_{crtl} = 10$, $n_{d1} = 10$, $n_{d3} = 10$, $n_{d5} = 10$), and the mean and SD ranges are given. ANOVA was used for the data in A and B.

Additional file 3: Influence of adrenaline, noradrenaline, dexamethasone and acetylcholine on intracellular NE and MPO in vitro. A: Intracellular MPO of granulocytes and monocytes of healthy donors treated with adrenaline, noradrenaline, dexamethasone or acetylcholine (n = 10). The mean and SD ranges are given. B: Intracellular NE of granulocytes and monocytes treated with adrenaline, noradrenaline, dexamethasone or acetylcholine (n = 10). The mean and SD ranges are given.

Additional file 4: Influence of adrenaline, noradrenaline, dexamethasone and acetylcholine on NE and MPO release in vitro. NE and MPO-ELISA of supernatants of PBMCs (of healthy donors) treated with 1×10^{-7} M (low) or 1×10^{-5} M (high) adrenaline and noradrenaline; 2.5×10^{-7} M (low) or 2.5×10^{-6} M (high) dexamethasone; and 5.5×10^{-6} M (low) or 5.5×10^{-4} M (high) acetylcholine. If the data failed a Gaussian distribution test by the D'agostino & Pearson omnibus normality test, the data were analysed by the Friedman test for repeated measures and Dunn's post hoc test. $^{*}p < 0.05$; $^{**}p < 0.01$. The medians are given (n = 10).

Additional file 5: Influence of adrenaline, noradrenaline, dexamethasone and acetylcholine on mean NET area. Effect of in vitro administration of 1×10^{-7} M or 1×10^{-5} M adrenaline (A) and noradrenaline (B); 2.5×10^{-7} M or 2.5×10^{-6} M dexamethasone (C); and 5.5×10^{-6} M or 5.5×10^{-4} M acetylcholine (D) on NET area was tested. After incubation of blood of healthy donors with hormones and acetylcholine for 4 h at room temperature, neutrophils were isolated, and NETs were induced using PMA or fMLP or left unstimulated ($n_{A,B} = 7$; $n_{C,D} = 6$). $^{*}p < 0.05$. The mean and SD ranges are given. ANOVA and Bonferroni comparisons as post hoc tests were used. Repeated measures tests were used within each of the three stimulation conditions.

Additional file 6: Influence of r-tPA on MPO and NE. PBMCs of healthy donors were incubated with 0.5 or 1 μg/ml r-tPA for 4 h at 37 °C in 5% CO_2. Afterwards, MPO and NE were measured intracellularly in granulocytes by flow cytometry (A, C), expressed in MFI, and in the supernatant using ELISA (B, D), expressed in ng/ml (n = 10). $^{*}p < 0.01$; $^{***}p < 0.005$. Mean and SD ranges are given. Repeated measures ANOVA and Bonferroni comparisons as post hoc tests were used.

Additional file 7: A: Influence of r-tPA on cytokine production with PHA stimulation. Production of INF-γ, IL-2, -4, -5, -6, -9, -13, -17A, -17 F, -21, -22 and TNF-α in the supernatants of PBMCs after 72 h of incubation with r-tPA. PBMCs were stimulated with PHA to induce cytokine production. IL-10 was not induced in any of the conditions and is not shown. As an example, the data from PBMCs isolated from venous blood of healthy donors anticoagulated with EDTA are shown. The results for heparin-anticoagulated venous blood were similar and are not shown. (n = 4). The means are given. B: Influence of r-tPA on cytokine production with anti-CD3/anti-CD28 stimulation. Production of INF-γ, IL-2, -10, -5, -6, -9, -13, -17A, -17 F, -21, -22 and TNF-α in supernatants of PBMC after 72 h of incubation with r-tPA. PBMCs of healthy donors were stimulated with anti-CD3/anti-CD28 to induce cytokine production. IL-4 was not induced in any of the conditions and is not shown. As an example, the data from PBMCs isolated from venous blood anticoagulated with EDTA are shown. The results for heparin-anticoagulated venous blood were similar and are not shown (n = 4). The means are given.

Abbreviations

Ach: Acetylcholine; APC: Allophycocyanin; Dexa: Dexamethasone; DNA: Deoxyribonucleic acid; *E. coli*: *Escherichia coli*; EDTA: Ethylenediaminetetraacetic acid; ELISA: Enzyme-linked immunosorbent assay; Epi: Adrenaline; FITC: Fluorescein isothiocyanate; fMLP: *N*-formylmethionine-leucyl-phenylalanine; HEPES: 4-(2-hydroxyethyl)-1-piperazineethanesulfonic acid; MFI: Mean fluorescence intensity; MPO: Myeloperoxidase; NE: Neutrophil elastase; NETs: Neutrophil extracellular traps; NIHSS: National Institute of Health Stroke Scale Score; Norepi: Noradrenaline; PBMC: Peripheral blood mononuclear cells; PE: Phycoerythrin; PMA: Phorbol 12-myristate 13-acetate; ROS: Reactive oxygen species; r-tPA: Recombinant tissue plasminogen activator; Unstim/US: Unstimulated conditions

Acknowledgements

English Language Editing was provided by the Springer Nature Author Services.

Funding

AV and AD received funding from the EU grant EnVision (FP7-REGPOT-2010, Grant-No 264143). JR and CL were funded by the Gerhard-Domagk-Program of the University Medicine Greifswald. The funders had no role in the study design, data collection and analysis, decision to publish or preparation of the article.

Authors' contributions

AV, JR and AD made substantial contributions to the conception and design, data analysis and interpretation of the data. CL, LB, GL, SL and SR made substantial contributions to the acquisition of data, data analysis and interpretation of the data. BMB was involved in drafting the manuscript and revising it critically for important intellectual content. All authors have read and approved the final manuscript.

Consent for publication

Not applicable.

Competing interests

The authors declare that they have no competing interests.

Author details

[1]Department of Neurology, University Medicine Greifswald, Fleischmannstraße 41, FC3, 17475 Greifswald, Germany. [2]Department of Immunology, University Medicine Greifswald, Greifswald, Germany. [3]Department of Diagnostic Radiology and Neuroradiology, University Medicine Greifswald, Greifswald, Germany. [4]Department of Neurology, Carl-Thiem Klinikum, Cottbus, Germany.

References

1. Ruhnau J, Schulze K, Gaida B, Langner S, Kessler C, Broker B, Dressel A, Vogelgesang A. Stroke alters respiratory burst in neutrophils and monocytes. Stroke. 2014;45:794–800.
2. Chamorro A, Meisel A, Planas AM, Urra X, van de Beek D, Veltkamp R. The immunology of acute stroke. Nat Rev Neurol. 2012;8:401–10.
3. Magnus T, Wiendl H, Kleinschnitz C. Immune mechanisms of stroke. Curr Opin Neurol. 2012;25:334–40.

4. Westendorp WF, Nederkoorn PJ, Vermeij JD, Dijkgraaf MG, van de Beek D. Post-stroke infection: a systematic review and meta-analysis. BMC Neurol. 2011;11:110.
5. Schulze J, Vogelgesang A, Dressel A. Catecholamines, steroids and immune alterations in ischemic stroke and other acute diseases. Aging Dis. 2014;5: 327–39.
6. Harms H, Reimnitz P, Bohner G, Werich T, Klingebiel R, Meisel C, Meisel A. Influence of stroke localization on autonomic activation, immunodepression, and post-stroke infection. Cerebrovasc Dis. 2011;32:552–60.
7. Chamorro A, Amaro S, Vargas M, Obach V, Cervera A, Gomez-Choco M, Torres F, Planas AM. Catecholamines, infection, and death in acute ischemic stroke. J Neurol Sci. 2007;252:29–35.
8. Vogelgesang A, May VE, Grunwald U, Bakkeboe M, Langner S, Wallaschofski H, Kessler C, Broker BM, Dressel A. Functional status of peripheral blood T-cells in ischemic stroke patients. PLoS One. 2010;5:e8718.
9. Fassbender K, Schmidt R, Mossner R, Daffertshofer M, Hennerici M. Pattern of activation of the hypothalamic-pituitary-adrenal axis in acute stroke. Relation to acute confusional state, extent of brain damage, and clinical outcome. Stroke. 1994;25:1105–8.
10. Engel O, Akyuz L, da Costa Goncalves AC, Winek K, Dames C, Thielke M, Herold S, Bottcher C, Priller J, Volk HD, et al. Cholinergic pathway suppresses pulmonary innate immunity facilitating pneumonia after stroke. Stroke. 2015;46:3232–40.
11. Prass K, Meisel C, Hoflich C, Braun J, Halle E, Wolf T, Ruscher K, Victorov IV, Priller J, Dirnagl U, et al. Stroke-induced immunodeficiency promotes spontaneous bacterial infections and is mediated by sympathetic activation reversal by poststroke T helper cell type 1-like immunostimulation. J Exp Med. 2003;198:725–36.
12. Brinkmann V, Zychlinsky A. Beneficial suicide: why neutrophils die to make NETs. Nat Rev Microbiol. 2007;5:577–82.
13. Papayannopoulos V, Metzler KD, Hakkim A, Zychlinsky A. Neutrophil elastase and myeloperoxidase regulate the formation of neutrophil extracellular traps. J Cell Biol. 2010;191:677–91.
14. Goto H, Fujisawa H, Oka F, Nomura S, Kajiwara K, Kato S, Fujii M, Maekawa T, Suzuki M. Neurotoxic effects of exogenous recombinant tissue-type plasminogen activator on the normal rat brain. J Neurotrauma. 2007;24:745–52.
15. Yepes M, Roussel BD, Ali C, Vivien D. Tissue-type plasminogen activator in the ischemic brain: more than a thrombolytic. Trends Neurosci. 2009;32:48–55.
16. Carbone F, Vuilleumier N, Bertolotto M, Burger F, Galan K, Roversi G, Tamborino C, Casetta I, Seraceni S, Trentini A, et al. Treatment with recombinant tissue plasminogen activator (r-TPA) induces neutrophil degranulation in vitro via defined pathways. Vascul Pharmacol. 2015;64:16–27.
17. Ansar S, Chatzikonstantinou E, Thiagarajah R, Tritschler L, Fatar M, Hennerici MG, Meairs S. Pro-inflammatory mediators and apoptosis correlate to rt-PA response in a novel mouse model of thromboembolic stroke. PLoS One. 2014;9:e85849.
18. Kablau M, Alonso A, Hennerici MG, Fatar M. Treatment with tPA predicts better outcome even if MCA occlusion persists. Int J Stroke. 2013;8:496–502.
19. Remijsen Q, Kuijpers TW, Wirawan E, Lippens S, Vandenabeele P, Vanden Berghe T. Dying for a cause: NETosis, mechanisms behind an antimicrobial cell death modality. Cell Death Differ. 2011;18:581–8.
20. Cojocaru IM, Cojocaru M, Iliescu I, Botnaru L, Gurban CV, Sfrijan F, Tanasescu R. Plasma myeloperoxidase levels in patients with acute ischemic stroke. Rom J Intern Med. 2010;48:101–4.
21. Vogelgesang A, Grunwald U, Langner S, Jack R, Broker BM, Kessler C, Dressel A. Analysis of lymphocyte subsets in patients with stroke and their influence on infection after stroke. Stroke. 2008;39:237–41.
22. Chua F, Laurent GJ. Neutrophil elastase: mediator of extracellular matrix destruction and accumulation. Proc Am Thorac Soc. 2006;3:424–7.
23. Lee WL, Downey GP. Leukocyte elastase: physiological functions and role in acute lung injury. Am J Respir Crit Care Med. 2001;164:896–904.
24. Si-Tahar M, Pidard D, Balloy V, Moniatte M, Kieffer N, Van Dorsselaer A, Chignard M. Human neutrophil elastase proteolytically activates the platelet integrin alphaIIbbeta3 through cleavage of the carboxyl terminus of the alphaIIb subunit heavy chain. Involvement in the potentiation of platelet aggregation. J Biol Chem. 1997;272:11636–47.
25. Carden D, Xiao F, Moak C, Willis BH, Robinson-Jackson S, Alexander S. Neutrophil elastase promotes lung microvascular injury and proteolysis of endothelial cadherins. Am J Physiol. 1998;275:H385–392.
26. Kavelaars A. Regulated expression of alpha-1 adrenergic receptors in the immune system. Brain Behav Immun. 2002;16:799–807.
27. Baschant U, Tuckermann J. The role of the glucocorticoid receptor in inflammation and immunity. J Steroid Biochem Mol Biol. 2010;120:69–75.
28. Zdanowski R, Krzyzowska M, Ujazdowska D, Lewicka A, Lewicki S. Role of alpha7 nicotinic receptor in the immune system and intracellular signaling pathways. Cent Eur J Immunol. 2015;40:373–9.
29. Razani-Boroujerdi S, Behl M, Hahn FF, Pena-Philippides JC, Hutt J, Sopori ML. Role of muscarinic receptors in the regulation of immune and inflammatory responses. J Neuroimmunol. 2008;194:83–8.

15

Cytokine production pattern of T lymphocytes in neonatal arterial ischemic stroke during the first month of life

Anna Bajnok[1,2], László Berta[2], Csaba Orbán[2], Tivadar Tulassay[2,3] and Gergely Toldi[1,2,4*]

Abstract

Background: The perinatal period carries the highest risk for stroke in childhood; however, the pathophysiology is poorly understood and preventive, prognostic, and therapeutic strategies are not available. A new pathophysiological model describes the development of neonatal arterial ischemic stroke (NAIS) as the combined result of prenatal inflammation and hypoxic–ischemic insult. Neuroinflammation and a systemic inflammatory response are also important features of NAIS. Identifying key players of the inflammatory system is in the limelight of current research.

Case presentation: We present four NAIS cases, in whom detailed analysis of intracellular and plasma cytokine levels are available from the first month of life. All neonates were admitted with the initial diagnosis of hypoxic ischemic encephalopathy (HIE); however, early MRI examination revealed NAIS. Blood samples were collected between 3 and 6 h of life, at 24 h, 72 h, 1 week, and 1 month of life. Peripheral blood mononuclear cells were assessed with flow cytometry and plasma cytokine levels were measured. Pooled data from the cohort of four NAIS patients were compared to infants with HIE.

At 6 and 72 h of age, the prevalence of IL10+ CD8+ lymphocytes remained lower in NAIS. At 6 h, CD8+ lymphocytes in NAIS produced more IL-17. At 72 h, CD8+ cells produced more IL-6 in severe HIE than in NAIS, but IL-6 production remained elevated in CD8 cells at 1 month in NAIS, while it decreased in HIE. At 1 week, the prevalence of TGF-β + lymphocytes prone to enter the CNS was elevated in NAIS. On the other hand, by 1 month of age, the prevalence of TGF-β + CD4+ lymphocytes decreased in NAIS compared to HIE. At 72 h, we found elevated plasma levels of IL-5, MCP-1, and IL-17 in NAIS. By 1 month, plasma levels of IL-4, IL-12, and IL-17 decreased in NAIS but remained elevated in HIE.

Conclusions: Differences in the cytokine network are present between NAIS and HIE. CD8 lymphocytes appear to shift towards the pro-inflammatory direction in NAIS. The inflammatory response appears to be more pronounced at 72 h in NAIS but decreases faster, reaching lower plasma levels of inflammatory markers at 1 month.

Keywords: Neonatal arterial ischemic stroke, Hypoxic ischemic encephalopathy, Inflammatory response, Cytokine network, T lymphocytes

* Correspondence: toldigergely@yahoo.com
[1]First Department of Obstetrics and Gynecology, Semmelweis University, Baross str. 27, Budapest H-1088, Hungary
[2]First Department of Pediatrics, Semmelweis University, Bókay János str. 53-54, Budapest H-1083, Hungary
Full list of author information is available at the end of the article

Background

The perinatal period carries the highest risk for stroke in the entire childhood, with almost similar incidence to that in the elderly population. "Perinatal stroke" is a broad term defining a group of heterogeneous conditions characterized by the focal disruption of cerebral blood flow, of which neonatal arterial ischemic stroke (NAIS) is one of the most common subtypes, with an incidence of 1/8000 live births. NAIS by definition is an arterial ischemic stroke, with clinical symptoms occurring in the neonatal period (within the first 28 days of life) which are supported by radiological evidence [1, 2]. NAIS generally occurs in term neonates and presents a major risk for life-long motor, cognitive, and/or behavioral disabilities ranging from fine motor impairments to unilateral cerebral palsy, which develops in around 20–30% of affected neonates. Thus NAIS is a leading cause of cerebral palsy [3].

Interestingly, in almost all cases of NAIS, the intra-cranial arteries developing from the carotid arterial tree are affected, i.e., the proximal parts of the anterior cerebral artery (ACA), the middle cerebral artery (MCA), and the posterior cerebral artery (PCA)—while the basilar artery and the extra-cranial arteries are left unaffected [4–6]. The area of the left MCA is the most common localization of the ischemic lesion, resulting in a higher incidence of right-sided congenital hemiplegia [1]. The clinical presentation of NAIS is often subtle and non-specific, the most frequent symptoms being seizures, general hypotonia, lethargy, and poor feeding, making the timely diagnosis of NAIS difficult [7]. Diagnosis of NAIS is often delayed, due to the prenatal onset or absence of specific signs; therefore, the primary focus regarding therapeutic interventions is focused on prevention and post-insult anti-inflammatory mechanisms [3]. Another challenge regarding the diagnosis of NAIS is the fact that the risk factors and clinical signs of global hypoxic-ischemic encephalopathy (HIE) due to perinatal asphyxia show a significant overlap with NAIS and the two often co-occur [7–9]. Differentiating between the two syndromes is a complex question, some studies list perinatal asphyxia as an independent risk factor for NAIS [10], while neuroinflammation following ischemia appears to be a common feature of the two.

The pathophysiology of NAIS is poorly understood, and disease-specific preventive measures, prognostic factors, and therapeutic strategies are not available. The risk factors of NAIS appear to be specific for the perinatal period and can be clearly distinguished from the risk factors of stroke in older children or adults. Major risk factors such as congenital heart disease or bacterial meningitis can be held accountable for approximately 30% of NAIS occurrences; however, in most of the cases, NAIS is thought to be multifactorial, and in 25–40% of cases, no identifiable risk factor is present [11, 12]. Only a few case-control studies have aimed to specify risk factors; however, the number of cases was relatively low and there is little consistency in the observed maternal, obstetric, and neonatal risk factors [7, 13, 14]. The only independent risk factor, which appeared in all case-control studies, was perinatal inflammation, while genetic prothrombotic disorders were not found to be associated with the frequency of NAIS [3].

According to the classic pathophysiological hypothesis, most ischemic lesions are a result of thromboembolic events, where the presumable source of the thrombi is the placenta or the umbilical vessels [15]. While in some instances this could be the case, this hypothesis does not give a plausible explanation to why NAIS is almost exclusively affecting the intracranial arterial territories developing from the carotid arterial tree, while the incidence of basilary arterial or extracerebral infarcts is negligible [15]. In addition, there is angiographic evidence indicating a possibility of local arterial wall defects and in situ thrombus generation [9, 16]. Based on these findings, Giraud et al. proposed a different pathomechanism, where maternofetal inflammation induces focal arteritis specific to the intracranial arteries developing from the carotid arterial tree, which are susceptible to NAIS [3]. Using a preclinical rat model of chorioamnionitis, they were able to demonstrate that classic prothrombotic stress applied alone to the MCA was not enough to induce NAIS; however, when combined with in utero exposure to inflammation-inducing agent (LPS), the same stress leads to the classical symptoms of NAIS and motor impairment. They also examined the walls of arteries susceptible to NAIS and found that the constitutive expression of certain pro-inflammatory cytokines, i.e., TNF-α and IL-1β, was higher in the susceptible intra-cerebral arteries compared to extra-cerebral arteries. Furthermore, pups born from LPS-exposed dams developed a specific cerebral arteritis with increased presence of inflammatory cells (macrophages) and elevated levels of pro-inflammatory cytokines IL-1β, TNF-α, and MCP-1 with increased IL-1/IL-1 receptor antagonist (ra) ratio in NAIS susceptible arteries, but not elsewhere. [5]

Based on preclinical findings, a new pathophysiological hypothesis is being raised, which considers the complex and bidirectional relationship of coagulation and inflammatory pathways [17]. It describes the development of NAIS as the result of a multiple hit mechanism, originating from both perinatal inflammation and hypoxia–ischemia (HI) [3]. Giraud et al. have identified three major risk factors, the combination of which could lead to NAIS: (i) materno-fetal inflammation leading to focal arteritis of arteries susceptible to NAIS, (ii) a window of susceptibility in the development of the neonatal brain, and (iii) the physiological pro-coagulatory state of the perinatal period aggravated by the inflammatory response [5]. Prenatal exposure to inflammation appears to sensitize the brain for postnatal HI injury [18–20]. The inflammation could be of maternal, placental, or fetal origin, which is in line with the proposed risk factors of NAIS (preeclampsia, chorioamnionitis, maternal fever, infection) [3, 10]. In addition, the initial hypoxic insult—as is now commonly recognized—is followed by a generalized neuroinflammatory response. The initial hypoxic insult leads to primary energy failure, necrosis, subsequent glutamate release, oxidative stress, and as a result excitotoxicity and widespread necrosis and necroptosis within the first 6 h of the insult [21–23]. Neural tissue damage could be aggravated by previous sensitization due to inflammation, which could lead to increased oxidative stress and an increased production of pro-inflammatory cytokines [19, 24–28]. The second phase of neuroinflammation occurs from 24 until 72 h after the initial HI insult and is characterized by the production of inflammatory cytokines, the migration of leukocytes into the brain tissue, and consequent apoptosis. By identifying the key players of the neuroinflammatory and apoptotic pathways, this second phase could be an important time for targeted intervention [3, 29, 30]. Inflammatory cells can be detected for weeks or even months following the HI insult [31], and this sustained inflammatory status can be considered the tertiary, latent phase of the inflammatory response, which could also be important regarding neurological outcome.

The primary aim of current research in the field of perinatal stroke is to gain a better understanding of the pathomechanism of the disease with specific regard to the activation of the inflammatory pathway that could present a possibility for more specific diagnosis, intervention, and even prevention [3]. Human experimental data on inflammatory markers is scarce; one case-control study is available, where they aimed to describe the levels of different cytokines in the plasma of NAIS patients. Elevated levels of TNF-α, IL-2, IL-6, and IL-8 were observed 6 months following acute ischemic stroke (AIS) compared to healthy controls. However, no differences were observed in soluble endothelial protein C receptor (sEPCR), IL-11, and FVIII median levels [32]. The limitation of this study is that they included both neonatal and pediatric stroke cases (from birth until 18 years of age), which are now viewed as clinically distinct syndromes. These results indicate that an ongoing inflammation could be observed up to 6 months following AIS; however, no information is available regarding the acute phase of NAIS.

The pivotal role of inflammatory pathways in ischemic brain injury is supported by recent years' research data. T lymphocytes appear to play a central role in ischemic infarct development; they appear in the brain tissue within hours of the hypoxic insult and can be detected for up to a month after the injury. T cell deficiency has been shown to result in smaller infarct size and improved neurological outcome in murine models [33, 34]. Several cytokines have been connected to acute ischemic stroke in adults. Pro-inflammatory cytokines IL-1β, IL-8, MCP-1, TNF-α, and IFN-γ appear to exacerbate cerebral injury in adults, whereas anti-inflammatory cytokines such as TGF-β and IL-10 appear to be neuroprotective [35–37]. Although the immune system of neonates shows many differences compared to adults, the inflammatory network appears to play a similarly critical role in ischemic brain injury; therefore, it is reasonable to hypothesize that the same cytokines might also influence the course of neuroinflammation in the neonatal brain.

In this paper, we present four NAIS cases, in whom detailed analysis of intracellular and plasma cytokine levels are available from immediately after birth until the first month of age. To our knowledge, no such information is available in humans in NAIS; therefore, the data presented could serve as a basis for future, larger-scale case-control studies.

Case presentation

Patients and methods

All neonates were admitted to the regional cooling center with the initial diagnosis of HIE, requiring therapeutic hypothermia. Eligibility for cooling was assessed according to the TOBY criteria [38], and hypothermia was initiated between 1 and 5 h of life. Rectal temperature was maintained between 33 and 34 °C for the 72-h intervention period. Clinical or culture-proven sepsis was not detected in any of the infants. All infants received regular preventive intravenous antibiotics, i.e., ampicillin and gentamicin during the hypothermic treatment. MRI data were interpreted by radiologists who were blinded to the clinical status of the neonates, based on criteria defined by Rutherford et al. [39, 40].

A total of 33 term neonates were enrolled with written parental consent in a study focusing on inflammatory changes in HIE (approved by the Hungarian Medical Research Council (TUKEB 6578-0/2011-EKU)). Four infants were diagnosed with NAIS after their MRI scans were completed. One infant was excluded due to suspected metabolic disease. In the HIE group, data from 28 neonates were analyzed and divided into two groups based on the severity of the hypoxic-ischemic encephalopathy. The groups were determined based on the initial amplitude-integrated EEG (aEEG) recordings and the recovery time during monitoring [37] together with the MRI scans, which were performed within the first week of life. The severe group ($n = 11$) was formed of newborns with moderate-to-severe HIE signs on the MRI scan AND burst-suppression or continuous extremely low voltage or flat tracing background activity on aEEG OR normalization of aEEG after the 48th hour of life or never, OR early death (< 28 days). Neonates that met none of the above-listed criteria constituted the moderate group ($n = 17$) (mild HIE signs on MRI scans AND continuous or discontinuous normal voltage background activity on aEEG OR normalization of aEEG activity before the 48th hour of life) [41]. Pooled data from the cohort of four NAIS patients were compared to infants with HIE. In the severe HIE group, three infants deceased before 1 month of age due to the severity of the insult. Available data from these neonates were included at the relevant time points within the severe group. Therefore, 72-h, 1-week, and 1-month data were missing in the case of two infants and 1-month data were missing from one infant. Clinical characteristics of infants are summarized in Table 1.

Two milliliters of venous blood was collected between 3 and 6 h of life (at admission), as well as at 24 h, 72 h, and 1 week of life, adjusted to blood sampling required by clinical care. A further venous blood sample was obtained at 1 month of age during a routine outpatient follow-up appointment.

Flow cytometry

Plasma was separated from peripheral blood samples by centrifugation. Plasma samples were aliquoted and immediately frozen and stored at − 80 °C for later determination of cytokine concentrations.

Remaining cells were resuspended in RPMI (Roswell Park Memorial Institute)-1640 medium (Sigma-Aldrich, St. Louis, MO, USA). Cells were incubated with PMA (phorbol 12-myristate 13-acetate) (50 ng/ml), ionomycin (1 μg/ml), and BFA (Brefeldin A) (10 μg/ml) for 6 h at 37 °C to allow intracellular accumulation of cytokines. For surface marker staining, samples were then incubated with the following fluorochrome-conjugated anti-human monoclonal antibodies: CD4 PE-Cy7 (phycoerythrin-cyanine 7) and CD8 APC-Cy7 (allophycocyanin-cyanine 7) (panel 1) or CD4 APC-Cy7 and CD49d PerCP (peridinin-chlorophyll-protein) (panel 2), according to the manufacturers' instructions (all from BioLegend, San Diego, CA, USA). Red blood cells were lysed and PBMCs were permeabilized using FACSLysing and FACSPermeabilizing solutions (BD Biosciences, San Jose, CA, USA). Cells were washed and resuspended in PBS (phosphate buffer saline) and divided into two equal aliquots and stained according to the manufacturers' instructions for intracellular cytokines using the following conjugated anti-human monoclonal antibodies or the appropriate isotype controls: IL-6 PE (phycoerythrin), IL-17A PerCP, IL-10 APC (allophycocyanin), and IFN-γ FITC (fluorescein isothiocyanate) (for panel 1), or TNF-α PE-Cy7, FoxP3 PE, TGF-β APC, and IL-1β FITC (for panel 2), respectively (all from BioLegend). Following labeling, cells were washed and resuspended in PBS for flow cytometry analysis. Samples were analyzed immediately on a FACSAria flow cytometer (BD Biosciences) equipped with 488- and 633-nm excitation lasers. Data were processed using the FACSDiVa software (BD Biosciences). One hundred thousand cells were recorded. Evaluators of flow cytometry data were blinded to the clinical status of the neonates.

Immunoassays

Plasma samples were stored at − 80 °C until analysis. The plasma levels of the following cytokines, chemokines, and growth factors were determined using Bio-Plex Pro Assays (Bio-Rad Laboratories, Hercules, CA, USA): IL-1β, IL-2, IL-4, IL-5, IL-6, IL-7, IL-8, IL-10, IL-12, IL-13, IL-17, IFN-γ, TNF-α, TGF-β, G-CSF,

Table 1 Clinical characteristics of neonates in the moderate and severe HIE and NAIS groups upon admission (within 12 h of age)

	Moderate HIE ($n = 17$)	Severe HIE ($n = 11$)	NAIS ($n = 4$)
Male gender (%)	10 (59%)	7 (64%)	2 (50%)
Birthweight (g)	3330 [2860–3605]	3000 [2490–3300]	3115 [2540–3885]
Gestational age (week)	39 [37–40]	38 [37–40]	39.5 [38.25–40]
No. of C-sections (%)	10 (59%)	8 (73%)	3 (75%)
Apgar at 1 min	3 [0.5–4.5]	1 [0–3]	4^{b} [3–5]
Apgar at 5 min	6 [5–7]	$2^{a, b}$ [0–4]	5.5^{b} [5, 6]
Apgar at 10 min	7 [5–8]	4^{a} [1.75–5.25]	7^{b} [6, 7]
Worst pH	7.03 [6.87–7.12]	6.86 [6.62–7.06]	6.94 [6.88–7.00]
Worst BD (mmol/L)	18.05 [16.65–21.28]	20.4 [19.38–23.5]	14^{b} [14–17]
S100 (μg/L)	7.5 [2.33–28.85]	21.8 [3.8–30.0]	3.6^{b} [1.88–18.35]
LDH (U/L)	2072 [1371–5274]	3335 [1879–5792]	1874 [1676–3187]

Data are presented as median and interquartile range; a = moderate vs severe HIE, $p < 0.05$; b = severe HIE vs NAIS, $p < 0.05$

GM-CSF, MCP-1, MIP-1b, and VCAM. Bio-Plex Pro Assays are immunoassays formatted on magnetic beads that utilize principles similar to those of a sandwich ELISA. Capture antibodies against the biomarker of interest are covalently coupled to the beads. A biotinylated detection antibody creates the sandwich complex, and the final detection complex is formed by the addition of a streptavidin-phycoerythrin (SA-PE) conjugate, where PE serves as the fluorescent reporter. Reactions are read using a Luminex-based reader.

Statistical analysis

Data are expressed as median and interquartile range. Comparisons between sample populations were performed with Mann-Whitney tests, as a test of normality (performed according to Kolmogorov-Smirnoff) indicated non-normal distribution of data. Comparisons between the paired values (samples collected at different time points) in the same population were made with Friedman tests. p values less than 0.05 were considered significant. Outliers were identified using Grubbs' tests and were excluded from analyses. Statistics were calculated using the GraphPad Prism 5 software (La Jolla, CA, USA).

NAIS case presentations

Case 1

The first patient was admitted following an emergency cesarean section performed due to oligohydramnios and fetal tachycardia on the 40th week of gestation. There was no maternal history of chorioamnionitis. However, the mother smoked during pregnancy. The amniotic fluid was stained with thick meconium. The neonate was born with an Apgar score of 5/6/7. She required intubation and ventilation at birth. Her first capillary blood gas showed lactic acidosis (pH 7.03, BE – 14 mmol/L, lactate 12.4 mmol/L), and she became irritable and had generalized increased muscle tone; thus, hypothermic treatment was initiated. On the second day of life, she presented with symptoms characteristic of pulmonary hypertension, which resolved after 1 day of NO inhalation and she was extubated on day 3 of life. Her early neurodevelopmental examination showed mild central hypotonia.

Cranial MRI with diffusion-weighted imaging was performed on day 4 of life, which showed a distinct, 5 × 7 mm area of ischemia with decreased diffusion in the left thalamus and no evidence of bleeding. MR spectroscopy showed a decrease in metabolites, correlating to minimal hypoxic-ischemic encephalopathy.

Case 2

The second neonate was admitted following an emergency cesarean section due to complete placental abruption on the 39th week of gestation. He was born with an Apgar score of 3/5/6/8. At the time of birth, he had a heartrate of 80/min, had no respiratory effort, and was hypotonic and pale. Following bag and mask ventilation, his heartrate normalized; however, only gasping could be observed, so he was intubated. He later became irritable. His initial blood gas showed severe metabolic acidosis (pH 6.99, BE – 14). A chest X-ray was performed, which showed a pneumothorax on the right side, which was drained and hypothermic treatment was initiated. Due to severe anemia and low blood pressure, he required blood transfusion on two occasions and inotropic support for 6 days, respectively. An early neurodevelopmental examination indicated grossly abnormal central and peripheral tone distribution.

Cranial MRI was performed on day 4 of life. Diffusion-weighted imaging showed a large area of ischemia with decreased diffusion in the area of the left middle cerebral artery, and several smaller lesions in the area of the right middle cerebral artery. The area of the left parietal cortex was blurred with hyperintensive signal subcortically. There were no signs of bleeding. TOF MRI angiography showed marked irregularity and significantly decreased blood flow in both, but particularly in the left MCA. No MRI signs of hypoxic-ischemic encephalopathy were present.

Case 3

The third neonate was born from an uncomplicated pregnancy on the 40th week of gestation, with an Apgar score of 5/5. The neonate was hypotonic and had no spontaneous breathing; therefore, she was intubated. The first gasping breaths were observed at 15 min after birth, but she remained generally hypotonic. The first blood gas showed severe lactic acidosis (pH 6.89, BE – 18 mmol/L, lactate 15 mmol/L). Therapeutic hypothermia was commenced. The initial aEEG recordings showed abnormal background activity; however, this normalized after a few hours. The early neurodevelopmental examination reported moderate generalized hypotonia.

Cranial MRI was performed on day 3 of life. Diffusion-weighted imaging showed a small (3 mm) ischemic lesion with decreased diffusion in the right thalamus. No other signs of ischemia and bleeding or signs of hypoxic ischemic encephalopathy could be observed.

Case 4

The fourth neonate was born from an uncomplicated pregnancy on the 38th week of gestation by emergency cesarean section due to imminent intrauterine asphyxia. He was born with an Apgar score of 3/6/7. He was flaccid with no signs of spontaneous breathing and a heart rate of 80/min. Following bag and mask ventilation, spontaneous breathing was noted after 5 min, but the neonate remained hypotensive and areflexive. He was intubated and hypothermic treatment was initiated. The aEEG recording showed no signs of seizures. The initial blood gas showed mixed acidosis (pH 6.875, BE − 14). The initial neurodevelopmental examination demonstrated abnormal central and peripheral tone distribution.

Cranial MRI was performed on day 1 of life. Diffusion-weighted imaging showed decreased diffusion indicating ischemia in the area of the right posterior cerebral artery. Smaller lesions were present in the right thalamus and the left parieto-occipital area. No signs of bleeding or hypoxic ischemic encephalopathy were present.

Results

Intracellular cytokine data

At 6 and 72 h of age, the prevalence of CD8+ IL10+ lymphocytes remained lower in NAIS than in the severe HIE group. Although the prevalence of CD8+ IL10+ lymphocytes remained consistently lower in NAIS, the difference did not reach a significant level at the 24-h time point. On the contrary, the prevalence of CD4+ IL-10+ was higher at 24 h in NAIS compared to moderate HIE. The prevalence of IFN-γ + CD4+ cells showed an elevated tendency from 24 h in NAIS; however, this value did not reach significance, which could be due to the small population. At 1 week, the prevalence of TGF-β + lymphocytes prone to enter the CNS (CD4+ TGF-β + CD49d + lymphocytes) was elevated in NAIS compared to both HIE groups, and also compared to all other time points within the NAIS group (Fig. 1). On the other hand, at 1 month of age, the prevalence of CD4+ TGF-β + lymphocytes decreased in NAIS compared to HIE. Data are shown in Table 2.

At 6 h, the prevalence of CD8+ IL17+ lymphocytes was higher in NAIS than in severe HIE and CD8 cells expressed higher levels of IL-17 in NAIS than moderate HIE. The level of IL-1β in CD4+ cells was highest at 6 h and decreased significantly by 72 h within the NAIS group. The mean fluorescence intensity (MFI) of IFN-γ in CD4+ lymphocytes in NAIS was highest at 24 h and decreased significantly by 72 h, when it reached a lower level in NAIS than in either of the HIE groups. The MFI of IL-6 in CD8+ cells was higher at 72 h in severe HIE than in NAIS. Interestingly, by 1 month, the MFI of IL-6 in CD8+ decreased in both HIE groups and rose in NAIS. Data are shown in Table 3.

We found no differences between NAIS and HIE in the intracellular production of IL-1β and TNF-α in CD4 or CD8 cells; however, these cytokines appear to be important in differentiating between the mild and severe form of HIE [41].

Plasma cytokine data

At 72 h, we found a marked inflammatory response in NAIS, characterized by elevated plasma levels of IL-5, IL-17, and MCP-1 compared to HIE. Plasma MCP-1 level was the highest at 72 h in NAIS. By 1 month, however, inflammatory response appears to be decreased in NAIS compared with HIE, indicated by decreased plasma levels of IL-4, IL-12, and IL-17 (Fig. 2). The level of IL-4 was lower at 1 month than 72 h in NAIS.

We found no alterations in NAIS in the plasma level of IL-1β, IL-2, IL-6, IL-7, IL8, IL-10, IL-13, IFN-γ, TNF-α, TGF-β, G-CSF, GM-CSF, MIP-1b, and VCAM when compared with HIE. Data are shown in Table 4.

Discussion

The contribution of T lymphocytes to ischemic brain injury now appears to be clear, with CD8+ and CD4+ T cells appearing in the CNS already a few hours after an ischemic insult. The accumulation of T cells peaks around 3–4 days following injury, and the inhibition of T cell trafficking to the CNS decreases the deleterious consequences of neuroinflammation [42, 43]. Data from murine stroke models showed persisting presence of T cells up to 7 weeks after the ischemic attack [44]. In our NAIS patients, CD8 lymphocytes appear to show a

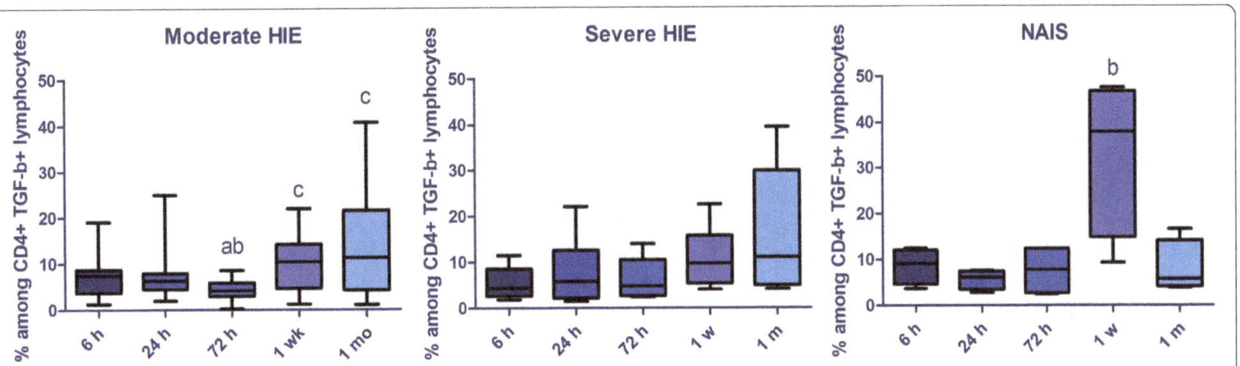

Fig. 1 Alterations of the prevalence of CD4+ TGF-β + CD49d + cells within the CD4+ population in the first month of life in moderate ($n = 17$) and severe ($n = 11$) hypoxic-ischemic encephalopathy (HIE) and in NAIS ($n = 4$). Horizontal line: median, box: interquartile range, whisker: range. $p < 0.05$ a vs 6 h, b vs 24 h, c vs 72 h

Table 2 Intracellular cytokines—cell prevalence data

% of parent population		Moderate HIE (n = 17)	Severe HIE (n = 11)	NAIS (n = 4)
IL-10+ CD8+ / CD8+	6 h	2.75 (1.19–4.12)	4.19 (1.94–6.91)	1.10 (0.40–1.36) b, p = 0.01
IL-10+ CD4+ / CD4+	24 h	2.88 (1.56–7.03)	4.52 (3.02–6.59)	9.47 (5.10–20.68) a, p = 0.03
IL-10+ CD8+ / CD8+	72 h	3.51 (1.85–5.12)	5.30 (2.41–6.08)	1.39 (0.52–2.99) b, p = 0.03
TGF-β + CD49d + CD4+ / CD4+	1 week	10.54 (4.77–14.28)	10.0 (5.46–15.20)	38.00 (14.93–46.78) a, p = 0.03; b, p = 0.05
TGF-β + CD4+ / CD4+	1 month	3.51 (1.46–4.47)	3.54 (2.47–6.27)	1.30 (0.54–2.49) b, p = 0.05
IL-17+ CD8+ / CD8+	6 h	3.89 (5.26–14.40)	2.30 (1.73–4.49) c, p = 0.02	5.04 (4.62–7.68) b, p = 0.03
IFN-γ + CD4+ / CD4+	72 h	6.40 (3.70–11.80)	6.17 (4.75–13.01)	17.50 (2.74–30.20)
IL-6+ CD8+ /CD8+	72 h	4.37 (3.26–6.29)	5.63 (2.68–8.80)	8.87 (4.75–10.52)
IL-6+ CD8+ /CD8+	1 month	4.02 (2.40–10.74)	3.70 (2.31–6.16)	4.47 (2.88–8.33)

The prevalence of T cells expressing various cytokines are shown as the percentage of the parent population

different cytokine production pattern than HIE with a more prominent pro-inflammatory response in NAIS. At 6 h, CD8 cells from NAIS patients produce higher levels of pro-inflammatory IL-17 than those from neonates with moderate HIE, and CD8+ IL17+ cells are more prevalent in NAIS than in severe HIE. At 72 h, CD8 cells of neonates with severe HIE produce higher levels of pro-inflammatory IL-6 than CD8 cells of NAIS patients. IL-6 is known to be an important factor in the early phase of HIE, and this difference could reflect an aggravated neuroinflammation in severe HIE. On the other hand, IL-6 has also been described to have neurotrophic, neuroregenerative, and anti-inflammatory properties within the brain [45–48]. The alteration in intracellular levels of IL-6 in CD8 cells becomes reversed by 1 month, when it remains elevated in NAIS, whereas it decreases in both HIE groups, indicating that a sustained level of IL-6 might be present for a longer time in NAIS, which is in line with literary data [32]. Therefore, IL-6 may exert its neuroprotective effects over a longer period of time in NAIS.

Plasma cytokine levels also indicate a difference between NAIS and HIE, with a higher level of pro-inflammatory response at 72 h in NAIS than in HIE. We found elevated IL-5, IL-17, and MCP-1 levels at 72 in NAIS (see Table 3 for details.) MCP-1 was found to be elevated following

Table 3 Intracellular cytokines—mean fluorescence intensity (MFI) data

Arbitrary unit		Moderate HIE (n = 17)	Severe HIE (n = 11)	NAIS (n = 4)
MFI IL-17 / CD8	6 h	1427 (661.5–2402)	1591 (1157–7047)	4855 (2618–8706) a, p = 0.01
MFI IFN-γ / CD4	72 h	455 (149.5–770)	887 (495.5–1427)	42.25 (28.13–438.5) a, p = 0.04; b, p = 0.01
MFI IL-6 /CD8	72 h	701 (364.8–1441)	1073 (795–2017)	646.5 (188.7–736.3) b, p = 0.03
MFI IL-6 / CD8	1 month	429 (101.7–617.0)	347 (83–491)	918.5 (638.3–1347) a, p = 0.01; b, p = 0.02
MFI IL-10 / CD8	6 h	1883 (512.5–5817)	1874 (1157–3415)	705 (280–3313)
MFI IL-10 / CD4	24 h	674.5 (177.8–2608)	1084 (203–1892)	666 (242.5–1063)
MFI IL-10 / CD8	72 h	2167 (1462–5964)	1505 (1055–3819)	443.5 (371–5977)
MFI TGF-β / CD4	1 week	4620 (2654–6647)	3129 (1238–5621)	3260 (1452–3680)
MFI TGF-β / CD4	1 month	811.5 (253–1740)	634 (259–1789)	330.5 (123–2283)

The intracellular level of certain cytokines in T cells is shown by the MFI of each cytokine. Data are expressed as median and interquartile range; a = moderate HIE vs NAIS, $p < 0.05$; b = severe HIE vs NAIS, $p < 0.05$

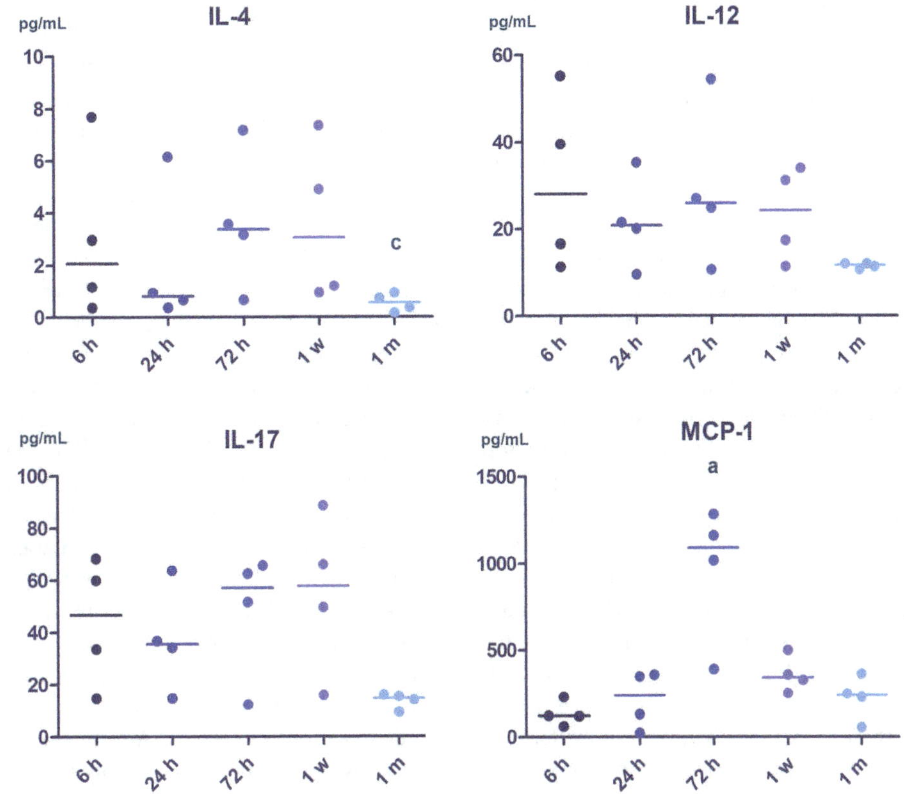

Fig. 2 Alterations of plasma cytokine levels in the first month of life in neonatal arterial ischemic stroke ($n = 4$). Horizontal line: median. $p < 0.05$ a vs 6 h, b vs 24 h, c vs 72 h

ischemic insult after in utero LPS exposure in a chorioamnionitis associated perinatal stroke murine model [5]. We found an elevation in the level of MCP-1 at 72 h compared to 6 h value in NAIS and to moderate HIE, which supports previous data emphasizing the role of in utero inflammation. Both the plasma levels of IL-17 and the prevalence of pro-inflammatory Th17 and γδ T cells are known to increase 1 week after adult acute ischemic stroke [49] and decrease by 1 month. In line with these findings, we found a higher level of IL-17 in the second

Table 4 Plasma cytokines

pg/mL		Moderate HIE ($n = 17$)	Severe HIE ($n = 11$)	NAIS ($n = 4$)
IL-5	72 h	1.37 (0.00–4.69)	0.20 (0.00–0.46)	3.42 (1.42–6.35) b, p = 0.01
IL-17	72 h	30.44 (26.65–51.62)	33.91 (29.16–48.02)	62.52 (51.62–645.7) a, p = 0.04, b, p = 0.05
MCP-1	72 h	251.9 (87.12–595.6)	678 (214–2311)	1090 (547.2–1254) a, p = 0.03
IL-4	1 month	1.68 (0.84–2.54)	1.52 (0.84–2.44)	0.55 (0.22–0.89) a, p = 0.04 b, p = 0.05
IL-12	1 month	18.11 (13.34–39.53)	21.52 (15.96–36.46)	11.74 (10.90–12.06) a, p = 0.05 b, p = 0.05
IL-17	1 month	32.58 (22.02–51.92)	31.11 (19.50–74.08)	14.75 (10.49–15.85) a, p = 0.02 b, p = 0.004

The plasma levels of cytokines are shown at different time points. Data are expressed as median and interquartile range; a = moderate HIE vs NAIS, $p < 0.05$; b = severe HIE vs NAIS, $p < 0.05$

phase (at 72 h) of neuroinflammation in NAIS compared with HIE. By 1 month, however, the level of IL-17 decreased in NAIS, while it remained elevated in HIE. We observed the same phenomenon with other cytokines such as IL-4 and IL-12. Overall, the plasma levels of several cytokines appear to decrease by 1 month of age in NAIS and appears to remain at a higher level in HIE.

We also found alterations in the anti-inflammatory pathways. IL-10 was thought to be primarily produced by CD4+ lymphocytes; however, Trandem et al. demonstrated in a murine model of virus encephalitis that the most highly activated and cytotoxic CD8+ T cells are also an important source of IL-10 at the peak of the inflammatory response. Their data suggests that CD8+ cells autoregulate their activation by IL-10 production when the inflammatory response reaches a certain level and that CD8-derived IL-10 has a primarily local effect to prevent tissue damage. IL-10 expression by CD8 cells rapidly decreased after 7 days, while CD4+ cells continued to express IL-10 for at least 42 days [50]. Our data showed a significantly higher prevalence of IL-10+ CD8 + lymphocytes in severe HIE than NAIS in the first 72 h of life. IL10-producing CD8 cells were also more prevalent in mild HIE than in NAIS; however, the difference was not significant. A lower prevalence of IL-10-producing CD8 cells, which at the same time produce more of pro-inflammatory cytokines such as IL-17, could lead to a more prominent pro-inflammatory and cytolytic response with decreased auto-regulatory IL-10 production in CD8 cells in NAIS in the first 72 h. Another interpretation could be that the decreased level of IL-10 production by CD8+ cells reflects an in utero inflammatory response that decreases by the time of birth. Supporting this hypothesis, in NAIS, we found elevated prevalence of IL10+ CD4+ lymphocytes, which are known to produce IL-10 for over a month following the insult. Altogether, it appears that IL-10 production is different in T cell subpopulations in NAIS and HIE and the manipulation of the IL-10 pathway could be interesting to explore from a neuroprotective point of view.

The prevalence of TGF-β-producing CD4+ cells, the majority of which are regulatory T (Treg) cells, was also different in NAIS and HIE. TGF-β is one of the most important cytokines regulating CNS repair. We found increased CD49d expression in this population in NAIS at 1 week compared to 24 h and both HIE groups, reflecting a higher capacity of these cells to enter the CNS. Meanwhile, the prevalence of the entire population decreased by 1 month in NAIS compared to HIE. This appears to be in line with plasma cytokine data, which showed an increased inflammatory response in NAIS in the second phase of neuroinflammation which could be followed by an earlier reparative phase and a decreasing inflammatory response by 1 month of age

Therapeutic hypothermia is currently the standard of care for term neonates with HIE. There is substantial evidence supporting the role of hypothermia in reducing mortality and improving neurological outcome [51] in infants with hypoxic ischemic encephalopathy. There is notable evidence in animal focal cerebral ischemia models supporting the role of hypothermia in the reduction of infarct size [52] and data suggesting that hypothermia might reduce the risk of seizures after perinatal stroke and thus improve outcome [53]. Therefore, there is intense discussion in the scientific community about extending guidelines to include new categories for therapeutic hypothermia such as preterm HIE and perinatal stroke; however, many issues remain to be addressed. Based on results from our previous study, one of the mechanisms behind the neuroprotective effect of hypothermia may be the reduction of systemic inflammatory response, seen in the reduced level of cytokines such as IL-6 and IL-4 in HIE patients treated with hypothermia compared to the normothermia group [54]. Therefore, it is likely that hypothermia may similarly reduce cytokine levels following NAIS.

The main limitation of these data is the small number of cases; however, they could provide a hypothesis for future, larger case-control studies. Another limitation is the lack of healthy control population; however, due to ethical considerations and the large number of blood sampling, enrolling healthy neonates was not possible. We also saw a notable variation in certain plasma cytokine levels, which is likely a result of the relative instability of plasma cytokine levels, which was the basis of primarily focusing on intracellular cytokine production in the current study. The value of the data from this study could lie in providing incentive for further clinical research on factors enabling differentiation between the two disorders which often present with similar symptoms at birth. Gaining a better understanding of the underlying pathophysiological factors is a main aim at the current stage of research in NAIS.

Conclusions

CD8 lymphocytes appear to show a shift in the pro-inflammatory direction in NAIS compared with HIE, with elevated production of pro-inflammatory IL-17 at 6 h, decreased auto-regulatory IL-10 production in the first 3 days, and elevated production of IL-6 at 1 month. Altogether, the inflammatory response appears to be higher at 72 h in NAIS than in HIE, but appears to decrease faster, indicated by lower levels of inflammatory markers at 1 month in NAIS than in HIE. Our data indicate similarities to observations in adult AIS and also support the hypothesis of an ongoing in utero inflammation prior to NAIS. Further clinical research in this area is pivotal, and a better understanding of the pathophysiology could lead to identifying specific factors to distinguish HIE from NAIS early and could open up new pathways for prevention and individualized care.

Abbreviations
ACA: Anterior cerebral artery; aEEG: Amplitude-integrated electroencephalography; AIS: Acute ischemic stroke; BFA: Brefeldin A; HIE: Hypoxic ischemic encephalopathy; MCA: Middle cerebral artery; MFI: Mean fluorescence intensity; NAIS: Neonatal arterial ischemic stroke; PCA: Posterior cerebral artery; PMA: Phorbol 12-myristate 13-acetate; Treg: Regulatory T cell

Funding
This work was supported by OTKA grant No. 109451.

Authors' contributions
GT was responsible for the study design, funding, and data interpretation and was a major contributor in writing the manuscript. AB performed flow cytometry measurements, analyzed the data, and was responsible for writing the manuscript. CO and LB performed flow cytometry measurements. TT made contributions to study conception and design and revised the manuscript critically. All authors read and approved the final manuscript.

Consent for publication
Written informed consent was obtained from parents of all participants.

Competing interests
The authors declare that they have no competing interests.

Author details
[1]First Department of Obstetrics and Gynecology, Semmelweis University, Baross str. 27, Budapest H-1088, Hungary. [2]First Department of Pediatrics, Semmelweis University, Bókay János str. 53-54, Budapest H-1083, Hungary. [3]MTA-SE Pediatrics and Nephrology Research Group, Budapest, Hungary. [4]Neonatal Unit, Birmingham Women's and Children's Hospital, Birmingham, UK.

References
1. Raju TN, Nelson KB, Ferriero D, Lynch JK. Ischemic perinatal stroke: summary of a workshop sponsored by the National Institute of Child Health and Human Development and the National Institute of Neurological Disorders and Stroke. Pediatrics. 2007;120(3):609–16.
2. Kirton A, Deveber G. Life after perinatal stroke. Stroke. 2013;44(11):3265–71.
3. Giraud A, Guiraut C, Chevin M, Chabrier S, Sebire G. Role of perinatal inflammation in neonatal arterial ischemic stroke. Front Neurol. 2017;8:612.
4. Nelson KB, Lynch JK. Stroke in newborn infants. Lancet Neurol. 2004; 3(3):150–8.
5. Guiraut C, Cauchon N, Lepage M, Sebire G. Perinatal arterial ischemic stroke is associated to materno-fetal immune activation and intracranial arteritis. Int J Mol Sci. 2016;17(12).
6. Osborn AG. Diagnostic cerebral angiography. Am J Neuroradiol. 1999;20(9):1767–9.
7. Kirton A, deVeber G. Paediatric stroke: pressing issues and promising directions. Lancet Neurol. 2015;14(1):92–102.
8. Ramaswamy V, Miller SP, Barkovich AJ, Partridge JC, Ferriero DM. Perinatal stroke in term infants with neonatal encephalopathy. Neurology. 2004; 62(11):2088–91.
9. Kirton A, Armstrong-Wells J, Chang T, Deveber G, Rivkin MJ, Hernandez M, Carpenter J, Yager JY, Lynch JK, Ferriero DM. Symptomatic neonatal arterial ischemic stroke: the international pediatric stroke study. Pediatrics. 2011; 128(6):e1402–10.
10. Chalmers EA. Perinatal stroke–risk factors and management. Br J Haematol. 2005;130(3):333–43.
11. Govaert P, Matthys E, Zecic A, Roelens F, Oostra A, Vanzieleghem B. Perinatal cortical infarction within middle cerebral artery trunks. Arch Dis Child Fetal Neonatal Ed. 2000;82(1):F59–63.
12. Lanthier S, Carmant L, David M, Larbrisseau A, de Veber G. Stroke in children: the coexistence of multiple risk factors predicts poor outcome. Neurology. 2000;54(2):371–8.
13. Darmency-Stamboul V, Chantegret C, Ferdynus C, Mejean N, Durand C, Sagot P, Giroud M, Bejot Y, Gouyon JB. Antenatal factors associated with perinatal arterial ischemic stroke. Stroke. 2012;43(9):2307–12.
14. Harteman JC, Groenendaal F, Kwee A, Welsing PM, Benders MJ, de Vries LS. Risk factors for perinatal arterial ischaemic stroke in full-term infants: a case-control study. Arch Dis Child Fetal Neonatal Ed. 2012;97(6):F411–6.
15. Bernson-Leung ME, Rivkin MJ. Stroke in neonates and children. Pediatr Rev. 2016;37(11):463–77.
16. Husson B, Hertz-Pannier L, Adamsbaum C, Renaud C, Presles E, Dinomais M, Kossorotoff M, Landrieu P, Chabrier S. MR angiography findings in infants with neonatal arterial ischemic stroke in the middle cerebral artery territory: a prospective study using circle of Willis MR angiography. Eur J Radiol. 2016; 85(7):1329–35.
17. Schouten M, Wiersinga WJ, Levi M, van der Poll T. Inflammation, endothelium, and coagulation in sepsis. J Leukoc Biol. 2008;83(3):536–45.
18. Larouche A, Roy M, Kadhim H, Tsanaclis AM, Fortin D, Sebire G. Neuronal injuries induced by perinatal hypoxic-ischemic insults are potentiated by prenatal exposure to lipopolysaccharide: animal model for perinatally acquired encephalopathy. Dev Neurosci. 2005;27(2–4):134–42.
19. Mallard C, Hagberg H. Inflammation-induced preconditioning in the immature brain. Semin Fetal Neonatal Med. 2007;12(4):280–6.
20. Wang X, Hagberg H, Nie C, Zhu C, Ikeda T, Mallard C. Dual role of intrauterine immune challenge on neonatal and adult brain vulnerability to hypoxia-ischemia. J Neuropathol Exp Neurol. 2007;66(6):552–61.
21. Davidson JO, Wassink G, van den Heuij LG, Bennet L, Gunn AJ. Therapeutic hypothermia for neonatal hypoxic-ischemic encephalopathy—where to from here? Front Neurol. 2015;6:198.
22. Kratzer I, Chip S, Vexler ZS. Barrier mechanisms in neonatal stroke. Front Neurosci. 2014;8:359.
23. Wang Q, Tang XN, Yenari MA. The inflammatory response in stroke. J Neuroimmunol. 2007;184(1–2):53–68.
24. Savard A, Lavoie K, Brochu ME, Grbic D, Lepage M, Gris D, Sebire G. Involvement of neuronal IL-1β in acquired brain lesions in a rat model of neonatal encephalopathy. J Neuroinflammation. 2013;10:110.
25. Savard A, Brochu ME, Chevin M, Guiraut C, Grbic D, Sébire G. Neuronal self-injury mediated by IL-1β and MMP-9 in a cerebral palsy model of severe neonatal encephalopathy induced by immune activation plus hypoxia-ischemia. J Neuroinflammation. 2015;12:111.
26. Eliwan HO, Watson RW, Aslam S, Regan I, Philbin B, O'Hare FM, O'Neill A, Preston R, Blanco A, Grant T, et al. Neonatal brain injury and systemic inflammation: modulation by activated protein C ex vivo. Clin Exp Immunol. 2015;179(3):477–84.
27. Stridh L, Smith PL, Naylor AS, Wang X, Mallard C. Regulation of toll-like receptor 1 and -2 in neonatal mice brains after hypoxia-ischemia. J Neuroinflammation. 2011;8:45.
28. Wang X, Stridh L, Li W, Dean J, Elmgren A, Gan L, Eriksson K, Hagberg H, Mallard C. Lipopolysaccharide sensitizes neonatal hypoxic-ischemic brain injury in a MyD88-dependent manner. J Immunol. 2009;183(11):7471–7.
29. Carlsson Y, Schwendimann L, Vontell R, Rousset CI, Wang X, Lebon S, Charriaut-Marlangue C, Supramaniam V, Hagberg H, Gressens P, et al. Genetic inhibition of caspase-2 reduces hypoxic-ischemic and excitotoxic neonatal brain injury. Ann Neurol. 2011;70(5):781–9.
30. Nijboer CH, Heijnen CJ, van der Kooij MA, Zijlstra J, van Velthoven CT, Culmsee C, van Bel F, Hagberg H, Kavelaars A. Targeting the p53 pathway to protect the neonatal ischemic brain. Ann Neurol. 2011;70(2):255–64.
31. Winerdal M, Winerdal ME, Kinn J, Urmaliya V, Winqvist O, Aden U. Long lasting local and systemic inflammation after cerebral hypoxic ischemia in newborn mice. PLoS One. 2012;7(5):e36422.
32. Yururer D, Teber S, Deda G, Egin Y, Akar N. The relation between cytokines, soluble endothelial protein C receptor, and factor VIII levels in Turkish pediatric stroke patients. Clin Appl Thromb Hemost. 2009;15(5):545–51.
33. Yilmaz G, Arumugam TV, Stokes KY, Granger DN. Role of T lymphocytes and interferon-gamma in ischemic stroke. Circulation. 2006;113(17):2105–12.
34. Vogelgesang A, Becker KJ, Dressel A. Immunological consequences of ischemic stroke. Acta Neurol Scand. 2014;129(1):1–12.
35. Siniscalchi A, Gallelli L, Malferrari G, Pirritano D, Serra R, Santangelo E, De

Sarro G. Cerebral stroke injury: the role of cytokines and brain inflammation. J Basic Clin Physiol Pharmacol. 2014;25(2):131–7.
36. Zhu Y, Yang GY, Ahlemeyer B, Pang L, Che XM, Culmsee C, Klumpp S, Krieglstein J. Transforming growth factor-beta 1 increases bad phosphorylation and protects neurons against damage. J Neurosci. 2002; 22(10):3898–909.
37. Spera PA, Ellison JA, Feuerstein GZ, Barone FC. IL-10 reduces rat brain injury following focal stroke. Neurosci Lett. 1998;251(3):189–92.
38. Azzopardi D, Brocklehurst P, Edwards D, Halliday H, Levene M, Thoresen M, Whitelaw A. The TOBY study. Whole body hypothermia for the treatment of perinatal asphyxial encephalopathy: a randomised controlled trial. BMC Pediatr. 2008;8:17.
39. Counsell SJ, Tranter SL, Rutherford MA. Magnetic resonance imaging of brain injury in the high-risk term infant. Semin Perinatol. 2010;34(1):67–78.
40. Rutherford M, Malamateniou C, McGuinness A, Allsop J, Biarge MM, Counsell S. Magnetic resonance imaging in hypoxic-ischaemic encephalopathy. Early Hum Dev. 2010;86(6):351–60.
41. Bajnok A, Berta L, Orban C, Veres G, Zadori D, Barta H, Meder U, Vecsei L, Tulassay T, Szabo M, et al. Distinct cytokine patterns may regulate the severity of neonatal asphyxia-an observational study. J Neuroinflammation. 2017;14(1):244.
42. Gelderblom M, Leypoldt F, Steinbach K, Behrens D, Choe CU, Siler DA, Arumugam TV, Orthey E, Gerloff C, Tolosa E, et al. Temporal and spatial dynamics of cerebral immune cell accumulation in stroke. Stroke. 2009;40(5):1849–57.
43. Liesz A, Zhou W, Mracsko E, Karcher S, Bauer H, Schwarting S, Sun L, Bruder D, Stegemann S, Cerwenka A, et al. Inhibition of lymphocyte trafficking shields the brain against deleterious neuroinflammation after stroke. Brain. 2011;134(Pt 3):704–20.
44. Selvaraj UM, Stowe AM. Long-term T cell responses in the brain after an ischemic stroke. Discov Med. 2017;24(134):323–33.
45. Sun L, Li Y, Jia X, Wang Q, Li Y, Hu M, Tian L, Yang J, Xing W, Zhang W, et al. Neuroprotection by IFN-γ via astrocyte-secreted IL-6 in acute neuroinflammation. Oncotarget. 2017;8(25):40065–78.
46. Loddick SA, Turnbull AV, Rothwell NJ. Cerebral interleukin-6 is neuroprotective during permanent focal cerebral ischemia in the rat. J Cereb Blood Flow Metab. 1998;18(2):176–9.
47. Hirota H, Kiyama H, Kishimoto T, Taga T. Accelerated nerve regeneration in mice by upregulated expression of interleukin (IL) 6 and IL-6 receptor after trauma. J Exp Med. 1996;183(6):2627–34.
48. Sébire G, Emilie D, Wallon C, Héry C, Devergne O, Delfraissy JF, Galanaud P, Tardieu M. In vitro production of IL-6, IL-1 beta, and tumor necrosis factor-alpha by human embryonic microglial and neural cells. J Immunol. 1993; 150(4):1517–23.
49. Hu Y, Zheng Y, Wu Y, Ni B, Shi S. Imbalance between IL-17A-producing cells and regulatory T cells during ischemic stroke. Mediat Inflamm. 2014;2014:813045.
50. Trandem K, Zhao J, Fleming E, Perlman S. Highly activated cytotoxic CD8 T cells express protective IL-10 at the peak of coronavirus-induced encephalitis. J Immunol. 2011;186(6):3642–52.
51. Azzopardi D, Strohm B, Marlow N, Brocklehurst P, Deierl A, Eddama O, Goodwin J, Halliday HL, Juszczak E, Kapellou O, et al. Effects of hypothermia for perinatal asphyxia on childhood outcomes. N Engl J Med. 2014;371(2):140–9.
52. Gancia P, Pomero G. Therapeutic hypothermia in the prevention of hypoxic-ischaemic encephalopathy: new categories to be enrolled. J Matern Fetal Neonatal Med. 2012;25(Suppl 4):94–6.
53. Harbert MJ, Tam EW, Glass HC, Bonifacio SL, Haeusslein LA, Barkovich AJ, Jeremy RJ, Rogers EE, Glidden DV, Ferriero DM. Hypothermia is correlated with seizure absence in perinatal stroke. J Child Neurol. 2011;26(9):1126–30.
54. Roka A, Beko G, Halasz J, Toldi G, Lakatos P, Azzopardi D, Tulassay T, Szabo M. Changes in serum cytokine and cortisol levels in normothermic and hypothermic term neonates after perinatal asphyxia. Inflamm Res. 2013; 62(1):81–7.

16

Arginine vasopressin altered the expression of monocarboxylate transporters in cultured astrocytes isolated from stroke-prone spontaneously hypertensive rats and congenic SHRpch1_18 rats

Kazuo Yamagata[1*], Natsumi Takahashi[1], Nozomi Akita[1] and Toru Nabika[2]

Abstract

Background: Astrocytes support a range of brain functions as well as neuronal survival, but their detailed relationship with stroke-related edema is not well understood. We previously demonstrated that the release of lactate from astrocytes isolated from stroke-prone spontaneously hypertensive rats (SHRSP/Izm) was attenuated under stroke conditions. The supply of lactate to neurons is regulated by astrocytic monocarboxylate transporters (MCTs). The purpose of this study was to examine the contributions of arginine vasopressin (AVP) and/or hypoxia and reoxygenation (H/R) to the regulation of MCTs and neurotrophic factor in astrocytes obtained from SHRSP/Izm and congenic SHRpch1_18 rats.

Methods: We compared AVP-induced lactate levels, MCTs, and brain-derived neurotrophic factor (BDNF) in astrocytes isolated from SHRSP/Izm, SHRpch1_18, and Wistar Kyoto rats (WKY/Izm). The expression levels of genes and proteins were determined by PCR and Western blotting (WB).

Results: The production of lactate induced by AVP was increased in astrocytes from all three strains. However, the levels of lactate were lower in SHRSP/Izm and SHRpch1_18 animals compared with the WKY/Izm strain. Gene expression levels of *Slc16a1*, *Slc16a4*, and *Bdnf* were lowered by AVP in SHRSP/Izm and SHRpch1_18 rats compared with WKY/Izm. The increase of MCT4 that was induced by AVP was blocked by the addition of a specific nitric oxide (NO) chelator, 2-(4-carboxyphenyl)-4,4,5,5-tetramethylimidazoline-1-oxyl-3-oxide (CPTIO). Furthermore, AVP increased the expression of iNOS and eNOS proteins in WKY/Izm and SHRSP/Izm rat astrocytes. However, the iNOS expression levels in SHRSP astrocytes differed from those of WKY/Izm astrocytes. The increase of MCT4 protein expression during AVP treatment was blocked by the addition of a specific NF-kB inhibitor, pyrrolidine dithiocarbamate (PDTC). The induction of MCT4 by AVP may be regulated by NO through NF-kB.

Conclusions: These results suggest that the expression of MCTs mediated by AVP may be regulated by NO. The data suggest that AVP attenuated the expression of MCTs in SHRSP/Izm and SHRpch1_18 astrocytes. Reduced expression of MCTs may be associated with decreased lactate production in SHRSP.

Keywords: Astrocytes, BDNF, SHRSP, MCT4

* Correspondence: kyamagat@brs.nihon-u.ac.jp
[1]Laboratory of Molecular Health of Food, Department of Food Bioscience and Biotechnology, College of Bioresource Sciences, Nihon University (NUBS), 1866, Kameino, Fujisawa, Kanagawa 252-8510, Japan
Full list of author information is available at the end of the article

Gene approved symbols MCT1; *SLC16A1*, MCT4; *SLC16A4*, BDNF; *Bdnf*

Background

Stroke-prone spontaneously hypertensive rats (SHRSP) develop severe hypertension and die of a stroke [1]. Following the induction of a stroke (ischemic conditions), neuronal cell death [2], and astrocytic edema [3] are observed in SHRSP/Izm animals (where "Izm" indicates the maintaining institution). In SHR brains, the expression of MCTs occurs after occlusion of the middle cerebral artery (MCAO) [4]. The SHRpch1_18 rat was produced by introducing the quantitative trait loci (QTLs) of chromosomes 1 and 18 from SHRSP/Izm into SHR/Izm [5]. SHRpch1_18 rats have salt sensitivity that may enhance stroke onset. In addition, we demonstrated that the release of lactate was significantly lower in astrocytes isolated from SHRSP/Izm rats than Wistar Kyoto rats/Izm (WKY/Izm) under ischemic conditions such as hypoxia and reoxygenation (H/R) [2, 6, 7].

Brain lactate is released from astrocytes under ischemic conditions. It is utilized as the sole energy substrate supporting neuronal functions [8]. A reduced supply of lactate from astrocytes under pathologic conditions, such as ischemia, is associated with neuronal cell death [9]. Following ischemic stimulation, the supply of lactate provided by astrocytes to neurons is regulated by several monocarboxylate transporters (MCTs) [10, 11]. MCTs are transporters of monocarboxylates such as lactate, pyruvate, and ketone bodies [12]. In the brain, three MCT isoforms have been identified: MCT1, MCT2, and MCT4. Within the brain, MCT1 is present in astrocytes, endothelial cells of blood vessels, and ependymocytes [12, 13]. In contrast, MCT2 is expressed by cultured brain neurons [12, 13]. MCT1 and MCT4 are strongly expressed by cortical astrocytes. These results suggest that astrocytes supply lactic acid to neuronal cells [12, 13]. Specifically, MCT1 and MCT4 regulate lactate release by astrocytes, whereas MCT2 regulates lactate uptake by neuronal cells [13]. On the other hand, dysfunction of these astrocytic MCTs may attenuate lactate production and increase neuronal injury [14].

Brain-derived neurotrophic factor (BDNF) regulates neuronal cell growth, neuronal synaptic plasticity, long-term memory, and neuronal cell survival [15]. Furthermore, in rats, BDNF enhances blood pressure in the hypothalamus (PVN) by angiotensin signaling [16]. In rat astrocytes, the anti-epileptic drug valproate enhances the expression of BDNF [17] and inducible nitric oxide synthase (iNOS), and they regulate inflammation and neuronal cell death under pathological conditions [18]. In addition, concentrations of BDNF are reduced in the acute phase of ischemic strokes, and it is associated with the risk of stroke onset [19]. In SHRSP strains, a mutation of the *TrkB* gene, which encodes the receptor for BDNF, has been found [20]. In particular, BDNF plays an important role in promoting neuronal survival [21, 22]. During ischemia, lactate and BDNF production may be regulated by astrocytes [23].

Arginine-vasopressin (AVP) induces production of inflammatory molecules after cerebral edema [24], and it is associated with disruption of the blood-brain barrier (BBB) [25]. In addition, AVP enhances ischemia-evoked edema in the cortex in ischemic strokes [26]. It was further demonstrated that the AVP V1 receptor inhibitor reduced ischemia-induced cerebral edema following stroke [27]. In particular, AVP influences astrocytic function, thereby contributing to the onset of stroke [28]. Under ischemic conditions, AVP might be related to augmented inflammation and serine production, and perhaps stroke in SHRSP/Izm rats [29, 30]. However, there is little understanding regarding AVP and MCT expression. For example, AVP-induced events (such as cerebral edema) are associated with stroke. However, in SHRSP astrocytes, the relationship between lactate control and BDNF expression by AVP is not known. We hypothesized that the reduction of lactate or BDNF expression by AVP might be related to the induction of stroke in the SHRSP/Izm rat strain. The purpose of this study was to examine the contributions of AVP and/or H/R to the regulation of MCTs and neurotrophic factor in astrocytes from SHRSP/Izm and congenic SHRpch1_18 rats. Here, we compared AVP-induced lactate levels, MCTs, and BDNF in astrocytes isolated from SHRSP/Izm and SHRpch1_18 and WKY/Izm rats.

Methods

Cell cultures and treatments

Primary dissociated astrocytes were isolated from fetal cerebral WKY/Izm, SHR/Izm, and SHRSP/Izm rats (Japan SLC, Inc., Tokyo, Japan) and the congenic rat strain, SHRpch1_18, as described previously [30, 31]. The SHRpch1_18 strain was produced by introducing the quantitative trait loci (QTL) for stroke sensitivity on chromosomes 1 and 18 of SHRSP/Izm into SHR/Izm [5]. Cultured cells consisted of > 95% astrocytes as determined by glial fibrillary acidic protein (GFAP, Doka Japan, Japan) staining. Astrocytes were plated on 90-mm culture dishes and cultured in Dulbecco's modified Eagle's medium (DMEM, Sigma, Japan) containing 10% fetal bovine serum (FBS, Sigma), penicillin (100 U/mL, Life Technologies, Japan), and streptomycin (100 μg/mL, Life Technologies, Sigma-Aldrich) until they reached confluence at 37 °C in a CO_2 incubator (95% air and 5% CO_2). The studies described here were approved by the Nihon University animal care and use committee (Approval number; AP15B068).

Astrocytes were seeded on 90-mm, 24-well culture plates (Sumitomo Bakelite Co., LTD, Tokyo, Japan) at an initial density of 40 × 10^4 cells per cm^2 and were grown in DMEM containing 10% FBS until confluence was reached.

For L-serine measurement, the confluent astrocytes were growth-arrested for 1 day in L-serine-free DMEM (GIBCO BRL, no. 61100) containing 0.2% FBS. Subsequently, the astrocytes' medium was changed to 100 nM AVP-supplemented (Sigma-Aldrich) or L-serine-free, 0.2% FBS-supplemented DMEM lacking AVP as a control. Hypoxia and reoxygenation stimulation exposed the cells to hypoxic conditions. Namely, the astrocytes were cultured in 1% O_2, 94% N_2, and 5% CO_2 in a CO_2 incubator (Wakenyaku, Co, Ltd., Japan) for 24 h. Subsequently, the astrocytes were stimulated in air (21% O_2) and 5% CO_2 for reoxygenation (30 min or 2 h), as indicated previously [2, 6, 7]. The confluent growth of astrocytes was treated with or without 2-(4-carboxyphenyl)-4,4,5,5-tetramethylimidazoline-1-oxyl-3-oxide (CPTIO, Dojindo Laboratories, Japan, 200 μM) or pyrrolidine dithiocarbamate (PDTC, Sigma-Aldrich) for 60 min before addition of AVP and 20 μM sodium nitroprusside (SNP, Wako Pure Chemical Inc., Japan).

Measurement of lactate contents in astrocyte-conditioned medium

The lactate content of astrocyte-conditioned medium was measured with an assay kit (Boehringer Mannheim, IN, USA). Protein levels were measured using the Bio-Rad protein assay kit (Bio-Rad, CA, USA), based on the Lowry method, with bovine serum albumin (BSA) as a standard.

Extraction of total RNA and cDNA synthesis

Total RNA was isolated from cultured astrocytes using TRIzol reagent (Life Technologies Japan Ltd., Tokyo, Japan). DNase I (Life Technologies Japan Ltd.) was added at room temperature for 20 min to remove genomic DNA. DNase I was treated for 15 min at 65 °C to inactivate enzyme activity. Synthesis of the first-strand cDNA was performed using the Superscript III kit (Life Technologies, Japan Ltd.).

Reverse transcription- polymerase chain reaction (PCR) and quantitative PCR

RT-PCR was carried out to analyze the expression of genes as described in our previous study [30]. After the reaction, gene amplicons were analyzed by 2% agarose electrophoresis (FMC Products, Rockland, ME, USA) and visualized with UV illumination after staining with ethidium bromide. Gene expression levels were evaluated relative to 18S ribosomal RNA (rRNA). Quantitative PCR was performed with the Sequence Detector System (Applied Biosystems, Foster City, CA) [32], as described previously [6]. Quantitative PCR was carried out for MCT1 (*Slc16A1*), MCT4 (*Slc16A4*), and BDNF (*Bdnf*) and to monitor the expression of a housekeeping gene, 18S rRNA (rRNA). Serial dilutions (1:5) of cDNA were used to create a standard curve for the quantitation of gene expression. Primers and TaqMan probes were designed with a primer design software, Primer Express (Applied Biosystems). The forward primer was 5′-TCGTTGGACCCCAGAGGT-3′ for *Slc16a1*, and the reverse primer was 5′-AGGACAGGACAAC ATTCCACA-3′. The primers for *Slc16a1* amplified a fragment of 67 bp. The sequence of the TaqMan probe was 5′-CAGTGCTGTGGGCTTGGTGACCA-3′ for *Slc16a1*. The forward primer for *Slc16a4* was 5′-CAGGTTTTTGG GATATGCCA-3′. The reverse primer for *Slc16a4* was 5′-TCCAGCCTGCT ATTGGTGG-3′. The primer sequence for *Slc16a4* amplified a fragment of 71 bp. The sequence of the TaqMan probe was 5′-TTTCTTTGCTGGGA TGGCTGTTCTTTC-3′ for *Slc16a4*. The forward primer chosen for *Bdnf* was 5′-CCATAAGGACGCGGACTTG-3′. The reverse primer was 5′-GAGCAGAGGAGGCTCC AAAG-3′. The primer sequence for *Bdnf* amplified a fragment of 73 bp. The sequence of the TaqMan probe was 5′-TCCCGGGTGATGCTCAGCAGTC-3′ for *Bdnf*. The details of quantitative PCR were outlined in our previous report [6] of RT-PCR were confirmed by quantitative PCR.

Evaluation of protein expression by Western blot

Astrocytes were lysed in RIPA buffer (Thermo Fisher Scientific K.K. Tokyo, Japan, 25 mM Tris-HCl pH 7.6, 150 mM NaCl, 1% NP-40, 1% sodium deoxycholate, and 0.1% SDS) containing a complete protease inhibitor cocktail (Roche Diagnostics). Cell lysates (30 μg protein/line) were assessed by SDS-PAGE and transferred to polyvinylidene difluoride membranes. Membranes were treated with a horseradish peroxidase-conjugated antibody (Life Technologies), and expression levels were examined using an enhanced chemiluminescence system (Life Technologies) with a C-Digit blot scanner (MS Techno Systems Inc. Tokyo, Japan). Antibodies for anti-MCT1 antibody (1: 200, Santa Cruz Biotechnology, USA: sc-50325), anti-MCT4 (1:200, Santa Cruz Biotechnology, USA: sc-50329), anti-iNOS (1:500, Abcam, ab 3523), anti-eNOS (1:1000, Cell Signaling Technology, The Netherlands: #32027), and β-actin (1:1000, Cell Signaling Technology: #4967) were used.

Statistical analysis

Data are presented as means ± SE. The significance of differences was determined using Fisher's protected least significant difference (PLSD) method following an analysis of variance (ANOVA).

Results

Effect of AVP on the production of lactate by astrocytes isolated from WKY/Izm, SHRSP/Izm, and SHRpch1_18h rats

Astrocytes provide lactate to neuronal cells for use as an energy substrate. Astrocytes isolated from WKY/Izm, SHRSP/Izm, and SHRpch1_18 strains were treated with AVP, and we determined the individual levels of lactate. In WKY/Izm, SHRSP/Izm, and SHRpch1_18 astrocytes, addition of 100 nM AVP enhanced the level of lactate production during the 24 h treatment (Fig. 1). However, the level of production of lactate was significantly ($p < 0.05$) lower in SHRSP/Izm and SHRpch1_18 strains than in WKY/Izm astrocytes at 100 nM AVP. Specifically, after 24 h, AVP-enhanced lactate production increased about 3.03-fold (WKY/Izm), 2.34-fold (SHRSP/Izm), and 2.44-fold (SHRpch1_18) above the control level in astrocytes isolated from WKY/Izm, SHRSP/Izm, and SHRpch1_18 rats, respectively. Effect of AVP on gene expression levels of Slc16a1, Slc16a4, and Bdnf in astrocytes isolated from WKY/Izm, SHRSP/Izm, and SHRpch1_18 rats.

Effect of AVP on Slc16a1, Slc16a4, and Bdnf gene expression in astrocytes from WKY/Izm, SHRSP/Izm, and SHRpch1_18 rats

The expression of a lactate transport gene (*Slc16a1*) was compared in astrocytes isolated from three strains (WKY/Izm, SHRSP/Izm, and SHRpch1_18h) following 8 h treatment with AVP (10, 50, and 100 μM). In astrocyte of three strains, AVP increased gene expression of *Slc16a1* (Fig. 2a). However, the gene expression level of *Slc16a1* in astrocytes was significantly lower ($p < 0.05$) in cells from SHRSP/Izm and SHRpch1_18 rats than in those from WKY/Izm rats at 10, 50, and 100 nM AVP ($p < 0.001$). In 100 nM AVP, enhanced gene expression was about 1.25-fold, 1.13-fold, and 1.12-fold the control level in astrocytes isolated from WKY/Izm, SHRSP/Izm, and SHRpch1_18 rats, respectively. Similarly, the expression of the *Slc16a4* gene was compared in astrocytes isolated from three strains following an 8 h treatment with AVP (10, 50, and 100 nM) (Fig. 2). In all astrocytes, AVP increased gene expression of *Slc16a4*. However, gene expression of *Slc16a4*

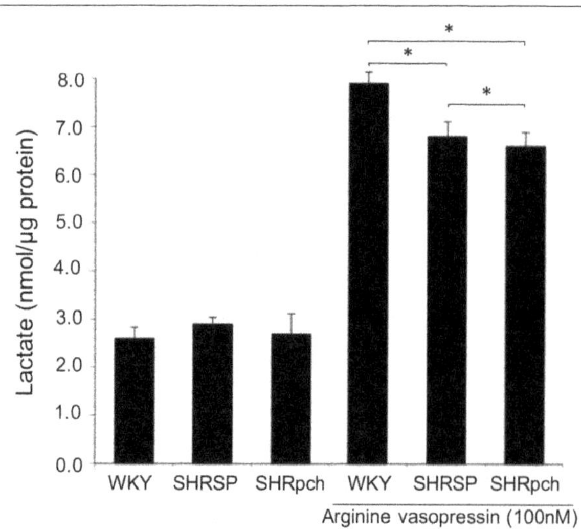

Fig. 1 Effect of AVP on lactate production by astrocytes isolated from WKY/Izm, SHRSP/Izm, and SHRpch1_18 rats. Confluent astrocytes isolated from WKY/Izm, SHRSP/Izm, and SHRpch1_18 rats were exposed to 0 or 100 nM AVP for 24 h. WKY, WKY/Izm; SHRSP, SHRSP/Izm; SHRpch; SHRpch1_18. Columns show means ± SE ($n = 4$). *$P < 0.05$

was significantly lower in SHRSP/Izm (1.0-, 1.12-, and 1.22-fold) and SHRpch1_18 (1.0-, 1.08-, and 1.1-fold) than in WKY/Izm (1.15-, 1.2-, and 1.37-fold) rat astrocytes at 10, 50, and 100 nM of AVP ($p < 0.05$). Furthermore, the expression levels of genes for neurotrophic factor *Bdnf* were compared in astrocytes isolated from the three strains after 8 h exposure to AVP (10, 50, and 100 μM) (Fig. 3). In astrocytes isolated from the three strains, gene expression levels of *Bdnf* were significantly increased by addition of AVP in a dose-dependent manner. In WKY/Izm astrocytes, increased levels were 1.16-, 1.24-, and 1.28-fold higher in 10, 50, and 100 nM AVP compared with basal levels, respectively (Fig. 2c). However, the gene expression levels of *Bdnf* were significantly lower in cells from the SHRSP/Izm (1.06-, 1.10-, and 1.24-fold) and SHRpch1_18 (1.01-, 1.15-, and 1.26-fold) strains than those from WKY/Izm (1.16-, 1.24-, and 1.28-fold) rat astrocytes at 10, 50, and 100 nM of AVP ($p < 0.05$). These results were confirmed by real-time PCR. Thus, the gene expression levels of *Slc16a1* and *Slc16a4* were significantly lower ($p < 0.05$) in cells from the SHRSP/Izm and SHRpch1_18 strains than those from WKY/Izm rat astrocytes at 50 and 100 nM AVP.

Effect of AVP during normoxia and hypoxia on Slc16a1 and Slc16a4 gene expression in astrocytes isolated from WKY/Izm and SHRpch1_18 rats

AVP and hypoxia induce astrocytic edema [33]. Therefore, cultured astrocytes isolated from WKY/Izm and SHRpch1_18 rats were exposed to 21% O_2 (normoxic conditions) or 1% O_2 (hypoxic conditions) for 24 h with or without 100 nM AVP. After 24 h normoxic conditions, *Slc16a1* gene expression levels in WKY/Izm astrocytes were significantly ($p < 0.05$) increased by AVP treatment compared to control cells, but this was not observed in SHRpch1_18 cells (Fig. 3a). Following 24 h hypoxic conditions, *Slc16a1* gene expression levels in WKY/Izm and SHRpch1_18 astrocytes were significantly ($p < 0.05$) increased by AVP treatment compared to control cells. However, expression of *Slc16a1* was significantly ($p < 0.05$) lower in SHRpch1_18 rat astrocytes than in WKY/Izm rat astrocytes in 100 nM AVP (Fig. 3a). In addition, the level of gene expression of *Slc16a1* was significantly ($p < 0.05$) lower in SHRpch1_18 astrocytes than WKY/Izm astrocytes under hypoxic conditions. Similarly, gene expression of *Slc16a4* was examined. As shown in Fig. 3b, after 24 h of normoxia, *Slc16a4* gene expression levels in WKY/Izm rat astrocytes were significantly ($p < 0.05$) increased by AVP treatment compared to control cells, but this did not occur in SHRpch1_18 cells. Under hypoxic conditions, *Slc16a4* gene expression in astrocytes isolated from WKY/Izm and SHRpch1_18 rats was significantly ($p < 0.05$) increased by AVP treatment compared to control cells. On the other hand, gene

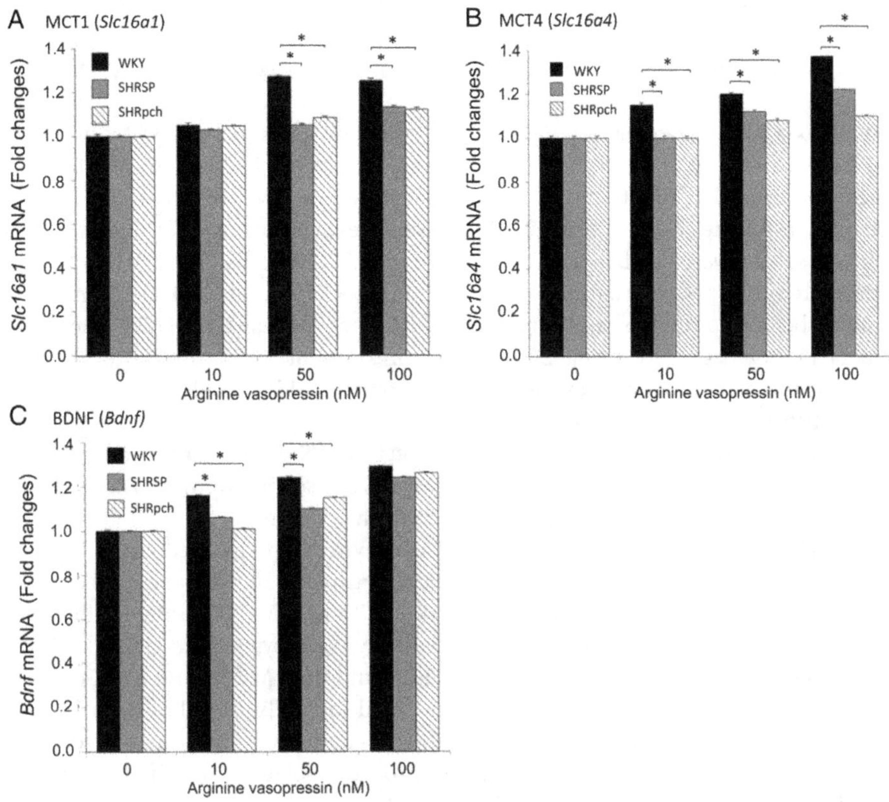

Fig. 2 Effect of AVP on *Slc16a1*, *Slc16a4*, and *Bdnf* gene expression in astrocytes from WKY/Izm, SHRSP/Izm, and SHRpch1_18 rats. Confluent astrocytes isolated from SHRSP/Izm, SHRpch1_18 rats, and WKY/Izm were exposed to 10, 50, or 100 nM AVP for 8 h, after which total cellular RNA was used for RT-PCR analysis. Comparison of **a** *Slc16a1*, **b** *Slc16a4*, and **c** *Bdnf* gene expression in astrocytes from all assayed rat strains. Gene expression levels were normalized to 18S ribosomal RNA. WKY WKY/Izm, SHRSP SHRSP/Izm, SHRpch SHRpch1_18. Columns show means ± SE ($n = 4$). $^*P < 0.05$

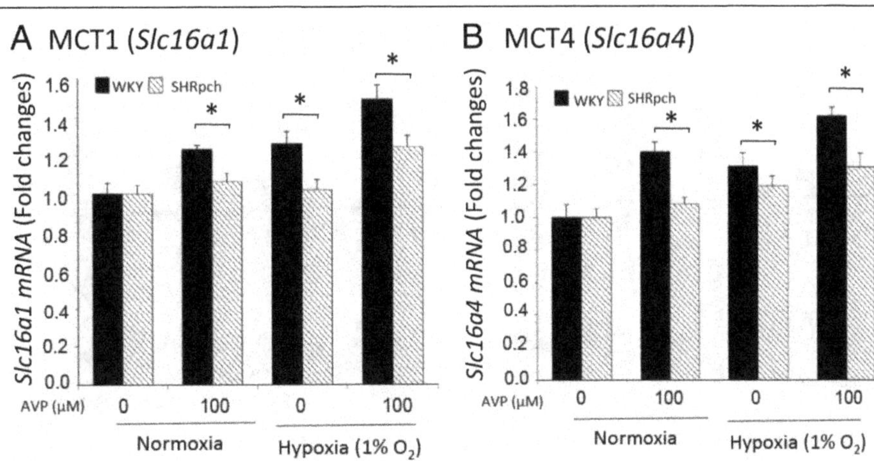

Fig. 3 Effect of AVP during normoxia and hypoxia on *Slc16a1* and *Slc16a4* gene expression in astrocytes isolated from WKY/Izm and SHRpch1_18 rats. Confluent astrocytes isolated from WKY/Izm and SHRpch1_18 rats were exposed to normoxic (21% O_2) or hypoxic (1% O_2) conditions for 24 h with or without 100 nM AVP. Total cellular RNA was isolated from the cultured astrocytes for RT-PCR, using primers for *Slc16a1* or *Slc16a4*. **a** *Slc16a1* and **b** *Slc16a4* gene expression from astrocytes from all assayed rat strains. Columns show means ± SE ($n = 4$). Normoxia 21% O_2, hypoxia 1% O_2. AVP arginine vasopressin. $^*P < 0.05$

expression of *Slc16a4* was significantly lower ($p < 0.05$) in SHRpch1_18 than in WKY/Izm rat cells at 100 nM AVP in normoxic and hypoxic conditions.

Effect of AVP during hypoxia and reoxygenation (H/R) on Slc16a1 and Slc16a4 gene expression in astrocytes isolated from WKY/Izm and SHRpch1_18 rats

In additional experiments, astrocytes isolated from WKY/Izm and SHRpch1_18 rat strains were incubated in 1% O_2 for 24 h and then transferred to 21% O_2 for 30 min or 2 h; 100 nM AVP was added before both hypoxia and reoxygenation. In 30 min of reoxygenation following 24 h of hypoxia, *Slc16a1* gene expression in astrocytes isolated from WKY/Izm and SHRpch1_18 rats was significantly ($p < 0.05$) increased by AVP treatment compared to control cells (without AVP) (Fig. 4a). However, in 100 nM AVP, expression of the *Slc16a1* gene was significantly ($p < 0.05$) lower in WKY/Izm cells than in those from the SHRpch1_18 strain. Furthermore, after 2 h of reoxygenation following 24 h of hypoxia, *Slc16a1* expression levels in WKY/Izm and SHRpch1_18 astrocytes were significantly ($p < 0.05$) increased by AVP treatment compared to control cells. Expression of *Slc16a1* was significantly lower ($p < 0.05$) in SHRpch1_18 than in WKY/Izm rat astrocytes in 100 nM AVP (Fig. 4a). Following the addition of AVP, gene expression of *Slc16a1* did not change compared with cells lacking AVP.

Similarly, expression of *Slc16a4* was examined with hypoxia and H/R conditions (Fig. 4b). Following 24 h of hypoxia and 30 min of reoxygenation, *Slc16a4* expression levels in astrocytes isolated from WKY/Izm and SHRpch1_18 rats were significantly ($p < 0.05$) increased by AVP treatment compared to control cells (without AVP) (Fig. 4a). However, expression of *Slc16a4* was significantly lower ($p < 0.05$) in SHRpch1_18 than in WKY/Izm rat cells in 100 nM AVP (Fig. 4b). Following 24 h of hypoxia and 2 h of reoxygenation, *Slc16a4* gene expression levels in astrocytes isolated from WKY/Izm and SHRpch1_18 rats were significantly ($p < 0.05$) increased by AVP treatment compared to control cells. Gene expression of *Slc16a4* was significantly lower ($p < 0.05$) in cells from SHRpch1_18 rats than those from WKY/Izm rats at 100 nM AVP. These results were confirmed in real-time PCR. Thus, AVP attenuated the expression of MCTs in SHRpch1_18 astrocytes during hypoxia and H/R conditions.

Effect of AVP on the expression of MCT4 protein in astrocytes isolated from WKY/Izm, SHRSP/Izm, and SHRpch1_18 rats

Astrocytes were isolated from WKY/Izm, SHRSP/Izm, and SHRpch1_18 rats, and we compared the expression of MCT1 and MCT4 proteins after culture in AVP. Specifically, astrocytes were treated with 100 nM AVP for 24 h, and then MCT1 and MCT4 protein levels were examined by WB. As shown in Fig. 5a, expression of MCT1 and MCT4 was increased by AVP treatment of astrocytes isolated from the three rat strains. In 100 nM AVP, astrocytes' expression of MCT1 protein was slightly lower in cells from SHRSP/Izm and SHRpch1_18 rats than in those from the WKY/Izm strain. Similarly, expression of MCT4 protein was slightly lower in astrocytes from the SHRSP/Izm and SHRpch1_18 strains than in those from WKY/Izm astrocytes.

We next determined whether AVP influenced the effects of MCT4 expression by pre-treating WKY/Izm astrocytes

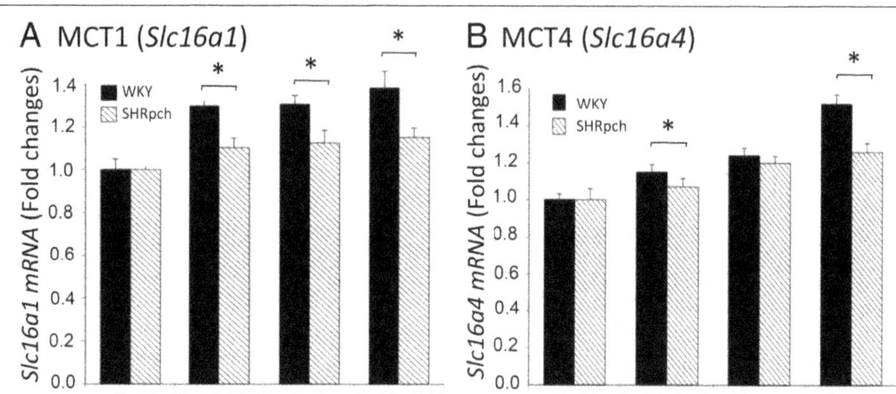

Fig. 4 Effect of AVP during hypoxia and reoxygenation (H/R) on *Slc16a1* and *Slc16a4* gene expression in astrocytes isolated from WKY/Izm and SHRpch1_18 rats. Confluent astrocytes isolated from WKY/Izm and SHRpch1_18 rats were exposed to hypoxic (1% O_2) conditions for 24 h with or without 100 nM AVP. After hypoxic culture, they were maintained under normoxic conditions for 30 min or for 2 h with or without 100 nM AVP. Total cellular RNA was isolated from the cultured astrocytes for RT-PCR, using primers for *Slc16a1* or *Slc16a4*. **a**. *Slc16a1* and **b**. *Slc16a4* gene expression from astrocytes from all assayed rat strains. Columns show means ± SE ($n = 4$). Re30, after hypoxic culture (1% O_2), cells were maintained in normoxic conditions (21% O_2) for 30 min; Re2h, after hypoxic culture (1% O_2), cells were maintained in normoxic conditions (21% O_2) for 2 h. AVP 100 nM arginine vasopressin. *$P < 0.05$

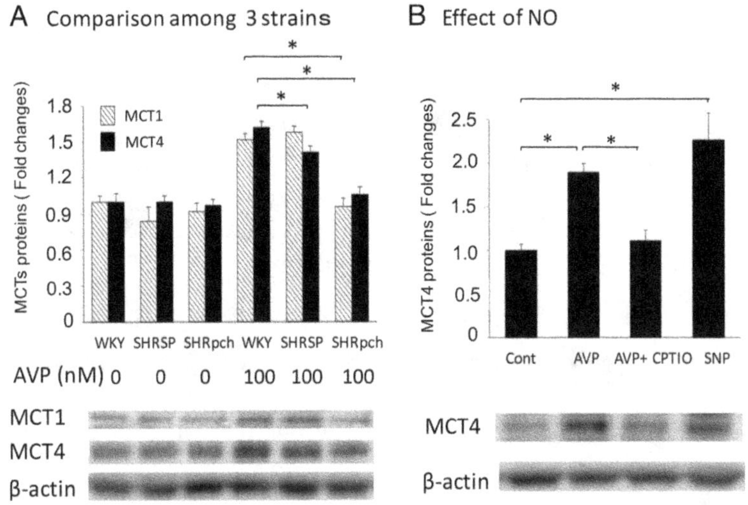

Fig. 5 Effect of AVP on expression of MCT4 protein in astrocytes isolated from WKY/Izm, SHRSP/Izm, and SHRpch1_18 rats. Astrocytes isolated from WKY/Izm, SHRSP/Izm, and SHRpch1_18 rats were exposed to 0 or 100 nM AVP for 24 h, after which MCT4 protein was assessed by WB analysis (**a**). In addition, astrocytes isolated from WKY/Izm were treated with or without AVP (100 nM), AVP plus CPTIO and SNP for 24 h (**b**). Astrocytes were exposed to CPTIO (200 μM) for 60 min before addition of AVP and 20 μM SNP. Total protein (30 μg) was analyzed by Western blot with an anti-MCT1 antibody or an anti-MCT4 antibody. AVP arginine vasopressin, WKY WKY/Izm, SHRSP SHRSP/Izm, SHRpch SHRpch1_18, AVP arginine vasopressin, SNP sodium nitroprusside. Columns show means ± SE (n = 4). $^*P < 0.05$

with or without an NO inhibitor. CPTIO is a chelator of NO that blocks the effect of NO [34]. In addition, SNP is a donor of NO that enhances levels of NO [35]. Thus, we investigated whether pre-treating WKY/Izm astrocytes with CPTIO or SNP affected AVP-induced expression of MCT4 protein. As shown in Fig. 5b, MCT4 protein expression in astrocytes was upregulated by 100 nM AVP treatment, and this increase could be inhibited by the addition of CPTIO. Furthermore, SNP treatment increased the expression of MCT4 protein. These results suggest that the expression of MCT4 is related to NO production.

Effect of AVP on the expression of iNOS and eNOS proteins in astrocytes isolated from WKY/Izm and SHRSP/Izm

We examined how AVP affected iNOS and eNOS protein expression in WKY/Izm and SHRSP/Izm astrocytes (Fig. 6). AVP significantly increased ($p < 0.05$) the expression of iNOS protein in WKY/Izm astrocytes (50 nM, 4.0-fold; 100 nM, 7.3-fold) and SHRSP astrocytes (50 nM, 10.6-fold; 100 nM, 16.3-fold) (Fig. 6). In addition, the iNOS expression levels in SHRSP/Izm astrocytes were elevated compared with WKY/Izm at 50 and 100 nM AVP. In WKY astrocytes, eNOS expression with AVP was significantly increased ($p < 0.05$) in a concentration-dependent manner (50 nM, 1.2-fold; 100 nM, 3.3-fold). However, eNOS expression in SHRSP/Izm was only slightly increased at 50 nM but significantly increased at 100 nM ($p < 0.05$) (Fig. 6d). The levels of eNOS expression in SHRSP/Izm were lower than in WKY/Izm.

Effects of PDTC on AVP-induced MCT4 and iNOS protein expression in astrocytes isolated from SHRSP/Izm rats

We investigated how AVP influenced the effects of MCT4 expression by pre-treating SHRSP/Izm astrocytes with or without an NF-kB inhibitor, PDTC [36]. As shown in Fig. 7, AVP increased the expression of iNOS protein in SHRSP astrocytes at 100 nM. The 60 min pretreatment with PDCT-inhibited expression of iNOS protein by AVP (0.79-fold). Also, the pretreatment with PDCT inhibited expression of MCT4 protein by AVP (0.60-fold).

Discussion

Brain ischemia-induced neuronal cell death is due to a shortage of oxygen and glucose [9, 37]. On the other hand, in the brain, lactate production increases with ischemia [38] and provides neuroprotection [9]. Lactate is produced by astrocytes via glycolysis and glycogenolysis and supports neuronal cells [39]. Regulation of lactate production and transport to neuronal cells by MCTs might reduce neuronal cell death after cerebral ischemia [40]. On the other hand, AVP affects astrocytic functions and regulates the onset of ischemic stroke [28]. For example, AVP induces ischemia-evoked brain edema in the setting of ischemic stroke [26]. Moreover, AVP induces production of inflammatory molecules after cerebral edema [24], and it subsequently enhances disruption of the BBB [25]. To better understand these findings, we compared AVP and/or H/R contributions to lactate production, expression of *Slc16a1*, *Slc16a4*, and *Bdnf* in cultured astrocytes isolated from SHRSP/Izm, SHRpch1_18, and WKY/Izm rats.

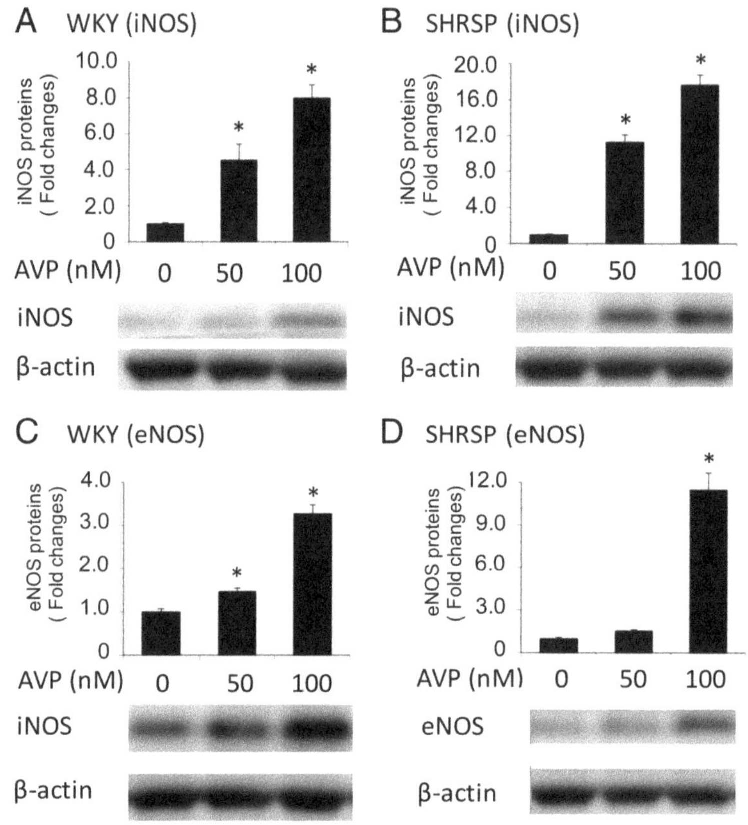

Fig. 6 Effect of AVP on expression of iNOS and eNOS proteins of astrocytes isolated from WKY/Izm and SHRSP/Izm rats. Astrocytes isolated from WKY/Izm and SHRSP/Izm rats were exposed to 0 or 100 nM AVP for 24 h, after which iNOS (**a**. WKY/Izm, **b**. SHRSP/Izm) and eNOS (**c**. WKY/Izm, **d**. SHRSP/Izm) protein was assessed by WB analysis. Total protein (30 μg) was analyzed by Western blot with an anti-iNOS or an anti-eNOS antibody. AVP arginine vasopressin, WKY WKY/Izm, SHRSP SHRSP/Izm. Columns show means ± SE (n = 4). *$P < 0.05$

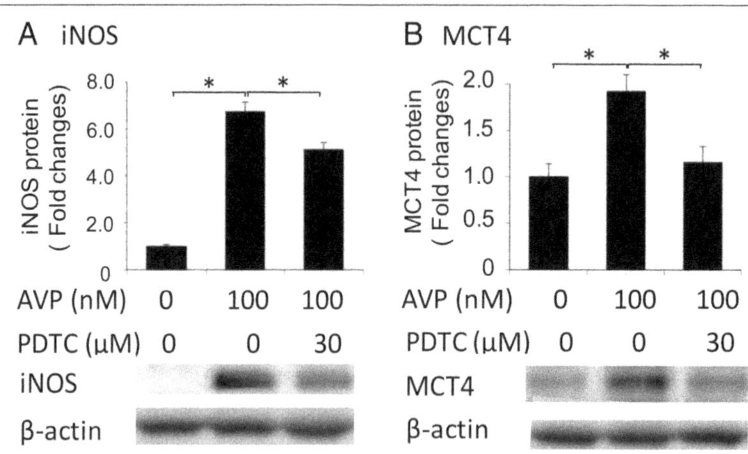

Fig. 7 Effects of PDTC on AVP-induced iNOS and MCT4 protein expression in astrocytes isolated from SHRSP/Izm rats. Astrocytes isolated from SHRSP/Izm rats were exposed to 0 or 100 nM AVP for 24 h, after which iNOS (**a**) and MCT4 (**b**) proteins were assessed by WB analysis. In addition, astrocytes isolated from SHRSP/Izm rats were treated with or without AVP (100 nM) or AVP plus PDCT. Astrocytes were exposed to PDCT (30 μM) for 60 min before addition of AVP. Total protein (30 μg) was analyzed by Western blot with an anti-iNOS antibody or an anti-MCT4 antibody. AVP arginine vasopressin. Columns show means ± SE (n = 4). *$P < 0.05$

A previous report demonstrated that following MCAO in SHR strain rats, the decrease in MCT expression coincided with neuronal cell death in the infarcted area [4]. However, the roles played by these MCTs in strokes in SHRSP strains are not clear. Therefore, in the present study, we assessed the AVP-induced gene expression of Slc16a1 and Slc16a4 in three strains of astrocytes. Expression of *Slc16a1* and *Slc16a4* in SHRSP/Izm and SHRpch1_18 was attenuated by AVP compared with WKY/Izm. These data indicate that the regulation of MCTs could be important for the supply of energy to neurons as well as the regulation of neurodegenerative diseases such as ischemic stroke. MCT1 and MCT4 enhance lactate release from astrocytes and regulate lactate uptake by neuronal cells [13]. Our results suggest that the reduced expression of *Slc16a4* by AVP regulates the supply of lactate to neurons in SHRSP/Izm and SHRpch1_18 rats.

Generally, ischemic conditions induce neurotoxicity and neuronal damage [41]. Importantly, lactate can assist the metabolic activity of hippocampal neuronal cells under hypoxic conditions [42]. Enhanced expression of MCT4 contributed to the resistance to hypoxic injury in astrocyte-neuron co-cultures [11]. In SHRSP strains, the reduced expression of MCT mediated by AVP may be associated with decreased lactate under ischemic conditions. For example, hypoxic and H/R conditions induce neuronal cell death in WKY/Izm and SHRSP/Izm rats [7]. The percentage of neuronal cells that undergo apoptosis during hypoxia-reperfusion is notably higher in SHRSP/Izm rats than in WKY/Izm rats [7]. A previous study analyzed the generation of hydroxyl radicals during hypoxia and reoxygenation in SHRSP rats [43]. In those animals, the generation of hydroxyl radicals was greater than that seen in the WKY strain. Moreover, there was greater oxidative stress, to which neurons are susceptible [2]. Furthermore, under ischemic conditions, AVP might enhance inflammation and attenuate serine production as well as stroke in SHRSP/Izm rats [29, 30]. Therefore, AVP-modulated expression of MCTs in WKY/Izm and SHRpch1_18 astrocytes was examined during hypoxia. In this study, hypoxia stimulation and AVP increased the expression of Slc16a1 and Slc16a4 in astrocytes. These results suggest that ischemic conditions enhanced lactate production that subsequently led to important responses associated with prevention of neuronal cell death. On the other hand, in the presence of AVP, both genes were expressed at significantly lower levels in SHRpch1_18 rat astrocytes than in those from WKY/Izm. These results suggest that ischemic conditions plus AVP addition exacerbated the astrocytic lactic acid supply and subsequently energy deficiency in neuronal cells.

In our study, the expression of *Slc16a1* and *Slc16a4* was examined under hypoxic and H/R conditions. After 30 min of hypoxia and 2 h of reoxygenation, the levels of *Slc16a1* and *Slc16a4* expression in WKY/Izm and SHRpch1_18 astrocytes were increased with and without treatment with AVP. However, the levels of *Slc16a1* and *Slc16a4* expression in AVP were lower in SHRpch1_18 rats than in WKY/Izm rats. On the other hand, it was reported that after the first few minutes of reoxygenation following brain ischemia, ROS (such as free radicals) induce cell damage [44, 45]. In other words, brain ischemia enhances HIF-1α and quickly produces large amounts of ROS, and the subsequent reactions cause cell and brain damage. In particular, in SHRSP/Izm rats, hydroxyl radicals are produced under H/R conditions [43]. In SHRSP/Izm and WKY/Izm rats, the generation of hydroxyl radicals in hippocampal neuronal cells peaked 20 min after the start of H/R. In addition, there was a significantly greater production of hydroxyl radicals in SHRSP/Izm compared with WKY/Izm cells. Our results and these reports appear to suggest sensitive differences for induced ROS production during H/R in SHRSP strains rats.

NO enhances glycolysis in astrocytes [46, 47]. Thus, the presence of NO may generate larger amounts of lactate from astrocytes. In the present study, we examined the contribution of NO to the expression of MCT4 induced by AVP in WKY/Izm cells. Namely, we examined whether AVP increased MCT4 protein expression after pre-treating astrocytes with CPTIO or SNP. In the presence of AVP, MCT4 protein expression in astrocytes was upregulated, and this increase could be inhibited by the addition of CPTIO. On the other hand, treatment with the NO donor, SNP increased the expression of MCT4 protein. One report demonstrated that NO induced the expression of MCT4 in cultured astrocytes [34]. Therefore, expression of MCT4 may be regulated by NO. We investigated whether AVP induced iNOS and eNOS protein expression in WKY/Izm and SHRSP/Izm rat astrocytes. We showed that AVP increased the expression of iNOS and eNOS proteins (Fig. 6). However, the level of expression of eNOS in SHRSP/Izm cells was lower than that in WKY/Izm. Furthermore, induction of MCT4 and iNOS by AVP was blocked by the NF-kB inhibitor PDCT (Fig. 7). Therefore, induction of MCT4 by AVP may be regulated by NO through NFkB. On the other hand, under hypoxic conditions, the increase of lactate production and MCTs may be induced through a transcription factor, hypoxia-inducible factor-1α (HIF-1α) [48]. NOSs may be associated with expression of MCT4 induced in hypoxia [34, 35]. Moreover, AVP, NF-kB, and HIF may be associated with these events. In SHRSP brains, NO production was high, which might explain the susceptibility to neuronal cell injury [49]. However, we previously demonstrated that gene expression of isoforms of 6-phosphofructo-2-kinase (PFK2), a master regulator of glycolysis, was reduced by SNP in SHRSP astrocytes [35]. Specifically, the SNP-induced gene expression of *PFK2.4* was more attenuated in astrocytes from SHRSP rats than in those from WKY. Induction of PFK2.4 by SNP attenuates the glycolytic system and lactate production may decrease. Therefore, in SHRSP cells, expression of MCT by NO may be less than in WKY. These features may be associated with changes in lactic acid, which decreased in SHRSP, although the exact mechanisms responsible for these alterations remain unclear.

BDNF decreases cortical neuronal cell death during post-MCAO ischemia in adult rats [50]. Similarly, BDNF plays a central role in neuronal recovery after cerebral ischemia [51]. Furthermore, 4 weeks after permanent occlusion of bilateral common carotid arteries (CCA), expression of BDNF was lower in SHRSP rats compared to WKY rats [52]. Therefore, we compared the effects of AVP on *Bdnf* gene expression in SHRSP/Izm, SHRpch1_18, and WKY/Izm astrocytes. Here, we showed that *Bdnf* expression in SHRSP/Izm and congenic SHRpch1_18 astrocytes was reduced compared with WKY/Izm rats. *Bdnf* expression in the presence of AVP may be lower in astrocytes from SHRSP/Izm and SHRpch1_18 rats than in astrocytes isolated from WKY/Izm rats. BDNF contributes to several functions such as neuronal cell growth, neuronal synaptic plasticity, long-term memory, and neuronal cell survival [15]. Recently, it was found that BDNF regulates blood pressure in the hypothalamus (PVN) with angiotensin signaling in rats [16]. We reason that the reduced expression of the *Bdnf* gene during AVP treatment may be associated with the attenuated nutritional support in the SHRSP/Izm strain, although the exact mechanisms responsible for these alterations remain unclear. However, these features of SHRSP/Izm and SHRpch1_18 rats may be important contributors to the attenuated neurotrophic supply in astrocytes.

In summary, we demonstrated that cultured astrocytes isolated from SHRSP/Izm and SHRpch1_18 rats differed from those obtained from the WKY/Izm strain in regard to their responsiveness to AVP or H/R conditions. Namely, we found that AVP attenuated lactate production in SHRSP/Izm and SHRpch1_18 astrocytes compared with WKY/Izm. Furthermore, we showed that the expression of MCT1 and MCT4 in astrocytes following AVP treatment or H/R stimulation was decreased. Induction of MCT4 by AVP and hypoxia may be regulated by NO through transcription factor NF-kB activation and HIFα [48]. Previously, we showed that SHRSP rat astrocyte gene expression for LDH and MCT was lower than that in WKY rats [6]. The in vivo study showed that expression of MCT increased in the brain following an ischemic insult [52]. These data might explain the alteration of MCT expression and low lactate production by SHRs strain rat cells in vivo. Thus, in SHRSP/Izm and SHRpch1_18 astrocytes subjected to AVP or H/R stimulation, the specific characteristics of these cells might explain the energy and nutritional deficiencies in neuronal cells.

Conclusions

The expression of MCTs mediated by AVP may be regulated by NO. AVP attenuated the expression of MCTs in SHRSP/Izm and SHRpch1_18 astrocytes. Attenuated expression of MCTs may be related with decreased lactate production in SHRSP. Reduced production of lactate may be associated with decreased neuronal energy supply in SHRSP/Izm rats. Furthermore, it may play an important role in post-ischemic neuronal recovery [48].

Abbreviations

AVP: Arginine vasopressin; BDNF: Brain-derived neurotrophic factor; H/R: Hypoxia and reoxygenation; MCT: Monocarboxylate transporter; SHRSP: Stroke-prone spontaneously hypertensive rats; WKY: Wistar Kyoto rats

Acknowledgements

Not applicable.

Funding

This work was supported by JSPS KAKENHI Grant Number 15K08321.

Authors' contributions

KY and TN conceived and designed the project; KY, NT, and NA performed the experiments; NT and NA performed statistical analysis of the data with inputs from NA. All authors read and approved the final manuscript.

Consent for publication

Not applicable.

Competing interests

The authors report no conflicts of interest.

Author details

[1]Laboratory of Molecular Health of Food, Department of Food Bioscience and Biotechnology, College of Bioresource Sciences, Nihon University (NUBS), 1866, Kameino, Fujisawa, Kanagawa 252-8510, Japan. [2]Department of Functional Pathology, Shimane University Faculty of Medicine, Matsue, Japan.

References

1. Yamori Y, Nagaoka A, Okamoto K. Importance of genetic factors in hypertensive cerebrovascular lesions: an evidence obtained by successive selective breeding of stroke-prone and-resistant SHR. Jpn Circ J. 1974;38:1095–100.
2. Tagami M, Yamagata K, Ikeda K, Nara Y, Fujino H, Kubota A, Numano F, Yamori Y. Vitamin E prevents apoptosis in cortical neurons during hypoxia and oxygen reperfusion. Lab Investig. 1998;78:1415–29.
3. Tagami M, Nara Y, Kubota A, Fujino H, Yamori Y. Ultrastructural changes in cerebral pericytes and astrocytes of stroke-prone spontaneously hypertensive rats. Stroke. 1990;21:1064–71.
4. Zhang F, Vannucci SJ, Philp NJ. Monocarboxylate transporter expression in the spontaneous hypertensive rat: effect of stroke. J Neurosci Res. 2005;79:139–45.
5. Gandolgor TA, Ohara H, Cui ZH, Hirashima T, Ogawa T, Saar K, Hubner N, Watanabe T, Isomura M, Nabika T. Two genomic regions of chromosomes 1 and 18 explain most of the stroke susceptibility under salt loading in stroke-prone spontaneously hypertensive rat/Izm. Hypertension. 2013;62:55–61.

6. Yamagata K, Tagami M, Ikeda K, Noguchi T, Yamori Y, Nara Y. Reduced production of lactate during hypoxia and reoxygenation in astrocytes isolated from stroke-prone spontaneously hypertensive rats. Neurosci Lett. 2000;296:113–6.
7. Tagami M, Ikeda K, Yamagata K, Nara Y, Fujino H, Kubota A, Numano F, Yamori Y. Vitamin E prevents apoptosis in hippocampal neurons caused by cerebral ischemia and reperfusion in stroke-prone spontaneously hypertensive rats. Lab Investig. 1999;79:609–15.
8. Galeffi F, Foster KA, Sadgrove MP, Beaver CJ, Turner DA. Lactate uptake contributes to the NAD(P)H biphasic response and tissue oxygen response during synaptic stimulation in area CA1 of rat hippocampal slices. J Neurochem. 2007;103:2449–61.
9. Banerjee A, Ghatak S, Sikdar SK. l-Lactate mediates neuroprotection against ischaemia by increasing TREK1 channel expression in rat hippocampal astrocytes in vitro. J Neurochem. 2016;138:265–81.
10. Gao C, Zhou L, Zhu W, Wang H, Wang R, He Y, Li Z. Monocarboxylate transporter-dependent mechanism confers resistance to oxygen- and glucose-deprivation injury in astrocyte-neuron co-cultures. Neurosci Lett. 2015a;594:99–104.
11. Gao C, Zhu W, Tian L, Zhang J, Li Z. MCT4-mediated expression of EAAT1 is involved in the resistance to hypoxia injury in astrocyte-neuron co-cultures. Neurochem Res. 2015b;40:818–28.
12. Pellerin L, Bergersen LH, Halestrap AP, Pierre K. Cellular and subcellular distribution of monocarboxylate transporters in cultured brain cells and in the adult brain. J Neurosci Res. 2005;79:55–64.
13. Pierre K, Pellerin L. Monocarboxylate transporters in the central nervous system:distribution, regulation and function. J Neurochem. 2005;94:1–14.
14. Bergersen LH. Is lactate food for neurons? Comparison of monocarboxylate transporter subtypes in brain and muscle. Neuroscience. 2007;145:11–9.
15. Leal G, Comprido D, Duarte CB. BDNF-induced local protein synthesis and synaptic plasticity. Neuropharmacology. 2014;76:Pt C639–56.
16. Erdos B, Backes I, McCowan ML, Hayward LF, Scheuer DA. Brain-derived neurotrophic factor modulates angiotensin signaling in the hypothalamus to increase blood pressure in rats. Am J Physiol Heart Circ Physiol. 2015;308:H612–22.
17. Chen PS, Peng GS, Li G, Yang S, Wu X, Wang CC, Wilson B, Lu RB, Gean PW, Chuang DM, Hong JS. Valproate protects dopaminergic neurons in midbrain neuron/glia cultures by stimulating the release of neurotrophic factors from astrocytes. Mol Psychiatry. 2006;11:1116–25.
18. Cardile V, Pavone A, Gulino R, Renis M, Scifo C, Perciavalle V. Expression of brain-derived neurotrophic factor (BDNF) and inducible nitric oxide synthase (iNOS) in rat astrocyte cultures treated with Levetiracetam. Brain Res. 2003;976:227–33.
19. Stanne TM, Aberg ND, Nilsson S. Low circulating acute brain-derived neurotrophic factor levels are associated with poor long-term functional outcome after ischemic stroke. Stroke. 2016;47:1943–5.
20. Kageyama H, Nemoto K, Nemoto F, Sekimoto M, Nara Y, Nabika T, Iwayama Y, Fukamachi K, Tomita I, Senba E, Forehand CJ, Hendley ED, Ueyama T. Mutation of the trkB gene encoding the high-affinity receptor for brain-derived neurotrophic factor in stroke-prone spontaneously hypertensive rats. Biochem Biophys Res Commun. 1996;229:713–8.
21. Almeida RD, Manadas BJ, Melo CV, Gomes JR, Mendes CS, Graos MM, Carvalho RF, Carvalho AP, Duarte CB. Neuroprotection by BDNF against glutamate-induced apoptotic cell death is mediated by ERK and PI3-kinase pathways. Cell Death Differ. 2005;12:1329–43.
22. Wu CL, Hwang CS, Yang DI. Protective effects of brain-derived neurotrophic factor against neurotoxicity of 3-nitropropionic acid in rat cortical neurons. Neurotoxicology. 2009;30:718–26.
23. Coco M, Caggia S, Musumeci G, Perciavalle V, Graziano AC, Pannuzzo G, Cardile V. Sodium L-lactate differently affects brain-derived neurothrophic factor, inducible nitric oxide synthase, and heat shock protein 70 kDa production in human astrocytes and SH-SY5Y cultures. J Neurosci Res. 2013;91:313–20.
24. Szmydynger-Chodobska J, Fox LM, Lynch KM, Zink BJ, Chodobski A. Vasopressin amplifies the production of proinflammatory mediators in traumatic brain injury. J Neurotrauma. 2010;27:1449–61.
25. O'Donnell ME, Duong V, Suvatne J, Foroutan S, Johnson DM. Arginine vasopressin stimulation of cerebral microvascular endothelial cell Na-K-Cl cotransporter activity is V1 receptor and [Ca] dependent. Am J Phys Cell Phys. 2005;289:C283–92.
26. Zhao XY, Wu CF, Yang J. Effect of arginine vasopressin on the cortex edema in the ischemic stroke of Mongolian gerbils. Neuropeptides. 2015;51:55–62.
27. Liu X, Nakayama S, Amiry-Moghaddam M, Ottersen OP, Bhardwaj A. Arginine-vasopressin V1 but not V2 receptor antagonism modulates infarct volume, brain water content, and aquaporin-4 expression following experimental stroke. Neurocrit Care. 2010;12:124–31.
28. Syed N, Martens CA, Hsu WH. Arginine vasopressin increases glutamate release and intracellular Ca2+ concentration in hippocampal and cortical astrocytes through two distinct receptors. J Neurochem. 2007;103:229–37.
29. Yamagata K, Yamamoto M, Kawakami K, Ohara H, Nabika T. Arginine vasopressin regulated ASCT1 expression in astrocytes from stroke-prone spontaneously hypertensive rats and congenic SHRpch1_18 rats. Neuroscience. 2014;267:277–85.
30. Yamagata K, Sone N, Suguyama S, Nabika T. Different effects of arginine vasopressin on high-mobility group box 1 expression in astrocytes isolated from stroke-prone spontaneously hypertensive rats and congenic SHRpch1_18 rats. Int J Exp Pathol. 2016;97:97–106.
31. McCarthy KD, de Vellis J. Preparation of separate astroglial and oligodendroglial cell cultures from rat cerebral tissue. J Cell Biol. 1980;85:890–902.
32. Rissoan MC, Soumelis V, Kadowaki N, Grouard G, Briere F, de Waal MR, Liu YJ. Reciprocal control of T helper cell and dendric cell differentiation. Science. 1999;5405:1183–6.
33. Rutkowsky JM, Wallace BK, Wise PM, O'Donnell ME. Effects of estradiol on ischemic factor-induced astrocyte swelling and AQP4 protein abundance. Am J Phys Cell Phys. 2011;301:C204–12.
34. Marcillac F, Brix B, Repond C, Johren O, Pellerin L. Nitric oxide induces the expression of the monocarboxylate transporter MCT4 in cultured astrocytes by a cGMP-independent transcriptional activation. Glia. 2011;59:1987–95.
35. Yamagata K, Tagami M, Yamori Y. Nitric oxide reduces astrocytic lactate production and induces neuronal vulnerability in stroke-prone spontaneously hypertensive rats. Glia. 2008;56:387–93.
36. Fan YH, Zhao LY, Zheng QS, Dong H, Wang HC, Yang XD. Arginine vasopressin increases iNOS-NO system activity in cardiac fibroblasts through NF-kappaB activation and its relation with myocardial fibrosis. Life Sci. 2007;81:327–35.
37. Quintard H, Patet C, Zerlauth JB, Suys T, Bouzat P, Pellerin L, Meuli R, Magistretti PJ, Oddo M. Improvement of neuroenergetics by hypertonic lactate therapy in patients with traumatic brain injury is dependent on baseline cerebral lactate/pyruvate ratio. J Neurotrauma. 2016;33:681–7.
38. Kalogeris T, Baines CP, Krenz M, Korthuis RJ. Cell biology of ischemia/reperfusion injury. Int Rev Cell Mol Biol. 2012;298:229–317.
39. Hertz L, Peng L, Dienel GA. Energy metabolism in astrocytes: high rate of oxidative metabolism and spatiotemporal dependence on glycolysis/glycogenolysis. J Cereb Blood Flow Metab. 2007;27:219–49.
40. Berthet C, Lei H, Thevenet J, Gruetter R, Magistretti PJ, Hirt L. Neuroprotective role of lactate after cerebral ischemia. J Cereb Blood Flow Metab. 2009;29:1780–9.
41. Descloux C, Ginet V, Clarke PG, Puyal J, Truttmann AC. Neuronal death after perinatal cerebral hypoxia-ischemia: focus on autophagy-mediated cell death. Int J Dev Neurosci. 2015;45:75–85.
42. Schurr A. Lactate: the ultimate cerebral oxidative energy substrate? J Cereb Blood Flow Metab. 2006;26:142–52.
43. Negishi H, Ikeda K, Nara Y, Yamori Y. Increased hydroxyl radicals in the hippocampus of stroke-prone spontaneously hypertensive rats during transient ischemia and recirculation. Neurosci Lett. 2001;306:206–8.
44. Bolli R. Oxygen-derived free radicals and myocardial reperfusion injury: an overview. Cardiovasc Drugs Ther Suppl. 1991;2:249–68.
45. Granger DN, Kvietys PR. Reperfusion injury and reactive oxygen species: The evolution of a concept. Redox Biol. 2015;6:524–51.
46. Almeida A, Moncada S, Bolanos JP. Nitric oxide switches on glycolysis through the AMP protein kinase and 6-phosphofructo-2-kinase pathway. Nat Cell Biol. 2004;6:45–51.
47. Rosafio K, Pellerin L. Oxygen tension controls the expression of the monocarboxylate transporter MCT4 in cultured mouse cortical astrocytes via a hypoxia-inducible factor-1α-mediated transcriptional regulation. Glia. 2014;62:477–90.
48. Ullah MS, Davies AJ, Halestrap AP. The plasma membrane lactate transporter MCT4, but not MCT1, is up-regulated by hypoxia through a HIF-1alpha-dependent mechanism. J Biol Chem. 2006;281:9030–7.
49. Ferrer I, Krupinski J, Goutan E, Marti E, Ambrosio S, Arenas E. Brain-derived neurotrophic factor reduces cortical cell death by ischemia after middle cerebral artery occlusion in the rat. Acta Neuropathol. 2001;101:229–38.
50. Bejot Y, Prigent-Tessier A, Cachia C, Giroud M, Mossiat C, Bertrand N, Garnier P, Marie C. Time-dependent contribution of non neuronal cells to BDNF production after ischemic stroke in rats. Neurochem Int. 2011;58:102–11.

51. Lee TH, Yang JT, Kato H, Wu JH. Hypertension downregulates the expression of brain-derived neurotrophic factor in the ischemia-vulnerable hippocampal CA1 and cortical areas after carotid artery occlusion. Brain Res. 2006;1116:31–8.
52. Rosafio K, Castillo X, Hirt L, Pellerin L. Cell-specific modulation of monocarboxylate transporter expression contributes to the metabolic reprograming taking place following cerebral ischemia. Neuroscience. 2016;317:108–20.

Mitochondrial dysfunction induces NLRP3 inflammasome activation during cerebral ischemia/reperfusion injury

Zhe Gong[1†], Jingrui Pan[1†], Qingyu Shen[1,2], Mei Li[1] and Ying Peng[1,2*]

Abstract

Background: Nod-like receptor protein 3 (NLRP3) inflammasome is a crucial factor in mediating inflammatory responses after cerebral ischemia/reperfusion (I/R), but the cellular location of NLRP3 inflammasome in cerebral I/R has yet come to a conclusion, and there is still no specific evidence to state the relationship between mitochondria and the NLRP3 inflammasome in cerebral I/R.

Methods: In the present study, we detected the cellular localization of NLRP3 inflammasomes in a transient middle cerebral artery occlusion (tMCAO) rat model and a transwell co-culture cell system under oxygen-glucose deprivation/reoxygenation (OGD/R) conditions. Then, we investigated the relationship between mitochondrial dysfunction and the activation of NLRP3 inflammasomes in different cell types after OGD/R and cerebral I/R injury.

Results: Our results showed that NLRP3 inflammasomes were first activated in microglia soon after cerebral I/R injury onset and then were expressed in neurons and microvascular endothelial cells later, but they were mainly in neurons. Furthermore, mitochondrial dysfunction played an important role in activating NLRP3 inflammasomes in microglia after OGD/R, and mitochondrial protector could inhibit the activation of NLRP3 inflammasomes in cerebral I/R rats.

Conclusion: Our findings may provide novel insights into the cell type-dependent activation of NLRP3 inflammasomes at different stages of cerebral I/R injury and the role of mitochondrial dysfunction in activating the NLRP3 inflammasome pathway.

Keywords: Stroke, NLRP3 inflammasome, Mitochondrial dysfunction, Microglia, Neuron

Background

Neuroinflammation is a crucial and complex pathophysiological process within the whole scheme of cerebral ischemia, spanning from early damage to post-ischemic tissue repair [1]. The exact molecular signaling pathways have not been fully clarified to date, leading to difficulty in clinical treatment. Recently, a novel inflammatory pathway, known as inflammasomes, was found in ischemic stroke, and several studies have highlighted that nod-like receptor protein 3 (NLRP3) inflammasomes may be crucial for mediating inflammatory responses and for inducing cellular damage and death after stroke [2–4]. NLRP3 inflammasomes are the most well-characterized members of the nod-like receptor family, which consists of NLRP3, apoptosis-associated speck-like protein containing a caspase activation recruitment domain (ASC) and precursor caspase-1 (pro-caspase1), and it plays great roles in ischemic stroke by triggering the release of IL-1β and IL-18 via caspase-1 activation [5, 6]. Subsequently, both IL-1β and IL-18 participate in the initiation and amplification of the inflammatory responses [7]. However, the specific cellular location and signaling pathway of NLRP3 inflammasomes in ischemic stroke remains unknown.

* Correspondence: 2353352460@qq.com
†Zhe Gong and Jingrui Pan contributed equally to this work.
[1]Department of Neurology, Sun Yat-sen Memorial Hospital, Sun Yat-sen University, Guangzhou 510120, China
[2]Guangdong Provincial Key Laboratory of Malignant Tumour Epigenetics and Gene Regulation, Sun Yat-sen Memorial Hospital, Sun Yat-sen University, Guangzhou, China

In addition, it has been reported that mitochondrial dysfunction activates NLRP3 inflammasomes in some inflammatory diseases, such as metabolic syndrome, diabetes, atherosclerosis, neurodegeneration, heart disease, and kidney disease [8]. However, there is still no specific evidence stating the relationship between mitochondria and NLRP3 inflammasomes in stroke.

In the present study, we aimed to clarify these questions, in the hope of revealing more details regarding neuroinflammation in mediating cerebral ischemia/reperfusion (I/R) injury in ischemic stroke.

Methods

Animals and substances

Healthy, male, 280–320 g Sprague-Dawley rats were obtained from the Laboratory Animal Center of Sun Yat-sen University, Guangzhou, China. The rats were housed in a temperature- (25 ± 2 °C) and humidity-controlled room. The animals were maintained under a 12:12-h light/dark cycle with free access to food and water.

Diazoxide, considered a highly selective mitochondrial ATP-sensitive potassium channel opener, was dissolved in sterile 0.1 M NaOH solution before being used. The concentration of diazoxide used in the cells was 100 μm, which was in accordance with a previous study reported [9].

Transient middle cerebral artery occlusion (tMCAO) model and drug treatment

The intraluminal suture MCAO method was used to induce tMCAO, as we previously described, in order to stimulate I/R injury in rats [10]. In brief, a midline incision was made in the neck to expose the right external carotid artery after each rat was anesthetized with 10% chloral hydrate. Then, a monofilament (Beijing Cinontech Co., Ltd.; China; 2838-A4) was inserted into the internal carotid artery, past the external carotid artery, until a mild resistance was felt, indicating that the filament was properly lodged in the proximal segment of the anterior cerebral artery and, thus, was blocking the blood flow to the middle cerebral artery. The monofilament was left in place for 120 min and then was withdrawn to induce reperfusion. When the rat regained consciousness, a successful model showed left foreleg paralysis or a circular motion, and infarct tissue without cerebral hemorrhage was observed when the brain was removed. A sham-operation was performed as a control, which included the same procedures as the tMCAO mentioned above but without the insertion of the monofilament and following reperfusion.

Rats were randomly divided into six groups: the sham-operation group (sham), the sham + diazoxide group, the 6 h after reperfusion group (I/R 6 h), the I/R 6 h + diazoxide group, the 24 h after reperfusion group (I/R 24 h), and the I/R 24 h + diazoxide group. The diazoxide was treated at 10 mg/kg intraperitoneally after reperfusion immediately as the previous studies [11, 12]. The diazoxide was dissolved in sterile 0.1 M NaOH solution, and diluted with saline to the concentration of 0.02 N NaOH solution before being used. The other animal group received equal volume of 0.02 N NaOH solution.

Immunofluorescence (IF)

The brains were removed after cardiac perfusion 6 h and 24 h after reperfusion in different groups and were fixed with 4% paraformaldehyde at 4 °C overnight. Frozen sectioning was performed after sucrose gradient dehydration. Then, the 10-μm thick coronal sections were blocked with 10% goat serum containing 0.5% Triton X-100 at room temperature for 30 min, followed by incubation with mouse anti-caspase-1 p20 (Santa-Cruz Biotechnology, sc-398,715, 1:50) antibody and rabbit anti-Iba1 antibody (Wako, 019–19,741, 1:250) or rabbit anti-NeuN antibody (Cell Signaling Technology, 24307S, 1:50) or rabbit anti-CD31 antibody (Abcam, ab222783, 1:100) (The antibody specificity was proved in Additional file 1: Figure S1) or rabbit anti-GFAP antibody (Abcam, ab33922, 1:250) at 4 °C overnight. The sections were washed for 3 × 10 min with PBS and then incubated with a mixture of Alexa Fluor 488-conjugated goat-anti mouse IgG (Beyotime, A0428, 1:500) and Alexa Fluor 555-conjugated donkey-anti rabbit IgG (Beyotime, A0453, 1:500) for 1 h at room temperature, followed by staining with DAPI for 5 min. After being washed with PBS three times, the sections were mounted with fluorescent mounting medium (Dako, S3023). An equal volume of PBS was used to replace the primary antibody as a negative control, and the other procedures remained unchanged. All images that were focused on the ischemic core cortex area [13] (Fig. 1f) were captured using a fluorescence microscope (lx71, OLYMPUS) at × 200 magnification and a 100-μm scale bar. The percentage of different cell types in caspase-1 p20-positive cells is equal to the counts of both cell markers and caspase-1 p20-positive cells/counts of caspase-1 p20-positive cells. The percentage of caspase-1 p20-positive cells in different cell type is equal to the counts of both cell markers and caspase-1 p20-positive cells/counts of different cell type.

Primary microglial cell culture

The method to isolate and cultivate primary microglial cells from C57BL/6 neonatal mice was according to a published protocol [14, 15]. Briefly, primary mixed glial cells were isolated from postnatal mice born within 24 h and then cultured in DMEM/F12 medium (Gibco, Invitrogen, 11,330–032) supplemented with 10% heat-inactivated fetal bovine serum (FBS) (Gibco, Invitrogen, 10,099–141) and 1% penicillin/streptomycin (HyClone, SV30010). On days

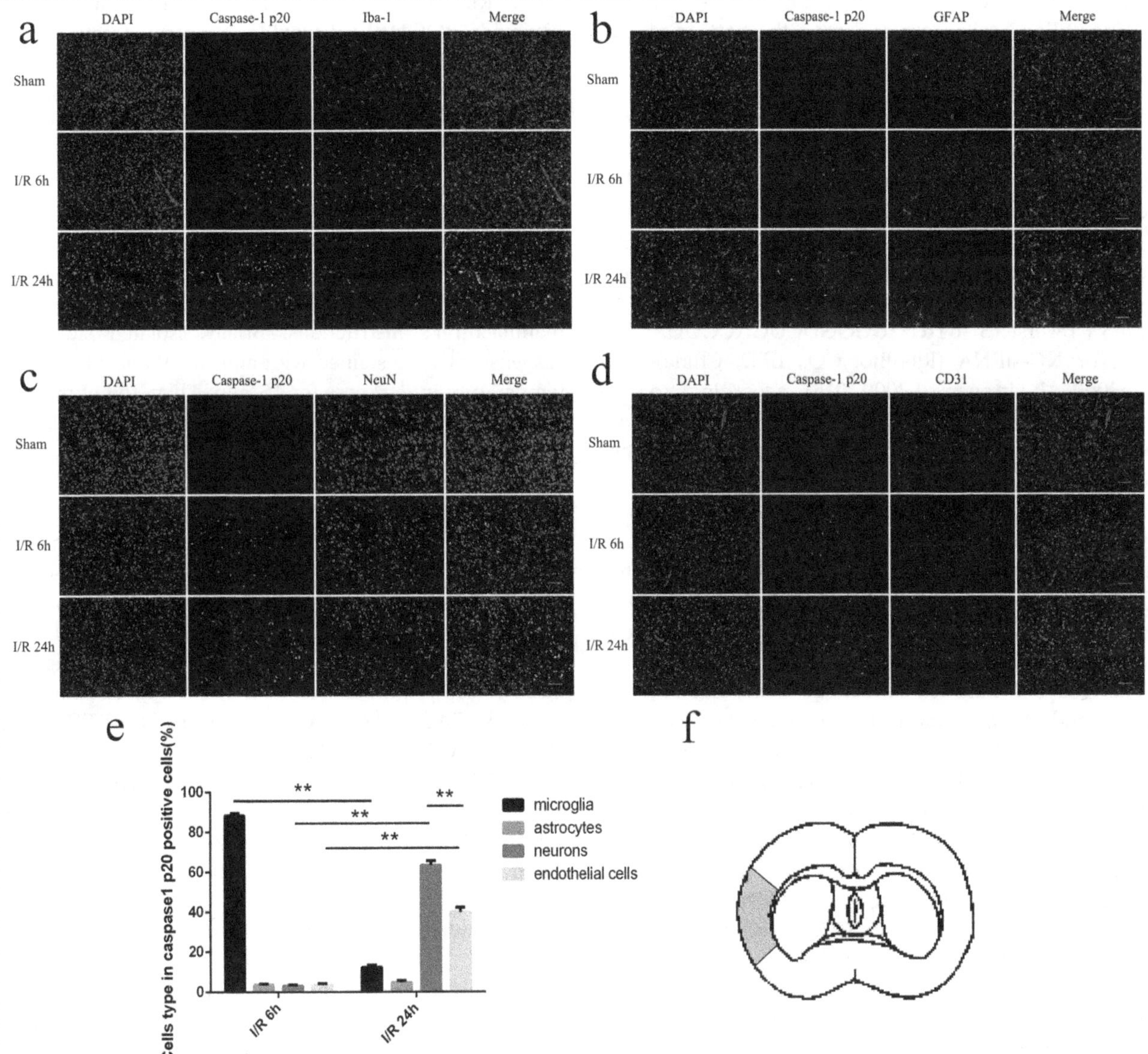

Fig. 1 Cellular localization of cleaved caspase-1 after ischemia/reperfusion (I/R) injury. **a–d** The expression of caspase-1 p20 in microglia, astrocytes, neurons, and endothelial cells in sham rats and after cerebral I/R at 6 h and 24 h. **e** The percentage of different cell types in caspase-1 p20-positive cells 6 h and 24 h after cerebral I/R. **f** The ischemic area where the cleaved caspsae-1 was richly expressed. Bar = 100 μm. *$p < 0.05$, **$p < 0.01$

12–14, microglial cells were harvested by shaking the cultures and collecting the floating cells. After centrifugation, cells were seeded into plastic tissue culture flasks and incubated at 37 °C for 12–24 h, followed by culture medium replacement. The purity of microglia was verified by immunofluorescence staining with Iba-1 (Wako, 019–19,741, Japan).

BV2 cells, PC12 cells, and bEnd3 cells were obtained from American Type Culture Collection (ATCC). BV2 cells were cultured in DMEM/F12 medium (Gibco, Invitrogen, 11,330–032), and the other cells were cultured in DMEM high glucose (HyClone, SH30243.01), supplemented with 10% heat-inactivated fetal bovine serum (Gibco, Invitrogen, 10,099–141) and 1% penicillin/streptomycin (HyClone, SV30010) in a humidified incubator at 37 °C, in the presence of 5% CO_2 in the air. For differentiation (Additional file 2: Figure S2), 100 ng/ml of nerve growth factor (NGF) (Sigma-Aldrich, N2513) was added to the culture medium of PC12 cells for 3 days, which was used for the following assays.

Transwell co-culture system

The transwell co-culture system was conducted as previously reported [11]: BV2 cells were cultured on the upper compartment of a two-chamber transwell system (0.4-mm pore size of polycarbonate membrane coated with poly-L-lysine; Corning, Corning, NY, USA), and PC12 or bEnd3 cells were grown on the bottom well of the chamber, cultured in DMEM/F12 medium [16].

siRNA transfection

Primary microglial cells, PC12 cells, bEnd3 cells, BV2 cells alone, and BV2 cells cultured in the upper chamber were transfected with NLRP3-siRNA (mouse) (forward, 5′-GUACUUAAAUCGUGAAACAdTdT-3′; reverse, 3′-dTdTCAUGAAUUUAGCACUUUGU-5′) or NLRP3-siR NA (rat) (forward, 5′-CAGCCAGAGUGGAAUG ACAd TdT-3′; reverse, 3′-dTdTGUCGGUCUCACCUUACUG U-5′) or NC-siRNA (RiboBio. CO., LTD, China) with Lipo3000 (Invitrogen, L3000–015) according to the manufacturer's instructions. After 24 h of transfection, the treated upper chambers were moved to the other wells with PC12 or bEND3 cells cultured in the bottom chambers. Similarly, the treated PC12 or bEnd3 cells in bottom chambers were co-cultured with BV2 cells cultured in upper chambers. Then, the siRNA-transfected primary microglial cells, PC12 cells, bEnd3 cells, BV2 cells, and transwell co-culture systems received oxygen-glucose deprivation/reoxygenation (OGD/R) treatment.

The groups in transwell co-culture system, siRNA transfection, and OGD/R treatment were as following: Control treatment in isolated culture (NC), OGD/R treatment in isolated culture (OGD/R), OGD/R treatment in isolated culture with NC-siRNA transfection (OGD/R + NC siRNA), OGD/R treatment in isolated culture with NLRP3-siRNA transfection (OGD/R + NLRP3 siRNA), control treatment in transwell co-culture (transwell NC), OGD/R treatment in transwell co-culture (transwell OGD/R), OGD/R treatment in transwell co-culture with NC-siRNA transfection (transwell OGD/R + NC siRNA), and OGD/R treatment in transwell co-culture with NLRP3-siRNA transfection (transwell OGD/R + NLRP3 siRNA).

Oxygen-glucose deprivation/reoxygenation (OGD/R) model and drug administration

The OGD/R model was generated by replacing the culture medium with glucose-free DMEM medium (Gibco, Invitrogen, 11,966–025), then placing the plate into a hypoxic incubator (MIC-101, Billups-Rothenberginc) that contained a gas mixture of 95% N_2 and 5% CO_2 for 4 h at 37 °C and then recovering normal gas and medium at the optimal time. The cell groups that needed drug treatment were treated with renewed normal medium with diazoxide after reoxygenation, and the other groups were treated with PBS as a control.

The groups in transwell co-culture system, drug treatment, and OGD/R treatment were as following: control treatment in isolated culture with PBS (NC), control treatment in isolated culture with diazoxide (NC + diazoxide), OGD/R treatment in isolated culture with PBS (OGD/R), OGD/R treatment in isolated culture with diazoxide (OGD/R + diazoxide), control treatment in transwell co-culture with PBS (transwell NC), OGD/R treatment in transwell co-culture with PBS (transwell OGD/R), and OGD/R treatment in transwell co-culture with diazoxide (transwell OGD/R + diazoxide).

Flow cytometry

The apoptotic rates of the PC12 cells were detected using flow cytometry with an annexin V-FITC/PI apoptosis detection kit (KeyGEN BioTECH, KGA107) according to the manufacturer's instructions. Briefly, isolated single-cell suspensions were stained with annexin-V and PI at room temperature in darkness for 15 min. Then, the number of cells was determined via flow cytometry (LSR II, BD).

Measurement of mitochondrial DNA (mtDNA) copy number and mtDNA damage

Genomic DNA from the cells was extracted using the Genomic DNA Miniprep Kit (TIANGEN, DP304–02). The mtDNA copy number was measured using real-time quantitative PCR (qPCR) and was normalized to the Hbb (β-globin) gene. The primer pairs for measuring the mtDNA copy number were as follows: mtDNA forward, GCCCATGACCAACATAACTG; reverse, CCTTGACGG CTATGTTGATG; Hbb (β-globin) forward, AGGCAGAG GCAGGCAGAT; reverse, GG CGGGAGGTTTGAGA CA. q-PCR reactions were performed in the LightCycler 480 II PCR System (LightCycler 480 II, Roche), using the All-in-One qPCR Mix kit (GeneCopoeia, AOPR-0200).

Measurement of the mitochondrial membrane potential (Δψm)

The Δψm was assayed using a JC-1 (5, 5′, 6, 6′-tetrach loro-1, 1′, 3, 3′-tetraethylbenzimidazolcarbocyanine iodide) staining Kit (Beyotime, C2006). Cells were incubated with 10 μg/ml JC-1 for 30 min at 37 °C, and images were captured with a fluorescence microscope. The ratio of JC-1 aggregates (red fluorescence) to monomers (green fluorescence) was calculated using Image-Pro Plus 6.0 (Media Cybernetics, lnc., USA). Loss of mitochondrial function by mPTP opening was indicated by a decrease in the ratio of the red/green fluorescence intensity [17].

RNA extraction and real-time quantitative PCR (qRT-PCR)

The PC12 or bEnd3 cells were prepared for total RNA extraction using TRIzol reagent (Takara, #9109), and cDNA was synthesized using the PrimeScript RT Reagent Kit (Takara, #RR037A) according to the manufacturer's instructions. The q-PCR reaction was performed in the LightCycler 480 II PCR System (LightCycler 480II, Roche, USA), using the All-in-One qPCR Mix kit (GeneCopoeia, AOPR-0200). Primers were provided as follows: IL-1β forward, TGCCACCTTTTGACAGTGATG and reverse,

AAGGTCCACGGGAAAGACAC; IL-18 forward, AGCA GTCCCAACTAAGCAGTA and reverse CAGCCAGTA GAGGATGCTGA; and β-actin forward GTGACGTTG ACATCCGTAAAGA and reverse GCCGGACTCATCGT ACTCC. The endpoint of qRT-PCR data is the comparative cycle threshold method (Ct). The relative changes in gene expression were quantified using the Livak method (also known as $2^{-\Delta\Delta Ct}$ method) after determining the Ct values for the reference and target genes in each sample set [18]. All reactions were repeated for three times.

Immunoprecipitation (IP)

The BV2 cell lysates (500 μg) were immunoprecipitated with 1 μg of anti-ASC antibody (Cell Signaling Technology, 67824S) for 1 h at 4 °C, and then were incubated with 20 μl of protein A agarose beads (Santa-Cruz, sc-2003) overnight at 4 °C, and centrifuged at 3000×*g* for 5 min. Protein complexes were washed five times with RIPA buffer, resuspended in × 2 loading buffer, and heated at 95 °C for 5 min. Then, the protein lysis buffers were used for western blot analysis with the following antibodies: rabbit anti-ASC (Cell Signaling Technology, 67824S, 1:1000), rabbit anti-NLRP3 (Cell Signaling Technology, #8242S, 1:1000), and mouse anti-caspase-1 (Santa-Cruz Biotechnology, sc-398,715, 1:100). Homophytic IgG was used as the negative control. SDS-PAGE and Western blot were used to analysis IP assay. The ASC protein was used as a loading control, and the loading quantities of precipitated materials were regulated according to the gray levels of ASC protein, to ensure brightness of reference bands were consistent. As the molecular weight of pro-caspase-1 and ASC were close to 50 kD or 25 kD, to avoid the influence of IgG light or heavy chain, the second antibodies used for pro-caspase-1 and ASC were anti-Mouse IgG Light Chain (Abbkine, A25012) and anti-Rabbit IgG Heavy Chain (Abbkine, A25222), respectively.

Western blotting

Western blotting was performed according to conventional protocols. Briefly, the ischemic cortex or the cells were prepared for protein lysates using total protein lysis buffer (Beyotime, P0013) or IP protein lysis buffer (Beyotime, P0027) and were analyzed using SDS-PAGE (12%). The membranes were incubated with primary antibodies against NLRP3 (Cell Signaling Technology, #8242S, 1:1000), ASC (Cell Signaling Technology, 67824S, 1:1000), caspase-1 (Santa-Cruz Biotechnology, sc-398,715, 1:100), IL-1β (Santa-Cruz Biotechnology, sc-7887, 1:100), IL-18 (Abcam, ab71495, 1:125), and GADPH (Cell Signaling Technology, #2118S, 1:1000) at 4 °C overnight, followed by incubation with anti-rabbit IgG (MultiSciences (LiankeBio), GAR007, 1:5000), or anti-mouse IgG (MultiSciences (LiankeBio), GAM007, 1:5000) for 1 h at room temperature. The epitopes were visualized using an ECL western blot detection kit (KeyGEN BioTECH, KGP1126).

Elisa

The supernatants were centrifuged and collected for ELISAs. The levels of the pro-inflammatory cytokines IL-1β (R&D Systems, MLB00C) and IL-18 (eBioscience, BMS618–3) were measured after OGD/R using commercial ELISA kits from eBioscience Systems. The procedures were performed according to the manufacturer's instructions using a microplate reader (Bio-Rad, CA, USA).

Statistical analysis

The Image-Pro Plus 6.0 (Media Cybernetics, Inc., USA) software was used to analyze the optical density of the western blot results and to calculate the number of caspase-1-positive cells or double staining cells and JC-1-stained cells. Statistical analyses were performed using the SPSS 19.0 (SPSS Inc., USA) software. Data were presented as the means ± SEM with the homogeneity of variance. Statistical analyses were performed with Student's *t* test between two groups or one-way ANOVA for multiple groups, followed by LSD for post hoc comparisons. Two-way ANOVA was used to compare the results among multiple groups according to the immunofluorescence in the brain slices. $p < 0.05$ was considered statistically significant.

Results

The cellular location where NLRP3 inflammasomes were activated changed dynamically in the process of ischemia/reperfusion (I/R) injury

It was observed in the ischemic core area (Fig. 1f) that cleaved caspase-1 was mainly expressed in microglia 6 h after the I/R injury (88.36 ± 1.102%) (Fig. 1a) and was rarely expressed in other cell types (Fig. 1b–d). Then, cleaved caspase-1 was mostly expressed in neurons (63.39 ± 2.219%) (Fig. 1c) and endothelial cells (39.97 ± 2.289%) (Fig. 1d) at 24 h, while limited expressed in microglia (12.21 ± 1.068%) (Fig. 1a) and astrocytes (4.67 ± 0.985%) (Fig. 1b) was observed. Therefore, the expression of cleaved caspase-1 gradually decreased in microglia between 6 h and 24 h but simultaneously increased in neurons and endothelial cells, particularly in neurons.

As cleaved caspase-1 was expressed in microglia first, we used primary microglia and BV2 cells to explore the pathway of caspase-1 activation. The purity of primary microglia was verified as 95% or higher (Fig. 2c). We found that the protein level of NLRP3 in BV2 cells increased over time after OGD/R, especially at 24 h, compared with the NC (all $p < 0.01$) (Fig. 2a). When NLRP3 expression was silenced by NLRP3-siRNA transfection in the primary microglia and BV2 cells, we observed that the expression levels of cleaved caspase-1, ASC, cleaved IL-1β, and cleaved IL-18 were significantly downregulated after OGD/R ($p < 0.05$) (Fig. 2b and d), indicating that the inflammasome pathway that was activated in microglia was mediated by NLRP3, and the activation of NLRP3 inflammasomes in BV2 cells after OGD/R could reflect the changes in primary microglia.

NLRP3 inflammasomes expressed in PC12 and bEnd3 cells after OGD/R were induced by co-cultured BV2 cells

PC12 and bEnd3 cells were used as alternative neurons and vascular endothelial cells, respectively. A transwell co-culture system, with BV2 cells in the upper chamber and PC12 or bEnd3 cells in the lower chamber, was used to explore the expression of NLRP3 inflammasomes in PC12 and bEnd3 cells. The results showed that the expression of NLRP3 was roughly upregulated in BV2 cells 2 h after OGD/R compared with the NC group in the transwell co-culture system of BV2 and PC12 cells ($p < 0.01$); this expression gradually decreased over time (all $p < 0.01$). In addition, the same trend was observed in ASC and cleaved caspase-1 in the BV2 cells co-cultured with PC12 cells (all $p < 0.05$) (Fig. 3a and b). In contrast, we found that the expression levels of NLRP3, ASC, and cleaved caspase-1 all increased over time in PC12 cells after OGD/R in the transwell co-culture system (all $p < 0.01$) (Fig. 3a, c). However, the activation of NLRP3 inflammasomes was not observed in PC12 cells cultured alone after OGD/R (Fig. 3a, d). Similarly, the expression levels of NLRP3, ASC, and cleaved caspase-1 were significantly upregulated in bEnd3 cells co-cultured with BV2 cells 24 h after OGD/R, compared with the transwell NC group, OGD/R group, and NC group (all $p < 0.01$). The above results indicated that NLRP3 inflammasome activation in PC12 and bEnd3 cells in the transwell co-culture system after OGD/R was induced by some stimulating factor released from BV2 cells.

Then, we transfected NLRP3-siRNA to block the production of NLRP3 in BV2 cells, followed by co-cultures with PC12 or bEnd3 cells and OGD/R treatment. It was observed that the expression levels of NLRP3, ASC, and cleaved caspase-1 in PC12 cells were significantly downregulated in the transwell OGD/R + NLRP3-siRNA group compared to the transwell OGD/R group and transwell OGD/R + NC-siRNA group (Fig. 4a and b) (all $p < 0.01$). Furthermore, the results from the qRT-PCR and ELISAs also revealed that the upregulation of IL-1β and IL-18 in the PC12 cells, and supernatants induced by OGD/R were both rescued by NLRP3-silencing in the BV2 cells (Fig. 4d) (all $p < 0.05$). The same trend was also observed in bEnd3 cells (Fig. 4a, c, e). These results indicated that the stimuli released from BV2 cells were originated from the activated NLRP3 inflammasome signaling pathway in BV2 cells.

To clarify the source of NLRP3 expressed in PC12 or bEnd3 cells, we transfected NLRP3-siRNA to block the production of NLRP3 in PC12 or bEnd3 cells, followed by co-cultures with BV2 cells and OGD/R treatment. The results show that the expression of NLRP3, ASC, and cleaved caspase-1 in PC12 (Fig. 5a and b) or bEnd3 cells (Fig. 5a, c) in the transwell OGD/R + NLRP3-siRNA group decreased significantly compared to the transwell OGD/R + NC-siRNA group, but were still higher than that in OGD/R + NLRP3-siRNA group (all $p < 0.05$). Such results reinforced the finding that the activation of NLRP3 inflammasomes in PC12 or bEnd3 cells was induced by BV2 cells, and revealed that the main source of NLRP3 inflammasomes expressed in PC12 or bEnd3 cells was from their own productions.

NLRP3 inflammasomes in BV2 cells after OGD/R were associated with BV2 cell-mediated PC12 cell damage

The results from the flow cytometry (Fig. 6a) showed that BV2 cells could significantly increase the apoptotic rate of PC12 cells after OGD/R (24.19 ± 1.948%), compared with the NC group (4.44 ± 0.348%). The apoptosis of PC12 cells in transwell co-cultures after OGD/R could be attenuated via NLRP3 knockdown in BV2 cells (13.43 ± 1.594%), indicating that the damage to PC12 cells was induced by the NLRP3 inflammasomes in BV2 cells after OGD/R (all $p < 0.01$) (Fig. 6b). Such results were not shown in isolated cultured PC12 cells after OGD/R.

Mitochondrial dysfunction could activate NLRP3 inflammasomes in primary microglia and BV2 cells after OGD/R

We found that the ratio of JC-1 aggregates to monomers and the mtDNA copy numbers significantly decreased in BV2 cells 24 h after OGD/R compared to the NC group (all $p < 0.01$) (Fig. 7a), which indicated damage to the mitochondria, including mitochondrial depolarization and mtDNA damage. In addition, this damage to the mitochondria was able to be rescued by the mitochondrial protector diazoxide (all $p < 0.01$) (Fig. 7a).

Next, we aimed to clarify the relationship between mitochondrial dysfunction and NLRP3 inflammasomes. For detecting the formation of NLRP3 inflammasome, which consists of NLRP3, ASC, and pro-caspase1, IP assay was performed, which was the direct evidence for protein interaction. The IP results revealed that the same amount of ASC in BV2 cells in OGD/R 24-h group could bind more NLRP3 and pro-caspase1 compared to the NC, indicating that the formation of the NLRP3 inflammasomes was obviously increased in BV2 cells after OGD/R, which could be inhibited by diazoxide (all $p < 0.01$) (Fig. 7b). In addition, diazoxide could also suppress the upregulation of NLRP3, ASC, and cleaved caspase-1induced by OGD/R in primary microglia and BV2

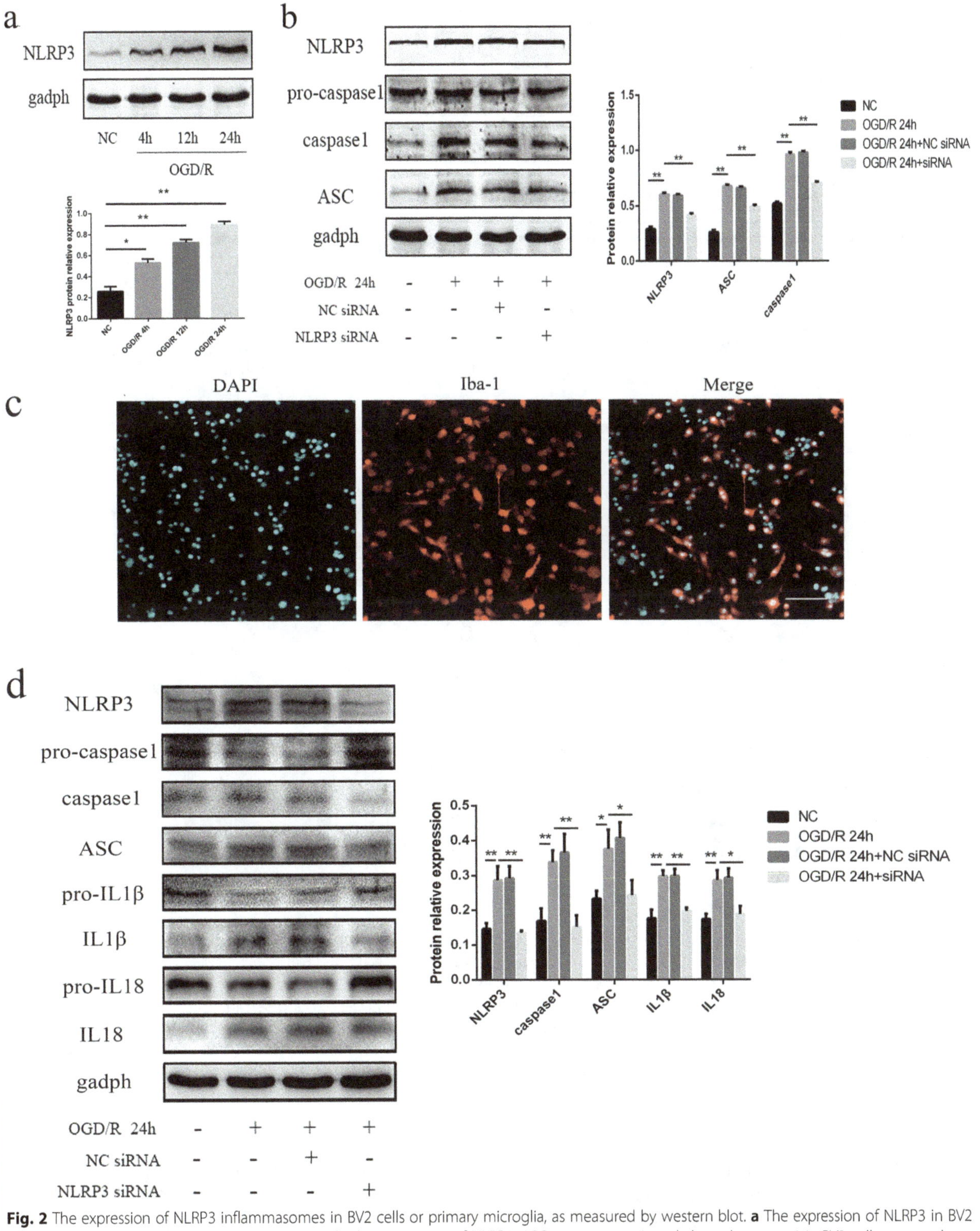

Fig. 2 The expression of NLRP3 inflammasomes in BV2 cells or primary microglia, as measured by western blot. **a** The expression of NLRP3 in BV2 cells at different time points after reoxygenation. **b** The expression of NLRP3, ASC, pro-caspase-1, and cleaved caspase-1 in BV2 cells among the different groups. **c** The purity of primary microglia. **d** The expression of NLRP3, ASC, pro-caspase-1, cleaved caspase-1, pro-IL1β, cleaved IL1β, pro-IL18, and cleaved IL18 in primary microglial cells among the different groups. OGD/R treatment was conducted at 24 h after siRNA transfection. Bar = 100 μm. $^{*}p < 0.05$, $^{**}p < 0.01$. OGD/R: oxygen-glucose deprivation/reoxygenation. The OGD continued for 4 h, followed by reoxygenation

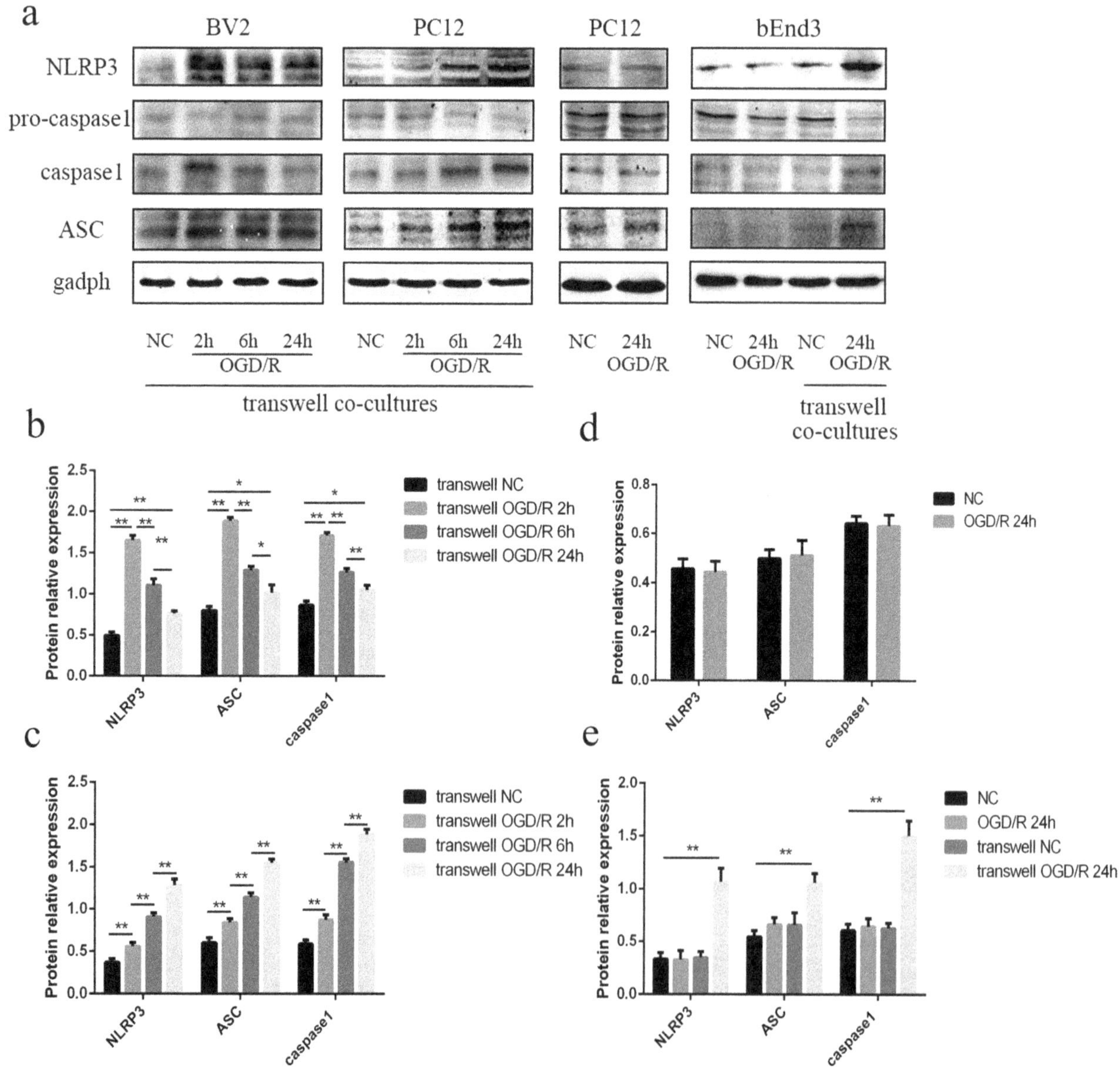

Fig. 3 NLRP3 inflammasome pathway expressed in PC12 and bEnd3 cells in the transwell co-culture system after OGD/R was induced by BV2 cells. **a** The expression levels of NLRP3, ASC, pro-caspase-1, and cleaved caspase-1 in BV2, PC12, and bEnd3 cells in different groups, as measured by western blot. **b** The changes of NLRP3, ASC, and cleaved caspase-1 in BV2 cells in the transwell co-culture with PC12 cells at different time points after reoxygenation, as measured by western blot. **c** The changes of NLRP3, ASC, and cleaved caspase-1 in PC12 cells in the transwell co-culture with BV2 cells at different time points after reoxygenation, as measured by western blot. **d** The changes of NLRP3, ASC, and cleaved caspase-1 in PC12 cells with isolated cultured between the two groups, as measured by western blot. **e** The changes of NLRP3, ASC, and cleaved caspase-1 in bEnd3 cells among the different groups, as measured by western blot. $^{*}p < 0.05$, $^{**}p < 0.01$. OGD/R: oxygen-glucose deprivation/reoxygenation. The OGD continued for 4 h, followed by reoxygenation

cells (Fig. 7c and d) (all $p < 0.01$). We also found that the upregulation of IL-1β and IL-18 24 h after OGD/R was suppressed by diazoxide in primary microglia and BV2 cells (all $p < 0.01$) (Fig. 7c and d). These results suggested that mitochondrial dysfunction was essential for the NLRP3 inflammasome formation and activation in primary microglia and BV2 cells after OGD/R. Also, the pathway in BV2 cells was same with primary microglia.

The mitochondrial protector could rescue the NLRP3 inflammasome pathway expressed in PC12 and bEnd3 cells in transwell co-cultures after OGD/R

The WB results revealed that the protein levels of NLRP3, ASC, and cleaved caspase-1 significantly decreased in PC12 (Fig. 8a and b) and bEnd3 cells (Fig. 8a, c) in the transwell OGD/R 24 h + diazoxide group, compared with the transwell OGD/R 24-h group (all $p < 0.05$). In addition, the

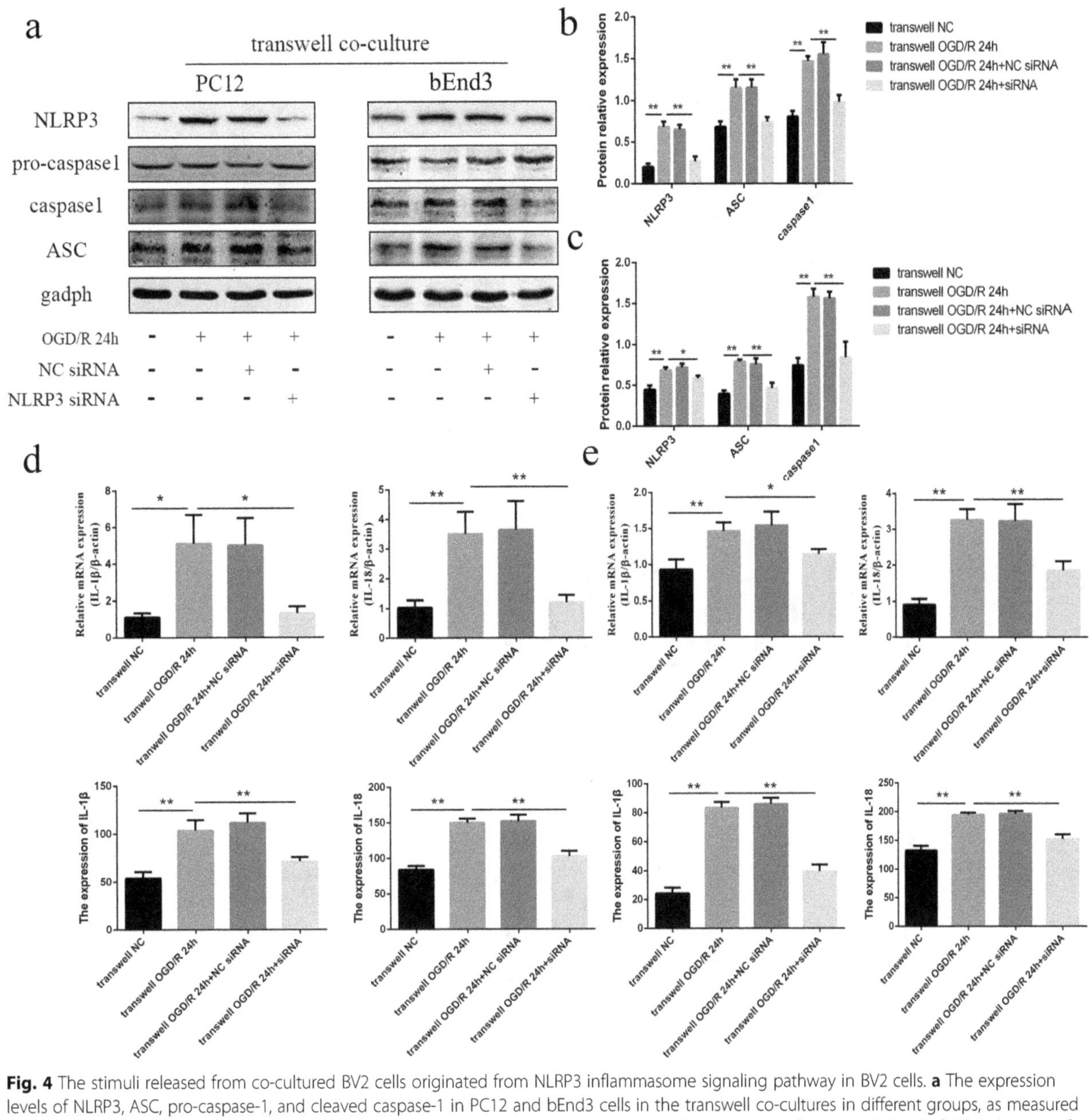

Fig. 4 The stimuli released from co-cultured BV2 cells originated from NLRP3 inflammasome signaling pathway in BV2 cells. **a** The expression levels of NLRP3, ASC, pro-caspase-1, and cleaved caspase-1 in PC12 and bEnd3 cells in the transwell co-cultures in different groups, as measured by western blot. OGD/R treatment of transwell co-culture system was conducted at 24 h after siRNA transfection in BV2 cells. **b** The changes of NLRP3, ASC, and cleaved caspase-1 in PC12 cells among the different groups, as measured by western blot. **c** The changes of NLRP3, ASC, and cleaved caspase-1 in bEnd3 cells among the different groups, as measured by western blot. **d** The expression levels of IL-1β and IL-18 in PC12 cells among the different groups, as measured by RT-PCR and ELISA. **e** The expression levels of IL-1β and IL-18 in bEnd3 cells among the different groups, as measured by RT-PCR and ELISA. *$p < 0.05$, **$p < 0.01$. OGD/R: oxygen-glucose deprivation/reoxygenation. The OGD continued for 4 h, followed by reoxygenation

results from the qRT-PCR and ELISA analyses also showed that the expression levels of IL-1β and IL-18 in PC12 (Fig. 8d) and bEnd3 cells (Fig. 8e) were all significantly downregulated in the transwell OGD/R 24 h + diazoxide group compared with the transwell OGD/R 24-h group (all $p < 0.01$). The other control groups showed no obvious changes compared with the NC groups. Such results indicated that the mitochondrial protector could effectively alleviate the NLRP3 inflammasome response in BV2, PC12, and bEnd3 cells after OGD/R.

The mitochondrial protector could inhibit the activation of NLRP3 inflammasome in cerebral I/R injury

The results of IF showed that the expression of cleaved caspase-1 was significantly decreased in microglia (12.72 ± 1.806% VS 69.9 ± 1.957%, Fig. 9a), neurons (11.87 ± 1.933%

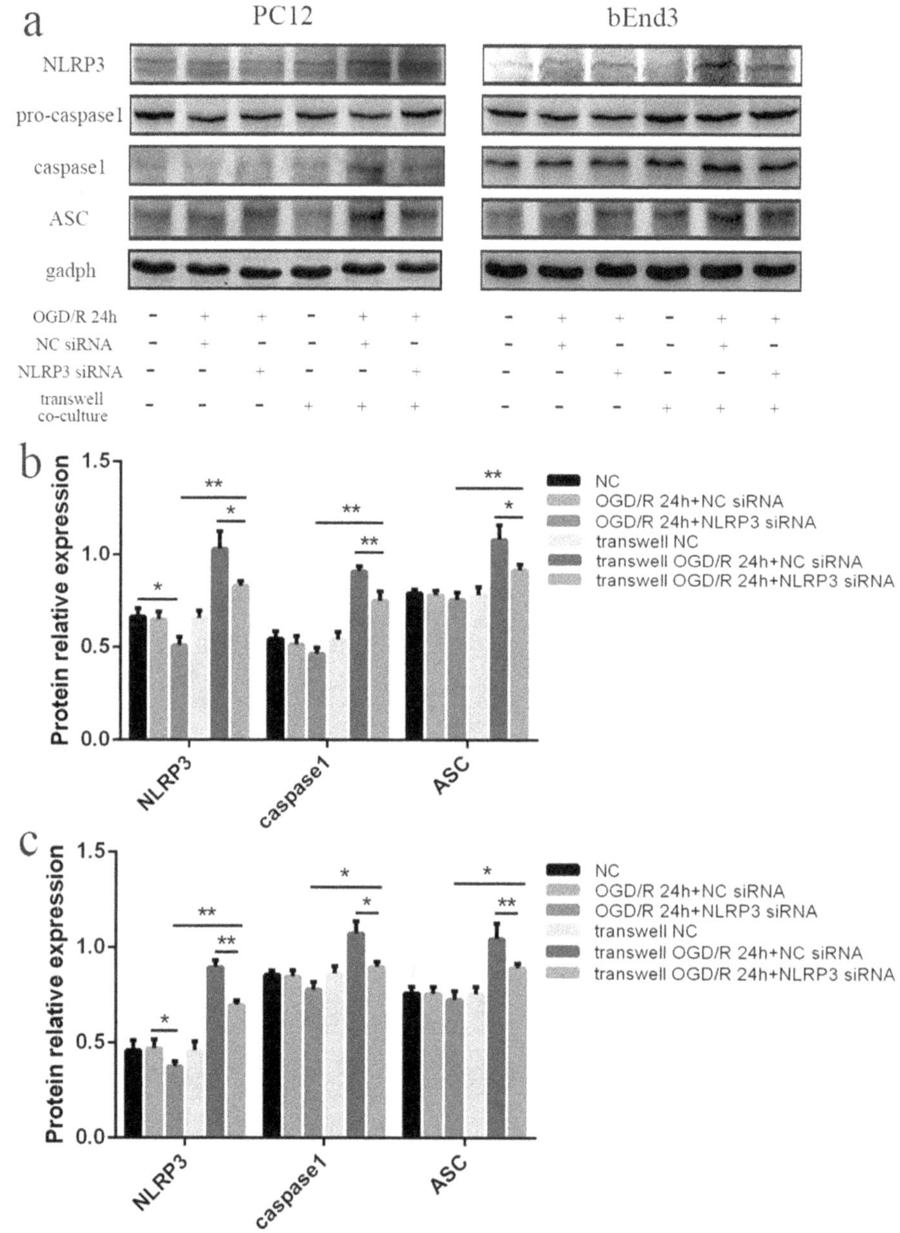

Fig. 5 The main source of NLRP3 inflammasomes expressed in PC12 or bEnd3 cells in transwell co-culture system was from their own productions. **a** The expression levels of NLRP3, ASC, pro-caspase-1, and cleaved caspase-1 in PC12 and bEnd3 cells in different groups, as measured by western blot. OGD/R treatment in isolated cultures or transwell co-cultures was conducted at 24 h after siRNA transfection in PC12 or bEnd3 cells. **b** The changes of NLRP3, ASC, and cleaved caspase-1 in PC12 cells among the different groups, as measured by western blot. **c** The changes of NLRP3, ASC, and cleaved caspase-1 in bEnd3 cells among the different groups, as measured by western blot. *$p < 0.05$, **$p < 0.01$. OGD/R: oxygen-glucose deprivation/reoxygenation. The OGD continued for 4 h, followed by reoxygenation

VS 70.76 ± 1.737%, Fig. 9b), and endothelial cells (9.12 ± 1.278% VS 57.76 ± 2.455%, Fig. 9c) in I/R + diazoxide groups at 6 h or 24 h after the cerebral I/R injury, compared with the I/R group (all $p < 0.01$).

The WB results revealed that the protein levels of NLRP3, ASC, cleaved caspase-1, cleaved IL-1β, and cleaved IL-18 significantly increased in I/R 24-h group, compared with the sham group (all $p < 0.01$) (Fig. 9d), and diazoxide could significantly inhibit the expression of NLRP3, ASC, cleaved caspase-1, cleaved IL-1β, and cleaved IL-18 (all $p < 0.01$) (Fig. 9d). These results showed that the mitochondrial protector could inhibit the activation of NLRP3 inflammasome in cerebral I/R injury, indicating that mitochondrial dysfunction played a great role in activating NLRP3 inflammasome in cerebral I/R injury.

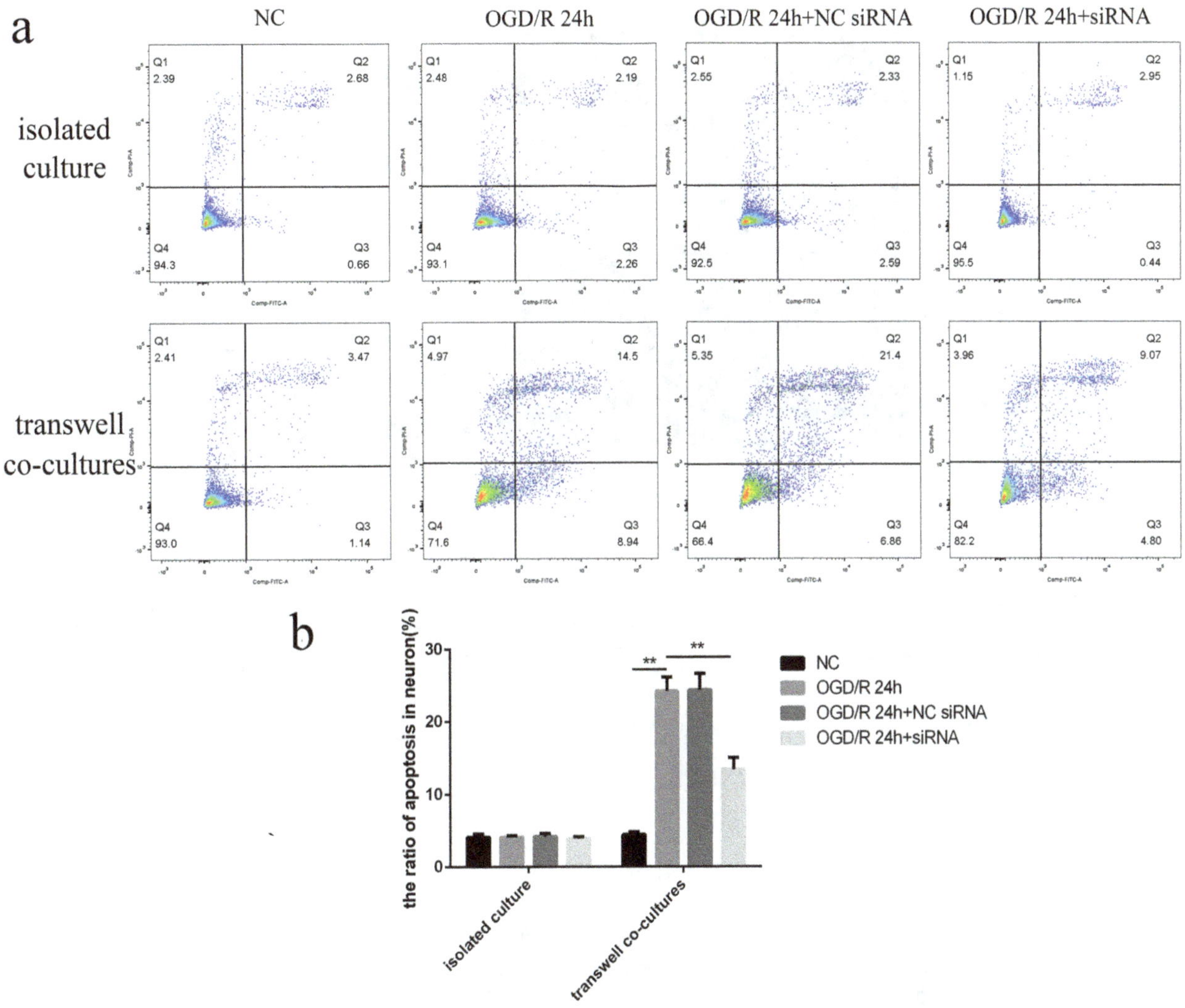

Fig. 6 NLRP3 knockdown in BV2 cells could inhibit the apoptosis of PC12 cells in the transwell co-cultures after OGD/R. **a, b** The rate of apoptotic PC12 cells among the different groups, as measured by flow cytometry. OGD/R treatment in isolated cultures or transwell co-cultures was conducted at 24 h after siRNA transfection. *$p < 0.05$, **$p < 0.01$. OGD/R: oxygen-glucose deprivation/reoxygenation. The OGD continued for 4 h, followed by reoxygenation

Discussion

Recently, NLRP3 inflammasomes have been found in some organs after I/R injury, such as the brain, heart, kidneys, and testes [19]. As has been reported, damage-associated molecular pattern (DAMP) is the critical initial stimulus to activate NLRP3 [20]. The oligomerization of NLRP3 recruits, ASC and ASC, could activate pro-caspase-1 to cleave into active fragments [21], and then cleaved caspase-1 induces the formation of mature pro-inflammatory cytokines, namely, IL-1β and IL-18 [22, 23]. These cytokines then initiate or amplify diverse downstream signaling pathways to drive pro-inflammatory processes [24], leading to cellular damage, such as autophagy and pyroptosis [22], which could release DAMPs to induce more inflammation [25].

In the mouse brain, it has been observed that NLRP3, ASC, and caspase-1 are expressed in microglia after LPS stimulation, which was not detected in astrocytes, indicating that microglia might be the main site involved in the formation of functional NLRP3 inflammasomes [4]. Moreover, Fann et al. and Wang et al. discovered that the levels of NLRP3 inflammasome proteins and of IL-1β and IL-18 were upregulated in primary cortical neurons under OGD/R conditions [5, 26]. In contrast, in a mouse model of middle cerebral artery occlusion (MCAO), Yang et al. demonstrated that NLRP3 was expressed in microglia and vascular endothelial cells but not in neurons [6]. Thus, the specific expression and distribution of NLRP3 inflammasomes in cerebral I/R injury have not led to a conclusion. In addition, the different models of ischemia, the durations of the ischemic insults, and the different interventions have been offered as possible explanations.

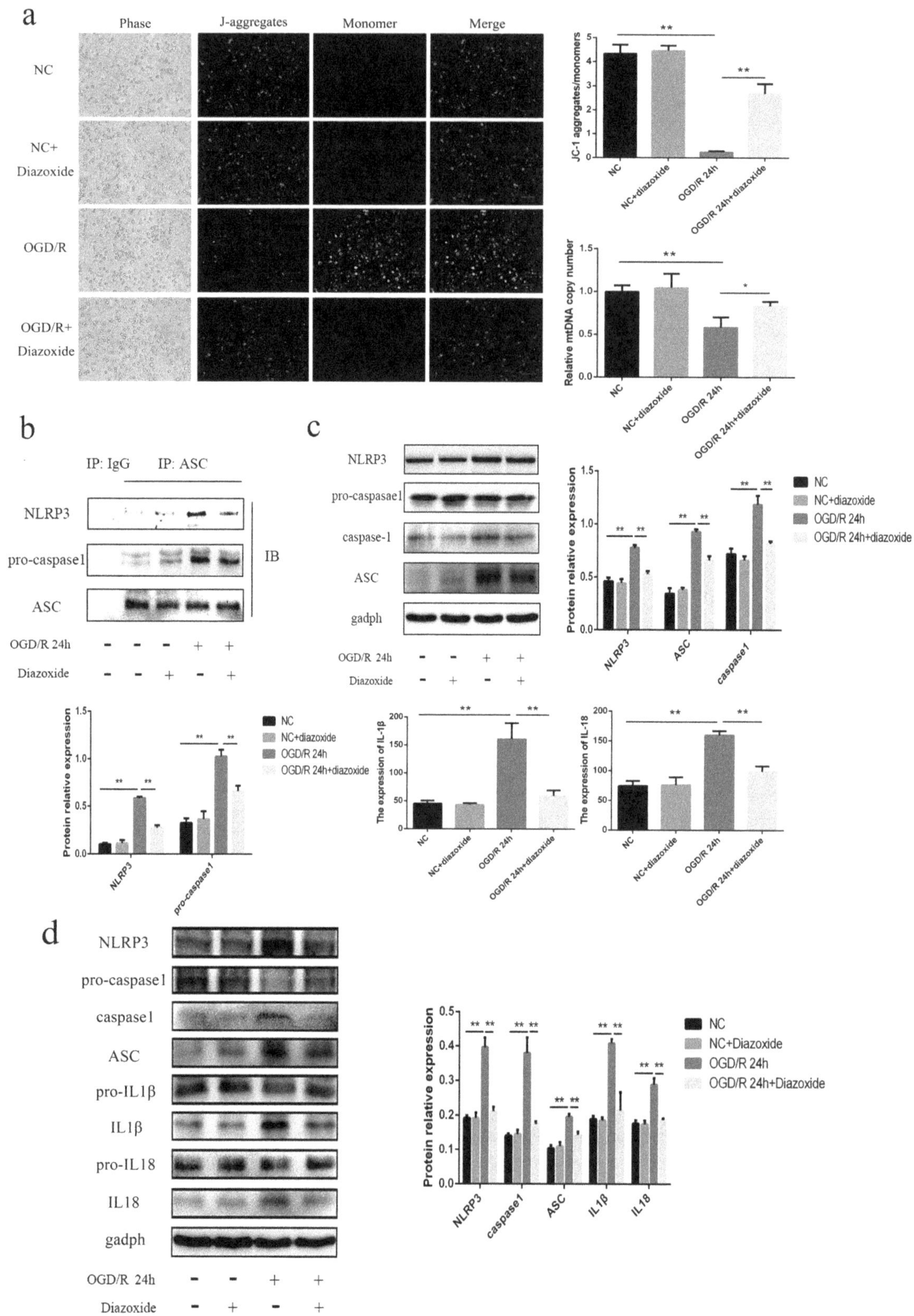

Fig. 7 (See legend on next page.)

(See figure on previous page.)

Fig. 7 Mitochondrial dysfunction could activate NLRP3 inflammasomes in BV2 cells after OGD/R. **a** Measurements of the Δψm and mtDNA copy numbers in BV2 cells among the different groups. The BV2 cells in OGD/R or OGD/R + diazoxide groups were measured at 24 h after reoxygenation. **b** The expression levels of NLRP3 and pro-caspase-1 physically associated with ASC in BV2 cells among the different groups, as measured by IP. Anti-ASC antibody was used to immunoprecipitate NLRP3 inflammasome. IB assay for ASC was used as a loading control. **c** The expression levels of NLRP3, ASC, cleaved caspase-1, IL-1β, and IL-18 in BV2 cells among the different groups, as measured by western blot and ELISA. **d** The expression of NLRP3, ASC, pro-caspase-1, cleaved caspase-1, pro-IL1β, cleaved IL1β, pro-IL18, and cleaved IL18 in primary microglial cells among the different groups. The 100 μm diazoxide was applied to the cells when got reoxygenation. Bar = 100 μm. $^{*}p < 0.05$, $^{**}p < 0.01$. OGD/R: oxygen-glucose deprivation/reoxygenation. The OGD continued for 4 h, followed by reoxygenation

In this study, we chose rats as the animal model because the genes of rats are relatively close to those of humans. In addition, it was the first time the cellular localization of the NLRP3 inflammasome pathway after I/R injury was observed dynamically. The cells used in vitro were primary microglia, BV2 microglia, PC12 neurons, and bEnd3 cerebral microvascular endothelial cells. We found that the cleaved caspase-1 in tMCAO rats was mainly expressed in ischemic core area within 24 h, which was the observed and counted area. Our results showed that activated inflammasomes were first formed in microglia after cerebral I/R injury, but not in astrocytes, and then they were mostly expressed in neurons and vascular endothelial cells at 24 h, particularly in neurons, mainly through the NLRP3 molecules. The results of this in vitro study revealed that the NLRP3 inflammasome pathway expressed in PC12 and bEnd3 cells in transwell co-culture systems after OGD/R was induced by BV2 cells, as the levels of NLRP3 inflammasomes were not changed in PC12 and bEnd3 cells only under OGD/R condition. Then, we used NLRP3-siRNA to knockdown the target gene in BV2 cells, which were cultured in a transwell co-culture system, thereby inducing a rough decrease in the level of NLRP3 inflammasomes and downstream inflammatory factors, such as caspase-1, IL-1β, and IL-18 in PC12 and bEnd3 cells in a transwell co-culture system after OGD/R. When we inhibited the expression of NLRP3 in PC12 or bEnd3 cells which were cultured in transwell co-culture system, the increase of NLRP3 inflammasomes in PC12 and bEnd3 cells in transwell co-culture system after OGD/R could be inhibited partly. These findings provided positive proof supporting that the NLRP3 inflammasomes that were expressed in PC12 and bEnd3 cells in transwell co-culture systems after OGD/R were activated by some stimulating factor originated from NLRP3 inflammasome signaling pathway in BV2 cells, and the main source of NLRP3 inflammasomes expressed in PC12 or bEnd3 cells was from their own productions. Furthermore, the apoptosis of PC12 cells was clearly activated when these cells were cultured with BV2 cells after OGD/R, which could be inhibited by NLRP3 knockdown in BV2 cells. A previous study revealed that NLRP3 inflammasomes induced caspase-1-dependent pyroptosis, which is an important event that may be an essential pathway involved in mitochondria-associated apoptosis in ketamine-induced hippocampal neurotoxicity [27]. These previous results were in accordance with our results. Taken together, it is reasonable to draw the conclusion that microglia are the main source of activated NLRP3 inflammasomes during the early stage after cerebral I/R injury, which could drive pro-inflammatory processes, leading to the cells death and disruption, which could release some stimuli (e.g., DAMPs and IL-1β) to trigger the activation of inflammasomes in surrounding cells [28, 29]. Thus, the NLRP3 inflammasomes are activated in neurons and microvascular endothelial cells over time and mainly gather in neurons during the late stage, which may induce neuronal death and blood-brain barrier (BBB) integrity dysfunction. Interestingly, we found that the expression of NLRP3 inflammasome in BV2 cells in co-culture system was gradually decreased over time, which was inconsistent with the results of isolated cultured BV2 cells. We thought the different cellular models were the main reason. In co-culture model, the released DAMP could be spread to the bottom chambers, which may result in the attenuation of activation of NLRP3 inflammasome in BV2 cells, compared to isolated culture model. Besides, the PC12 cells in co-culture model, expressing NLRP3 inflammasome later, may release some negative feedback regulator, which may inhibit the expression of NLRP3 inflammasome in BV2 cells. Of course, the specific reason still needs further studies.

As we know, microglia and astrocytes are the main cells inducing immunoreaction to cerebral I/R injury. In our results, the quantity of microglia and astrocytes in ischemic core area showed a severe decrease, especially at 24 h after cerebral I/R injury, but the microglia were activated significantly. Some studies have revealed that a specific loss of GFAP immunolabeling in protoplasmic astrocytes occurred in the area with total depletion of regional CBF (rCBF) levels, associated with advanced disintegration of cytoplasmic elements and loss of ATP in the ischemic core, whereas "classical" astrogliosis was observed in areas with remaining rCBF [30, 31], which was in accordance with our results. Also, the findings in the ischemic core, the round Iba1-positive cells appeared from 24 h and reached a peak at 4 to 7 days [32], could support our results, and degeneration of microglia in the ischemic core after prolonged MCAO was also reported by other studies [33, 34].

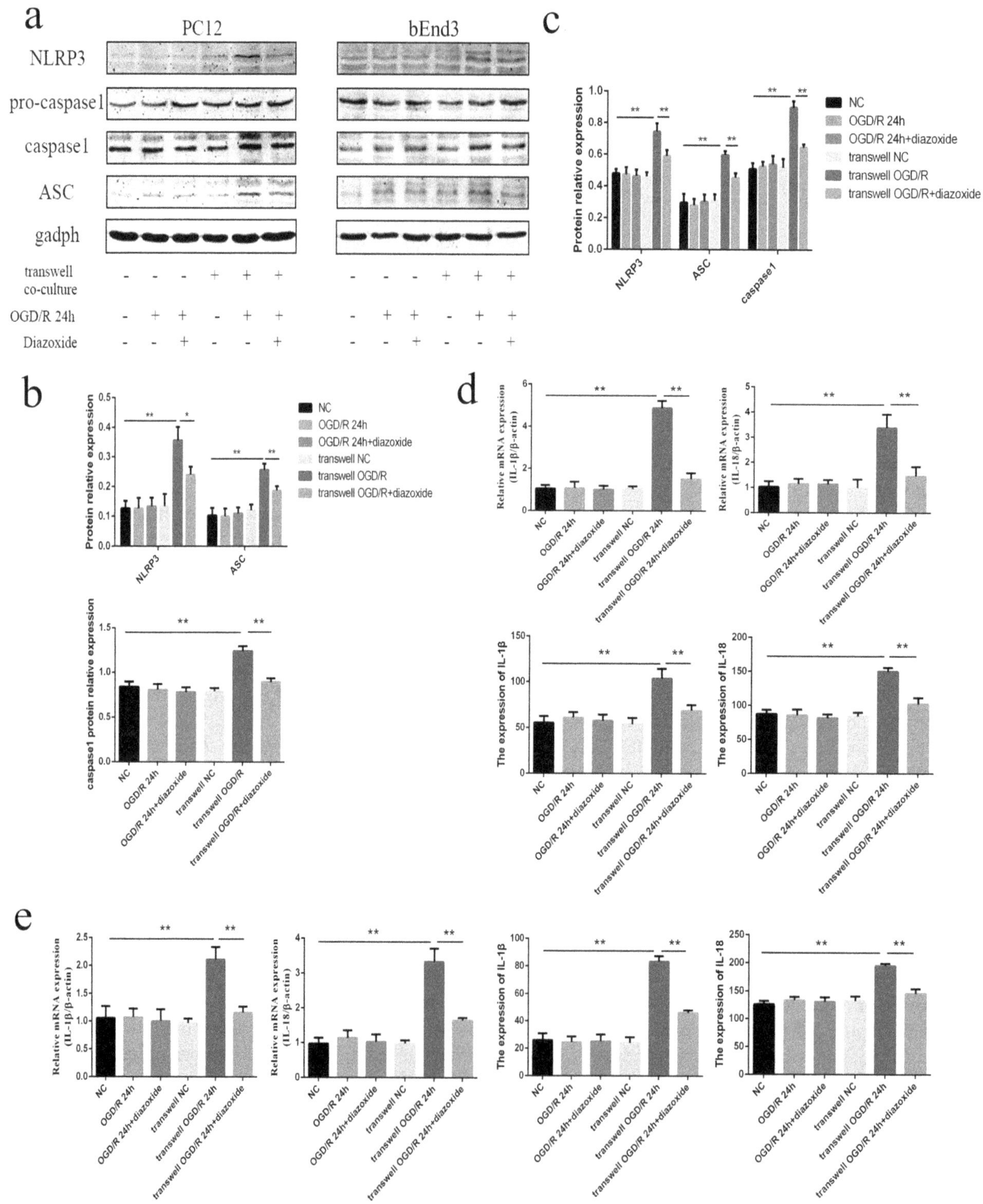

Fig. 8 (See legend on next page.)

A series of studies have demonstrated that NLRP3 inflammasomes are activated by three mechanisms: the potassium efflux [35], the release of mitochondrial reactive oxygen species (mtROS) [36], and lysosomal damage [37]. However, it has been suggested that these three models could be integrated and associated with the production of oxidized mitochondrial DNA (mtDNA) [38, 39]. Zhou et al. reported that ROS that were generated

(See figure on previous page.)

Fig. 8 Mitochondrial protector could rescue the NLRP3 inflammasome pathway expressed in PC12 and bEnd3 cells in the transwell co-cultures after OGD/R. **a** The expression levels of NLRP3, ASC, pro-caspase-1, and cleaved caspase-1 in PC12 and bEnd3 cells among the different groups, as measured by western blot. **b** The changes of NLRP3, ASC, and cleaved caspase-1 in PC12 cells among the different groups, as measured by western blot. **c** The changes of NLRP3, ASC, and cleaved caspase-1 in bEnd3 cells among the different groups, as measured by western blot. **d** The expression levels of IL-1β and IL-18 in PC12 cells among the different groups, as measured by RT-PCR and ELISA. **e** The expression levels of IL-1β and IL-18 in bEnd3 cells among the different groups, as measured by RT-PCR and ELISA. The 100 μm diazoxide was applied to the cells when got reoxygenation. $^*p < 0.05$, $^{**}p < 0.01$. OGD/R: oxygen-glucose deprivation/reoxygenation. The OGD continued for 4 h, followed by reoxygenation

following mitochondrial dysfunction, which manifested as a decrease in the mitochondrial membrane potential (Δψm), induced by the opening of the mitochondrial permeability transition pore (mPTP), could promote NLRP3 inflammasome activation [40]. In addition to the mtROS, mtDNA released into the cytoplasm from the damaged mitochondria has also been proposed to act as a mitochondrial danger signal, promoting the activation of NLRP3 inflammasomes [38, 41]. Similarly, we found that the function of mitochondria in BV2 cells after OGD/R

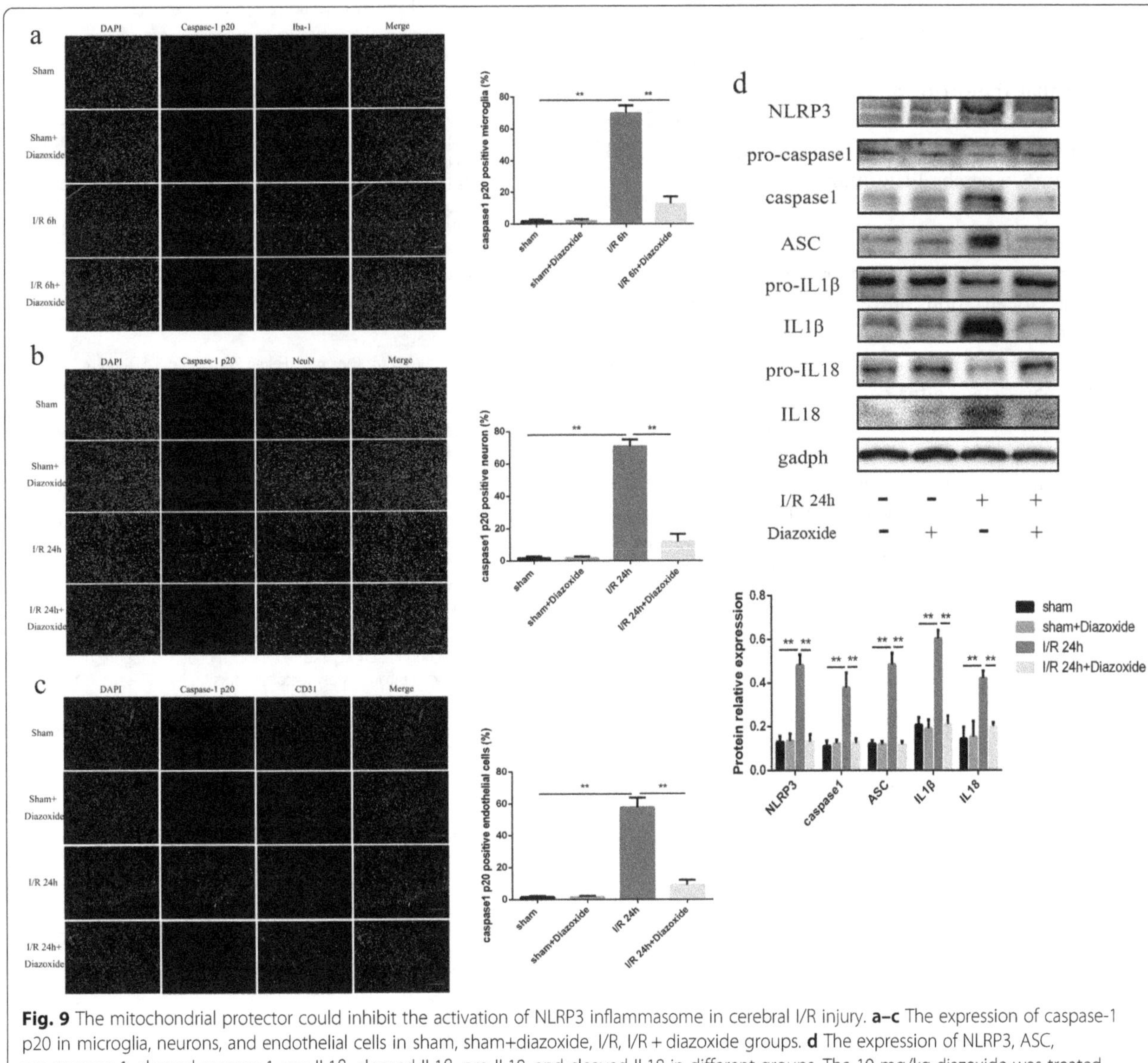

Fig. 9 The mitochondrial protector could inhibit the activation of NLRP3 inflammasome in cerebral I/R injury. **a–c** The expression of caspase-1 p20 in microglia, neurons, and endothelial cells in sham, sham+diazoxide, I/R, I/R + diazoxide groups. **d** The expression of NLRP3, ASC, pro-caspase-1, cleaved caspase-1, pro-IL1β, cleaved IL1β, pro-IL18, and cleaved IL18 in different groups. The 10 mg/kg diazoxide was treated intraperitoneally when the rats got reperfusion. Bar = 100 μm. $^*p < 0.05$, $^{**}p < 0.01$

was damaged and included mitochondrial depolarization and mtRNA damage. In addition, diazoxide was shown to be able to protect the function of mitochondria by preventing mitochondrial depolarization and mtRNA damage, which aligned with previous studies that discovered that diazoxide could prevent the opening of the mPTP and mitochondrial depolarization in cardiac hypertrophy and in an oxidatively stressed ischemic environment [42, 43]. Thus, we used diazoxide to determine the relationship between mitochondrial dysfunction and NLRP3 inflammasomes in primary microglia and BV2 cells. The results indicated that mitochondrial dysfunction played a substantial role in the activation of the NLRP3 inflammasome pathway in primary microglia and BV2 cells after OGD/R, and that diazoxide could effectively alleviate the NLRP3 inflammasome response in primary microglia and BV2 cells, transwell co-cultured PC12, and bEnd3 cells after OGD/R. Then we detected the activation of NLRP3 inflammsome pathway in rats during cerebral I/R injury, and found that the diazoxide could inhibit the activation of NLRP3 inflammasome, which indicated that mitochondrial dysfunction played a great role in activating NLRP3 inflammasome in cerebral I/R injury.

Conclusion

Our study was the first to find the dynamic change in the cellular localization of the NLRP3 inflammasome pathway after cerebral I/R injury, showing that microglia are the main source of activated NLRP3 inflammasomes during the early stage after cerebral I/R injury, and then the NLRP3 inflammasomes were activated in neurons and microvascular endothelial cells over time and mainly gathered in neurons during the late stage. Furthermore, mitochondrial dysfunction was essential for the activation of NLRP3 inflammasomes in microglia, and a mitochondrial protector could effectively alleviate the NLRP3 inflammasome response in microglia, neurons, and microvascular endothelial cells after OGD/R and cerebral I/R injury.

Abbreviations

Δψm: Mitochondrial membrane potential; ASC: Apoptosis-associated speck-like protein containing a caspase activation recruitment domain; BBB: Blood-brain barrier; I/R: Ischemia/reperfusion; IF: Immunoprecipitation; mPTP: Mitochondrial permeability transition pore; mtDNA: Mitochondrial DNA; mtROS: Mitochondrial reactive oxygen species; NLRP3: Nod-like receptor protein 3; OGD/R: Oxygen-glucose deprivation/reoxygenation; pro-caspase1: Precursor caspase-1; qPCR: Real-time quantitative PCR; tMCAO: Transient middle cerebral artery occlusion

Funding

This work was supported by the National Natural Science Foundation of China [NSFC 81572481 to YP], the key project of production, study and research of Guangzhou city [No. 201508020058 to YP], the International Collaboration Program of Universities in Guangdong Province Grant [No. 2012 gjhz001 to Y.P.], the Science & Technique Plan fund of Guangdong Province [2009B060700040 to YP], the Sun Yat-Sen Scientific Research Sailing Project [YXQH201702 to J.Pan], the Guangdong Natural Science Foundation [2017A030313655 to J. Pan], and the Science &Technique Plan fund of Guangdong Province [2013B021800098 to M.Li].

Authors' contributions

ZG and JP carried out the experiments, performed the analysis, and wrote the manuscript. QS collaborated with us and facilitated the equipment and software to perform the biochemical experiments. ML analyzed the data and imaging. YP designed the study and contributed to writing and editing the manuscript. All authors read and approved the final manuscript.

Consent for publication

Not applicable.

Competing interests

The authors declare that they have no competing interests,

References

1. Palencia G, Medrano JA, Ortiz-Plata A, Farfan DJ, Sotelo J, Sanchez A, et al. Anti-apoptotic, anti-oxidant, and anti-inflammatory effects of thalidomide on cerebral ischemia/reperfusion injury in rats. J Neurol Sci. 2015;351:78–87.
2. de Abulafia DP, Rivero Vaccari JP, Lozano JD, Lotocki G, Keane RW, Dietrich WD. Inhibition of the inflammasome complex reduces the inflammatory response after thromboembolic stroke in mice. J Cereb Blood Flow Metab. 2009;29:534–44.
3. Savage CD, Lopez-Castejon G, Denes A, Brough D. NLRP3- inflammasome activating DAMPs stimulate an inflammatory response in glia in the absence of priming which contributes to brain inflammation after injury. Front Immunol. 2012;3:288.
4. Gustin A, Kirchmeyer M, Koncina E, Felten P, Losciuto S, Heurtaux T, et al. NLRP3 inflammasome is expressed and functional in mouse brain microglia but not in astrocytes. PLoS One. 2015;10:e0130624.
5. Fann DY, Lee SY, Manzanero S, Tang SC, Gelderblom M, Chunduri P, et al. Intravenous immunoglobulin suppresses NLRP1 and NLRP3 inflammasome-mediated neuronal death in ischemic stroke. Cell Death Dis. 2013;4:e790.
6. Yang F, Wang Z, Wei X, Han H, Meng X, Zhang Y, et al. NLRP3 deficiency ameliorates neurovascular damage in experimental ischemic stroke. J Cereb Blood Flow Metab. 2014;34:660–7.
7. Latz E. The inflammasomes: mechanisms of activation and function. Curr Opin Immunol. 2010;22:28–33.
8. Yu JW, Lee MS. Mitochondria and the NLRP3 inflammasome: physiological and pathological relevance. Arch Pharm Res. 2016;39:1503–18.
9. Liu X, Wu JY, Zhou F, Sun XL, Yao HH, Yang Y, et al. The regulation of rotenone-induced inflammatory factor production by ATP-sensitive potassium channel expressed in BV-2 cells. Neurosci Lett. 2006;394:131–5.
10. Pan JR, Li Y, Pei Z, Li XP, Peng Y, Wang YD. Hypoxic tissues are associated with microvessel density following brain ischemia-reperfusion. Neurol Sci. 2010;31:765–71.
11. Wu H, Wang P, Li Y, Wu M, Lin J, Huang Z. Diazoxide attenuates postresuscitation brain injury in a rat model of asphyxial cardiac arrest by opening mitochondrial ATP-sensitive potassium channels. Biomed Res Int. 2016;2016:1253842.
12. Yang Z, Chen Y, Zhang Y, Jiang Y, Fang X, Xu J. Sevoflurane postconditioning against cerebral ischemic neuronal injury is abolished in diet-induced obesity: role of brain mitochondrial KATP channels. Mol Med Rep. 2014;9:843–50.
13. Ashwal S, Tone B, Tian HR, Cole DJ, Pearce WJ. Core and penumbral nitric oxide synthase activity during cerebral ischemia and reperfusion. Stroke. 1998;29:1037–47.
14. Ni M, Aschener M. Neonatal rat primary microglia: isolation, culturing and selected applications. Curr. Protoc. Toxicol. 2010;Chapter 12:Unit 12.17.
15. Pan JR, He L, Li XP, Li M, Zhang XN, Venesky J, et al. Activating autophagy in hippocampal cells alleviates the morphine-induced memory impairment. Mol Neurobiol. 2017;54:1710–24.

16. Zujovic V, Taupin V. Use of cocultured cell systems to elucidate chemokine-dependent neuronal/microglial interactions: control of microglial activation. Methods. 2003;29:345–50.
17. Chen Y, Veenman L, Singh S, Ouyang F, Liang J, Huang W, et al. 2-Cl-MGV-1 ameliorates apoptosis in the thalamus and hippocampus and cognitive deficits after cortical infarct in rats. Stroke. 2017;48:3366–74.
18. Gong Z, Zhao S, Zhang J, Xu X, Guan W, Jing L, et al. Initial research on the relationship between let-7 family members in the serum and massive cerebral infarction. J Neurol Sci. 2016;361:150–7.
19. Guo Z, Yu S, Chen X, Ye R, Zhu W, Liu X. NLRP3 is involved in ischemia/reperfusion injury. CNS Neurol Disord Drug Targets. 2016;15:699–712.
20. Hornung V, Latz E. Critical functions of priming and lysosomal damage for NLRP3 activation. Eur J Immunol. 2010;40:620–3.
21. Rubartelli A. Redox control of NLRP3 inflammasome activation in health and disease. J Leukoc Biol. 2012;92:951–8.
22. Schroder K, Tschopp J. The inflammasomes. Cell. 2010;140:821–32.
23. Zheng Q, Ren Y, Reinach PS, She Y, Xiao B, Hua S, et al. Reactive oxygen species activated NLRP3 inflammasomes prime environment-induced murine dry eye. Exp Eye Res. 2014;125:1–8.
24. Niu L, Zhang S, Wu J, Chen L, Wang Y. Upregulation of NLRP3 inflammasome in the tears and ocular surface of dry eye patients. PLoS One. 2015;10:e0126277.
25. Lamkanfi M, Dixit VM. Manipulation of host cell death pathways during microbial infections. Cell Host Microbe. 2010;8:44–54.
26. Wang CP, Zhang LZ, Li GC, Shi YW, Li JL, Zhang XC, et al. Mulberroside a protects against ischemic impairment in primary culture of rat cortical neurons after oxygen-glucose deprivation followed by reperfusion. J Neurosci Res. 2014;92:944–54.
27. Ye Z, Li Q, Guo Q, Xiong Y, Guo D, Yang H, et al. Ketamine induces hippocampal apoptosis through a mechanism associated with the caspase-1 dependent pyroptosis. Neuropharmacology. 2017;128:63–75.
28. Kono H, Kimura Y, Latz E. Inflammasome activation in response to dead cells and their metabolites. Curr Opin Immunol. 2014;30:91–8.
29. Gao L, Dong Q, Song Z, Shen F, Shi J, Li Y. NLRP3 inflammasome: a promising target in ischemic stroke. Inflamm Res. 2017;66:17–24.
30. Lukaszevicz AC, Sampaïo N, Guégan C, Benchoua A, Couriaud C, Chevalier E, et al. High sensitivity of protoplasmic cortical astroglia to focal ischemia. J Cereb Blood Flow Metab. 2002;22:289–98.
31. Mu S, Liu B, Ouyang L, Zhan M, Chen S, Wu J, et al. Characteristic changes of astrocyte and microglia in rat striatum induced by 3-NP and MCAO. Neurochem Res. 2016;41:707–14.
32. Ito D, Tanaka K, Suzuki S, Dembo T, Fukuuchi Y. Enhanced expression of Iba1, ionized calcium-binding adapter molecule 1, after transient focal cerebral ischemia in rat brain. Stroke. 2001;32:1208–15.
33. Denes A, Vidyasagar R, Feng J, Narvainen J, McColl BW, Kauppinen RA, et al. Proliferating resident microglia after focal cerebral ischaemia in mice. J Cereb Blood Flow Metab. 2007;27:1941–53.
34. Davies CA, Loddick SA, Stroemer RP, Hunt J, Rothwell NJ. An integrated analysis of the progression of cell responses induced by permanent focal middle cerebral artery occlusion in the rat. Exp Neurol. 1998;154:199–212.
35. Petrilli V, Papin S, Dostert C, Mayor A, Martinon F, Tschopp J. Activation of the NALP3 inflammasome is triggered by low intracellular potassium concentration. Cell Death Differ. 2007;14:1583–9.
36. Dostert C, Petrilli V, Van Bruggen R, Steele C, Mossman BT, Tschopp J. Innate immune activation through Nalp3 inflammasome sensing of asbestos and silica. Science. 2008;320:674–7.
37. Hornung V, Bauernfeind F, Halle A, Samstad EO, Kono H, Rock KL, et al. Silica crystals and aluminum salts activate the NALP3 inflammasome through phagosomal destabilization. Nat Immunol. 2008;9:847–56.
38. Shimada K, Crother TR, Karlin J, Dagvadori J, Chiba N, Chen S, et al. Oxidized mitochondrial DNA activates the NLRP3 inflammasome during apoptosis. Immunity. 2012;36:401–14.
39. Gurung P, Lukens JR, Kanneganti TD. Mitochondria: diversity in the regulation of the NLRP3 inflammasome. Trends Mol Med. 2015;21:193–201.
40. Zhou R, Yazdi AS, Menu P, Tschopp J. A role for mitochondria in NLRP3 inflammasome activation. Nature. 2011;469:221–5.
41. Nakahira K, Haspel JA, Rathinam VA, Lee SJ, Dolinay T, Lam HC, et al. Autophagy proteins regulate innate immune responses by inhibiting the release of mitochondrial DNA mediated by the NALP3 inflammasome. Nat Immunol. 2011;12:222–30.
42. Lucas AM, Caldas FR, da Silva AP, Ventura MM, Leite IM, Filgueiras AB, et al. Diazoxide prevents reactive oxygen species and mitochondrial damage, leading to anti-hypertrophic effects. Chem Biol Interact. 2017;261:50–5.
43. Chen W, Liu Y, Xue G, Zhang L, Zhang L, Shao S. Diazoxide protects L6 skeletal myoblasts from H2O2-induced apoptosis via the phosphatidylinositol-3 kinase/Akt pathway. Inflamm Res. 2016;65:53–60.

A review of the role of cav-1 in neuropathology and neural recovery after ischemic stroke

Qianyi Huang, Wei Zhong, Zhiping Hu and Xiangqi Tang*

Abstract

Ischemic stroke starts a series of pathophysiological processes that cause brain injury. Caveolin-1 (cav-1) is an integrated protein and locates at the caveolar membrane. It has been demonstrated that cav-1 can protect blood–brain barrier (BBB) integrity by inhibiting matrix metalloproteases (MMPs) which degrade tight junction proteins. This article reviews recent developments in understanding the mechanisms underlying BBB dysfunction, neuroinflammation, and oxidative stress after ischemic stroke, and focuses on how cav-1 modulates a series of activities after ischemic stroke. In general, cav-1 reduces BBB permeability mainly by downregulating MMP9, reduces neuroinflammation through influencing cytokines and inflammatory cells, promotes nerve regeneration and angiogenesis via cav-1/VEGF pathway, reduces apoptosis, and reduces the damage mediated by oxidative stress. In addition, we also summarize some experimental results that are contrary to the above and explore possible reasons for these differences.

Keywords: Ischemic stroke, Cav-1, BBB permeability, Neurogenesis, Angiogenesis, Neuroinflammation, Apoptosis, Oxidative stress

Introduction

Stroke is a common cerebrovascular event and is one of the leading causes of mortality and morbidity worldwide. Ischemic stroke (IS) and hemorrhagic stroke are the two major categories of stroke, and IS is more common, accounting for 87% of all strokes [1]. IS is caused by a blocked blood vessel as a result of a thrombus or embolus and leads to hypoxia and loss of glucose in the cerebral tissue that survives [2]. Intensive basic and clinical studies have revealed a variety of stroke risk factors and elucidated many mechanisms of ischemic brain injury. Cerebral ischemia initiates multiple pathophysiological processes, including vasogenic edema, excitotoxicity, disruption of the blood–brain barrier (BBB), oxidative stress, cerebral inflammation, and neuronal death [3, 4]. Although significant progress has been made in understanding the pathophysiology of IS, patients with acute brain ischemia still lack treatment options.

Administration of tissue plasminogen activator (tPA) is the most effective treatment option for cerebral ischemia several years ago [5], but its use is limited to a narrow window after the onset of stroke, as the risk of hemorrhagic transformation increases over time, causing increased brain damage. Since 2015, mechanical thrombectomy has become the first-line treatment for anterior circulation stroke with proximal large-artery occlusion. However, only about 20% of stroke patients have large-artery occlusion and it is a challenge to deliver treatment to them within the 24-h time window because the procedure can only be performed in highly specialized centers [6]. In general, for more patients who cannot accept thrombolysis or mechanical thrombectomy, it is essential to elucidate the molecular mechanisms underlying IS and explore potential therapeutic targets to restore function after stroke.

The caveolae of the cell membrane are invaginations of the plasma membrane with an omega shape and a diameter of 60–80 nm which are rich in cholesterol and glycosphingolipids [7]. The caveolin family of proteins, which includes caveolin-1 (cav-1), caveolin-2, and caveolin-3, are located in cell membrane caveolae [8]. Cav-1 is the major component, is a specific marker of caveolae, and is generally distributed in smooth muscle cells, endothelial cells, skeletal myoblasts, fibroblasts, and adipocytes [9]. Cav-1 modulates a wide range of cellular events such as proliferation, lipid metabolism, cellular tracking, and signal transduction [10]. Cav-1 has also demonstrated a beneficial

* Correspondence: txq6633@csu.edu.cn
Department of Neurology, The Second Xiangya Hospital, Central South University, Renmin Road 139#, Changsha 410011, Hunan, China

role in IS. In this review, we discuss how caveolins modulate BBB permeability and the relationships between cav-1 and a series of processes including neurogenesis, angiogenesis, neuroinflammation, apoptosis, and oxidative stress in IS.

Pathophysiological mechanisms in IS: BBB damage, inflammation, and free radicals

In acute IS, an embolic or thrombotic event usually results in a rapid reduction in blood supply to a specific brain region, temporarily or permanently. The glucose and oxygen supply to the brain decreases, causing a rapid decline in ATP and a subsequent large movement of Ca^{2+} from the extracellular to the intracellular space [11]. Because of a lack of energy, the membrane ion pump which includes the Na^+-K^+-ATPase fails to efflux intracellular sodium and this is a fundamental reason for cytotoxic edema [12]. BBB damage further exacerbates brain edema and cerebral injury [13]. Middle cerebral artery occlusion (MCAO) with reperfusion leads to a biphasic disruption of the BBB [14]. The initial opening is reversible and is associated with the activation of MMP-2. The second opening of the BBB is mediated by MMP-3 and MMP-9 which are induced by inflammatory cytokines [15]. Matrix metalloproteases (MMPs) are a group of endopeptidases that cleave protein substrates including fibronectin, laminin, proteoglycans, and type-IV collagen based on Zn^{2+} ion [16]. The early degradation of tight junction (TJ) proteins appears to be associated with MMP-2 in the early period of ischemia, and direct injection of MMP-2 into the rat brain disrupts the BBB [17]. However, MMP-2 knockout did not provide neuroprotection in a rodent MCAO stroke model [18]. This may indicate that MMP-2 is not the major deleterious enzyme in the MMP response to ischemic stroke. In contrast, knockout of the MMP-9 gene demonstrates significant neuroprotection in an MCAO animal model [19]. Although inhibition or knockout of MMP-9 attenuates early degradation of the BBB in MCAO models, it is ineffective in preventing later opening of the BBB at 48 h after IS, and MMP-9 is thought to be beneficial in later stroke recovery, especially in promoting angiogenesis and neurogenesis [8, 20]. Therefore, it remains a challenge to identify agents that restore the integrity of the BBB and prevent brain edema without intervening in recovery.

Post-ischemic inflammation is another critical factor in the evolution of cerebral damage in IS models. In the first few hours after IS, microglial cells resident in the brain are activated and release toxic proinflammatory cytokines. These cytokines enable leukocytes to transmigrate across the endothelium and exacerbate brain infarction [21, 22]. Following microglial activation, peripheral macrophages, lymphocytes, and dendritic cells migrate to the site of injury, which precedes a neutrophil influx [23]. The infiltrating neutrophils promote BBB breakdown, resulting in deteriorating stroke outcomes. Inhibiting the upregulation of neutrophil integrins can ameliorate inflammatory responses and BBB dysfunction after ischemia [24]. It has been shown that neutrophils in the infarct core produce MMP-9 after IS and MMP-9 can further promote leukocyte recruitment. This positive feedback contributes to serious BBB breakdown and neuronal injury [25]. In terms of lymphocytes, Yilmaz et al. has shown that $CD4^+$ (helper T cells, Th) and $CD8^+$ T cells (cytotoxic T cells, Tc) are promotors of brain infarction and contributors to inflammatory responses after IS [26]. Previous studies have found that $CD4^+$ Th1 cells secrete pro-inflammatory cytokines, such as interferon gamma, and lymphotoxin alpha in stroke, whereas $CD4^+$ Th2 produce anti-inflammatory cytokines including IL-4, IL-10, and IL-13 [27]. Contrary to Th cells, the role of regulatory cells (Tregs) after ischemia is controversial. Liesz et al. found an increase in delayed brain damage in Treg-deficient mice, but less secondary infarct growth after the re-expression of Treg cells [28]. However, Kleinschnitz et al. showed that knockout of endogenous Tregs can reduce the cerebral volume of infarction and improve functional outcomes [29]. Another study has clearly demonstrated that depletion of B cells profoundly increases infarct volumes and mortality and impairs neurological function [30].

Free radicals and reactive species are thought to play major roles in cerebral ischemia reperfusion (I/R) injury. Reactive species include reactive oxygen species (ROS) and reactive nitrogen species (RNS). Huge quantities of ROS are produced following ischemia reperfusion, and they can increase brain damage through different mechanisms. For instance, ROS can destroy some cellular macromolecules contributing to autophagy, apoptosis, and necrosis [31]. ROS enhance inflammatory responses by activating inflammation factors and promoting leucocyte infiltration [32]. Furthermore, free radicals can affect BBB permeability through different ways. For example, ROS can oxidize and peroxidize proteins and lipids, and peroxidation of membrane lipids can directly damage BBB integrity [33]. ROS can also activate ProMMPs which degrade TJ proteins, further inducing BBB hyperpermeability. Reduction of ROS through the knockdown of NADPH oxidase blocks the upregulation of MMP-9 by inhibiting nuclear factor-κB (NF-κB)-dependent MMP-9 promoter activity [34]. ROS produced by the xanthine/xanthine oxidase system can directly redistribute TJ proteins by acting on the Rho, PI3K, and PKB pathways [35]. RNS, typically including NO and peroxynitrite, mediate BBB damage and functional deficits following IS. Physiological concentrations of NO are essential for a variety of processes, including neuronal communication, vascular tone regulation, and synaptic transmission [36, 37]. High concentrations of NO can induce inflammation and apoptotic cell death, resulting in a larger infarction size, which is detrimental to the ischemic brain tissue [38, 39]. RNS also mediate MMP activation in cerebral I/R injury [40]. Thus, reducing free radicals could be an effective mechanism for protection in acute ischemic stroke.

Caveolae and caveolins

Caveolae were first observed by Palade and Yamada independently in the 1950s [41]. Caveolins and cavins have been found to be critical for the caveolae formation. Cavin, which is also termed polymerase I and transcript release factor, is an adapter protein that forms oligomers and assists in membrane curvature [42]. Caveolins are 22–24 kDa integral membrane proteins which are divided into three groups, caveolin-1, caveolin-2, and caveolin-3, with an NH_2-terminal membrane attachment domain and a COOH-terminal membrane attachment domain that bind to membranes with high affinity, and both the N- and C-termini face the cytoplasm [43, 44]. Cav-1 and cav-2 are ubiquitously distributed, while cav-3 is primarily expressed in vascular smooth muscle, skeletal, and cardiac muscle cells. However, cav-3 has also been detected in astrocytes, neurons, and microglial cells [45, 46]. In the brain, cav-1 and cav-2 are primarily expressed in endothelial cells, and cav-3 is expressed in astrocytes [47, 48]. Human cav-1 and human cav-3 share 65% sequence identity and 85% sequence similarity and display similar activities [49]. Cav-2 shares 38% sequence identity and 58% sequence similarity with cav-1 [50], but unlike cav-1, cav-2 is not essential for caveolae formation. In cav-2-deficient mice, although the expression of cav-1 is decreased, the formation of caveolae is not affected [51]. Caveolins contain several separate domains: an N-terminal domain (residues 1–53), a caveolin-scaffolding domain (CSD) (residues 54–73), a transmembrane domain (residues 74–106), and a C-terminal domain (residues 107–151) [52]. Cav-1 and cav-3 interact with many proteins through the CSD. The CSD binds to caveolin-binding motifs (CBDs). This binding motif is characterized by the amino acid sequence: ΦXΦXXXXΦ, ΦXXXXΦXXΦ, ΦXΦXXXXΦXXΦ, where Φ is an aromatic residue, such as tyrosine, tryptophan, or phenylalanine, and X is any amino acid [53]. The CSD functions as a docking site for many intracellular signaling proteins. For example, CBD binding to the CSD usually inhibits a diverse range of proteins, such as eNOS, epithelial growth factor receptor, PKA, PKC, G proteins, and Src family proteins. Moreover, the CSD has also been described as an activator of insulin receptor signaling [54, 55].

Functionally, caveolae are important in endocytosis, oncogenesis, and phagocytosis [56]. Caveolins can bind and regulate proteins with the CBD including NOS, MMP2, and epidermal growth factor receptor (EGFR), and they are involved in numerous cellular activities such as apoptosis [57], cholesterol transport [58], and cancer metastasis [59, 60]. Cav-1, a well-established major structural protein of caveolae, has been suggested as playing an important role in the regulation of multiple cellular processes, including cell growth, differentiation, endocytosis, cholesterol trafficking, and cellular senescence [61]. Interestingly, it has been shown that cav-1 regulates the anti-atherogenic properties of macrophage, but cav-1 promotes atherosclerosis in endothelial cells [62, 63]. In the cerebrum, cav-1 regulates neuronal signaling and promotes dendritic growth [64]. Changes in cav-1 can sequentially induce a series of alterations in BBB permeability, neuroinflammation, cerebral angiogenesis, apoptosis, and oxidative stress, which we will discuss in detail.

Important role of cav-1 in IS

Recently, it has been shown that cav-1 has a beneficial role in cerebral ischemia. Overexpression (OE) of cav-1 decreased brain edema following photothrombosis and MCAO in rats [65]. Knockout (KO) of the cav-1-encoding gene in mice produced an enlargement in infarction size, impaired angiogenesis, and increased apoptotic cell death compared with wild-type (cav-1(+/+)) mice and cav-2-deficient (cav-2(−/−)) mice [66]. Recently, Choi et al. found that cav-1 KO mice showed a dramatic increase in the extent of BBB disruption compared with wild-type mice, and this effect was inhibited by lentiviral-mediated re-expression of cav-1 [67]. However, some researchers believe that the protective effects in brain ischemia of several natural active compounds are related to the reduced expression of cav-1. Zhang et al. showed that green tea polyphenols could reduce BBB permeability and brain edema, and this neuroprotection effect may be related to the downregulation of cav-1 and phosphorylated ERK1/2 [68]. Huang et al. also found that post-infarct treatment with Cerebralcare Granule significantly decreased the elevated BBB permeability in the ischemic region, which was associated with the inhibition of cav-1 in the endothelial cells [69]. The discrepancy is probably due to the multifaceted role of natural objects and different stroke models. Their protective role in ischemic stroke is not necessarily due to the reduction of cav-1, and there is no further intervention on cav-1. Further studies are still needed to confirm if reduced cav-1 is one of the mechanisms of the protective effects of natural compounds. The following discussion is about the role of cav-1 in ischemic stroke.

Cav-1 regulates BBB permeability in stroke (Fig. 1)

It is well established that cav-1 is closely related to BBB permeability in stroke. Experimental models of cerebral ischemia indicate that the downregulation of cav-1 membrane protein results in increased BBB permeability [70]. In a clinical study, low serum levels of caveolin-1 were considered to be a predictor of symptomatic

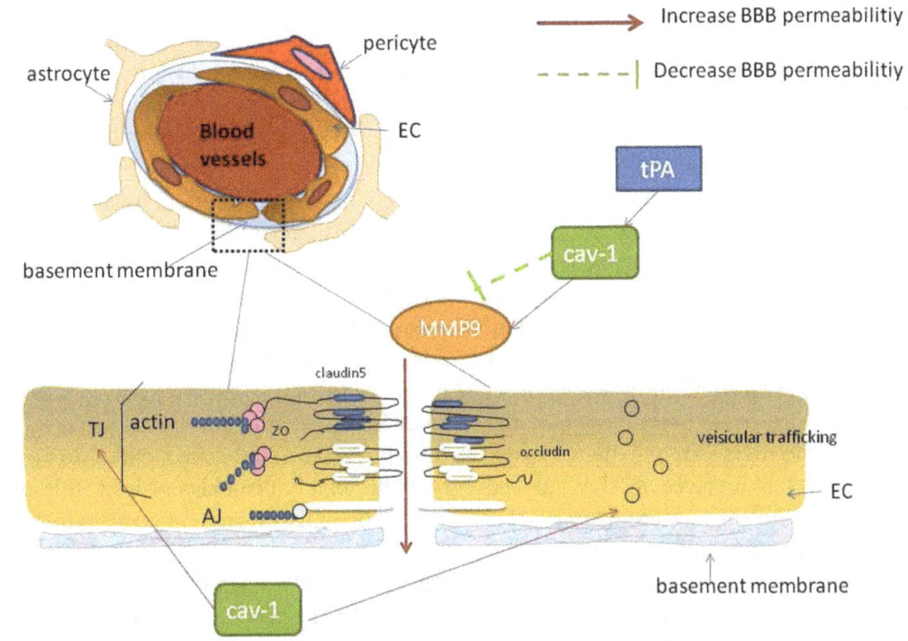

Fig. 1 Effect of caveolin-1 (cav-1) on the blood-brain barrier (BBB). Cav-1 increases the BBB permeability via caveolae-based transcytosis and translocation of tight junction (TJ) protein. Cav-1 inhibits matrix metalloproteinase-9 (MMP-9) which disrupts TJ proteins and basement membrane under ischemic stroke condition, while cav-1 appears to promote MMP-9 upregulation by tPA. However, cav-1 (–/–) mice demonstrated higher MMP activity and BBB permeability than cav-1(+/+) mice in a focal cerebral ischemia-reperfusion model, which means that cav-1 may mainly protects BBB integrity after IS. Endothelial cell (EC), ischemic stroke (IS), tight junction (TJ): actin ZO claudin 5 occludin

hemorrhagic transformation (sHT). sHT is related to increased endothelial permeability after r-tPA administration [71].

Cav-1 predominantly regulates BBB permeability through transcellular and paracellular routes. There are 14-fold fewer vesicles in the brain endothelium than in the endothelium of non-neural vessels, which demonstrates the unique properties of central nervous system (CNS) endothelial cells: their limited vesicular transport (transcytosis). Numerous macromolecules, including albumin, lipoproteins, insulin, and transferrin, have been shown to be transendothelially delivered through caveolae [72]. *Phoneutria nigriventer* spider venom-induced BBB opening is relevant to increased expression of cav-1α [73]. Cav-1 KO mice showed defects in the uptake and transport of albumin from the blood to the interstitium [74]. Co-administration of focused ultrasound and a dose of microbubbles resulted in a high expression of cav-1 and increased BBB permeability through a caveolae-mediated transcellular mechanism [75]. Feng et al. demonstrated that vascular endothelial growth factor (VEGF) enhanced retinal endothelial cell permeability via eNOS-dependent transcytosis in caveolae [76]. Knowland et al. showed that the increased endothelial caveolae number and transcytosis rate account for early BBB hyperpermeability after MCAO [77]. Therefore, it is considered that cav-1 can increase the BBB permeability via caveolae-based transcytosis.

Caveolae-mediated transport is regulated by Src-mediated phosphorylation. To regulate caveola formation and fission, it is essential to orchestrate the localization and activity of proteins of the endocytic machinery [78]. Src-mediated phosphorylation of caveolin-1 at Tyr14 initiates plasmalemmal vesicle fission and transendothelial vesicular transport [79]. Sun et al. observed that phosphorylation of cav-1 is crucial in H_2O_2 exposure-induced pulmonary vascular hyperpermeability, which occurs through transcellular and paracellular pathways [80]. In terms of the regulatory mechanism of cav-1 phosphorylation, Takeuchi et al. showed that oxidative stress-induced cav-1 phosphorylation and endocytosis was inhibited by the activation of AMPK, in part by suppressing the dissociation between c-Abl and Prdx1 proteins [81]. Andreone et al. reported the regulation of CNS endothelial cell lipid composition specifically inhibited the caveolae-mediated transcytosis [82].

Decreased levels of TJs typically increase BBB permeability. Cav-1 affects paracellular permeability by controlling MMPs. Cav-1-deficient mice showed higher MMP proteolytic activity and breakdown of TJ proteins than wild type mice, and the opposite effects were observed following re-expression of cav-1 [67]. Downregulation of cav-1 led to decreased expression of TJ-associated proteins, proteolysis of TJs, and opening of the blood–tumor barrier (BTB), whereas cav-1 OE restored the expression of TJ-associated proteins [83]. Gu et al. found that cav-1 in the ischemic region was reduced after focal cerebral ischemia with reperfusion. The decreased cav-1 was associated with enhanced activities of MMP-2 and MMP-9 activity, downregulation of zonula occludens-1 expression, and increased BBB permeability. The researchers used two methods, including cav-1 knockdown in cultured brain microvascular endothelial cells (BMECs) and a cav-1 gene KO mouse model. Cav-1 knockdown resulted in high MMP activity and BMEC hyperpermeability. Cav-1(−/−) mice demonstrated higher MMP activity and BBB permeability than cav-1 (+/+) mice in a focal cerebral ischemia-reperfusion model [70]. Interestingly, cav-1 seems to play a role in tPA-induced MMP-9 activation in the ischemic brain, which exaggerates brain infarction and increases the risk of symptomatic cerebral hemorrhage. To determine whether cav-1 is involved in tPA-induced MMP-9 upregulation, cultured BMECs were treated using cav-1 siRNA. It was shown that knockdown of cav-1 blocked tPA-induced MMP-9 mRNA increases and increases in MMP-9 protein levels in the conditioned media, but did not affect decreased MMP-9 levels in cellular extracts. It means that cav-1 may not affect MMP-9 secretion from the endothelial cells [84]. However, Song et al. reported that cav-1 s-nitrosylation is involved in the secretion of MMP-2 and MMP-9 from tPA-treated ischemic endothelial cells. In the context of tPA-induced ERK activation, oxygen-glucose deprivation (OGD)-triggered cav-1 s-nitrosylation can enhance MMP-2 and MMP-9 secretion and subsequently promote extracellular matrix (ECM) degradation [85]. Taken together, cav-1 inhibits MMP-9 under ischemic stroke condition. In contrast, cav-1 appears to promote MMP-9 upregulation by tPA. These findings give us a hint that the effect of cav-1 may be stimulus-dependent. And more work is needed to clarify the signaling mechanisms.

Cav-1 is also connected with the distribution of TJ proteins. Liu et al. found that MMP-2 was responsible for OGD-induced occludin degradation, and in vitro, cav-1 mediated claudin-5 redistribution in OGD [86]. They further investigated the fate of translocated claudin-5 and the mechanisms through which OGD promoted cav-1 translocation, and their data demonstrate that NO promotes the delivery of claudin-5 to the autophagosome for autophagy-lysosome-dependent degradation which is mediated by cav-1 [87]. Caveolae also mediate the internalization of TJ proteins, including occludin and claudin-5, when brain endothelial cells are exposed to chemokine (C-C motif) ligand 2 (CCL2) which induces TJ remodeling [88].

Contrary to the view that cav-1 is neuroprotective in cerebral ischemia, there are a host of studies demonstrating that cav-1 may damage the BBB. To simulate this situation, three models of high BBB permeability were established, including MCAO insult, lipopolysaccharide (LPS) treatment, and cold injury. In these models, the expression of both claudin-5 and VE-cadherin was reduced, whereas cav-1 protein expression was increased [89]. In rats with cerebral ischemia-reperfusion injury, Xie et al. demonstrated that inhibiting transient receptor potential vanilloid 4 ameliorated BBB disruption through reducing the expression of cav-1 and cav-2 [90]. Pretreatment with electroacupuncture profoundly ameliorated the elevated BBB permeability and reduced brain edema in a focal I/R rat model, and it was related to the decreased degradation of TJ proteins and downregulation of the expression of p-cav-1 in endothelial cells [91]. The discrepancy in previous studies may arise from different ischemia models, different time of ischemia-reperfusion, or different sample sources. In general, cav-1 can increase BBB permeability through caveolae-mediated endocytosis and translocation of TJ protein, but can also protect BBB integrity by inhibiting MMP activity during ischemic stroke.

Cav-1 and angiogenesis (Fig. 2)

Angiogenesis refers to the sprouting of new microvessels from existing vasculature. It is a process of endothelial proliferation, migration, and differentiation and is often stimulated by hypoxia [92]. Both in humans and rodents, angiogenesis takes place in the area surrounding a brain infarction, starting 3–4 days after the ischemic insult [93, 94]. Upon the onset of ischemia, NO and VEGF lead to vasodilation and increased vascular permeability, resulting in extravasation of plasma proteins. Subsequently, these proteins lay down a temporary scaffold for the migration of endothelial cells which is necessary for vascular sprouting [95], and then angiopoietin-2 dissociates smooth muscle cells and loosens the ECM [96]. Following complete restructuring of the ECM, ECM tracts are formed [92]. ECM tracts are used to establish new capillary buds. Angiogenesis is tightly controlled through a balance between angiogenic (pro-angiogenic) and angiostatic (anti-angiogenic) factors. VEGF is considered to be the major angiogenic factor [97]. Activation of the vascular endothelial growth factor receptor 1 (VEGFR-1) and VEGFR-2 promotes endothelial cell proliferation and migration and exacerbates ECM degradation through different mechanisms including the PI3K/Akt and MEK/ERK protein kinase pathways [98]. NO, miRNAs, and Ang also have important roles in mediating angiogenesis. NO can increase the expression of VEGF in endothelial cells and increase vascular permeability in the ischemic brain. Ang can stabilize and remodel nascent blood vessels by binding to Tie-2 receptors. miR-210 and miR-140-5p modulate angiogenesis via upregulation of VEGFA expression, whereas it has been reported that miR-15a and miR-150 reduced vascular density in the infarct region in a rat model of MCAO [98].

Treadmill exercise has been demonstrated to promote angiogenesis in the infarct penumbra of animal brains,

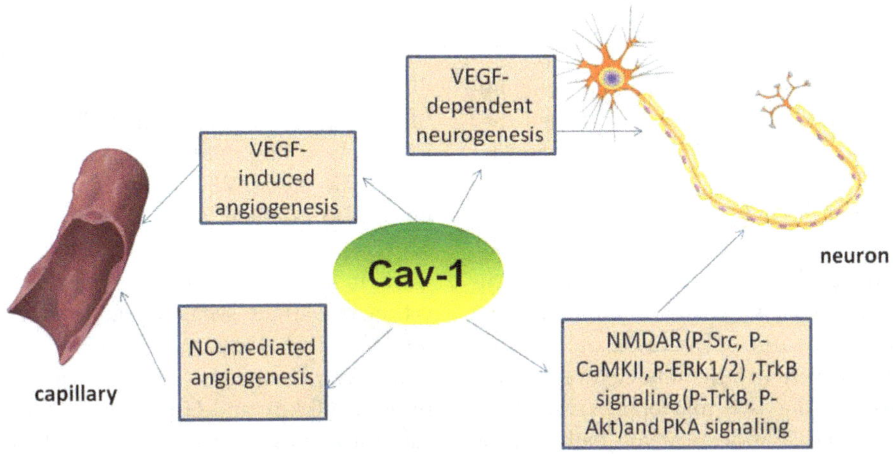

Fig. 2 The role of cav-1 in angiogenesis and neurogenesis. Cav-1 is essential for NO-mediated angiogenesis and VEGF-induced angiogenesis. VEGF can promote NO production and NO can increase the expression of VEGF. Cav-1/VEGF-dependent pathway is important for neurogenesis, and cav-1 enhances NMDAR (P-Src, P-CaMKII, P-ERK1/2), TrkB signaling (P-TrkB, P-Akt), and PKA signaling, and augments dendritic growth and arborization. Methyl-D-aspartate receptor (NMDAR), calcium/calmodulin-dependent protein kinase II (CaMKII), phosphorylated (P)-extracellular signal-regulated kinase (ERK), tyrosine kinase B receptor (TrkB), cAMP-dependent protein kinase (PKA)

and an exercise group showed significantly higher expression of cav-1 and VEGF protein, better neurological recovery, and a smaller cerebral volume of infarction than a non-exercise group. And rats received the injection of the cav-1 inhibitor, daidzein, showed decreased expression of VEGF compared with the exercise group, which probably means that cav-1 pathway is involved in the regulation of VEGF after treadmill exercise [99]. Treatment using apigenin upregulated the expression of cav-1, VEGF, and eNOS compared with a control group, and cav-1 silencing counteracted apigenin-induced angiogenesis in vitro by promoting the tube formation ability of human umbilical vein endothelial cells (HUVECs) [100]. Genetic ablation of the cav-1 in mice resulted in impaired angiogenesis and increased apoptotic cell death in the ischemic brain. In vitro, adenoviral-mediated OE of caveolin-1 clearly accelerated endothelial cell differentiation/tubule formation and led to an upregulation in the number of capillary-like tubular structures. Conversely, knockdown of cav-1 using an antisense adenoviral gene delivery system reduced the number of capillary-like tubules, which demonstrates that cav-1 plays a positive role in the regulation of endothelial cell differentiation [101]. These findings suggest that cav-1 may promote angiogenesis in IS. More specifically, in the process of angiogenesis, it appears that cav-1 negatively regulates endothelial cell proliferation and promotes cell differentiation [79]. Cav-1 inhibited endothelial cell proliferation by arresting cell cycle at the G0/G1 phase [102]. PD98059 is a specific inhibitor of mitogen-activated protein kinase and can suppress angiogenesis. PD98059 can also block decreases in cav-1 expression. Therefore, it is quite reasonable to consider that decreased cav-1 expression may play a significant role in the signaling required for endothelial cell proliferation [103].

Cav-1 has been shown to interact with certain angiogenic (pro-angiogenic) factors. Treatment of a HUVEC line (ECV 304) with some well-known angiogenic growth factors (VEGF, basic fibroblast growth factor, or hepatocyte growth factor/scatter factor) contributed to a dramatic reduction in cav-1 expression [103]. VEGFR-2 is localized in endothelial caveolae, and OE of cav-1 inhibits the activity of VEGFR-2 [104]. However, cav-1 also activates VEGFR-2 via a VEGF-dependent pathway, and the removal of caveolin and VEGFR-2 from caveolae leads to the inhibition of endothelial cell migration [104]. Re-expression of cav-1 in cav-1-deficient endothelial cells resulted in the relocation of VEGFR-2 in caveolar membranes and restored the VEGF-induced ERK and eNOS activation [105]. Cav-1 is also essential for NO-mediated angiogenesis. VEGF promotes the production of NO and the formation of capillary-like tubules. Antisense cav-1 oligonucleotides were transfected into HUVECs, and this resulted in a significant decrease in capillary-like tubules, and NO production did not respond to the addition of VEGF and NG-nitro-L-arginine methyl ester (L-NAME), a nonselective NOS inhibitor [106]. Although some angiogenic growth factors inhibit cav-1, cav-1 is important for VEGF or NO-mediated-angiogenesis. Cav-1 is a potential therapeutic target to improve angiogenesis for the treatment of stroke.

Cav-1 and neurogenesis (Fig. 2)

Similar to the angiogenic process, neurogenesis includes the proliferation, migration, and differentiation of neural stem cells (NSCs), which can differentiate into a variety of cells, including neurons, ependymal cells, astrocytes, and oligodendrocytes [107].

For instance, in neurogenesis in the olfactory bulb, initially, NSCs differentiate into neuroblasts, and then they migrate to the olfactory bulb and differentiate into periglomerular or granule neurons [108]. After stroke, if endogenous NSCs are not injured, NSCs will migrate to the ischemic region and differentiate into astrocytes [109]. Studies have demonstrated that adult NSCs in the subventricular zone (SVZ) of the lateral ventricle and the dentate gyrus of the hippocampus can be activated and produce neuroblasts which will recruit to the infarcted region and participate in repairing the ischemic brain tissue [110, 111]. The PI3K pathway, Wnt/beta-catenin pathway, the Notch pathway, and the Sonic Hedgehog pathway have been reported as affecting neurogenesis, as discussed in a review written by Koh and Park [107].

As mentioned earlier, treadmill exercise promotes angiogenesis in the infarcted penumbra via a cav-1/VEGF-dependent pathway. Recently, a research group observed that the upregulation of both cav-1 and VEGF protein expression following treadmill exercise was consistent with improved recovery in neurological function which correlated with the proliferation, migration, and differentiation of SVZ-derived NSCs in the brain tissue. Furthermore, knockdown of cav-1 by a cav-1 inhibitor remarkably inhibited the treadmill exercise-induced upregulation in VEGF expression, improved neurological recovery, and decrease in the cerebral volume of infarction [112]. In addition, the cav-1/VEGF signaling pathway was found to play a role in basic fibroblast growth factor-induced angiogenesis and neurogenesis following treadmill exercise after acute IS [113]. This evidence suggests that cav-1 plays a positive role in neurogenesis. However, Li et al. found that in the hippocampal dentate gyrus (DG), cav-1 (−/−) mice displayed significantly higher levels of VEGF expression and more abundant formation of newborn neurons than cav-1 (+/+) mice. Cav-1 peptide markedly inhibited neuronal differentiation [114]. It has been reported that cav-1 can regulate synaptic plasticity. Decreased expression of hippocampal caveolin-1 caused synaptic plasticity deficits in aged rats [115]. Cav-1 knockdown inhibited the morphine-induced upregulation of neurite outgrowth [116]. Neuron-targeted cav-1 overexpression enhanced dendritic arborization within the apical dendrites of hippocampal and granule cell neurons in adult and aged mice [117]. Similarly, Egawa et al. showed that neuron-targeted OE of cav-1 (SynCav1) promoted ultrastructural and functional hippocampal synaptic plasticity [118]. Head et al. showed that cav-1 OE, achieved using a synapsin-driven cav-1 vector, upregulated the formation of lipid rafts and the expression of neurotransmitter and neurotrophin receptors in primary neurons [119]. In conclusion, cav-1 promotes neurogenesis and neuroplasticity after ischemic stroke, but some studies demonstrate that cav-1 inhibits neural progenitor cells differentiation under normoxic and hypoxic conditions through the downregulation of VEGF signaling. One feasible explanation could be the paradox phenomenon between cav-1 and VEGF: cav-1 can downregulate VEGF, but is also essential for VEGF signaling. The relationship between cav-1 and VEGF signaling still needs further work. In neurons, pro-survival signals occur after the activation of various synaptic signaling receptors, including the *N*-methyl-D-aspartate (NMDA) glutamate receptor (NMDAR), the neurotrophin-activated tyrosine kinase B receptor (TrkB), and G-protein coupled receptors. These survival signals converge via intracellular protein kinases (CaMKII, Src, Akt, cAMP) to phosphorylate extracellular signal-regulated kinase 1/2 (ERK1/2), initiating the transcription of pro-survival and pro-growth genes. These receptors are distributed in regions enriched in caveolins. Cav-1 OE enhanced NMDAR (P-Src, P-CaMKII, P-ERK1/2) and TrkB signaling (P-TrkB, P-Akt) and augmented dendritic growth and arborization [120]. On glial cell line-derived neurotrophic factor stimulation, expression of cav-1 is increased in mesencephalic dopaminergic neurons, and modulation of genes which are correlated with neuronal plasticity and survival is mediated in part by ERK and cAMP-dependent protein kinase (PKA) signaling [121]. Increased p-ERK1/2 was almost diminished by the inhibition of caveolin and vice versa [120]. Therefore, cav-1 is essential for ERK activation and appears to be important in pro-survival signaling. Thus, cav-1 could be a novel therapeutic target protein for promoting neurogenesis after ischemic stroke.

Cav-1 and neuroinflammation (Fig. 3)

The role of caveolins in many aspects of the inflammatory response, including angiogenesis, leukocyte recruitment, pathogen invasion, the production of inflammatory mediators, and fibrosis, has been extensively demonstrated in the literature [122]. Severe BBB breakdown occurs several hours after ischemic attack and is followed by a massive infiltration of polymorphonuclear (PMN) leukocytes [123]. This event not only results in brain edema formation but also induces the activation of brain microglia which produce pro-inflammatory cytokines and ROS exacerbating the brain injury. Thus, we logically address that cav-1 inhibits inflammation via maintaining the integrity of BBB under brain ischemia condition. Niesman et al. illustrate that cav-1 regulates neuroinflammatory responses after traumatic brain injury (TBI), as cav-1 KO mice exhibited a significant increase in cytokine/chemokine production in a controlled cortical impact model of TBI [124]. Moreover, cavtratin, a cell permeable peptide of cav-1, has previously been shown to inhibit the

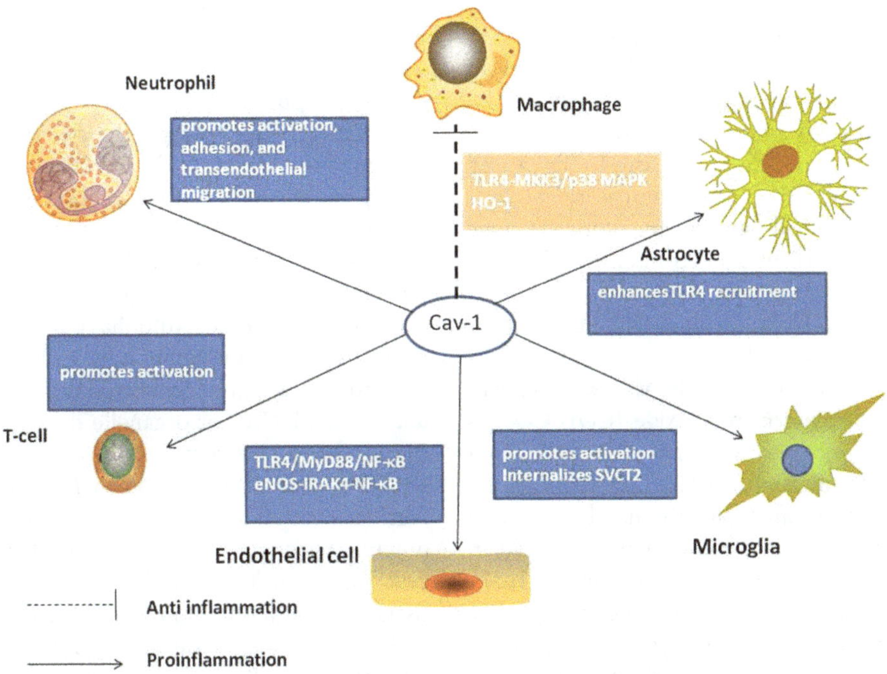

Fig. 3 Schematic illustrating the role of cav-1 in different cell. In endothelial cells, after exposure to LPS, cav-1 interacts with toll-like receptor 4 (TLR4), and then TLR4 promotes activation of MyD88, leading to NF-κB activation and the generation of proinflammatory cytokines. Under normal condition, cav-1 inhibits eNOS. If eNOS is activated, NO will nitrate IRAK4 which is a signaling factor required for NF-κB activation. And cav-1 in microglia can induce the internalization of SVCT2 which is the primary mediator of vitamin C uptake in neurons, triggering a proinflammatory phenotype in microglia and inducing microglia activation. Whereas in macrophages, cav-1decreases proinflammatory cytokine production and augments anti-inflammatory production through the TLR4/MKK3/p38 MAPK pathway. Besides, TLR4 activation by LPS also stimulates HO-1 transporting to the caveolae and producing CO which has anti-inflammatory effects and augments the cav-1/TLR4 interaction in murine macrophages. Toll-like receptor 4 (TLR4), interleukin-1 receptor associated kinase 4 (IRAK4), heme oxygenase-1 (HO-1), carbon oxide (CO), plasma membrane sodium-vitamin C cotransporter 2 (SVCT2)

transmigration and viability of macrophages and microglia via the JNK pathway and reduce inflammation in ocular neovascularization [125]. Cavtratin also reduces inflammatory cell infiltration, contributing to the improvement in BBB function in an immunologic mouse model of multiple sclerosis [126]. It is noteworthy that in healthy situation, cav-1 may as well inhibit inflammation, as systemic administration of cav-1 CSD to mice suppressed acute inflammation and vascular leak to the same extent as a glucocorticoid [127]. Caveolae have been reported as important in the internalization and later fate of several pathogens. For example, by targeting caveolae as an endocytic pathway, pathogens such as simian virus 40 and certain strains of *Escherichia coli* can be transported directly to the Golgi and/or ER, avoiding disruption in lysosomes and ensuring their intracellular survival [128]. However, cav-1 promotes the ability of macrophages to phagocytose both *E. coli* and apoptotic cells in vitro [129].

In the endothelium, after exposure to LPS, cav-1 was phosphorylated at Tyr(14) which resulted in interaction between cav-1 and toll-like receptor 4 (TLR4), and then TLR4 promoted activation of MyD88, leading to NF-κB activation and the generation of proinflammatory cytokines [130]. Cav-1 OE dose-dependently increased monocyte chemoattractant protein-1 (MCP-1), vascular cell adhesion molecule-1 (VCAM-1), and plasminogen activator inhibitor-1 (PAI-1) mRNA levels in human umbilical vein ECs. Pigment epithelium-derived factor binding to cav-1 could inhibit the pro-inflammatory effects of cav-1 in endothelial cells [131]. Cav-1 can affect NF-κB to influence the inflammatory response. Signaling by the pro-inflammatory cytokine interleukin-1β (IL-1β) is dependent on ROS, because after IL-1β binding to its receptor (IL-1R1), ROS generated by Nox2 is responsible for the downstream recruitment of IL-1R1 effectors (IRAK, TRAF6, IkappaB kinase kinases) and ultimately for activation of NF-κB. Lipid rafts and cav-1 coordinate IL-1β-dependent activation of NF-κB. Inhibiting cav-1-mediated endocytosis can prevent NF-κB activation [132]. Cav-1 gene KO lungs displayed suppression of NF-κB activity and reduced transcription of iNOS and intercellular adhesion molecule 1 (ICAM-1) [133]. Secondary to the loss of cav-1, eNOS is activated, which inhibits the innate immune response to LPS through interleukin-1 receptor-associated kinase 4 (IRAK4) nitration. IRAK4 is a signaling factor required for NF-κB activation and innate immunity. Cav-1 KO can impair the activity of NF-κB and reduce LPS-induced lung injury [134]. Cav-1 appears to have different roles in different cells. In macrophages, the interaction of cav-1 with TLR4 has an opposite outcome compared with that in endothelium, whereby overexpression of cav-1 decreased LPS-induced TNF-α and IL-6 proinflammatory cytokine production and augmented anti-inflammatory cytokine IL-10 production. Cav-1 regulates LPS-induced inflammatory cytokine production through the MKK3/p38 MAPK pathway [135]. It is valuable to mention that TLR4 activation by LPS also stimulates heme oxygenase-1 (HO-1) transporting to the caveolae by a p38 MAPK-dependent mechanism and producing carbon oxide (CO). CO has anti-inflammatory effects and augments the cav-1/TLR4 interaction in murine macrophages [136]. In PMN leukocytes, cav-1 appears to promote activation, adhesion, and transendothelial migration and shows a positive role in PMN activation-induced lung and vascular injury [137]. Cav-1 also plays a key role in antigen-presenting cells, leading to the activation of T lymphocytes [138]. Furthermore, apoptosis of thymocytes in cav-1-deficient mice was higher than that in wild type mice, indicating that cav-1 is a key regulator of thymocyte apoptosis during inflammation [139]. In addition, cav-1 has a possible role in microglial activation. Cav-1 was remarkably reduced and localized in the plasmalemma and cytoplasmic vesicles of inactive microglia, whereas active (amoeboid-shaped) microglia exhibited increased cav-1 expression [46]. Recently, Portugal et al. found that cav-1 in microglia induced the internalization of plasma membrane sodium-vitamin C cotransporter 2 (SVCT2), triggering a proinflammatory phenotype in microglia and inducing microglia activation [140]. Besides, cav-1 transfection into Fatty acid-binding proteins-KO astrocytes remarkably enhanced TLR4 recruitment into lipid raft and tumor necrosis factor-α production after LPS stimulation [141]. Together, in non-pathological states or after LPS stimulation, cav-1 in endothelial cells increases proinflammatory cytokines, while cav-1 inhibits LPS-induced inflammatory effects in murine macrophages. Cav-1 is involved in activation of microglia, PMN, and T lymphocytes.

Apart from the LPS-eNOS-TLR4-NFκB, MKK3/p38 MAPK, and IL-1β-IL-1R1 pathways which we have already mentioned, cav-1 participates in additional inflammatory signaling pathways [142]. Cyclooxygenase (COX)-2 is pivotal in post-ischemic brain damage, and the selective inhibition of the COX-2 enzyme inhibited subsequent prostaglandin E2 (PGE2) production, ischemic BBB leakage, leukocyte infiltration, and edema formation [143]. In cav-1-null mice, COX-2 protein levels are higher. Cav-1 binds COX-2 in the endoplasmic reticulum (ER) and modulates its degradation through an ER-dependent mechanism [144]. This suggests that cav-1 can regulate inflammatory responses by controlling COX-2 expression.

Cav-1 and apoptosis

Apoptosis is morphologically characterized by a programmed cell death [145]. However, necrosis is a process of physico-chemical cell destruction and involves cellular plasma membrane disruption [146]. Autophagy is mainly triggered by cell starvation, and cells orchestrate self-digestion of long-lived proteins and damaged organelles in the lysosome. Autophagy might principally serve for cell survival, but sometimes leads to cell death [147]. Apoptosis is a highly conserved cellular response to cellular stress, DNA-, or organelle damage, but also plays a crucial role in the removal of superfluous cells. The destruction of one cell can be beneficial: the removal of superfluous cells is necessary for the development of functioning organs, and the removal of injured or aged cells that have lost their function can help to maintain tissue vitality [148]. Apoptosis can be initiated via two main routes: the extrinsic and intrinsic pathways. The intrinsic apoptotic pathway is usually triggered by stimuli, including DNA damage, organelle dysfunction of either mitochondria or the ER, the accumulation of unfolded proteins, growth factor withdrawal, or hyperthermia. The extrinsic pathway is triggered when ligands bind their trans-membrane death receptors. The extrinsic pathway not only directly leads to the activation of proteases which cause cell death, but also promotes the release of pro-apoptotic factors from mitochondria, which are linked with the intrinsic pathway [148].

Caveolins are directly connected with both the intrinsic and extrinsic cell death pathways. The key to the extrinsic pathway is the expression of transmembrane receptors, called death receptors, including TNF-receptor 1, Fas/CD95, and the TNF-related apoptosis-inducing ligand receptors. A potential cav-1 binding motif (G53LHHDGQFCH) has been identified in the human death receptor Fas sequence [149]. Cav-1 KO disrupted death-induced signaling complex formation following colocalization and interaction between cav-1 and Fas [150]. Recently, Glukhova et al. found that the deletion of both caveolin-binding sites (which bind the N-terminal domain and B-terminal domain of cav-1) in the Fas-ligand attenuated extrinsic cell death pathway-associated cytotoxicity, demonstrating that the relationship between the Fas-ligand and cav-1 provides a molecular basis for the location of the ligand to lipid rafts and Fas-ligand-dependent apoptosis [151]. As for the intrinsic apoptosis pathway, mitochondrial outer membrane permeabilization is the central event of the intrinsic pathway: in response to apoptotic stimuli, mitochondria release intermembrane space proteins, such as cytochrome C and apoptosis-inducing factor, which exert a cryptic cytotoxic activity following their mitochondrial release [152]. And mitochondrial dysfunction is considered as a hallmark of intrinsic apoptosis. In E11 podocytes, cav-1 OE attenuated H_2O_2-induced oxidative stress responses and preserved mitochondrial function, as well as significantly suppressing apoptosis [153]. Moreover, various cav-1-deficient cells have displayed mitochondrial dysfunction including impaired energy generation, and increased mitochondrial ROS production [154–156]. Based on the abovementioned findings, we speculate that cav-1 could relay apoptotic signaling via allowing Fas multimerization, but also attenuates apoptosis through preventing mitochondrial dysfunction.

Additionally, cav-1 plays a different role in regulating apoptosis in different cell types. In HEK293T cells, cav-1 was shown to reduce survivin, which inhibits apoptosis through a pathway involving diminished beta-catenin-Tcf/Lef-dependent transcription. This suggests that cav-1 has pro-apoptotic properties [157]. However, there is also evidence to suggest that cav-1 suppresses apoptosis. In hypoxic human SK-N-MC neuroblastoma cells, iNOS-induced NO production reduces the expression of cav-1. OE of cav-1, either through cav-1 transfection or administration of a cav-1 CSD peptide, decreased the production of NO and impaired apoptotic cell death in hypoxic SK-N-MC cells [158]. Yue et al. demonstrated that cav-1 could suppress ER stress-induced macrophage apoptosis in vitro, and one of the underlying mechanisms may be associated with the activation of the p38 MAPK pro-survival pathway [159]. Cav-1 KO macrophages were more susceptible to apoptosis and more prone to induce inflammation than wild-type macrophages. Decreased cav-1 protein levels mediated I/R injury-induced liver damage by inhibiting sphingosine kinase 2/sphingosine-1-phosphate receptor 2 signaling and enhancing apoptosis [160].

The anti-apoptotic role of cav-1 in ischemic stroke is suggested by Jasmin et al.; they showed increased apoptotic cell death in cav-1 KO ischemic brains, as compared with WT ischemic brains. But the underlying mechanisms are still not clear. Recently, it was found that downregulation of cav-1 using cav-1 small interfering RNA remarkably worsened astrocyte cell damage, while overexpression of cav-1 using a cav-1 CSD peptide attenuated OGD-induced cell apoptosis via Ras/Raf/ERK pathway [161]. This may partly explain why cav-1 inhibits apoptosis in IS.

Cav-1 and free radicals (Fig. 4)

As discussed in previous sections, ROS and RNS play important roles in IS. Cav-1 has been shown to reduce ROS production in endothelial cells. Mitochondrial ROS production was increased in endothelial cells following cav-1 knockdown. Chen et al. observed that cav-1 inhibited the activity of NADPH oxidases, a major source of cellular ROS [162]. Cav-1-targeted treatments could scavenge reactive species in cancer cells [163]. Src homology 2-containing protein tyrosine phosphatase 2 (SHP-2)

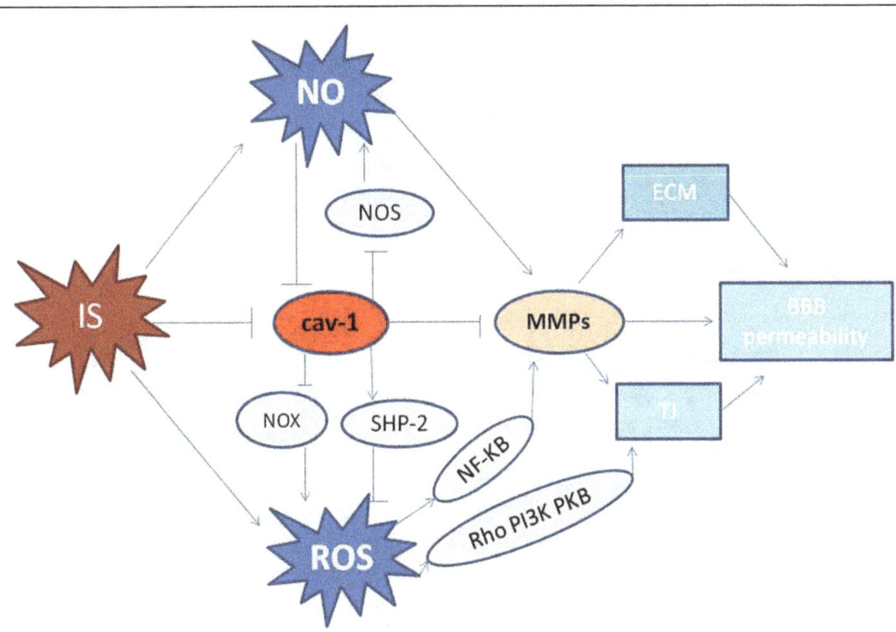

Fig. 4 Relationship between cav-1 and free radicals. On one hand, cav-1 directly binds to NOS and decreases NO; on the other hand, NO negatively regulates cav-1 expression. Cav-1 reduces the production of ROS via inhibiting the activity of NADPH oxidases (NOX) and (or) promoting SHP-2 activation. NO and ROS can activate MMP-2 and MMP-9, disrupting TJ and ECM, finally inducing BBB hyperpermeability. Thus, cav-1 can inhibit the activity of MMP2 and MMP9 through reducing NO and ROS. Ischemic stroke (IS), NADPH oxidases (NOX), Src homology 2-containing protein tyrosine phosphatase 2 (SHP-2)

provided neuroprotection in a stroke model. Cav-1 protected astrocytes from ROS-induced oxidative stress via SHP-2 activation [164]. According to the aforementioned findings that ROS can induce and/or activate MMPs, we propose that cav-1 protects the BBB from disruption by reduction of ROS and inhibition of MMPs activity.

NO can inhibit the expression of cav-1, but cav-1 can inhibit NO production through binding with NO synthase (NOS) and inhibition of cav-1 promotes the activation of NOS and increases NO levels. Glutathione S-transferase (GST) pull-down using purified proteins confirmed that direct binding of cav-1 and NOS occurred between residues 82–101 [165] and that F92 is the key residue to mediate endothelial NO synthase (eNOS) inhibition by cav-1 [166]. High NO concentrations decrease cav-1 abundance and alter its cellular distribution in endothelial cells [167]. NO decreased the expression of cav-1 after IS, and NOS inhibitors prevented the loss of cav-1 in the core and penumbra of the ischemic brain [168]. It is interesting to note that positive regulation of cav-1 by NO is found in tumor cells. The NO donor diethylenetriamine (DETA)/NO upregulated cav-1 in hypoxic human SK-N-MC neuroblastoma cells [33]. Thus, the role of NO in the modulation of cav-1 expression appears to be different in different cell types. Incubation of pure eNOS with peptides derived from the CSD of cav-1 and cav-3 led to inhibition of eNOS, inducible NO synthase (iNOS), and neuronal NO synthase (nNOS) activity [169]. And overexpression of caveolin markedly decreased eNOS enzyme activity in endothelial cells [170]. In addition, delivery of the cav-1 CSD inhibited NO synthesis and inflammation [127]. Loss of cav-1 leads to persistent eNOS activation and high levels of NO in cells, through the loss of cav-1 inhibitory effects on eNOS [171]. It has also been shown that pharmacological blockade or genetic deletion of eNOS prevents many of the physiological changes observed in cav-1 KO mice [172]. Based on the literature, it seems that the interaction of cav-1 and NO partly explains why cav-1 protects BBB integrity from IS. Cav-1 KO mice had increased eNOS activity and NO production; subsequently, NO production directly contributed to MMP activation and BBB disruption. L-NAME preserved the expression of cav-1, inhibited MMPs activity, and reduced BBB permeability.

Conclusion (Fig. 5)

IS is a major cause of death and long-lasting disability worldwide. In this review, we have introduced several major pathophysiological mechanisms in IS, such as BBB damage, inflammation, and free radicals, and summarized the role of T cells in IS. In addition, we discussed evidence

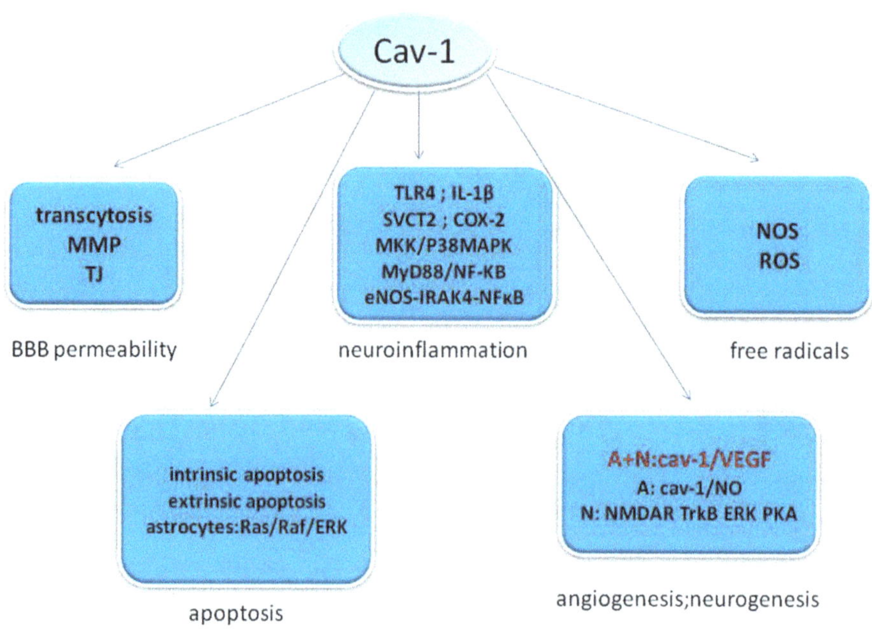

Fig. 5 Schematic representation illustrating the role of caveolin-1 in regulating BBB permeability, neuroinflammantion, free radicals, apoptosis, angiogenesis, and neurogenesis and showing some of the signaling pathways coupling caveolae/caveolins with IS. Changing BBB permeability via transcytosis, MMP, and TJ; regulating neuroinflammantion via TLR4, IL-1β, SVCT2, COX2, MKK/P38MAPK, MyD88/NF-KB, and eNOS-IRAK4-NFκB pathway; altering free radicals via reducing NOS and ROS; influencing apoptosis through intrinsic apoptotic pathway and extrinsic apoptotic pathway and protecting astrocytes from apoptosis via Ras/Raf/ERK pathway; promoting angiogenesis through cav-1/VEGF and cav-1/NO pathway; and promoting neurogenesis via cav-1/VEGF pathway and neuroplasticity through NMDAR, TrkB, ERK, and PKA pathway. Interleukin-1β (IL-1β), cyclooxygenase-2 (COX-2), mitogen-activated protein kinase (MAPK), reactive nitrogen species (RNS), reactive oxygen species (ROS), extracellular signal-regulated kinase (ERK), vascular endothelial growth factor (VEGF), *N*-methyl-D-aspartate receptor (NMDAR)

that cav-1 may serve to promote neuroprotection after stroke and also listed some opposing results. Cav-1 OE decreases brain edema in a rat MCAO model, and cav-1 KO increases brain infarction volume. However, some natural active compounds, such as green tea polyphenols, show a protective role in brain ischemia which is correlated with a decrease in cav-1. In angiogenesis, cav-1 negatively regulates endothelial cell proliferation, while promoting differentiation. Cav-1 is necessary for VEGFR-2 to undergo VEGF-dependent activation, but OE of cav-1 inhibits VEGFR-2 activity. As for neurogenesis, treadmill exercise-mediated improved neurological recovery is significantly inhibited when cav-1 is reduced. Cav-1 also enhances pro-survival signaling (NMDAR, TrkB, ERK signaling) and promotes dendritic growth and arborization. It is worth noting that in the hippocampal DG, cav-1 KO mice showed more newborn neurons than the wild-type mice. Cav-1 plays a pro-inflammatory role in endothelial cells, neutrophils, lymphocytes, and microglia, but has an opposing role in macrophages. Cav-1 connects with both the intrinsic and extrinsic apoptotic pathways. Interaction of Fas-ligand and cav-1 provides a molecular basis for the induction of Fas-ligand-dependent cell death. Cav-1 exerts anti-apoptotic action in the intrinsic apoptotic pathway. Using different cell or animal models may help to fully elucidate the role of cav-1 in IS, and we should explore more to answer the controversy.

Abbreviations

BBB: Blood–brain barrier; BMECs: Brain microvascular endothelial cells; BTB: Blood-tumor barrier; Cav: Caveolin; CBD: Caveolin-binding motifs; CO: Carbon oxide; COX-2: Cyclooxygenase-2; CSD: Caveolin scaffolding domain; DG: Dentate gyrus; ECM: Extracellular matrix; eNOS: Endothelial NO synthase; ER: Endoplasmic reticulum; ERK: Extracellular signal-regulated kinase; H_2O_2: Hydrogen peroxide; HO-1: Heme oxygenase-1; ICAM-1: Intercellular adhesion molecule 1; IL-1: Interleukin-1; iNOS: Inducible NO synthase; IS: Ischemic stroke; KO: Knockout; L-NAME: NG-nitro-L-arginine methyl ester; LPS: Lipopolysaccharide; MCAO: Middle cerebral artery occlusion; MCP-1: Monocyte chemoattractant protein-1; MMPs: Matrix metalloproteases; NMDAR: *N*-methyl-D-aspartate receptor; nNOS: neuronal NO synthase; NSCs: Neural stem cells; OE: Overexpression; OGD: Oxygen-glucose deprivation; PAI-1: Plasminogen activator inhibitor-1; PKA: cAMP-dependent protein kinase; PMN: Polymorphonuclear; RNS: Reactive nitrogen species; ROS: Reactive oxygen species; sHT: Symptomatic hemorrhagic transformation; SVCT2: Plasma membrane sodium-vitamin C cotransporter 2; SVZ: Subventricular zone; TBI: Traumatic brain injury; Tc: Cytotoxic T cells/CD8 + T cells; Th: Helper T cells/CD4+T cells; TJs: Tight junctions; tPA: Tissue plasminogen activator; Tregs: Regulatory cells; TrkB: Tyrosine kinase B receptor; VCAM-1: Vascular cell adhesion molecule-1; VEGF: Vascular endothelial growth factor; VEGFR: Vascular endothelial growth factor receptor

Acknowledgements

Not applicable

Funding

This work was supported by the National Natural Science Foundation of China (Grant no. 81271298).

Authors' contributions

This work was primarily written by QH. WZ contributed to the acquisition or analysis of literature for the work. Figures were produced by ZH and QH. ZH also contributed to editing the review. XT supervised the work, helped with summarizing the paper, and contributed to the review revision. All authors read and approved the final manuscript.

Consent for publication

Not applicable

Competing interests

The authors declare that they have no competing interests.

References

1. Benjamin EJ, Virani SS, Callaway CW, Chamberlain AM, Chang AR, Cheng S, Chiuve SE, Cushman M, Delling FN, Deo R, et al. Heart disease and stroke statistics-2018 update: a report from the American Heart Association. Circulation. 2018;137:e67–e492.
2. Lakhan SE, Kirchgessner A, Tepper D, Leonard A. Matrix metalloproteinases and blood-brain barrier disruption in acute ischemic stroke. Front Neurol. 2013;4:32.
3. Dirnagl U, Iadecola C, Moskowitz MA. Pathobiology of ischaemic stroke: an integrated view. Trends Neurosci. 1999;22:391–7.
4. Allen CL, Bayraktutan U. Oxidative stress and its role in the pathogenesis of ischaemic stroke. Int J Stroke. 2009;4:461–70.
5. Powers WJ, Rabinstein AA, Ackerson T, Adeoye OM, Bambakidis NC, Becker K, Biller J, Brown M, Demaerschalk BM, Hoh B, et al. Guidelines for the early management of patients with acute ischemic stroke: a guideline for healthcare professionals from the American Heart Association/American Stroke Association. Stroke. 2018;2018(49):e46–e110.
6. Henderson SJ, Weitz JI, Kim PY. Fibrinolysis: strategies to enhance the treatment of acute ischemic stroke. J Thromb Haemost. 2018;16:1932–40.
7. Echarri A, Del Pozo MA. Caveolae. Curr Biol. 2012;22:R114–6.
8. Nag S, Kapadia A, Stewart DJ. Review: molecular pathogenesis of blood-brain barrier breakdown in acute brain injury. Neuropathol Appl Neurobiol. 2011;37:3–23.
9. Anderson RG. The caveolae membrane system. Annu Rev Biochem. 1998;67: 199–225.
10. Liu P, Rudick M, Anderson RGW. Multiple functions of caveolin-1. J Biol Chem. 2002;277:41295–8.
11. Sims NR. Calcium, energy metabolism and the development of selective neuronal loss following short-term cerebral ischemia. Metab Brain Dis. 1995; 10:191–217.
12. Deb P, Sharma S, Hassan KM. Pathophysiologic mechanisms of acute ischemic stroke: an overview with emphasis on therapeutic significance beyond thrombolysis. Pathophysiology. 2010;17:197–218.
13. Wang S, Head BP. Caveolin-1 in stroke neuropathology and neuroprotection: a novel molecular therapeutic target for ischemic-related injury. Curr Vasc Pharmacol. 2019;17:41–49.
14. Kuroiwa T, Ting P, Martinez H, Klatzo I. The biphasic opening of the blood-brain barrier to proteins following temporary middle cerebral artery occlusion. Acta Neuropathol. 1985;68(2):122–9.
15. Rosenberg GA. Neurological diseases in relation to the blood-brain barrier. J Cereb Blood Flow Metab. 2012;32:1139–51.
16. Klein T, Bischoff R. Physiology and pathophysiology of matrix metalloproteases. Amino Acids. 2011;41:271–90.
17. Rosenberg GA, Kornfeld M, Estrada E, Kelley RO, Liotta LA, Stetler-Stevenson WG. TIMP-2 reduces proteolytic opening of blood-brain barrier by type IV collagenase. Brain Res. 1992;576:203–7.
18. Asahi M, Sumii T, Fini ME, Itohara S, Lo EH. Matrix metalloproteinase 2 gene knockout has no effect on acute brain injury after focal ischemia. Neuroreport. 2001;12:3003–7.
19. Asahi M, Asahi K, Jung JC, del Zoppo GJ, Fini ME, Lo EH. Role for matrix metalloproteinase 9 after focal cerebral ischemia: effects of gene knockout and enzyme inhibition with BB-94. J Cereb Blood Flow Metab. 2000;20: 1681–9.

20. Bazzoni G, Dejana E. Endothelial cell-to-cell junctions: molecular organization and role in vascular homeostasis. Physiol Rev. 2004;84:869–901.
21. Wang Q, Doerschuk CM. The signaling pathways induced by neutrophil-endothelial cell adhesion. Antioxid Redox Signal. 2002;4:39–47.
22. Jin R, Yang G, Li G. Inflammatory mechanisms in ischemic stroke: role of inflammatory cells. J Leukoc Biol. 2010;87:779–89.
23. Gelderblom M, Leypoldt F, Steinbach K, Behrens D, Choe C, Siler DA, Arumugam TV, Orthey E, Gerloff C, Tolosa E, Magnus T. Temporal and spatial dynamics of cerebral immune cell accumulation in stroke. Stroke. 2009;40:1849–57.
24. Jiang X, Andjelkovic AV, Zhu L, Yang T, Bennett MVL, Chen J, Keep RF, Shi Y. Blood-brain barrier dysfunction and recovery after ischemic stroke. Prog Neurobiol. 2018;163–164:144–71.
25. Gidday JM, Gasche YG, Copin J, Shah AR, Perez RS, Shapiro SD, Chan PH, Park TS. Leukocyte-derived matrix metalloproteinase-9 mediates blood-brain barrier breakdown and is proinflammatory after transient focal cerebral ischemia. Am J Physiol Heart Circ Physiol. 2005;289:H558–68.
26. Yilmaz G, Arumugam TV, Stokes KY, Granger DN. Role of T lymphocytes and interferon-gamma in ischemic stroke. Circulation. 2006;113:2105–12.
27. Gu L, Jian Z, Stary C, Xiong X. T cells and cerebral ischemic stroke. Neurochem Res. 2015;40:1786–91.
28. Liesz A, Suri-Payer E, Veltkamp C, Doerr H, Sommer C, Rivest S, Giese T, Veltkamp R. Regulatory T cells are key cerebroprotective immunomodulators in acute experimental stroke. Nat Med. 2009;15:192–9.
29. Kleinschnitz C, Kraft P, Dreykluft A, Hagedorn I, Gobel K, Schuhmann MK, Langhauser F, Helluy X, Schwarz T, Bittner S, et al. Regulatory T cells are strong promoters of acute ischemic stroke in mice by inducing dysfunction of the cerebral microvasculature. Blood. 2013;121:679–91.
30. Offner H, Hurn PD. A novel hypothesis: regulatory B lymphocytes shape outcome from experimental stroke. Transl Stroke Res. 2012;3:324–30.
31. Rodrigo R, Fernandez-Gajardo R, Gutierrez R, Matamala JM, Carrasco R, Miranda-Merchak A, Feuerhake W. Oxidative stress and pathophysiology of ischemic stroke: novel therapeutic opportunities. CNS Neurol Disord Drug Targets. 2013;12:698–714.
32. Emerich DF, Dean RLR, Bartus RT. The role of leukocytes following cerebral ischemia: pathogenic variable or bystander reaction to emerging infarct? Exp Neurol. 2002;173:168–81.
33. Gu Y, Dee CM, Shen J. Interaction of free radicals, matrix metalloproteinases and caveolin-1 impacts blood-brain barrier permeability. Front Biosci (Schol Ed). 2011;3:1216–31.
34. Shinohara M, Adachi Y, Mitsushita J, Kuwabara M, Nagasawa A, Harada S, Furuta S, Zhang Y, Seheli K, Miyazaki H, Kamata T. Reactive oxygen generated by NADPH oxidase 1 (Nox1) contributes to cell invasion by regulating matrix metalloprotease-9 production and cell migration. J Biol Chem. 2010;285:4481–8.
35. Schreibelt G, Kooij G, Reijerkerk A, van Doorn R, Gringhuis SI, van der Pol S, Weksler BB, Romero IA, Couraud P, Piontek J, et al. Reactive oxygen species alter brain endothelial tight junction dynamics via RhoA, PI3 kinase, and PKB signaling. FASEB J. 2007;21:3666–76.
36. Lundberg JO, Weitzberg E, Gladwin MT. The nitrate-nitrite-nitric oxide pathway in physiology and therapeutics. Nat Rev Drug Discov. 2008;7: 156–67.
37. Kiss JP, Vizi ES. Nitric oxide: a novel link between synaptic and nonsynaptic transmission. Trends Neurosci. 2001;24:211–5.
38. Murphy S, Gibson CL. Nitric oxide, ischaemia and brain inflammation. Biochem Soc T. 2007;35:1133–7.
39. Matsui T, Nagafuji T, Kumanishi T, Asano T. Role of nitric oxide in pathogenesis underlying ischemic cerebral damage. Cell Mol Neurobiol. 1999;19:177–89.
40. Chen H, Chen X, Li W, Shen J. Targeting RNS/caveolin-1/MMP signaling cascades to protect against cerebral ischemia-reperfusion injuries: potential application for drug discovery. Acta Pharmacol Sin. 2018;39:669–82.
41. Yamada E. The fine structure of the gall bladder epithelium of the mouse. J Biophys Biochem Cytol. 1955;1:445–58.
42. Busija AR, Patel HH, Insel PA. Caveolins and cavins in the trafficking, maturation, and degradation of caveolae: implications for cell physiology. Am J Physiol Cell Physiol. 2017;312:C459–77.
43. Arbuzova A, Wang L, Wang J, Hangyas-Mihalyne G, Murray D, Honig B, McLaughlin S. Membrane binding of peptides containing both basic and aromatic residues. Experimental studies with peptides corresponding to the scaffolding region of caveolin and the effector region of MARCKS. Biochemistry-Us. 2000;39:10330–9.
44. Schlegel A, Lisanti MP. A molecular dissection of caveolin-1 membrane attachment and oligomerization. Two separate regions of the caveolin-1 C-terminal domain mediate membrane binding and oligomer/oligomer interactions in vivo. J Biol Chem. 2000;275:21605–17.
45. Shin T, Kim H, Jin J, Moon C, Ahn M, Tanuma N, Matsumoto Y. Expression of caveolin-1, -2, and -3 in the spinal cords of Lewis rats with experimental autoimmune encephalomyelitis. J Neuroimmunol. 2005;165(1–2):11–20. https://doi.org/10.1016/j.jneuroim.2005.03.019.
46. Niesman IR, Zemke N, Fridolfsson HN, Haushalter KJ, Levy K, Grove A, Schnoor R, Finley JC, Patel PM, Roth DM, et al. Caveolin isoform switching as a molecular, structural, and metabolic regulator of microglia. Mol Cell Neurosci. 2013;56:283–97.
47. Ikezu T, Ueda H, Trapp BD, Nishiyama K, Sha JF, Volonte D, Galbiati F, Byrd AL, Bassell G, Serizawa H, et al. Affinity-purification and characterization of caveolins from the brain: differential expression of caveolin-1, -2, and -3 in brain endothelial and astroglial cell types. Brain Res. 1998;804:177–92.
48. Virgintino D, Robertson D, Errede M, Benagiano V, Tauer U, Roncali L, Bertossi M. Expression of caveolin-1 in human brain microvessels. Neuroscience. 2002;115:145–52.
49. Tang Z, Scherer PE, Okamoto T, Song K, Chu C, Kohtz DS, Nishimoto I, Lodish HF, Lisanti MP. Molecular cloning of caveolin-3, a novel member of the caveolin gene family expressed predominantly in muscle. J Biol Chem. 1996;271(4):2255–61.
50. Scherer PE, Okamoto T, Chun M, Nishimoto I, Lodish HF, Lisanti MP. Identification, sequence, and expression of caveolin-2 defines a caveolin gene family. Proc Natl Acad Sci U S A. 1996;93(1):131–5.
51. Razani B, Wang XB, Engelman JA, Battista M, Lagaud G, Zhang XL, Kneitz B, Hou HJ, Christ GJ, Edelmann W, Lisanti MP. Caveolin-2-deficient mice show evidence of severe pulmonary dysfunction without disruption of caveolae. Mol Cell Biol. 2002;22:2329–44.
52. Gazzerro E, Sotgia F, Bruno C, Lisanti MP, Minetti C. Caveolinopathies: from the biology of caveolin-3 to human diseases. Eur J Hum Genet. 2010;18: 137–45.
53. Couet J, Li S, Okamoto T, Ikezu T, Lisanti MP. Identification of peptide and protein ligands for the caveolin-scaffolding domain. Implications for the interaction of caveolin with caveolae-associated proteins. J Biol Chem. 1997; 272:6525–33.
54. Okamoto T, Schlegel A, Scherer PE, Lisanti MP. Caveolins, a family of scaffolding proteins for organizing "preassembled signaling complexes" at the plasma membrane. J Biol Chem. 1998;273:5419–22.
55. Yamamoto M, Toya Y, Schwencke C, Lisanti MP, Myers MGJ, Ishikawa Y. Caveolin is an activator of insulin receptor signaling. J Biol Chem. 1998;273: 26962–8.
56. Pelkmans L. Secrets of caveolae- and lipid raft-mediated endocytosis revealed by mammalian viruses. Biochim Biophys Acta. 2005;1746:295–304.
57. Gargalovic P, Dory L. Cellular apoptosis is associated with increased caveolin-1 expression in macrophages. J Lipid Res. 2003;44:1622–32.
58. Fielding CJ, Fielding PE. Caveolae and intracellular trafficking of cholesterol. Adv Drug Deliv Rev. 2001;49:251–64.
59. Burgermeister E, Liscovitch M, Rocken C, Schmid RM, Ebert MPA. Caveats of caveolin-1 in cancer progression. Cancer Lett. 2008;268:187–201.
60. Goetz JG, Lajoie P, Wiseman SM, Nabi IR. Caveolin-1 in tumor progression: the good, the bad and the ugly. Cancer Metastasis Rev. 2008;27:715–35.
61. Nguyen KCT, Cho KA. Versatile functions of caveolin-1 in aging-related diseases. Chonnam Med J. 2017;53:28–36.
62. Pavlides S, Gutierrez-Pajares JL, Katiyar S, Jasmin J, Mercier I, Walters R, Pavlides C, Pestell RG, Lisanti MP, Frank PG. Caveolin-1 regulates the anti-atherogenic properties of macrophages. Cell Tissue Res. 2014;358:821–31.
63. Fernandez-Hernando C, Yu J, Suarez Y, Rahner C, Davalos A, Lasuncion MA, Sessa WC. Genetic evidence supporting a critical role of endothelial caveolin-1 during the progression of atherosclerosis. Cell Metab. 2009;10:48–54.
64. Stary CM, Tsutsumi YM, Patel PM, Head BP, Patel HH, Roth DM. Caveolins: targeting pro-survival signaling in the heart and brain. Front Physiol. 2012;3:393.
65. Choi KH, Kim HS, Park MS, Lee EB, Lee JK, Kim JT, Kim JH, Lee MC, Lee HJ, Cho KH. Overexpression of caveolin-1 attenuates brain edema by inhibiting tight junction degradation. Oncotarget. 2016;7:67857–67.
66. Jasmin J, Malhotra S, Singh Dhallu M, Mercier I, Rosenbaum DM, Lisanti MP. Caveolin-1 deficiency increases cerebral ischemic injury. Circ Res. 2007;100(5): 721–9. https://doi.org/10.1161/01.RES.0000260180.42709.29 Epub 2007 Feb 9.
67. Choi K, Kim H, Park M, Kim J, Kim J, Cho K, Lee M, Lee H, Cho K. Regulation

of caveolin-1 expression determines early brain edema after experimental focal cerebral ischemia. Stroke. 2016;47:1336–43.
68. Zhang S, Liu Y, Zhao Z, Xue Y. Effects of green tea polyphenols on caveolin-1 of microvessel fragments in rats with cerebral ischemia. Neurol Res. 2010; 32:963–70.
69. Huang P, Zhou C, Qin-Hu LY, Hu B, Chang X, Zhao X, Xu X, Li Q, Wei X, et al. Cerebralcare Granule(R) attenuates blood-brain barrier disruption after middle cerebral artery occlusion in rats. Exp Neurol. 2012;237:453–63.
70. Gu Y, Zheng G, Xu M, Li Y, Chen X, Zhu W, Tong Y, Chung SK, Liu KJ, Shen J. Caveolin-1 regulates nitric oxide-mediated matrix metalloproteinases activity and blood-brain barrier permeability in focal cerebral ischemia and reperfusion injury. J Neurochem. 2012;120:147–56.
71. Castellanos M, van Eendenburg C, Gubern C, Kadar E, Huguet G, Puig J, Sobrino T, Blasco G, Serena J, Sanchez JM. Low levels of caveolin-1 predict symptomatic bleeding after thrombolytic therapy in patients with acute ischemic stroke. Stroke. 2018;49:1525–7.
72. Preston JE, Joan Abbott N, Begley DJ. Transcytosis of macromolecules at the blood-brain barrier. Advances in pharmacology (San Diego, Calif). 2014;71: 147–63.
73. Soares ES, Mendonca MCP, Irazusta SP, Coope A, Stavale LM, da Cruz-Hofling MA. Evidences of endocytosis via caveolae following blood-brain barrier breakdown by Phoneutria nigriventer spider venom. Toxicol Lett. 2014;229:415–22.
74. Schubert W, Frank PG, Razani B, Park DS, Chow CW, Lisanti MP. Caveolae-deficient endothelial cells show defects in the uptake and transport of albumin in vivo. J Biol Chem. 2001;276:48619–22.
75. Deng J, Huang Q, Wang F, Liu Y, Wang Z, Wang Z, Zhang Q, Lei B, Cheng Y. The role of caveolin-1 in blood-brain barrier disruption induced by focused ultrasound combined with microbubbles. J Mol Neurosci. 2012;46:677–87.
76. Feng Y, Venema VJ, Venema RC, Tsai N, Behzadian MA, Caldwell RB. VEGF-induced permeability increase is mediated by caveolae. Invest Ophthalmol Vis Sci. 1999;40:157–67.
77. Knowland D, Arac A, Sekiguchi KJ, Hsu M, Lutz SE, Perrino J, Steinberg GK, Barres BA, Nimmerjahn A, Agalliu D. Stepwise recruitment of transcellular and paracellular pathways underlies blood-brain barrier breakdown in stroke. Neuron. 2014;82:603–17.
78. Sverdlov M, Shajahan AN, Minshall RD. Tyrosine phosphorylation-dependence of caveolae-mediated endocytosis. J Cell Mol Med. 2007;11:1239–50.
79. Xu L, Guo R, Xie Y, Ma M, Ye R, Liu X. Caveolae: molecular insights and therapeutic targets for stroke. Expert Opin Ther Tar. 2015;19:633–50.
80. Sun Y, Hu G, Zhang X, Minshall RD. Phosphorylation of caveolin-1 regulates oxidant-induced pulmonary vascular permeability via paracellular and transcellular pathways. Circ Res. 2009;105:676–85 15-685.
81. Takeuchi K, Morizane Y, Kamami-Levy C, Suzuki J, Kayama M, Cai W, Miller JW, Vavvas DG. AMP-dependent kinase inhibits oxidative stress-induced caveolin-1 phosphorylation and endocytosis by suppressing the dissociation between c-Abl and Prdx1 proteins in endothelial cells. J Biol Chem. 2013; 288:20581–91.
82. Andreone BJ, Chow BW, Tata A, Lacoste B, Ben-Zvi A, Bullock K, Deik AA, Ginty DD, Clish CB, Gu C. Blood-brain barrier permeability is regulated by lipid transport-dependent suppression of caveolae-mediated transcytosis. Neuron. 2017;94:581–94.
83. Li Y, Liu L, Ma T, Wang P, Xue Y. Effect of caveolin-1 on the expression of tight junction-associated proteins in rat glioma-derived microvascular endothelial cells. Int J Clin Exp Pathol. 2015;8:13067–74.
84. Jin X, Sun Y, Xu J, Liu W. Caveolin-1 mediates tissue plasminogen activator-induced MMP-9 up-regulation in cultured brain microvascular endothelial cells. J Neurochem. 2015;132:724–30.
85. Song H, Cheng Y, Bi G, Zhu Y, Jun W, Ma W, Wu H. Release of matrix metalloproteinases-2 and 9 by S-nitrosylated caveolin-1 contributes to degradation of extracellular matrix in tPA-treated hypoxic endothelial cells. PLoS One. 2016;11:e149269.
86. Liu J, Jin X, Liu KJ, Liu W. Matrix metalloproteinase-2-mediated occludin degradation and caveolin-1-mediated claudin-5 redistribution contribute to blood-brain barrier damage in early ischemic stroke stage. J Neurosci. 2012; 32(9):3044–57. https://doi.org/10.1523/JNEUROSCI.6409-11.2012.
87. Liu J, Weaver J, Jin X, Zhang Y, Xu J, Liu KJ, Li W, Liu W. Nitric oxide interacts with caveolin-1 to facilitate autophagy-lysosome-mediated claudin-5 degradation in oxygen-glucose deprivation-treated endothelial cells. Mol Neurobiol. 2016;53:5935–47.
88. Stamatovic SM, Keep RF, Wang MM, Jankovic I, Andjelkovic AV. Caveolae-mediated internalization of occludin and claudin-5 during CCL2-induced tight junction remodeling in brain endothelial cells. J Biol Chem. 2009;284:19053–66.
89. Liu W, Wang Z, Wang Y, Tong L, Li Y, Wei X, Luan P, Li L. Increasing the permeability of the blood-brain barrier in three different models in vivo. CNS Neurosci Ther. 2015;21:568–74.
90. Xie H, Lu W. Inhibition of transient receptor potential vanilloid 4 decreases the expressions of caveolin-1 and caveolin-2 after focal cerebral ischemia and reperfusion in rats. Neuropathology. 2018. https://doi.org/10.1111/neup.12469. [Epub ahead of print].
91. Zou R, Wu Z, Cui S. Electroacupuncture pretreatment attenuates bloodbrain barrier disruption following cerebral ischemia/reperfusion. Mol Med Rep. 2015;12:2027–34.
92. del Zoppo GJ, Mabuchi T. Cerebral microvessel responses to focal ischemia. J Cereb Blood Flow Metab. 2003;23:879–94.
93. Krupinski J, Kaluza J, Kumar P, Kumar S, Wang JM. Role of angiogenesis in patients with cerebral ischemic stroke. Stroke. 1994;25:1794–8.
94. Hayashi T, Noshita N, Sugawara T, Chan PH. Temporal profile of angiogenesis and expression of related genes in the brain after ischemia. J Cereb Blood Flow Metab. 2003;23:166–80.
95. Carmeliet P, Collen D. Molecular basis of angiogenesis. Role of VEGF and VE-cadherin. Ann N Y Acad Sci. 2000;902:249–62.
96. Feng Y, Vom Hagen F, Wang Y, Beck S, Schreiter K, Pfister F, Hoffmann S, Wagner P, Seeliger M, Molema G, et al. The absence of angiopoietin-2 leads to abnormal vascular maturation and persistent proliferative retinopathy. Thromb Haemost. 2009;102:120–30.
97. Yang J, Liu H, Liu X. VEGF promotes angiogenesis and functional recovery in stroke rats. J Investig Surg. 2010;23(3):149–55. https://doi.org/10.3109/08941930903469482.
98. Seto S, Chang D, Jenkins A, Bensoussan A, Kiat H. Angiogenesis in ischemic stroke and angiogenic effects of Chinese herbal medicine. Journal of clinical medicine. 2016;5(6):56.
99. Gao Y, Zhao Y, Pan J, Yang L, Huang T, Feng X, Li C, Liang S, Zhou D, Liu C, et al. Treadmill exercise promotes angiogenesis in the ischemic penumbra of rat brains through caveolin-1/VEGF signaling pathways. Brain Res. 2014;1585:83–90.
100. Tu F, Pang Q, Chen X, Huang T, Liu M, Zhai Q. Angiogenic effects of apigenin on endothelial cells after hypoxia-reoxygenation via the caveolin-1 pathway. Int J Mol Med. 2017;40:1639–48.
101. Liu J, Wang XB, Park DS, Lisanti MP. Caveolin-1 expression enhances endothelial capillary tubule formation. J Biol Chem. 2002;277:10661–8.
102. Fang K, Fu W, Beardsley AR, Sun X, Lisanti MP, Liu J. Overexpression of caveolin-1 inhibits endothelial cell proliferation by arresting the cell cycle at G0/G1 phase. Cell Cycle. 2007;6(2):199–204. https://doi.org/10.4161/cc.6.2.3740 Epub 2007 Jan 20.
103. Liu J, Razani B, Tang S, Terman BI, Ware JA, Lisanti MP. Angiogenesis activators and inhibitors differentially regulate caveolin-1 expression and caveolae formation in vascular endothelial cells. Angiogenesis inhibitors block vascular endothelial growth factor-induced down-regulation of caveolin-1. J Biol Chem. 1999;274:15781–5.
104. Labrecque L, Royal I, Surprenant DS, Patterson C, Gingras D, Beliveau R. Regulation of vascular endothelial growth factor receptor-2 activity by caveolin-1 and plasma membrane cholesterol. Mol Biol Cell. 2003;14:334–47.
105. Sonveaux P, Martinive P, DeWever J, Batova Z, Daneau G, Pelat M, Ghisdal P, Gregoire V, Dessy C, Balligand J, Feron O. Caveolin-1 expression is critical for vascular endothelial growth factor-induced ischemic hindlimb collateralization and nitric oxide-mediated angiogenesis. Circ Res. 2004;95:154–61.
106. Pan Y, Yao Y, Zhu Z, Sun X, Qiu Y, Ding Y. Caveolin-1 is important for nitric oxide-mediated angiogenesis in fibrin gels with human umbilical vein endothelial cells. Acta Pharmacol Sin. 2006;27:1567–74.
107. Koh S, Park H. Neurogenesis in stroke recovery. Transl Stroke Res. 2017;8:3–13.
108. Sakaguchi M, Okano H. Neural stem cells, adult neurogenesis, and galectin-1: from bench to bedside. Dev Neurobiol. 2012;72:1059–67.
109. Faiz M, Sachewsky N, Gascon S, Bang KWA, Morshead CM, Nagy A. Adult neural stem cells from the subventricular zone give rise to reactive astrocytes in the cortex after stroke. Cell Stem Cell. 2015;17:624–34.
110. Zhang RL, Zhang ZG, Zhang L, Chopp M. Proliferation and differentiation of progenitor cells in the cortex and the subventricular zone in the adult rat after focal cerebral ischemia. Neuroscience. 2001;105:33–41.
111. Jin K, Minami M, Lan JQ, Mao XO, Batteur S, Simon RP, Greenberg DA. Neurogenesis in dentate subgranular zone and rostral subventricular zone after focal cerebral ischemia in the rat. P Natl Acad Sci Usa. 2001; 98:4710–5.

112. Zhao Y, Pang Q, Liu M, Pan J, Xiang B, Huang T, Tu F, Liu C, Chen X. Treadmill exercise promotes neurogenesis in ischemic rat brains via caveolin-1/VEGF signaling pathways. Neurochem Res. 2017;42:389–97.
113. Pang Q, Zhang H, Chen Z, Wu Y, Bai M, Liu Y, Zhao Y, Tu F, Liu C, Chen X. Role of caveolin-1/vascular endothelial growth factor pathway in basic fibroblast growth factor-induced angiogenesis and neurogenesis after treadmill training following focal cerebral ischemia in rats. Brain Res. 2017;1663:9–19.
114. Li Y, Luo J, Lau W, Zheng G, Fu S, Wang T, Zeng H, So K, Chung SK, Tong Y, et al. Caveolin-1 plays a crucial role in inhibiting neuronal differentiation of neural stem/progenitor cells via VEGF signaling-dependent pathway. PLoS One. 2011;6:e22901.
115. Liu Y, Liang Z, Liu J, Zou W, Li X, Wang Y, An L. Downregulation of caveolin-1 contributes to the synaptic plasticity deficit in the hippocampus of aged rats. Neural Regen Res. 2013;8:2725–33.
116. Cui W, Ren Y, Wang S, Zeng M, Han S, Li J, Han R. The role of caveolin-1 in morphine-induced structural plasticity in primary cultured mouse cerebral cortical neurons. Neurosci Lett. 2018;665:38–42.
117. Mandyam CD, Schilling JM, Cui W, Egawa J, Niesman IR, Kellerhals SE, Staples MC, Busija AR, Risbrough VB, Posadas E, et al. Neuron-targeted caveolin-1 improves molecular signaling, plasticity, and behavior dependent on the hippocampus in adult and aged mice. Biol Psychiatry. 2017;81:101–10.
118. Egawa J, Zemljic-Harpf A, Mandyam CD, Niesman IR, Lysenko LV, Kleschevnikov AM, Roth DM, Patel HH, Patel PM, Head BP. Neuron-targeted caveolin-1 promotes ultrastructural and functional hippocampal synaptic plasticity. Cerebral cortex (New York, NY : 1991). 2017:1–12.
119. Head BP, Hu Y, Finley JC, Saldana MD, Bonds JA, Miyanohara A, Niesman IR, Ali SS, Murray F, Insel PA, et al. Neuron-targeted caveolin-1 protein enhances signaling and promotes arborization of primary neurons. J Biol Chem. 2011;286:33310–21.
120. Head BP, Patel HH, Tsutsumi YM, Hu Y, Mejia T, Mora RC, Insel PA, Roth DM, Drummond JC, Patel PM. Caveolin-1 expression is essential for N-methyl-D-aspartate receptor-mediated Src and extracellular signal-regulated kinase 1/2 activation and protection of primary neurons from ischemic cell death. FASEB J. 2008;22:828–40.
121. Consales C, Volpicelli F, Greco D, Leone L, Colucci-D'Amato L, Perrone-Capano C, di Porzio U. GDNF signaling in embryonic midbrain neurons in vitro. Brain Res. 2007;1159:28–39.
122. de Almeida CJG. Caveolin-1 and Caveolin-2 can be antagonistic partners in inflammation and beyond. Front Immunol. 2017;8:1530.
123. Sifat AE, Vaidya B, Abbruscato TJ. Blood-brain barrier protection as a therapeutic strategy for acute ischemic stroke. AAPS J. 2017;19:957–72.
124. Niesman IR, Schilling JM, Shapiro LA, Kellerhals SE, Bonds JA, Kleschevnikov AM, Cui W, Voong A, Krajewski S, Ali SS, et al. Traumatic brain injury enhances neuroinflammation and lesion volume in caveolin deficient mice. J Neuroinflammation. 2014;11:39.
125. Jiang Y, Lin X, Tang Z, Lee C, Tian G, Du Y, Yin X, Ren X, Huang L, Ye Z, et al. Critical role of caveolin-1 in ocular neovascularization and multitargeted antiangiogenic effects of cavtratin via JNK. P Natl Acad Sci Usa. 2017;114:10737–42.
126. Argaw AT, Asp L, Zhang J, Navrazhina K, Pham T, Mariani JN, Mahase S, Dutta DJ, Seto J, Kramer EG, et al. Astrocyte-derived VEGF-A drives blood-brain barrier disruption in CNS inflammatory disease. J Clin Invest. 2012;122:2454–68.
127. Bucci M, Gratton JP, Rudic RD, Acevedo L, Roviezzo F, Cirino G, Sessa WC. In vivo delivery of the caveolin-1 scaffolding domain inhibits nitric oxide synthesis and reduces inflammation. Nat Med. 2000;6:1362–7.
128. Harris J, Werling D, Hope JC, Taylor G, Howard CJ. Caveolae and caveolin in immune cells: distribution and functions. Trends Immunol. 2002;23:158–64.
129. Li J, Scherl A, Medina F, Frank PG, Kitsis RN, Tanowitz HB, Sotgia F, Lisanti MP. Impaired phagocytosis in caveolin-1 deficient macrophages. Cell Cycle. 2005;4:1599–607.
130. Jiao H, Zhang Y, Yan Z, Wang Z, Liu G, Minshall RD, Malik AB, Hu G. Caveolin-1 Tyr14 phosphorylation induces interaction with TLR4 in endothelial cells and mediates MyD88-dependent signaling and sepsis-induced lung inflammation. J Immunol. 2013;191:6191–9.
131. Matsui T, Higashimoto Y, Taira J, Yamagishi S. Pigment epithelium-derived factor (PEDF) binds to caveolin-1 and inhibits the pro-inflammatory effects of caveolin-1 in endothelial cells. Biochem Bioph Res Co. 2013;441:405–10.
132. Oakley FD, Smith RL, Engelhardt JF. Lipid rafts and caveolin-1 coordinate interleukin-1beta (IL-1beta)-dependent activation of NFkappaB by controlling endocytosis of Nox2 and IL-1beta receptor 1 from the plasma membrane. J Biol Chem. 2009;284:33255–64.
133. Garrean S, Gao X, Brovkovych V, Shimizu J, Zhao Y, Vogel SM, Malik AB. Caveolin-1 regulates NF-kappaB activation and lung inflammatory response to sepsis induced by lipopolysaccharide. J Immunol. 2006;177:4853–60.
134. Mirza MK, Yuan J, Gao X, Garrean S, Brovkovych V, Malik AB, Tiruppathi C, Zhao Y. Caveolin-1 deficiency dampens Toll-like receptor 4 signaling through eNOS activation. Am J Pathol. 2010;176:2344–51.
135. Wang XM, Kim HP, Song R, Choi AMK. Caveolin-1 confers antiinflammatory effects in murine macrophages via the MKK3/p38 MAPK pathway. Am J Resp Cell Mol. 2006;34:434–42.
136. Wang XM, Kim HP, Nakahira K, Ryter SW, Choi AMK. The heme oxygenase-1/carbon monoxide pathway suppresses TLR4 signaling by regulating the interaction of TLR4 with caveolin-1. J Immunol. 2009;182:3809–18.
137. Hu G, Ye RD, Dinauer MC, Malik AB, Minshall RD. Neutrophil caveolin-1 expression contributes to mechanism of lung inflammation and injury. Am J Physiol Lung Cell Mol Physiol. 2008;294:L178–86.
138. Ohnuma K, Inoue H, Uchiyama M, Yamochi T, Hosono O, Dang NH, Morimoto C. T-cell activation via CD26 and caveolin-1 in rheumatoid synovium. Mod Rheumatol. 2006;16:3–13.
139. Feng H, Guo L, Song Z, Gao H, Wang D, Fu W, Han J, Li Z, Huang B, Li X. Caveolin-1 protects against sepsis by modulating inflammatory response, alleviating bacterial burden, and suppressing thymocyte apoptosis. J Biol Chem. 2010;285:25154–60.
140. Portugal CC, Socodato R, Canedo T, Silva CM, Martins T, Coreixas VSM, Loiola EC, Gess B, Rohr D, Santiago AR, et al. Caveolin-1-mediated internalization of the vitamin C transporter SVCT2 in microglia triggers an inflammatory phenotype. Sci Signal. 2017;10. https://doi.org/10.1126/scisignal.aal2005.
141. Kagawa Y, Yasumoto Y, Sharifi K, Ebrahimi M, Islam A, Miyazaki H, Yamamoto Y, Sawada T, Kishi H, Kobayashi S, et al. Fatty acid-binding protein 7 regulates function of caveolae in astrocytes through expression of caveolin-1. Glia. 2015; 63:780–94.
142. Feng H, Guo W, Han J, Li X. Role of caveolin-1 and caveolae signaling in endotoxemia and sepsis. Life Sci. 2013;93:1–6.
143. Candelario-Jalil E, Gonzalez-Falcon A, Garcia-Cabrera M, Leon OS, Fiebich BL. Post-ischaemic treatment with the cyclooxygenase-2 inhibitor nimesulide reduces blood-brain barrier disruption and leukocyte infiltration following transient focal cerebral ischaemia in rats. J Neurochem. 2007;100:1108–20.
144. Chen S, Liou J, Huang T, Lin Y, Yeh A, Tam K, Tsai T, Wu KK, Shyue S. Caveolin-1 facilitates cyclooxygenase-2 protein degradation. J Cell Biochem. 2010;109:356–62.
145. Kerr JF, Wyllie AH, Currie AR. Apoptosis: a basic biological phenomenon with wide-ranging implications in tissue kinetics. Brit J Cancer. 1972;26: 239–57.
146. Festjens N, Vanden Berghe T, Vandenabeele P. Necrosis, a well-orchestrated form of cell demise: signalling cascades, important mediators and concomitant immune response. Biochim Biophys Acta. 2006;1757:1371–87.
147. Codogno P, Meijer AJ. Autophagy and signaling: their role in cell survival and cell death. Cell Death Differ. 2005;12(Suppl 2):1509–18.
148. Hellwig CT, Passante E, Rehm M. The molecular machinery regulating apoptosis signal transduction and its implication in human physiology and pathophysiologies. Curr Mol Med. 2011;11:31–47.
149. Quest AFG, Lobos-Gonzalez L, Nunez S, Sanhueza C, Fernandez J, Aguirre A, Rodriguez D, Leyton L, Torres V. The caveolin-1 connection to cell death and survival. Curr Mol Med. 2013;13:266–81.
150. Zhang W, Yokota H, Xu Z, Narayanan SP, Yancey L, Yoshida A, Marcus DM, Caldwell RW, Caldwell RB, Brooks SE. Hyperoxia therapy of pre-proliferative ischemic retinopathy in a mouse model. Invest Ophthalmol Vis Sci. 2011;52: 6384–95.
151. Glukhova XA, Trizna JA, Proussakova OV, Gogvadze V, Beletsky IP. Impairment of Fas-ligand-caveolin-1 interaction inhibits Fas-ligand translocation to rafts and Fas-ligand-induced cell death. Cell Death Dis. 2018;9:73.
152. Tait SWG, Green DR. Mitochondria and cell death: outer membrane permeabilization and beyond. Nat Rev Mol Cell Biol. 2010;11:621–32.
153. Chen Y, Lin W, Liu C, Su S. H2O2 induces caveolin1 degradation and impaired mitochondrial function in E11 podocytes. Mol Med Rep. 2017;16:7841–7.
154. Shiroto T, Romero N, Sugiyama T, Sartoretto JL, Kalwa H, Yan Z, Shimokawa H, Michel T. Caveolin-1 is a critical determinant of autophagy, metabolic switching, and oxidative stress in vascular endothelium. PLoS One. 2014;9:e87871.
155. Bosch M, Mari M, Herms A, Fernandez A, Fajardo A, Kassan A, Giralt A, Colell A, Balgoma D, Barbero E, et al. Caveolin-1 deficiency causes cholesterol-

dependent mitochondrial dysfunction and apoptotic susceptibility. Curr Biol. 2011;21:681–6.
156. Volonte D, Liu Z, Shiva S, Galbiati F. Caveolin-1 controls mitochondrial function through regulation of m-AAA mitochondrial protease. Aging. 2016; 8:2355–69.
157. Torres VA, Tapia JC, Rodriguez DA, Parraga M, Lisboa P, Montoya M, Leyton L, Quest AFG. Caveolin-1 controls cell proliferation and cell death by suppressing expression of the inhibitor of apoptosis protein survivin. J Cell Sci. 2006;119:1812–23.
158. Shen J, Lee W, Li Y, Lau CF, Ng KM, Fung ML, Liu KJ. Interaction of caveolin-1, nitric oxide, and nitric oxide synthases in hypoxic human SK-N-MC neuroblastoma cells. J Neurochem. 2008;107:478–87.
159. Yue W, Yao S, Zhou X, Si Y, Sang H, Wang J, Shang Z. Inhibitory effect of caveolin-1 on endoplasmic reticulum stress-induced apoptosis in macrophages via p38 MAPK pathway. Sheng Li Xue Bao. 2012;64(2):149–54.
160. Kang J, Lee S. Impaired expression of caveolin-1 contributes to hepatic ischemia and reperfusion injury. Biochem Bioph Res Co. 2014;450:1351–7.
161. Xu L, Wang L, Wen Z, Wu L, Jiang Y, Yang L, Xiao L, Xie Y, Ma M, Zhu W, et al. Caveolin-1 is a checkpoint regulator in hypoxia-induced astrocyte apoptosis via Ras/Raf/ERK pathway. Am J Physiol Cell Physiol. 2016;310:C903–10.
162. Chen F, Barman S, Yu Y, Haigh S, Wang Y, Black SM, Rafikov R, Dou H, Bagi Z, Han W, et al. Caveolin-1 is a negative regulator of NADPH oxidase-derived reactive oxygen species. Free Radic Biol Med. 2014;73:201–13.
163. Wang S, Wang N, Zheng Y, Zhang J, Zhang F, Wang Z. Caveolin-1: an oxidative stress-related target for cancer prevention. Oxidative Med Cell Longev. 2017;2017:7454031.
164. Yun JH, Park SJ, Jo A, Kang JL, Jou I, Park JS, Choi YH. Caveolin-1 is involved in reactive oxygen species-induced SHP-2 activation in astrocytes. Exp Mol Med. 2011;43:660–8.
165. Ju H, Zou R, Venema VJ, Venema RC. Direct interaction of endothelial nitric-oxide synthase and caveolin-1 inhibits synthase activity. J Biol Chem. 1997; 272:18522–5.
166. Bernatchez PN, Bauer PM, Yu J, Prendergast JS, He P, Sessa WC. Dissecting the molecular control of endothelial NO synthase by caveolin-1 using cell-permeable peptides. P Natl Acad Sci Usa. 2005;102:761–6.
167. Phillips PG, Birnby LM. Nitric oxide modulates caveolin-1 and matrix metalloproteinase-9 expression and distribution at the endothelial cell/tumor cell interface. Am J Physiol Lung Cell Mol Physiol. 2004;286:L1055–65.
168. Shen J, Ma S, Chan P, Lee W, Fung PCW, Cheung RTF, Tong Y, Liu KJ. Nitric oxide down-regulates caveolin-1 expression in rat brains during focal cerebral ischemia and reperfusion injury. J Neurochem. 2006;96:1078–89.
169. Garcia-Cardena G, Martasek P, Masters BS, Skidd PM, Couet J, Li S, Lisanti MP, Sessa WC. Dissecting the interaction between nitric oxide synthase (NOS) and caveolin. Functional significance of the nos caveolin binding domain in vivo. J Biol Chem. 1997;272:25437–40.
170. Michel JB, Feron O, Sacks D, Michel T. Reciprocal regulation of endothelial nitric-oxide synthase by Ca2+-calmodulin and caveolin. J Biol Chem. 1997; 272:15583–6.
171. Chidlow JHJ, Sessa WC. Caveolae, caveolins, and cavins: complex control of cellular signalling and inflammation. Cardiovasc Res. 2010;86:219–25.
172. Zhao Y, Zhao YD, Mirza MK, Huang JH, Potula HSK, Vogel SM, Brovkovych V, Yuan JX, Wharton J, Malik AB. Persistent eNOS activation secondary to caveolin-1 deficiency induces pulmonary hypertension in mice and humans through PKG nitration. J Clin Invest. 2009;119:2009–18.

19

Inflammation is correlated with severity and outcome of cerebral venous thrombosis

Liyan Wang[1], Jiangang Duan[2*], Tingting Bian[1], Ran Meng[1], Longfei Wu[1], Zhen Zhang[1], Xuxiang Zhang[3], Chunxiu Wang[4] and Xunming Ji[1*]

Abstract

Background: Few studies have suggested a relationship between inflammation and cerebral venous thrombosis (CVT). This retrospective study aimed to explore the changes in inflammation in different CVT stages and the correlation between inflammation and severity and outcome of CVT.

Methods: In total, 95 suitable patients with CVT and 41 controls were compared. Patients with CVT were divided into three groups. The inflammatory factors studied included hypersensitive C-reactive protein (Hs-CRP), interleukin-6 (IL-6), and neutrophil-to-lymphocyte ratio (NLR) in the peripheral blood and immunoglobulin A (IgA), immunoglobulin M (IgM), and immunoglobulin G (IgG) in the cerebrospinal fluid (CSF). The severity of CVT was evaluated with the modified Rankin Scale (mRS), the National Institutes of Health Stroke Scale (NIHSS), fundus condition, intracranial pressure (ICP), and complications on admission. The short-term outcome was evaluated with the mRS at discharge.

Results: The following results were obtained: (1) Inflammatory factor levels in patients with CVT were higher than those in the controls. (2) Inflammatory factor levels in the acute and subacute stages were significantly higher than those in the chronic stage (all $P < 0.05$). (3) Serum NLR and CSF IgM levels were positively related to baseline degree of disability (odds ratio [OR], 1.279, 95% confidence interval [CI] 1.009–1.621, $P = 0.042$; OR 1.402, 95% CI 1.036–1.896, $P = 0.028$). The Hs-CRP level was positively correlated with the baseline occurrence of seizure (OR 1.040, 95% CI 1.001–1.080, $P = 0.043$). The baseline serum NLR ($r = 0.244$, $P = 0.017$), CSF IgA ($r = 0.615$, $P < 0.001$), CSF IgM ($r = 0.752$, $P < 0.001$), and CSF IgG ($r = 0.248$, $P = 0.015$) levels were positively associated with NIHSS. (4) The baseline NLR was significantly associated with high risk of poor outcome at discharge (OR 1.339, 95% CI 1.097–1.784, $P = 0.007$). Moreover, the ROC showed that NLR ≥ 4.205 could better predict the poor outcome at discharge. The data were analyzed using SPSS.

Conclusions: Inflammation may develop after CVT and gradually decrease during the course. Inflammation was significantly correlated with severity on admission and short-term poor outcome at discharge in CVT.

Keywords: Cerebral venous thrombosis, Inflammation, Stage, Severity, Outcome

Background

Unlike artery ischemic stroke, cerebral venous thrombosis (CVT) is an uncommon type of stroke mainly developing in the young and middle-aged population, especially women [1]. Currently, the incidence of CVT is higher than 1.3–1.6/100,000 in Western countries and probably even higher in Asia and the Middle East [2]. The risk factors could be divided into inflammatory factors including infection or nonspecific inflammation of the head and face or other sites and non-inflammatory factors such as hypercoagulability, blood stasis, vascular wall injury, and intracranial hypotension [3]. The current main medical treatments of CVT include anticoagulation, etiological treatment, and symptomatic therapy [1]. Over the past decades, the mortality has declined because of improved diagnostics and early treatment with anticoagulation. However, many patients recovering without evident physical disability may have residual chronic symptoms consisting of headache or neuropsychological problems and the like [2]. Hence, we want to explore some undefined

* Correspondence: djg333@163.com; jixm@ccmu.edu.cn
[2]Emergency Department of Xuanwu Hospital Capital Medical University, Changchun street 45, Xicheng District, Beijing, China
[1]Neurosurgery Department of Xuanwu Hospital Capital Medical University, Changchun st 45, Xicheng District, Beijing, China
Full list of author information is available at the end of the article

therapeutic targets and potential treatments to improve the prognosis of CVT.

Anecdotal evidences have showed the extensive cross-talk between inflammatory cytokines and coagulation factors, indicating that inflammation and coagulation are correlative [4]. Numerous studies have found that inflammation plays vital roles in many thromboembolic diseases such as acute ischemic stroke (AIS), deep venous thrombosis (DVT), and pulmonary embolism (PE) [5–7]. Furthermore, inflammation can be the cause of CVT [8]. However, the relationship between inflammation and CVT in patients without definite inflammatory diseases remains unknown.

Recently, a number of studies have focused on determining the appropriate inflammatory factors to predict the outcome of patients with various thromboembolic diseases. As clinically easily available inflammatory factors, the increased hypersensitive C-reactive protein (Hs-CRP), interleukin-6 (IL-6) levels, and neutrophil-to-lymphocyte ratio (NLR) in the peripheral blood have been confirmed to be correlated with poor outcome in AIS, DVT, and PE [6, 9, 10]. CRP is a blood biomarker produced by the liver representing acute-phase systemic inflammation. Hs-CRP can accurately detect low-grade inflammation and is widely used in clinical practice particularly in cerebrovascular and cardiovascular diseases [11, 12]. IL-6 is a significant inflammatory factor produced by various cells including endothelial cells. Previous animal and clinical experiments have revealed that IL-6 participates in inflammation during coagulation partly through provoking stimulation of acute-phase reactants or chemoattractants [13, 14]. Moreover, IL-6 was correlated with venous thrombosis [15]. Recently, the NLR, which was associated with poor outcome in various vascular diseases of the heart and brain, also turns out to be a relatively reliable indicator of ongoing destructive inflammation [16–18]. Moreover, NLR was believed to be more stable and valuable than single changes in neutrophil or lymphocyte [19].

CVT is a type of cerebrovascular disease. Hence, evaluating inflammation of the brain is necessary. Cerebrospinal fluid (CSF) is produced in the brain, circulates throughout the central nervous system (CNS), and is located between the brain and skull [20]. The CSF can reflect the biochemical changes occurring in the brain because of its direct contact with the extracellular space of the brain [21]. It is well known that the significant elevation of CSF immunoglobulin (Ig) could indicate inflammatory reaction in the CNS [22].

To investigate the changes in inflammation in different stages of CVT and the correlation between inflammation and severity and outcome of CVT, we conducted this study and selected the above inflammatory biomarkers as research indicators. Hopefully, we could provide evidence for potential anti-inflammatory treatment on patients with CVT without definite inflammatory diseases to improve the outcome.

Methods

Study design

We retrospectively identified 95 newly diagnosed patients with CVT and 41 age- and sex-matched individuals for the control group admitted to our hospital from March 2015 to March 2018. Inclusion criteria for our study were newly diagnosed CVT on magnetic resonance imaging (MRI), magnetic resonance venography (MRV), computed tomographic venography (CTV), or conventional digital subtraction angiography (DSA) [1, 23]. The age and sex were unlimited. The individuals in the control group were those who were admitted to our hospital with suspicious CVT but diagnosed with other non-inflammatory diseases at discharge. Patients and control individuals were excluded if they have the following conditions [9]: AIS, acute myocardial infarction, renal or hepatic failure, malignancy, DVT and PE; definite immune diseases such as connective tissue diseases, rheumatic diseases; definite acute or chronic infection; use of anti-inflammatory medication within 4 weeks prior to blood collection; and refusal of blood sampling and lumbar puncture. All patients received the formal anticoagulation treatment. All protocols were approved by the Institutional Review Board.

Data collection

The following data of included patients with CVT were obtained at baseline in the study: demographics; risk factors for CVT; dates of onset of symptoms; symptoms and signs from onset to diagnosis; the features of imaging; the National Institutes of Health Stroke Score (NIHSS); modified Rankin Scale (mRS); the fundus condition; the intracranial pressure (ICP) [cerebrospinal fluid (CSF) opening pressure obtained by lumbar puncture in recumbent position)]; CVT-related complications, including intracranial hemorrhage, cerebral venous infarction and seizure; levels of D-dimer, hypersensitive C-reactive protein (Hs-CRP), interleukin-6 (IL-6), and the neutrophil-to-lymphocyte ratio (NLR) in peripheral blood and immunoglobulin A (IgA), immunoglobulin M (IgM), and immunoglobulin G (IgG) in CSF measured within 24 h after admission. The mRS score at discharge was also collected. Additionally, the mRS score, the fundus condition, and ICP at 3 to 12 months after the discharge were also documented. The data on age, sex, and six abovementioned inflammatory factors were also collected in the control group.

Clinical assessment

The severity of CVT on admission was assessed by NIHSS, mRS, presence of papilledema, intracranial hypertension (IH), cerebral venous infarction, intracranial hemorrhage, and seizure. The mRS ≤ 1 was defined as good condition and mRS > 1 was defined as poor condition [24]. Fundus photography detected the presence of papilledema. An ICP of more than 200 mmH2O was defined as intracranial hypertension.

The short-term outcome of CVT was evaluated with mRS at discharge [25]. The mRS ≤ 1 was defined as good outcome and mRS > 1was defined as poor outcome. The long-term outcome of CVT was assessed by mRS, presence of papilledema, and IH at 3 to 12 months after discharge.

Statistical analysis

All statistical analyses were performed by SPSS. Quantitative variables with a normal distribution were specified as mean ± standard deviation, and those with an abnormal distribution were expressed as median with interquartile range (IQR). Categorical variables were specified with number and percentage (%) values. Student's *t* test or Mann–Whitney test was used for continuous data, while χ^2 or Fisher's exact test was used for categorical data. The independent variables associated with the severity and outcome of CVT were analyzed by logistic regression analysis. Possible confounding factors were tested in a univariable regression analysis, and then, confounders with a *P* value < 0.05 were tested in a multivariable logistic regression analysis. The correlation between baseline NIHSS and inflammatory factors were assessed by Spearman's correlation coefficients. The receiver operating characteristic (ROC) curve was used to demonstrate the sensitivity and specificity of significant variables and the optimal cutoff values for predicting the outcome. A difference between the groups was considered significant if *P* < 0.05.

Results

Patients

A total of 95 patients with CVT (mean age, 38.93 ± 13.53 years, and 60.0% were female) and 41 controls (mean age, 40.90 ± 16.70 years, and 63.41% were female) were included in the study. In patients with CVT, 23.16% were in the acute stage, 32.63% in the subacute stage, and 44.21% in the chronic stage; 41.05% of patients were in poor condition (mRS > 1), 68.35% had IH, 60.56% had papilledema, 38.95% had cerebral venous infarction, 25.26% had seizure, and 11.58% had intracerebral hemorrhage. Of the patients, 30.53% had incomplete follow-up information and were removed from the follow-up data analysis.

Inflammation between patients with CVT and controls

Compared with the controls, the patients with CVT had higher Hs-CRP (3.3 [0.7, 11.73] vs 0.5[0.26, 1.6],*P* < 0.001), IL-6 (9.49 [5.76, 14.94] vs 4.32 [3.01, 5.02], *P* = 0.003), NLR (2.84 [1.86, 3.73] vs 2.05 [1.77, 2.59], *P* < 0.001), CSF IgA (0.4 [0.24, 0.81] vs 0.2 [0.13, 0.23], *P* < 0.001), CSF IgM (1.3 [0.5, 2.6] vs 0.04 [0.02, 0.08], *P* < 0.001), and CSF IgG (3.48 [2.22, 5.56] vs 2.54 [1.98, 2.88], *P* = 0.001) (Table 1).

Inflammation and stages of CVT

The levels of most inflammatory factors between acute and subacute stages have no difference (*P* > 0.05). The Hs-CRP level in the acute stage was higher than that in the subacute stage. The levels of all inflammatory factors in the acute and sub-acute stages were higher compared with those in the chronic stage (Hs-CRP, 14.03 [4.93, 28.42] vs 1.16 [0.26, 2.95], *P* < 0.001, and 6.83 [1.51, 14.15] vs 1.16 [0.26, 2.95], *P* < 0.001; NLR, 3.58 [2.63, 5.24] vs 2.56 [1.66, 3.15], *P* = 0.003, and 3.08 [2.15, 4.65] vs 2.56 [1.66, 3.15], *P* = 0.043; IL-6, 14.58 [8.93, 14.94] vs 6.82 [4.81, 8.01], *P* < 0.001, and 14.63 [6.73, 16.14] vs 6.82 [4.81, 8.01], *P* = 0.001; CSF IgA, 0.47 [0.25, 0.91] vs 0.31 [0.15, 0.48], *P* = 0.046, and 0.60 [0.29, 1.01] vs 0.31 [0.15, 0.48], *P* = 0.001; CSF IgM, 0.16 [0.03, 0.53] vs 0.05 [0.03, 0.09], *P* = 0.026, and 0.17 [0.10, 0.24] vs 0.05 [0.03, 0.09], *P* < 0.001; CSF IgG, 4.45 [2.50, 7.61] vs 2.36 [1.61, 3.19], *P* = 0.002, and 4.60 [3.05, 5.85] vs 2.36 [1.61, 3.19], *P* < 0.001) (Fig. 1).

Inflammation and the severity of CVT

Spearman's correlation analysis showed that the level of serum NLR (*r* = 0.244, *p* = 0.017), CSF IgA (*r* = 0.615, *p* < 0.001), CSF IgM (*r* = 0.752, *p* < 0.001), and CSF IgG (*r* = 0.248, *p* = 0.015) were positively associated with baseline NIHSS. We conducted a logistic regression analysis on the correlation between inflammation and degree of disability defined by mRS, IH, papilledema, cerebral venous infarction, seizure, and intracranial hemorrhage. The independent variables were the levels of six inflammatory factors, age, and sex. The results were as follows: the serum NLR [adjusted odds ratio (OR), 1.279; 95% confidence interval (*CI*) 1.009–1.621, *P* = 0.042], and CSF IgM (adjusted OR, 1.402; 95% *CI* 1.036–1.896, *P* = 0.028) level

Table 1 The clinical features of the two groups

	CVT patients *n* = 95	Control individuals *n* = 41	*P* value
Age, years	38.93 ± 13.53	40.90 ± 16.70	0.469
Gender (female, %)	60	63.41	0.708
Hs-CRP	3.3 (0.7, 11.73)	0.5 (0.26, 1.6)	< 0.001
IL-6	9.49 (5.76, 14.94)	4.32 (3.01, 5.02)	0.003
NLR	2.84 (1.86, 3.73)	2.05 (1.77, 2.59)	< 0.001
CSF IgA	0.4 (0.24, 0.81)	0.2 (0.13, 0.23)	< 0.001
CSF IgM	1.3 (0.5, 2.6)	0.04 (0.02, 0.08)	< 0.001
CSF IgG	3.48 (2.22, 5.56)	2.54 (1.98, 2.88)	0.001

CVT cerebral venous thrombosis, *Hs-CRP* hypersensitive C-reactive protein, *Il-6* interleukin-6, *NLR* the neutrophil to lymphocyte ratio, *IgA* immunoglobulin A, *IgM* immunoglobulin M, *IgG* immunoglobulin G, *CSF* cerebrospinal fluid

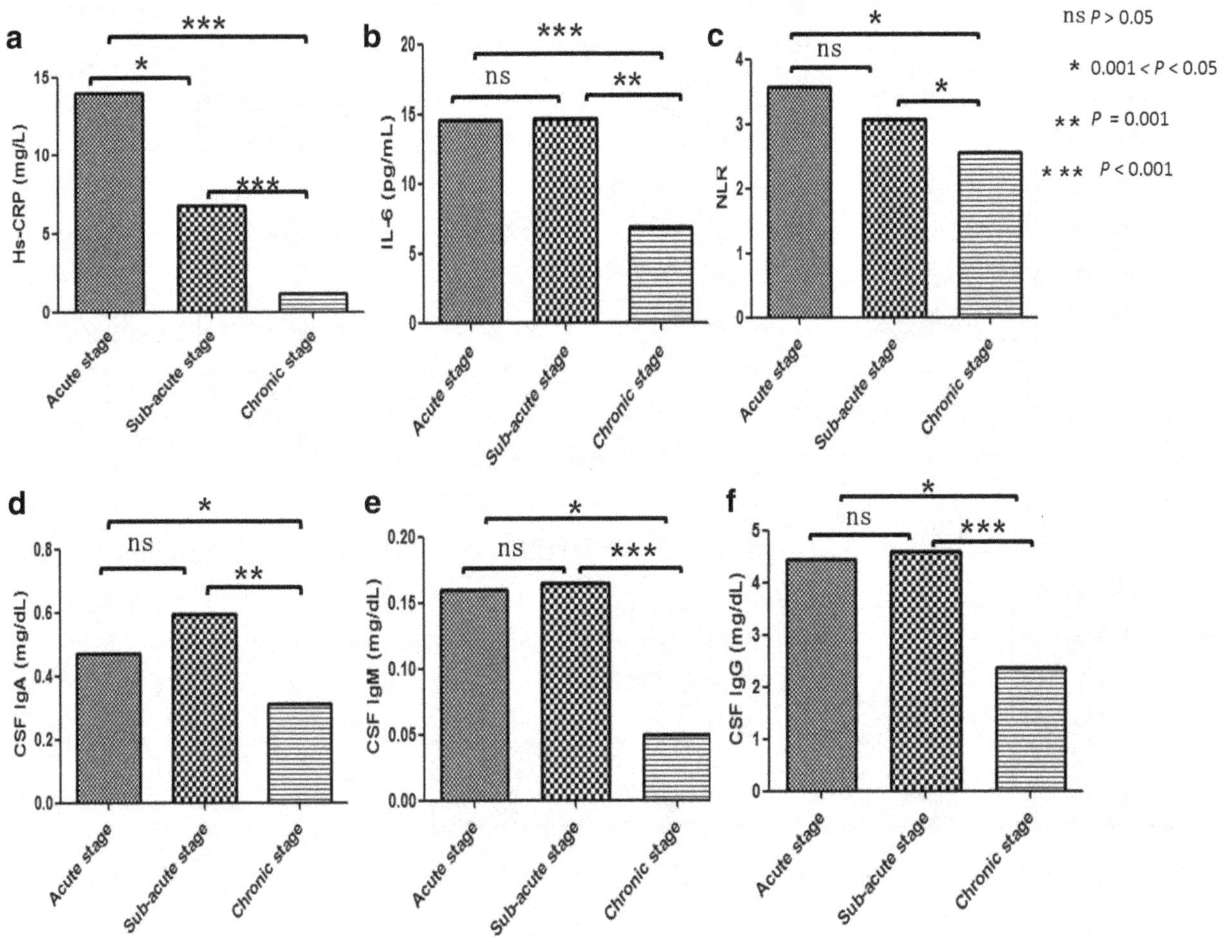

Fig. 1 **a** The Hs-CRP level in the acute and sub-acute stages were higher than that in the chronic stage, and its level in the acute stage was higher than that in the subacute stage. **b** The IL-6 level in the acute and sub-acute stages were significantly higher than that in the chronic stage. **c** The NLR level in the acute and sub-acute stages were higher than that in the chronic stage. **d** The CSF IgA level in the acute and sub-acute stages were higher than that in the chronic stage. **e** The CSF IgM level in the acute and sub-acute stages were higher than that in the chronic stage. **f** The CSF IgG level in the acute and sub-acute stages were higher than that in the chronic stage

were positively associated with baseline degree of disability. The Hs-CRP level was positively associated with the development of seizure at baseline (adjusted OR 1.040; 95% *CI* 1.001–1.080, $P = 0.043$). All 95 patients were grouped respectively based on mRS and seizure on admission: patients with good and poor condition and those with and without seizure. The NLR and CSF IgM level were significantly higher in patients with poor condition compared with those with good condition (3.45 [2.31, 5.29] vs 2.45 [1.72, 3.14], $P = 0.001$; and 1.90 [0.60, 3.00] vs 0.95 [0.40, 2.02], $P = 0.005$) (Fig. 2a, b). The Hs-CRP level was higher in patients with seizure than that in patients without seizure (6.64 [0.94, 35.72] vs 3.12 [0.54, 9.22], $P = 0.034$) (Fig. 2c).

Although the univariate logistics analysis revealed the correlation between baseline cerebral venous infarction and serum Hs-CRP (OR 1.053; 95% *CI* 1.016–1.092, $P = 0.005$), CSF IgM (OR 1.377, 95% *CI* 1.049–1.809, $P = 0.021$), and CSF IgG levels (OR 1.291, 95% *CI* 1.071–1.556, $P = 0.007$), the multivariate logistics analysis found no relationship between them (all $P > 0.05$). However, there was no significant relationship between inflammatory factors and baseline IH and papilledema (all $P > 0.05$).

Inflammation and outcome of CVT

All 95 patients were divided into two groups based on mRS at discharge: patients with good outcome and poor outcome. Baseline characteristics of the patients in two groups are shown in Table 2. There was no statistical difference between the two groups with regard to age, sex, stages, duration of hospital stay, and serum Hs-CRP, IL-6, CSF IgA, and CSF IgG levels (all $P > 0.05$). Compared with patients with good outcome, patients with poor outcome had higher NIHSS score (median 2.00 [1.00, 7.50] vs 0.00 [0.00, 1.00], $p < 0.001$), NLR (median 5.29 [3.00, 7.26] vs

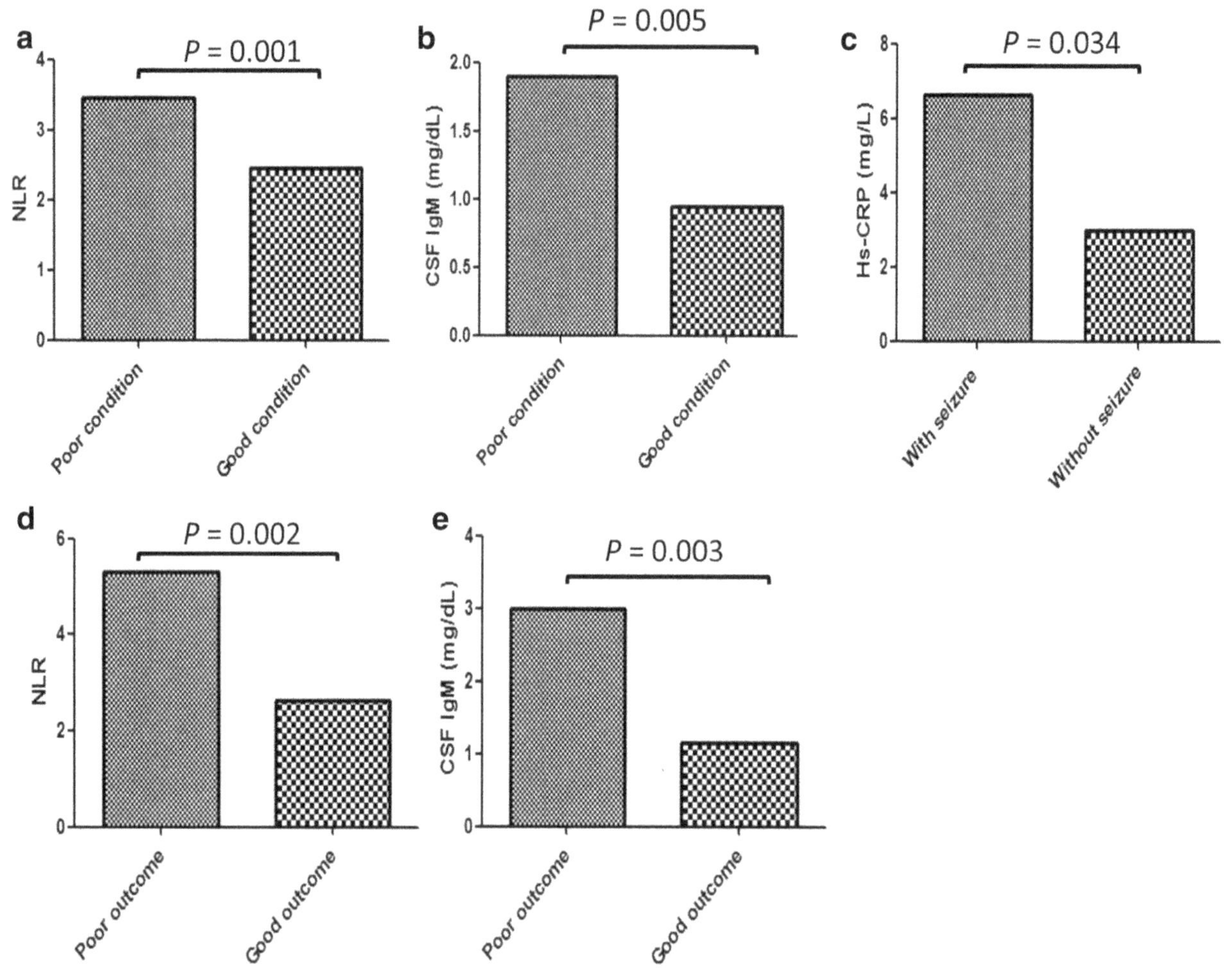

Fig. 2 **a**, **b** The difference in NLR and CSF IgM level between patients with good condition and those with poor condition. **c** The difference in Hs-CRP level between patients with seizure and those without seizure. **d**, **e** The difference in NLR and CSF IgM level between patients with good outcome and those with poor outcome

Table 2 Data of patients with good and poor condition on admission

	Poor condition $n = 39$	Good condition $n = 56$	P value
Female (%)	27/39 (69.23%)	30/56 (53.57%)	0.142
Male (%)	12/39 (30.77%)	26/56 (46.43%)	0.142
Age, years	37.62 ± 11.67	39.84 ± 14.72	0.434
Serum Hs-CRP (mg/L)	4.88 (0.86, 20.42)	3.06 (0.65, 6.74)	0.194
Serum NLR	3.45 (2.31, 5.29)	2.45 (1.72, 3.14)	0.001
Serum IL-6 (pg/ml)	11.87 (6.50, 14.94)	8.01 (4.98, 14.94)	0.451
CSF IgA (mg/dl)	0.46 (0.21, 0.90)	0.38 (0.38, 0.74)	0.617
CSF IgM (mg/dl)	1.90 (0.60, 3.00)	0.95 (0.40, 2.02)	0.005
CSF IgG (mg/dl)	4.16 (1.87, 6.80)	3.22 (2.29, 4.96)	0.423

CVT cerebral venous thrombosis, *Hs-CRP* hypersensitive C-reactive protein, *Il-6* interleukin-6, *NLR* the neutrophil to lymphocyte ratio, *IgA* immunoglobulin A, *IgM* immunoglobulin M, *IgG* immunoglobulin G, *CSF* cerebrospinal fluid

2.62 [1.79, 3.44], $p = 0.002$), and CSF IgM level (median 3.00 [1.65, 6.22] vs 1.15 [0.48, 2.33], $p = 0.003$) (Fig. 2d, e).

Logistic regression was used to study the value of inflammatory factors in predicting the outcomes at discharge. The independent variables were the baseline levels of six inflammatory factors, age, sex, and NIHSS score. The multivariate logistics analysis found that the baseline NLR was significantly associated with high risk of disability at discharge (adjusted OR, 1.339; 95% *CI* 1.097–1.784, $P = 0.007$).

The ROC curve demonstrated the predicting power of baseline serum NLR on the short-term outcome with an area under the curve value of 0.774 ($P = 0.002$, 95% *CI* 0.620–0.928) (Fig. 3). The optimal cutoff is 4.205 (positive predictive value 61.5%, negative predictive value 86.6%, + likelihood ratio [LR] 1.60, − LR 0.15). To further estimate the significance of baseline NLR on predicting the outcome of CVT, patients were divided into two groups according to the cutoff value of NLR (NLR < 4.205

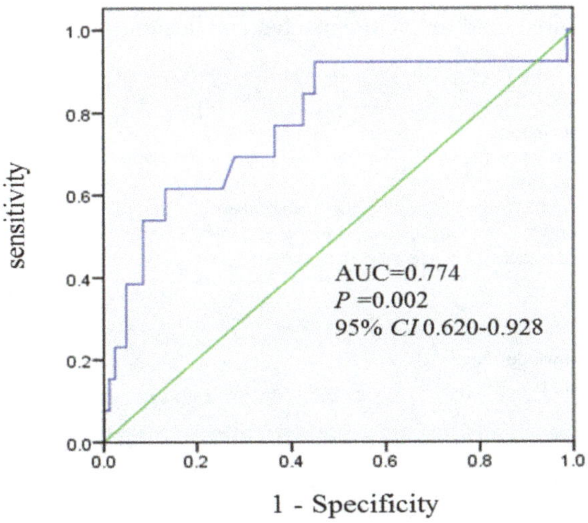

Fig. 3 Receiver operating characteristic (ROC) curve for serum NLR on predicting short-term outcome of non-inflammatory CVT. CVT, cerebral venous thrombosis; AUC, area under the curve; CI, confidence interval; NLR, neutrophil-to-lymphocyte ratio

and ≥ 4.025), and the details are shown in Table 3. The results revealed that the group with NLR ≥ 4.205 had higher NIHSS scores (median 2.00 [0.00, 7.00] vs 0.00 [0.00, 1.00], $P < 0.001$) and poor outcome (42.11% vs 6.58%, $P < 0.001$).

During the follow-up, 69.47% (66/95) of patients completed the telephone follow-up, and 53.68% (51/95) underwent lumbar puncture and fundus examination. The IL-6 level (OR, 1.063; 95% *CI* 1.008–1.122, $P = 0.025$) and NIHSS score (OR, 1.264; 95% *CI* 1.001–1.596, $P = 0.049$) were associated with high risk of poor outcome in the univariable model. However, the multivariate logistics analysis found no significant relationship (all $P > 0.05$). Moreover, the levels of these inflammatory factors were not correlated with the prognosis of non-inflammatory CVT including the development of IH and papilledema (all $P > 0.05$).

Discussion

It is well known that inflammation plays vital roles in artery stroke, which not only participates in the development of stroke but also plays a continuing role during the various stages of stroke and influences the outcome [26–29]. Similarly, inflammation could act as the cause of CVT, which has been demonstrated by numerous previous studies [8]. However, whether the inflammation develops after CVT and is associated with its severity and outcome is not yet presently defined.

As clinically easily available inflammatory biomarkers, Hs-CRP, IL-6, and NLR in the peripheral blood and Ig (A, M, G), in the CSF were used in our study to represent the inflammatory response. According to our results, the levels of abovementioned six inflammatory factors were higher in patients with CVT compared with those in the controls. Furthermore, these inflammatory factors including Hs-CRP, IL-6, and NLR in the peripheral blood and IgA, IgM, and IgG in the CSF increased significantly during the acute and subacute stages and decreased during the chronic stage. It indicated that inflammation may develop soon after CVT and gradually decrease during the course. In other words, the degree of inflammation may change with the course of the disease. As in DVT, the IL-6 and CRP levels were higher on admission and then gradually declined during the subsequent days [30].

Moreover, the serum NLR and CSF IgM level were positively correlated with baseline degree of disability on admission. The Hs-CRP level was positively correlated with the development of seizure at baseline. The baseline serum NLR and CSF IgA, CSF IgM, and CSF IgG levels were positively associated with NIHSS. Although the multivariate logistics analysis found no relationship between inflammatory factors and cerebral venous infarction at baseline, the univariate logistics analysis revealed the correlation between cerebral venous infarction at

Table 3 Data of patients classified according to NLR subgroup

	NLR < 4.205 *n* = 76	NLR ≥ 4.205 *n* = 19	*P* value
Male (%)	28/76 (36.84)	10/19 (52.63)	0.209
Female (%)	48/76 (63.16)	9/19 (47.37)	0.209
Age, years(mean ± SD)	38.01 ± 13.23	42.58 ± 14.45	0.190
NIHSS score on admission (median, IQR)	0.00 (0.00, 1.00)	2.00 (0.00, 7.00)	< 0.001
Seizure (%)	17/76 (22.37)	7/19 (36.84)	0.194
Infarction (%)	28/76 (36.84)	9/19 (47.37)	0.400
Intracerebral hemorrhage (%)	7/76 (9.21)	4/19 (21.05)	0.149
Papilledema (%)	33/76 (43.42)	9/19 (47.37)	0.757
Intracranial hypertension (%)	53/76 (69.74)	13/19 (68.42)	0.911
Poor outcome (%)	5/76 (6.58)	8/19 (42.11)	< 0.001

NIHSS the National Institutes of Health Stroke Score, *IQR* interquartile range

baseline and serum Hs-CRP, CSF IgM, and CSF IgG levels. Hence, it is suggested that a significant correlation between inflammation and severity of CVT may exist. Previous studies have also found the correlation between Hs-CRP level and disability and neurological deficit in cerebrovascular diseases [11, 12]. Currently, Nagai et al. also demonstrated that blood-brain barrier disruption and encephala edema after CVT are linked to the leukocyte–endothelial cell adhesion [31].

Furthermore, the baseline NLR was significantly associated with high risk of poor outcome at discharge. The ROC curve showed that an NLR ≥ 4.205 could better predict poor outcome at discharge, suggesting that baseline inflammation could influence and predict the short-term outcome of CVT. Recently, a retrospective study on the usefulness of NLR in predicting the presence of cerebral venous sinus thrombosis (CVST) found that higher NLRs were significantly and independently related to the presence of CVST, showing that inflammation may play an important role in CVST [8], which was consistent with our findings. Therefore, it is suggested that anti-inflammation probably improves the outcome of CVT in patients without definite inflammatory diseases. Although the use of steroids in CVT is not recommended in the current guideline, it does not mean the denial of the effect of immunoregulation in CVT. This study on steroids aimed at proving its function of decreasing vasogenic edema rather than anti-inflammation [32]. However, the study found no association between baseline inflammation and long-term outcome of these patients.

Our study has some important limitations. First, as a retrospective study, there are some missing data, and we cannot evaluate the outcome at a fixed time point. Second, some patients failed to be followed up due to various reasons. Third, the number of studied inflammatory factors was too small to obtain the ideal conclusion. Lastly, there was not enough study population. However, perhaps the limitations above could partly account for the fact that we did not find a correlation between inflammation and long-term outcome of CVT. Unfortunately, the underlying mechanism of inflammation acting on CVT cannot be precisely explained by this type of clinical study. Therefore, further exploration on this aspect using animal experiments is needed.

Conclusions

Inflammation may develop soon after the development of CVT and changes with the course of the disease. Moreover, inflammation is correlated with severity and short-term outcome of CVT. Therefore, inflammation may be a promising therapeutic target for CVT in patients without definite inflammatory diseases. However, given the limitations of the study, we need to increase the sample size, explore more inflammatory factors, and conduct a prospective randomized controlled study so that we could draw an expected conclusion.

Abbreviations

CI: Confidence interval; CSF: Cerebrospinal fluid; Hs-CRP: Hypersensitive C-reactive protein; ICP: Intracranial pressure; Ig: Immunoglobulin; IL-6: Interleukin-6; IQR: Interquartile range; mRS: The modified Rankin Scale; NIHSS: The National Institutes of Health Stroke Score; NLR: The Neutrophil to Lymphocyte ratio; OR: Odds ratio; ROC: Receiver operating characteristic curve

Acknowledgements

Not applicable.

Funding

This study was supported by The Scientific and Technological plan of Beijing Municipal Commission of Science and Technology (Z181100001918026).

Authors' contributions

LW coordinated the study, collected and analyzed the data, and drafted the manuscript. TB, RM, LW, ZZ, and XZ collected data and helped to modify the manuscript. CW participated in the statistical analysis. XJ and JD have equally contributed to this work as corresponding authors and participated in its design and coordination and helped to draft the manuscript. All authors read and approved the final manuscript.

Consent for publication

The authors agree to publish.

Competing interests

The authors declare that they have no competing interests.

Author details

[1]Neurosurgery Department of Xuanwu Hospital Capital Medical University, Changchun st 45, Xicheng District, Beijing, China. [2]Emergency Department of Xuanwu Hospital Capital Medical University, Changchun street 45, Xicheng District, Beijing, China. [3]Ophtalmology Department of Xuanwu Hospital Capital Medical University, Changchun street 45, Xicheng District, Beijing, China. [4]Evidence-based Medicine Department of Xuanwu Hospital Capital Medical University, Changchun street 45, Xicheng District, Beijing, China.

References

1. Gustavo Saposnik MD, et al. Diagnosis and management of cerebral venous thrombosis. Stroke. 2011;42:1158–92.
2. Suzanne MS, de Sousa DA, José MF, et al. Cerebral venous thrombosis. Neurology. 2017;13:555–65.
3. Chinese society of neurology. The guidance of diagnosis and treatment for cerebral venous thrombosis in China 2015. Chin J Neurol. 2015;48:819–29.
4. Levi M, van der Poll T, Büller HR. Bidirectional relation between inflammation and coagulation. Circulation. 2004;109(22):2698–704.
5. Iadecola C, Anrather J. The immunology of stroke: from mechanisms to translation. Nat Med. 2011;17:796–808.
6. Varma MR, Varga AJ, Knipp BS, et al. Neutropenia impairs venous thrombosis resolution in the rat. J Vasc Surg. 2003;38:1090–8.
7. van Aken BE, den Heijer M, Bos GM, et al. Recurrent venous thrombosis and markers of inflammation. Thromb Haemost. 2000;83:536–9.

8. Gupta R, Patadia D, Velayudhan V, et al. Orbital cellulitis, cavernous sinus thrombosis, internal jugular vein thrombus, and clival osteomyelitis secondary to acute sinusitis. Am J Respir Crit Care Med. 2017;195(4):533.
9. Qun S, Tang Y, Sun J, et al. Neutrophil-to-lymphocyte ratio predicts 3-month outcome of acute ischemic stroke. Neurotox Res. 2017;31:1–9.
10. Bisoendial RJ, Kastelein JJ, Levels JH, et al. Activation of inflammation and coagulation after infusion of C-reactive protein in humans. Circ Res. 2005;96: 714–6.
11. Pandey A, Shrivastava AK, Saxena K. Neuron specific enolase and C-reactive protein levels in stroke and its subtypes: correlation with degree of disability. Neurochem Res. 2014;39:1426–32.
12. Yongjing Z, Wei H, et al. Hs-CRP in stroke: a meta-analysis. Clin Chim Acta. 2016;453:21–7.
13. Van der Poll T, Levi M, Hack CE, et al. Elimination of IL-6 attenuates coagulation in experimental endotoxemia in chimpanzees. J Exp Med. 1994; 179:1253–9.
14. Stouthard JM, Levi M, Hack CE, et al. Interleukin-6 stimulates coagulation, not fibrinolysis, in humans. Thromb Haemost. 1996;76:738–42.
15. Vormittag R, Hsieh K, Kaider A, et al. Interleukin-6 and interleukin-6 promoter polymorphism (-174) G > C in patients with spontaneous venous thromboembolism. Thromb Haemost. 2006;95(5):802–6.
16. Çiçek G, Açıkgoz SK, Bozbay M, et al. Neutrophil-lymphocyte ratio and platelet-lymphocyte ratio combination can predict prognosis in patients with ST-segment elevation myocardial infarction undergoing primary percutaneous coronary intervention. Angiology. 2015;66:441–7.
17. Wang F, Hu S, Ding Y, et al. Neutrophil-to-lymphocyte ratio and 30-day mortality in patients with acute intracerebral hemorrhage. J Stroke Cerebrovasc Dis. 2016;25(1):182–7.
18. Azab B, Shah N, Akerman M, et al. Value of platelet/lymphocyte ratio as a predictor of all-cause mortality after non-ST-elevation myocardial infarction. J Thromb Thrombolysis. 2016;34:326–34.
19. Akboga YE, Bektas H, Anlar O. Usefulness of platelet to lymphocyte and neutrophil to lymphocyte ratios in predicting the presence of cerebral venous sinus thrombosis and in-hospital major adverse cerebral events. J Neurol Sci. 2017;380:226–9.
20. Khasawneh AH, Garling RJ, Harris CA. Cerebrospinal fluid circulation: what do we know and how do we know it? Brain Circ. 2018;4:14–8.
21. Domenico N, et al. Inflammatory mediators as biomarkers in brain disorders. Inflammation. 2014;37(3):639–48.
22. Prasad R. Immunoglobulins in certain CNS disorders: a study of CSF Ig classes G, A, M, D, and E concentrations. Am J Clin Pathol. 1985;83(2):190.
23. Alshoabi SA. Cerebral venous sinus thrombosis: a diagnostic challenge in a rare presentation. Brain Circ. 2017;3:227–130.
24. Arauz A, et al. Time to recanalisation in patients with cerebral venous thrombosis under anticoagulation therapy. J Neurol Neurosurg Psychiatr. 2015;0:1–5.
25. Hu Y, Meng R, Zhang X, et al. Serum neuron specific enolase may be a marker to predict the severity and outcome of cerebral venous thrombosis. J Neurol. 2017;265(Suppl 1):1–6.
26. Rust R, Hofer AS, Schwab ME. Stroke promotes systemic endothelial inflammation and atherosclerosis. Trends Mol Med. 2018;24(7):593–5.
27. Arenillas JF. Intracranial atherosclerosis and inflammation: lessons from the East and the West. Brain Circ. 2015;1:47–52.
28. Khoyetsyan A, Kacimi R, Tsakanova G, et al. Activated complement protein C5a does not affect brain-derived endothelial cell viability and zonula occludens-1 levels following oxygen-glucose deprivation. Brain Circ. 2017;3:14–20.
29. Zhao H, Li G, Ma Q, et al. MicroRNA-99a-5p in circulating immune cells as a potential biomarker for the early diagnosis of ischemic stroke. Brain Circ. 2017;3:21–8.
30. Roumen-Klappe EM, den Heijer M, van Uum SH, et al. Inflammatory response in the acute phase of deep vein thrombosis. J Vasc Surg. 2002; 35(04):701–6.
31. Nagai M, Terao S, Yilmaz G, et al. Roles of inflammation and the activated protein C pathway in the brain edema associated with cerebral venous sinus thrombosis. Stroke. 2010;41:147–52.
32. Canhão P, Cortesão A, Cabral M, et al. Are steroids useful to treat cerebral venous thrombosis? Stroke. 2008;39:105–10.

Permissions

All chapters in this book were first published in JNI, by BioMed Central; hereby published with permission under the Creative Commons Attribution License or equivalent. Every chapter published in this book has been scrutinized by our experts. Their significance has been extensively debated. The topics covered herein carry significant findings which will fuel the growth of the discipline. They may even be implemented as practical applications or may be referred to as a beginning point for another development.

The contributors of this book come from diverse backgrounds, making this book a truly international effort. This book will bring forth new frontiers with its revolutionizing research information and detailed analysis of the nascent developments around the world.

We would like to thank all the contributing authors for lending their expertise to make the book truly unique. They have played a crucial rôle in the development of this book. Without their invaluable contributions this book wouldn't have been possible. They have made vital efforts to compile up to date information on the varied aspects of this subject to make this book a valuable addition to the collection of many professionals and students.

This book was conceptualized with the vision of imparting up-to-date information and advanced data in this field. To ensure the same, a matchless editorial board was set up. Every individual on the board went through rigorous rounds of assessment to prove their worth. After which they invested a large part of their time researching and compiling the most relevant data for our readers.

The editorial board has been involved in producing this book since its inception. They have spent rigorous hours researching and exploring the diverse topics which have resulted in the successful publishing of this book. They have passed on their knowledge of decades through this book. To expedite this challenging task, the publisher supported the team at every step. A small team of assistant editors was also appointed to further simplify the editing procedure and attain best results for the readers.

Apart from the editorial board, the designing team has also invested a significant amount of their time in understanding the subject and creating the most relevant covers. They scrutinized every image to scout for the most suitable representation of the subject and create an appropriate cover for the book.

The publishing team has been an ardent support to the editorial, designing and production team. Their endless efforts to recruit the best for this project, has resulted in the accomplishment of this book. They are a veteran in the field of academics and their pool of knowledge is as vast as their experience in printing. Their expertise and guidance has proved useful at every step. Their uncompromising quality standards have made this book an exceptional effort. Their encouragement from time to time has been an inspiration for everyone.

The publisher and the editorial board hope that this book will prove to be a valuable piece of knowledge for researchers, students, practitioners and scholars across the globe.

List of Contributors

Teruyo Hosoya, Takatoshi Ueki and Kohji Sato
Department of Neuroanatomy and Neuroscience, Hamamatsu University School of Medicine, 1-20-1 Handayama, Higashi-ku, Hamamatsu 431-3192, Japan

Dai Fukumoto, Takeharu Kakiuchi, Shingo Nishiyama, Shigeyuki Yamamoto, Hiroyuki Ohba and Hideo Tsukada
Central Research Laboratory, Hamamatsu Photonics KK, 5000 Hirakuchi, Hamakita-ku, Hamamatsu 434-8601, Japan

Yasuomi Ouchi
Department of Biofunctional Imaging, Preeminent Medical Photonics Education & Research Center, Hamamatsu University School of Medicine, 1-20-1 Handayama, Higashi-ku, Hamamatsu 431-3192, Japan

Hilary A. Seifert
Neuroimmunology Research R&D-31 Veterans Affairs Portland Health Care System, 3710 SW US Veterans Hospital Rd, Portland, OR 97239, USA
Department of Neurology, Oregon Health and Science University, Portland, OR, USA

Halina Offner
Department of Anesthesiology and Perioperative Medicine, Oregon Health and Science University, Portland, OR, USA
Neuroimmunology Research R&D-31 Veterans Affairs Portland Health Care System, 3710 SW US Veterans Hospital Rd, Portland, OR 97239, USA
Department of Neurology, Oregon Health and Science University, Portland, OR, USA

Shuang Chen, Zhiping Dong, Man Cheng, Yaqian Zhao, Mengying Wang, Na Sai, Xuan Wang, Huan Liu, Guowei Huang and Xumei Zhang
Department of Nutrition and Food Science, School of Public Health, Tianjin Medical University, Tianjin 300070, China

Hiramani Dhungana, Mikko T. Huuskonen, Merja Jaronen, Sighild Lemarchant, Humair Ali, Velta Keksa-Goldsteine, Gundars Goldsteins, Katja M. Kanninen, Jari Koistinaho and Tarja Malm
A.I. Virtanen Institute for Molecular Sciences, University of Eastern Finland, Finland

Yan Feng, Shiwei Liao, Changjuan Wei, Dongmei Jia, Qiang Liu, Fu-Dong Shi and Wei-Na Jin
Department of Neurology, Tianjin Neurological Institute, Tianjin Medical University General Hospital, Tianjin 300052, China

Yan Feng, Fu-Dong Shi and Wei-Na Jin
Center for Neuroinflammation, Beijing TianTan Hospital, Beijing 100070, China

Kristofer Wood, Qiang Liu, Fu-Dong Shi and Wei-Na Jin
Department of Neurology, Barrow Neurological Institute, St. Joseph's Hospital and Medical Center, Phoenix 85013, AZ, USA

Xiaoying Wang
Neuroprotection Research Laboratory, Departments of Radiology and Neurology, Massachusetts General Hospital, Harvard Medical School, Boston 02129, MA, USA

Benjarat Changyaleket, Zhao Zhong Chong, Randal O. Dull and Danop Nanegrungsunk
Department of Anesthesiology, University of Illinois at Chicago, Chicago, IL, USA

Haoliang Xu
Department of Pathology, University of Illinois at Chicago, 840 South Wood Street, Chicago, IL 60612, USA

Lianhua Zhao, Wei Zhao and Zaiyu Guo
Department of Neurology, Tianjin TEDA Hospital, Tianjin, China

Lianhua Zhao, Shengpan Chen, Prativa Sherchan, Yan Ding, Jing Yu, Jiping Tang and John H. Zhang
Department of Physiology and Pharmacology, Loma Linda University, 11041 Campus St, Loma Linda, CA 92354, USA

Shengpan Chen
Department of Neurosurgery, Affiliated Haikou Hospital, Xiangya School of Medicine, Central South University, Haikou, China

Hans Worthmann, Meike Dirks, Ramona Schuppner and Karin Weissenborn
Department of Neurology, Hannover Medical School, 30623 Hannover, Germany

Na Li
Department of Neurology, Beijing Tiantan Hospital, Capital Medical University, Beijing, China

Jens Martens-Lobenhoffer and Stefanie M. Bode-Böger
Department of Clinical Pharmacology, Otto-von-Guericke-University of Magdeburg, University Hospital, Magdeburg, Germany

Ralf Lichtinghagen
Department of Clinical Chemistry, Hannover Medical School, Hannover, Germany

Jan T. Kielstein
Department of Nephrology and Hypertension, Hannover Medical School, Hannover, Germany
Medical Clinic V, Academic Teaching Hospital Braunschweig, Braunschweig, Germany

Peter Raab and Heinrich Lanfermann
Institute of Diagnostic and Interventional Neuroradiology, Hannover Medical School, Hannover, Germany

Heba A. Ahmed, Bindu Pillai, Abdelrahman Y. Fouda, Mohammed A. Sayed, Wael Eldahshan, Adviye Ergul and Susan C. Fagan
Program in Clinical and Experimental Therapeutics, Charlie Norwood VA Medical Center and University of Georgia College of Pharmacy, HM Bldg., 1120 15th St, Augusta, GA 30912, USA

Tauheed Ishrat
Department of Anatomy and Neurobiology, College of Medicine, Neuroscience Institute, University of Tennessee Health Science Center, Memphis, TN, USA

Adviye Ergul
Department of Physiology, Augusta University, Augusta, GA, USA

Susan C. Fagan
Department of Neurology, Augusta University, Augusta, GA, USA

Jennifer L. Waller
Department of Biostatistics and Epidemiology, Augusta University, Augusta, GA, USA

Mengni Yi, Tianjiao Wei, Qin Lu, Gaoxian Chen, Xiaoling Gao, Hongzhuan Chen and Zhihua Yu
Department of Pharmacology, Institute of Medical Sciences, Shanghai Jiao Tong University School of Medicine, Shanghai 200025, China

Yanxia Wang
Experimental Teaching Center of Basic Medicine, School of Medicine, Shanghai Jiao Tong University, Shanghai 200025, China

Herbert M. Geller
Developmental Neurobiology Section Division of Intramural Research, National Heart, Lung, and Blood Institute, National Institutes of Health, Bethesda, MD 20892, USA

Ruimin Ge, Daniel Tornero, Masao Hirota, Emanuela Monni, Cecilia Laterza, Olle Lindvall and Zaal Kokaia
Laboratory of Stem Cells and Restorative Neurology, Lund Stem Cell Center, University Hospital, SE-221 84 Lund, Sweden

Miaodan Li, Shumin Chen, Xue Shi, Chenfei Lyu, Yongfang Zhang, Miaoqin Tan, Chen Wang, Nailiang Zang, Xiaoxi Liu, Yafang Hu, Liang Zhou and Yong Gu
Department of Neurology, Nanfang Hospital, Southern Medical University, Guangzhou, Guangdong 510515, People's Republic of China

Jiangang Shen
School of Chinese Medicine, The University of Hong Kong, Hong Kong, People's Republic of China

Dong Bin Back, Kyoung Ja Kwon, Seol-Heui Han and Hahn Young Kim
Department of Neurology, Konkuk University School of Medicine, Research Institute of Medical Science, Seoul, Republic of Korea

Kyoung Ja Kwon and Dong-Hee Choi
Department of Medicine, Konkuk University School of Medicine, Seoul, Republic of Korea

Chan Young Shin
Department of Pharmacology, Konkuk University School of Medicine, Seoul, Republic of Korea

Jongmin Lee
Department of Rehabilitation Medicine, Konkuk University School of Medicine, Seoul, Republic of Korea

Hahn Young Kim
Konkuk University Medical Center, 120-1 Neungdong-ro, Gwangjin-gu, Seoul 05030, Republic of Korea

Anna Bajnok and Gergely Toldi
First Department of Obstetrics and Gynecology, Semmelweis University, Baross str. 27, Budapest H-1088, Hungary

Anna Bajnok, László Berta, Csaba Orbán, Tivadar Tulassay and Gergely Told
First Department of Pediatrics, Semmelweis University, Bókay János str. 53-54, Budapest H-1083, Hungary

Tivadar Tulassay
MTA-SE Pediatrics and Nephrology Research Group, Budapest, Hungary

Gergely Toldi
Neonatal Unit, Birmingham Women's and Children's Hospital, Birmingham, UK

Kazuo Yamagata, Natsumi Takahashi and Nozomi Akita
Laboratory of Molecular Health of Food, Department of Food Bioscience and Biotechnology, College of Bioresource Sciences, Nihon University (NUBS), 1866, Kameino, Fujisawa, Kanagawa 252-8510, Japan

Toru Nabika
Department of Functional Pathology, Shimane University Faculty of Medicine, Matsue, Japan

Zhe Gong, Jingrui Pan, Qingyu Shen, Mei Li and Ying Peng
Department of Neurology, Sun Yat-sen Memorial Hospital, Sun Yat-sen University, Guangzhou 510120, China

Qingyu Shen and Ying Peng
Guangdong Provincial Key Laboratory of Malignant Tumour Epigenetics and Gene Regulation, Sun Yat-sen Memorial Hospital, Sun Yat-sen University, Guangzhou, China

Qianyi Huang, Wei Zhong, Zhiping Hu and Xiangqi Tang
Department of Neurology, The Second Xiangya Hospital, Central South University, Renmin Road 139#, Changsha 410011, Hunan, China

Liyan Wang, Tingting Bian, Ran Meng, Longfei Wu, Zhen Zhang and Xunming Ji
Neurosurgery Department of Xuanwu Hospital Capital Medical University, Changchun st 45, Xicheng District, Beijing, China

Jiangang Duan
Emergency Department of Xuanwu Hospital Capital Medical University, Changchun street 45, Xicheng District, Beijing, China

Xuxiang Zhang
Ophtalmology Department of Xuanwu Hospital Capital Medical University, Changchun street 45, Xicheng District, Beijing, China

Chunxiu Wang
Evidence-based Medicine Department of Xuanwu Hospital Capital Medical University, Changchun street 45, Xicheng District, Beijing, China

Index

www.ingramcontent.com/pod-product-compliance
Lightning Source LLC
LaVergne TN
LVHW080905210926
848485LV00004B/598
* 9 7 8 1 6 3 9 2 7 3 2 9 4 *